Movement Disorders 3

Butterworth-Heinemann International Medical Reviews

Neurology

Published titles

1 **Clinical Neurophysiology**
Erik Stålberg and Robert R. Young

2 **Movement Disorders**
C. David Marsden and Stanley Fahn

3 **Cerebral Vascular Disease**
Michael J. G. Harrison and Mark L. Dyken

4 **Peripheral Nerve Disorders**
Arthur K. Asbury and R. W. Gilliatt

5 **The Epilepsies**
Roger J. Porter and Paolo L. Morselli

6 **Multiple Sclerosis**
W. I. McDonald and Donald H. Silberger

7 **Movement Disorders 2**
C. David Marsden and Stanley Fahn

8 **Infections of the Nervous System**
Peter G. E. Kennedy and Richard T. Johnson

9 **The Molecular Biology of Neurological Disease**
Roger N. Rosenberg and A. E. Harding

10 **Pain Syndromes in Neurology**
Howard L. Fields

11 **Principles and Practice of Restorative Neurology**
Robert R. Young and Paul J. Delwaide

12 **Stroke: Populations, Cohorts, and Clinical Trials**
Jack P. Whisnant

13 **Movement Disorders 3**
C. David Marsden and Stanley Fahn

14 **Mitochondrial Disorders in Neurology**
A. H. V. Schapira and S. DiMauro

Movement Disorders 3

Edited by

C. David Marsden, FRS, DSc, MB, BS, MRCPsych, FRCP
Professor of Neurology, Institute of Neurology, The National Hospital for Neurology and Neurosurgery, Queen Square, London, UK

and

Stanley Fahn, MD
H Houston Merritt Professor of Neurology, Columbia University College of Physicians and Surgeons, Neurological Institute, New York, USA

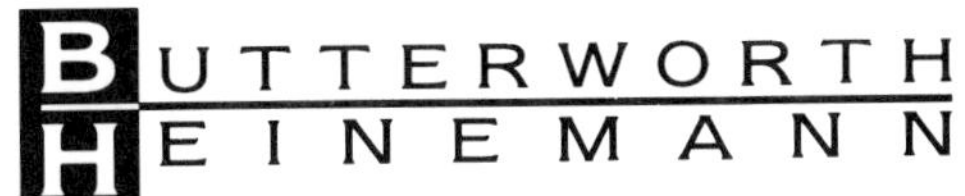

Butterworth-Heinemann Ltd
Linacre House, Jordan Hill, Oxford OX2 2DP

A member of the Reed Elsevier group

OXFORD LONDON BOSTON
MUNICH NEW DELHI SINGAPORE SYDNEY
TOKYO TORONTO WELLINGTON

First published 1994

British Library Cataloguing in Publication Data
Movement Disorders. – Vol. 3 –
Butterworths International Medical
Reviews. Neurology; Vol. 12)
I. Marsden, C. David II. Fahn, Stanley
III. Series
616.8

ISBN 0 7506 1412 9

Library of Congress Cataloguing in Publication Data
Movement disorders 3/edited by C. David Marsden and Stanley Fahn.
p. cm. – (Butterworth-Heinemann international medical reviews. Neurology; 12)
Includes bibliographical references and index.
ISBN 0 7506 1412 9
1. Movement disorders. I. Marsden, C. David. II. Fahn, Stanley, 1933– . III. Title: Movement disorders three. IV. Series.
[DNLM: 1. Movement Disorders. 2. Parkinson Disease. WL 390 M93572 1994]
RC376.5.M683 1994
616.8'3–dc20 93–19893
CIP

Typeset by P&R Typesetters, Salisbury, UK

Printed and bound in Great Britain at the University Press, Cambridge

Contents

Series Preface

For almost a quarter of a century (1951–1975), subjects of topical interest were written about in the periodic volumes of our predecessor, *Modern Trends in Neurology*. The legacy continues with the present Butterworth-Heinemann series in Neurology. As was the case with *Modern Trends*, the current volumes are intended for use by physicians who grapple with the problems of neurological disorders on a daily basis, be they neurologists, neurologists in training, or those in related fields such as neurosurgery, internal medicine, psychiatry, and rehabilitation medicine.

Our purpose is to produce annually a monograph on a topic in clinical neurology in which progress through research has brought about new concepts of patient management. The subject of each monograph is selected by the Series Editors using two criteria: first, that there has been significant advance in knowledge in that area and, second, that such advances have been incorporated into new ways of managing patients with the disorders in question. This has been the guiding spirit behind each volume, and we expect it to continue. In effect we emphasize research, both in the clinic and in the experimental laboratory, but principally to the extent that it changes our collective attitudes and practices in caring for those who are neurologically afflicted.

C. D. Marsden
A. K. Asbury
Series Editors

Preface

The first volume of *Movement Disorders* in this series was published in 1982. We stated then: "This book is not a textbook on movement disorders and does not encompass all that has been written on the subject in recent years." We selected topics that appeared to have "reached a stage that warrants definitive discussion". The second volume on movement disorders in this series was published in 1987. This included chapters on topics previously discussed in which there had been major advances in the previous five years, and chapters on new topics not covered in the first volume. We have followed the same principle in the third volume in the series on movement disorders.

As before, we have selected a number of areas for discussion, and invited as authors those with particular expertise on these subjects to present their personal viewpoints. Our editing of all chapters makes us share equally with the authors any responsibility for errors, omissions or misinterpretations.

This volume is introduced by five general chapters. The first two update current knowledge on the anatomy of the basal ganglia (Alice Flaherty and Ann Graybiel) and on experimental models of basal ganglia diseases (Michael Sambrook, Alan Crossman and Ian Mitchell). The next three deal with the genetic aspects of movement disorders (Anita Harding), functional imaging (David Brooks) and eye movement abnormalities (Rick Stell and Adolfo Bronstein). As before, the remainder of the book is divided into two halves. The first deals with aspects of Parkinsonism, the second with various dyskinesias. Each of these halves is prefaced by an introductory chapter in which we discuss our reasons for including the subjects dealt with by the invited authors, and we also give brief reviews of other items which may be of practical interest to the reader. We hope that this book will be of value to neurologists in training, and to those in research and in practice. We trust that its clinical content will again help in the practical management of patients with movement disorders, while its more scientific sections may aid in understanding of the background to the field.

We wish to thank the publishers for preparing this volume, the authors for sharing our enthusiasm for the need for this third volume, and for their timely cooperation and patience, and our wives for their understanding.

C. D. Marsden
S. Fahn

Contributors

Dr M. F. Brin
Department of Neurology, Neurological Institute, 710 West 168th Street, New York, USA

Dr A. Blitzer
Professor of Clinical Otolaryngology and Acting Chairman, Columbia University College of Physicians and Surgeons, 603 West 168th Street, New York, USA

Dr A. M. Bronstein
Medical Research Council Human Movement and Balance Unit, Institute of Neurology, The National Hospital, Queen Square, London, UK

Dr D. J. Brooks
MRC Cyclotron Unit, Hammersmith Hospital, Ducane Road, London, UK

Dr P. Brown
The National Hospital for Neurology and Neurosurgery, Queen Square, London, UK

Dr T. N. Chase
National Institute of Neurological Disorders and Stroke, National Institutes of Health, Building 10, Room 5C103, 9000 Rockville Pike, Bethesda, Maryland, USA

Dr L. Cleeves
The National Hospital for Neurology and Neurosurgery, Queen Square, London, UK

Dr A. R. Crossman
University of Manchester School of Biological Sciences, Department of Cell and Structural Biology, Stopford Building, Oxford Road, Manchester, UK

Dr S. Fahn
Professor of Neurology, Columbia University College of Physicians and Surgeons, Neurological Institute, New York, USA

Dr A. W. Flaherty
Department of Brain and Cognitive Sciences, Massachusetts Institute of Technology E25-618, 45 Carleton Street, Cambridge, Massachusetts, USA

Dr L. J. Findley
Honorary Senior Lecturer, Institute of Neurology, The National Hospital for Neurology and Neurosurgery, Queen Square, London, UK

Dr D. R. Fish
The National Hospital for Neurology and Neurosurgery, Queen Square, London, UK

Dr W. R. G. Gibb
University Department of Neurology, Institute of Psychiatry, DeCrespigny Park, Denmark Hill, London, UK

Dr A. Graybiel
Department of Brain and Cognitive Sciences, Massachusetts Institute of Technology E25-618, 45 Carleton Street, Cambridge, Massachusetts, USA

Dr P. Greene
Department of Neurology, Neurological Institute, 710 West 168th Street, New York, USA

Dr M. Hallett
Clinical Director, National Institute of Neurological Disorders and Stroke, National Institutes of Health, Building 10, Room 5N226, Bethesda, Maryland, USA

Professor A. E. Harding
Department of Clinical Neurology, Institute of Neurology, Queen Square, London, UK

Dr J. Jankovic
Professor of Neurology, Department of Neurology, Baylor College of Medicine, Houston, Texas, USA

Dr A. J. Lees
PDS Brain Bank, Institute of Neurology, 1 Wakefield Street, London, UK

Professor O. Lindvall
Restorative Neurology Unit, Department of Neurology, University Hospital S-221 85, Lund, Sweden

Professor C. D. Marsden
Professor of Neurology, Institute of Neurology, The National Hospital for Neurology and Neurosurgery, Queen Square, London, UK

Dr J. Matsumoto
Department of Neurology, Mayo Clinic, Rochester, Minnesota, USA

Dr I. J. Mitchell
University of Manchester School of Biological Sciences, Department of Cell and Structural Biology, Stopford Building, Oxford Road, Manchester, UK

Dr M. M. Mouradian
Experimental Therapeutics Branch, National Institute of Neurological Disorders and Stroke, National Institutes of Health, Bethesda, Maryland, USA

Dr S. S. Mirra
Veterans Affairs Medical Center and Department of Pathology and Laboratory Medicine, Emory University School of Medicine, Atlanta, Georgia, USA

Dr N. Quinn
Senior Lecturer in Neurology, University Department of Clincal Neurology, The Institute of Neurology and Honorary Consultant Neurologist, The National Hospital for Neurology and Neurosurgery, Queen Square, London, UK

Dr E. P. Richardson Jr
Charles S. Kubik Laboratory of Neuropathology and Neurology Service, Massachusetts General Hospital and Harvard Medical School, Boston, Massachusetts, USA

Dr M. A. Sambrook
Consultant Neurologist, Withington Hospital, West Didsbury, Manchester, UK

Dr J. R. Sladek
Department of Neuroscience, University of Health Sciences, The Chicago Medical School, North Chicago, Illinois, USA

Dr K. Steece-Collier
Department of Neurology, University of Rochester School of Medicine and Dentistry, Rochester, New York, USA

Dr R. Stell
Department of Neurology, Sir Charles Gairdner Hospital, Queen Elizabeth II Medical Centre, Perth, Western Australia

Dr I. Shoulson
Louis C Lasagna Professor of Experimental Therapeutics, Departments of Neurology and Pharmacology, University of Rochester Medical Center, Rochester, New York, USA

Dr C. Tanner
Parkinson's Institute, 1170 Morse Avenue, Sunnyvale, California, USA

Dr P. D. Thompson
Medical Research Council Human Movement and Balance Unit and University Department of Clinical Neurology, Institute of Neurology, National Hospital for Neurology and Neurosurgery, Queen Square, London, UK

Dr R. Watts
Department of Neurology, Emory University School of Medicine, 401 Woodruff Memorial Building, Atlanta, Georgia, USA

Part I

General

1
Anatomy of the basal ganglia

Alice W. Flaherty and Ann M. Graybiel

The functional organization of the basal ganglia has long interested neurologists studying extrapyramidal movement disorders. None the less, links between structure and function in the basal ganglia are less well-understood than are those in the cerebral cortex – in part because the basal ganglia and their allied nuclei, buried deep in the forebrain, are less accessible than the cortex, and because the basal ganglia are not as clearly linked to sensation and behaviour as are sensory and motor areas of the cortex. However, four technical innovations have recently advanced basal ganglia neurobiology. Firstly, axon transport methods with markers such as horseradish peroxidase, lectins, and radiolabelled and fluorescent molecules have clarified the connections of the basal ganglia. Secondly, chemoanatomical methods such as immunohistochemistry, receptor binding, microdialysis, and *in situ* hybridization have allowed study of neurotransmitters in the basal ganglia. Thirdly, computed tomography (CT), magnetic resonance imaging (MRI) and positron emission tomography (PET) scanning methods have permitted observation of the living human brain. Fourthly, the methods of molecular biology and genetics have illuminated cellular mechanisms in both normal and dysfunctional basal ganglia.

Studies with these four methods have helped confirm and extend the classic hypothesis that many movement disorders are associated with highly specific damage to particular nuclei – or specific groups of neurons within particular nuclei – in the basal ganglia and allied regions. They have also provided unexpected evidence for a role of the basal ganglia in neuropsychiatric disorders such as depression, obsessive-compulsive disorder and schizophrenia (Carlsson and Carlsson, 1990; Sedvall, 1990). We will review some of the recent discoveries in basal ganglia neuroanatomy, emphasizing functional and neurochemical subdivisions of the basal ganglia and their allied nuclei. We will focus on the parts of the basal ganglia most clearly identified with movement disorders, although there are also provocative findings about the ventral part of the basal ganglia, a region thought to be related to motivation and limbic functions (Alheid and Heimer, 1988).

The chief nuclei of the basal ganglia are the striatum and the pallidum or globus pallidus. Each nucleus is itself divided into parts. The term striatum, especially in clinical discussions, often connotes the caudate nucleus and putamen, together called the dorsal striatum. However, the striatum also includes the ventral striatum: the region at the base of the caudate–putamen complex that lies mainly anterior to the anterior commissure. The ventral striatum contains the ventral continuations of the caudate nucleus and putamen, the nucleus accumbens septi and parts of the olfactory tubercle. The globus pallidus has an external segment (GPe), an internal segment (GPi) and a region known as the ventral pallidum. Strictly speaking, the amygdala is part of the basal ganglia. It is now generally discussed separately, but it does have direct connections with the striatum, especially with the ventral striatum.

Two other nuclei, the subthalamic nucleus and the substantia nigra, are closely allied to the basal ganglia. The substantia nigra has two main parts: the dopamine-rich pars compacta (SNpc), and the non-dopaminergic pars reticulata (SNpr). In many respects, the SNpr can be considered a caudal extension of the GPi. But it differs from the GPi in having a special link with the dopamine-rich SNpc: many dopamine-containing dendrites, and some dopamine-containing cell bodies, extend from the SNpc into the SNpr. Other regions that are important for basal ganglia function include cortical motor, somatosensory, and premotor areas; thalamic ventral anterior (VA), ventral lateral (VL), and centre median-parafascicular (CM-PF) nuclei; midbrain monoamine-containing cell groups near the SNpc (including the ventral tegmental area, retrorubral area and dorsal raphe nuclei); and the tegmental pedunculopontine nucleus.

Basal ganglia circuitry is notoriously complicated (Fig. 1.1), but the current model of basal ganglia function simplifies it by focusing on only two of the pathways. Both of them, the direct pathway through GPi and SNpr, and the indirect pathway through GPe and the subthalamic nucleus, can be interpreted as cortical feedback loops in which information from the entire neocortex is sent in sequence through the dorsal striatum, pallidum and thalamus, and then back from the thalamus to the cortex, especially the frontal cortex. A related circuit goes through the ventral basal ganglia: the hippocampal formation and related allocortex project to the ventral striatum, then the ventral pallidum and substantia nigra, thalamus and cortex.

In this model, a series of inhibitory projections in the direct pathway create a double inhibition that results in a net positive feedback loop: the cortex sends excitatory inputs to the striatum, the striatum sends inhibitory inputs to the pallidum, the pallidum inhibits the thalamus, and the thalamus sends excitatory inputs to the frontal cortex. The net effect of cortical activity via these pathways is to trigger the striatum to release the thalamus from pallidal inhibition, thus allowing thalamic outputs to excite the cortex (Fig. 1.2). This double inhibition is not simply the result of taking the negative of a negative to make a positive; the two successive stages of inhibition in these output pathways need not necessarily have added up to net excitation. For instance, the striatum can release the thalamus from pallidal inhibition only because the pallidal neurons are tonically active. If pallidal neurons normally had low firing rates – as do those in the striatum – then inhibition from the striatum might not change the firing rate of pallidal outputs to the thalamus. In other words, whether double inhibition adds up to net release empirically depends on the exact neuronal connections and physiological characteristics of each stage of the circuit.

Moreover, net effects of the direct pathway are influenced by alternative pathways through the basal ganglia. Some of these, notably the GPe-subthalamic loop discussed below, may result in triple, rather than double, inhibition. If the influence of such other pathways is dominant, then the net effect of the basal ganglia on the thalamus and cortex will be negative feedback, not release. There is an interesting possibility, however, that basal ganglia inhibition of cortical activity might not inhibit movement, but facilitate it, by selectively inhibiting muscles antagonistic to the desired movement (Mink and Thach, 1991a,b). Thus the direct and indirect pathways through the basal ganglia may not be working in opposition, but in tandem.

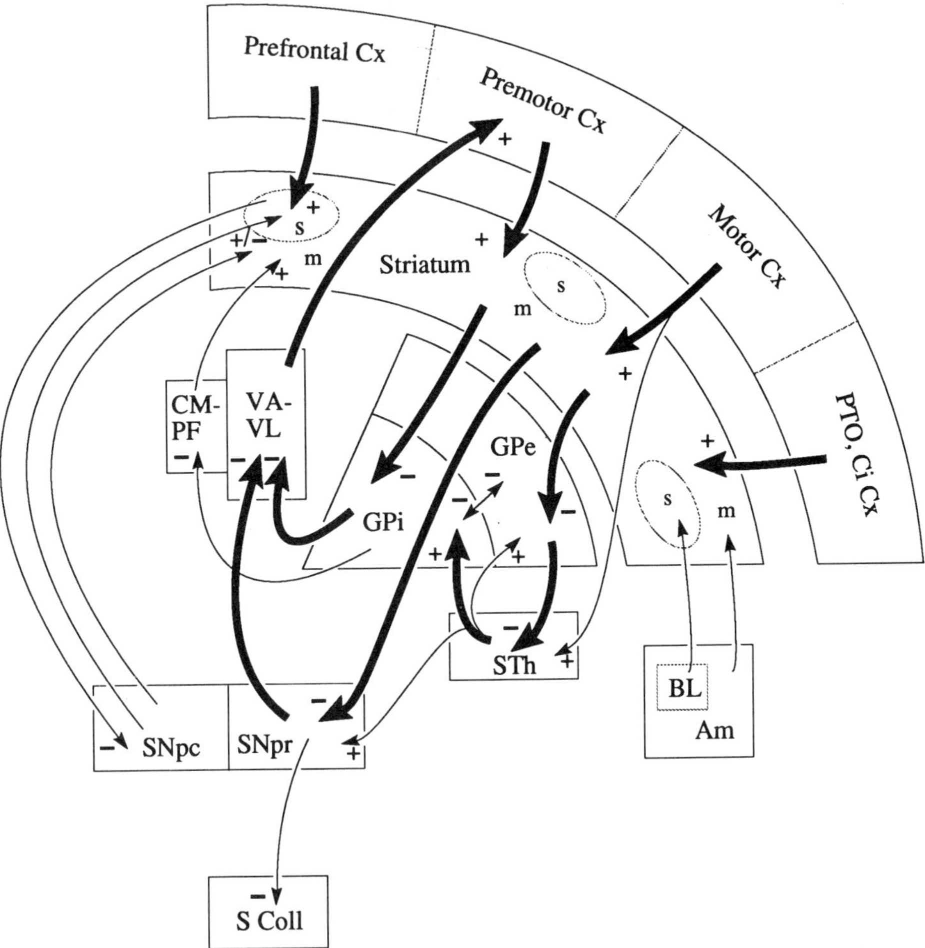

Figure 1.1 A diagram of basic basal ganglia pathways. What is thought to be the primary flow of cortical information is shown with thick arrows. Excitatory and inhibitory inputs are indicated with plus and minus signs. The connections of the limbic system-associated ventral striatum and ventral pallidum are not shown. Am = Amygdala; BL = basolateral nucleus of the amygdala; Ci = cingulate; CM-PF = centre median and parafascicular thalamic complex; Cx = cortex; GPe = external pallidal segment; GPi = internal pallidal segment; m = matrix; PTO = parietotemporo-occiptal; s = striosome; SColl = superior colliculus; SNpc = substantia nigra, pars compacta; SNpr = substantia nigra, pars reticulata; STh = subthalamic nucleus; VA-VL = ventral anterior and ventral lateral thalamic nuclei.

This model has been effective in integrating anatomy and electrophysiology with the symptoms of basal ganglia disorders (Albin *et al.*, 1989), but it is not without drawbacks. For instance, although it is convenient to think of basal ganglia processing as a sequence of inhibitory stages, it may also be misleading: electrophysiological studies of movement-related activity in the motor cortex and the striatum suggest that the two regions may control movement in parallel, rather than creating a strict hierarchy (Crutcher and Alexander, 1990). Moreover, although the main sources and ultimate targets of the basal ganglia are cortical, there are other important inputs from within and without the extended basal ganglia system. Activity in the direct

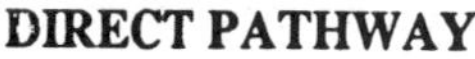

INDIRECT PATHWAYS

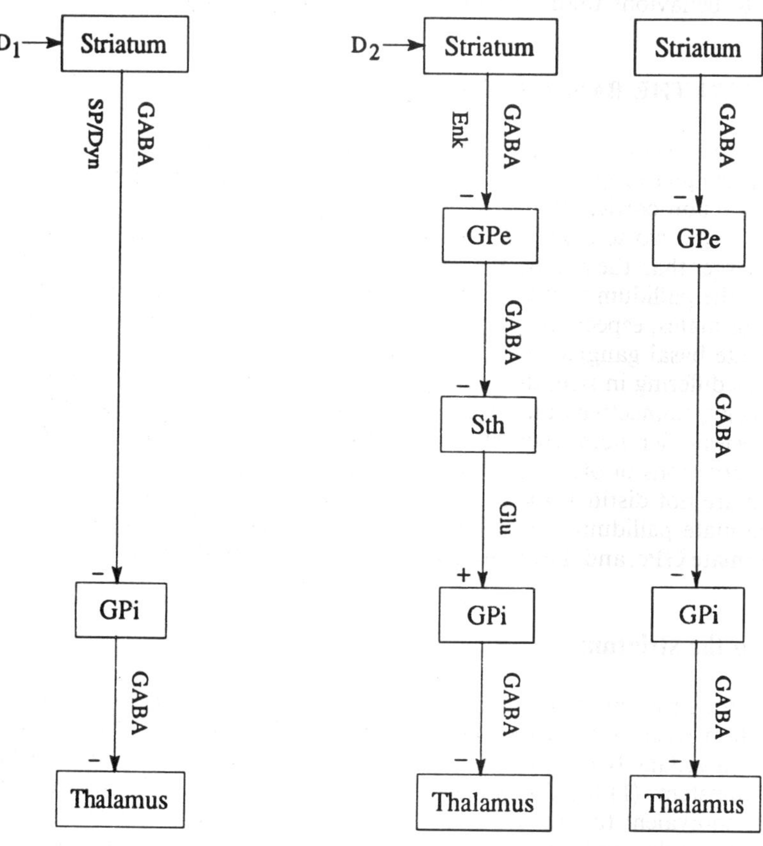

NET RELEASE **NET INHIBITION**

Figure 1.2 Direct and indirect pathways through the basal ganglia are thought to have opposite effects on the thalamus and cortex. On the left, the doubly inhibitory pathway through the internal pallidal segment (GPi) has the net effect of releasing the thalamus from pallidal inhibition. At centre, the pathway through the external pallidal segment (GPe) and the subthalamic nucleus contains three inhibitory steps, resulting in thalamic inhibition. On the right, a projection linking GPe and GPi via the subthalamic nucleus also contains three inhibitory steps, producing thalamic inhibition. The neurotransmitter and neuropeptide co-transmitters used in these projections differ in the three pathways. D_1 = D_1-type dopamine receptor; D_2 = D_2-type dopamine receptor; Dyn = dynorphin; Enk = encephalin; GABA = gamma-aminobutyric acid; Glu = glutamate; SP = substance P; Sth = subthalamic nucleus.

pathway may be modulated by side-loops that connect the striatal and pallidal stages of the primary circuit to the substantia nigra, the subthalamic nucleus, the CM-PF thalamic nuclei, and the tegmental pedunculopontine nucleus. The debilitating movement disorders that result from damage to the substantia nigra and the subthalamic nucleus demonstrate the important influence these accessory loop nuclei can have on basal ganglia processing. Indeed, it is a problem for the current model of basal ganglia processing that lesions of the modulatory side-loops seem to do more damage to behaviour than do lesions in the direct pathway.

INPUTS TO THE BASAL GANGLIA

Inputs to the striatum and the pallidum differ greatly. The striatum is the region in the basal ganglia loop that receives the majority of cortical inputs, and it receives most of the non-cortical inputs as well. The pallidum, by contrast, receives most of its inputs from two sources: the striatum and the subthalamic nucleus. The straitum is much larger than the pallidum; it is the largest subcortical cell mass in the forebrain. But both the pallidum and the striatum, like the neocortex, are proportionally very large in primates, especially humans. It is tempting to suppose that the large size of the primate basal ganglia reflects the primate specialization for fine motor control. As well as differing in size, the basal ganglia of primates differ from non-primates in morphology, connectivity and regional specialization. It is important to keep in mind these species differences when attempting to make inferences about human diseases from observations of other species. In the rat, for instance, the caudate nucleus and putamen are not distinct nuclei, and the apparent homologues of the two segments of the primate pallidum are split into two nuclei: the globus pallidus, homologous to the primate GPe, and the entopeduncular nucleus, homologous to the primate GPi.

Inputs to the striatum

Inputs to the striatum are summarized in Table 1.1. Besides receiving cortical afferents, the striatum receives robust inputs from the CM-PF complex of the thalamus and from the amygdala. It also receives fibre projections from three monoaminergic regions of the brainstem: (1) the dopamine-containing midbrain nuclei, including the SNpc (roughly equivalent to cell group A9), its caudal extension in the retrorubral region (cell group A8), and the ventral tegmental area (cell group A10); (2) the serotonin-containing dorsal raphe nucleus; and (3) the noradrenaline-containing locus coeruleus, which projects mainly to the ventral striatum. Dopamine, serotonin and noradrenaline make up only a small subset of the many neurotransmitters found in the striatum, which is noted for its high concentration and diversity of neurotransmitters (Graybiel, 1990).

Long lists of interconnections are a frustrating aspect of basal ganglia neurobiology, in part because they give no information about the relative strengths of the different fibre projections. But anatomical strength may not be the best index of functional relevance. For instance, studies of Parkinson's disease demonstrate that the dopamine-containing nigrostriatal pathway is crucial functionally, yet nigrostriatal synapses are thought to make up only a small percentage of all striatal afferent synapses. Thus, it is possible that the sparse inputs to the striatum from the subthalamic nucleus, pallidum and tegmental pedunculopontine nucleus are more important then their numbers suggest.

CORTICOSTRIATAL INPUTS

Given the plentiful subcortical inputs to the striatum, what justifies the traditional emphasis on the cortical inputs to the striatum? Firstly, in the context of motor processing, the cerebral cortex – and especially the sensorimotor cortex, which has

Table 1.1 Connections of the striatum

Inputs	Outputs
CAUDATE NUCLEUS AND PUTAMEN	
Inputs From neocortex (glutamate) To matrix from sensorimotor cortex To putamen from primary and supplementary motor cortex, somatosensory cortex To caudate nucleus from frontal and medial eye fields, posterior association cortex To striosomes from frontal cortex From thalamus (glutamate) To matrix from CM-PE: CM to sensorimotor Outamen, PF to association areas of caudate nucleus and putamen From SNpc and ventral tegmental area (dopamine) To matrix from cell group A8 and parts of SNpc To striosomes from some SNpc From amygdala To striosomes from basolateral nucleus To matrix from other amygdaloid nuclei From dorsal raphe nucleus to matrix (serotonin) From subthalamic nucleus (glutamate) From pallidum (GABA) From pedunculopontine nucleus	*Outputs (GABA, neuropeptides)* To pallidum mainly from matrix To Gpe (GABA and encephalin) To GPi (GABA, substance P, dynorphin; some encephalin to inner GPe) To substantia nigra To SNpr from matrix, mainly from caudate nucleus (GABA, substance P, dynorphin) To SNpc from striosomes (GABA, substance P, dynorphin)
VENTRAL STRIATUM	
Inputs From limbic cortex: hippocampus; piriform, cingulate and temporal cortex (glutamate) From thalamus: midline nuclei (glutamate) From SNpc and ventral tegmental area (dopamine) From amygdala From dorsal raphe nucleus (serotonin) From locus coeruleus (noradrenaline)	*Outputs (GABA)* To ventral pallidum To ventral tegmental area To lateral hypothalamus To substantia nigra To medial thalamus To bed nuclei of stria terminalis To pedunculopontine nucleus To brainstem

CM = Centre median; GABA = gamma-aminobutyric acid; GPe = external globus pallidus; GPi = pallidus internal globus; PF = parafascicular; SNpc = substantia nigra pars compacta; SNpr = substantia nigra pars reticulata.

a massive fibre projection to the striatum – is the one region projecting to the striatum that is known to have an executive role in the control of movement. Secondly, because the entire cortex projects to the striatum, fibre projections from cortex carry as a whole a broader array of information to the striatum than do those from non-cortical regions. Thirdly, functional domains in the striatum seem to be strongly influenced by the types of cortical input they receive. Behavioural experiments have shown that lesions within a particular striatal zone produce deficits similar to the deficits produced by lesions in the cortical area projecting to that zone (Dunnett and Iversen, 1980, 1982).

The dopamine-, serotonin- and noradrenaline-containing inputs seem to have a different role in striatal processing than the informational inputs that the striatum receives from the neocortex. The current best guess at the function of these monoaminergic inputs is that they are modulators of corticostriatal processing, rather than themselves carrying detailed information about the sensorimotor periphery. Clues to the nature of this modulation will be discussed below. The functions of the inputs from the thalamus and amygdala to the striatum are unclear. The CM-PF nuclei of the thalamus may be important in feedback or even feedforward motor control, for they receive dense inputs from motor cortex (to CM) and premotor cortex (to PF). These nuclei project to the same regions of the striatum as do the motor and premotor cortices themselves. A more limbic function, related to affect and memory, is proposed for the amygdala's projection to the ventral striatum and to the striosomes within the dorsal striatum (see below).

Corticostriatal fibres use glutamate or aspartate as their neurotransmitter, and are thought to excite striatal output neurons. It is not certain whether the other forebrain inputs to the striatum are excitatory as well, nor have their neurotransmitters been identified. All of these inputs are thought to terminate, at least in part, directly on the output neurons of the striatum. Excitatory amino acids such as glutamate may play a role in the striatal cell death of Huntington's disease (DiFiglia, 1990), and the interactions of glutamate and dopamine effects on striatal neurons may have implications for Parkinson's disease; for instance, the substantia nigra is protected by antagonists to the glutamate NMDA receptor in one model of drug-induced parkinsonism (Turski *et al*., 1991).

The corticostriatal projection is highly ordered topographically. The neocortex primarily innervates the dorsal striatum, whereas the allocortex (especially the hippocampal formation) innervates the ventral striatum. Within the striatum, the neocortical projection is broadly systematic, with the zones of densest input following a front-to-front and back-to-back topography. Frontal cortex projects most strongly to the head of the caudate nucleus, sensorimotor and parietal cortex to the putamen, temporal cortex to the medial and caudal putamen and caudate nucleus, and occipital cortex to the tail of the caudate nucleus. However, any given cortical area projects not only to such a single circumscribed striatal region, but to an elongated, patchy zone that can extend nearly the entire length of the striatum. Because of this divergent projection, any particular part of the striatum receives inputs from multiple discrete regions of cortex.

Projections from different cortical regions diverge or converge in the striatum depending on their areas of origin. This suggests that the striatum processes certain inputs along independent, parallel channels while integrating other cortical inputs. Determining the topography and interaction of corticostriatal projections is important because of the roles cortical inputs play in determining the function of their striatal targets.

Sensorimotor inputs from the cortex to the striatum. One of the strongest cortical inputs to the striatum comes from the sensorimotor cortex (Brodmann areas 1–4). The location of fibre projections from these areas defines the sensorimotor-recipient striatum. The striatal zone that receives inputs from motor and somatosensory cortex is almost entirely within the putamen, supporting the view that the putamen is the motor nucleus of the striatum. Physiological evidence supports a role of the putamen in motor function: neurons that fire during limb movement are more common in the putamen than in the caudate nucleus, and electrical stimulation of discrete zones of the putamen produces limb movement (Alexander and DeLong, 1985). By contrast, the caudate nucleus receives dense projections from the prefrontal cortex. It is thought to have fewer direct ties to movement execution and a greater role in the planning, memory-based and psychological aspects of basal ganglia function.

The sensorimotor-recipient zone of the putamen is somatotopically organized. The body maps of motor cortex and somatosensory cortex all are projected in register onto the lateral putamen (Künzle, 1975, 1977; Jones *et al.*, 1977; Fotuhi *et al.*, 1989; Flaherty and Graybiel, 1991). Cortical regions with representations of the foot project most dorsally, and cortical regions representing trunk, arm, hand and face project successively more ventrally. This somatotopic organization may account for focal extrapyramidal movement disorders, such as parkinsonian tremors restricted to a single body part, and focal dystonias.

There is a major exception to the generalization that the putamen is the sensorimotor part of the striatum: oculomotor functions are prominently represented in the caudate nucleus. Eye movement-related regions in the frontal lobes – notably the frontal eye fields and medial (supplementary) eye fields – project mainly to the caudate nucleus (Stanton *et al.*, 1988; Huerta and Kaas, 1990; Parthasarathy *et al.*, 1992), and many neurons firing in relation to saccadic eye movements are found there (Hikosaka and Sakamoto, 1986). This striatal region appears to influence the midbrain's control of eye movements, as we will discuss below.

There is evidence that functional deficits in disorders of the basal ganglia reflect these corticostriatal projection patterns. In the early stages of idiopathic Parkinson's disease, more dopamine is lost from the putamen than from the caudate nucleus (Kish *et al.*, 1988). This differential loss may help account for the early appearance in Parkinson's disease of its characteristic motor deficits. In Huntington's disease, early degeneration is prominent in the caudate nucleus (Vonsattel *et al.*, 1985), and cognitive and eye movement abnormalities are common (Kennard and Lueck, 1989).

Local compartmentalization of corticostriatal inputs. The striatum has local modules within it, much as the cortex has layers and columns. The most extensively studied modules in the striatum are the neurochemically specialized striosomes (striatal bodies) that form branched three-dimensional labyrinths in the striatum. These regions have attracted interest because their boundaries govern the distribution of nearly every neurotransmitter-related compound in the striatum, and because of their connections with the limbic system. In tissue sections striosomes appear as differentially stained ellipses and rings, about 0.5 mm wide, having a higher or lower level of a given transmitter-related compound than does the surrounding extrastriosomal matrix. For instance, neurons in striosomes have higher levels of mu opiate receptors, D_1 dopamine receptors, and neuropeptides such as dynorphin and substance P. The extrastriosomal matrix is enriched in D_2 dopamine receptors, cholinergic markers such as acetylcholinesterase, and encephalin-containing neuropil. Striosomes are not distributed uniformly: they are especially evident in the head of the caudate nucleus and rostral putamen, and also in the most caudal sectors of these nuclei. The sensorimotor-recipient region of the putamen apparently has few striosomes, at least as detected with current methods.

Striosomes and matrix have different inputs and outputs. Striosomes receive inputs from much of the prefrontal, insular and temporal cortex. By contrast, the extrastriosomal matrix receives inputs from the sensorimotor cortex, from much of the parietal-temporal-occipital association cortex, and from the cingulate gyrus. Most subcortical inputs are governed by striosomal boundaries as well: the CM-PF complex of the thalamus projects to the matrix, whereas the midline nuclei of the thalamus and basolateral amygdala project to striosomes. Striosomes in different regions of the striatum receive different inputs, just as the matrix does, and these regional differences in corticostriatal projections are anatomically 'rule-driven'. For instance, cortical association areas in the cat can be placed in a simple hierarchy according to their patterns of striosome-matrix projections (Ragsdale and Graybiel, 1990), and, in the rat, cells in different cortical layers project preferentially to striosomes or to matrix (Gerfen, 1989). Such patterns have not yet been studied in primates.

It is thought that motor signals in the striatum are processed primarily in the matrix: projections from both motor and somatosensory cortex innervate the extrastriosomal matrix and avoid striosomes, and indirect evidence indicates that physiologically identified movement-related neurons are also in the matrix. Moreover, the matrix projects strongly to the pallidum and the SNpr, sites thought to be the main outputs of the basal ganglia motor system. Striosomes, by contrast, project primarily to the SNpc or to the immediately adjacent part of SNpr.

Because striosomes interdigitate with the surrounding matrix, matrix–striosome borders may serve as interfaces where the sensorimotor systems of the matrix interact with the striosomial processing of prefrontal and other inputs. Some striatal cell types send dendrites across striatal boundaries, and could presumably mediate striosome–matrix interactions, but it is interesting that the dendrites of certain other striatal cell types obey striosomal boundaries, and do not cross them (Bolam *et al.*, 1988; Kawaguchi *et al.*, 1990; Penny *et al.*, 1988). In humans and other primates, but not in non-primates, these border regions are distinguished by rings of neurochemically distinct tissue (Graybiel, 1984; Dragunow *et al.*, 1990a). The neurochemical differences between striosomes and matrix make it possible that new drugs could selectively target either striosomal or matrix neurons. Disease processes, too, might have such selective targets. In the striatal degeneration seen in Huntington's disease, for instance, there are reports that striosomes and matrix are differentially affected (Ferrante and Kowall, 1987; Seto-Ohshima *et al.*, 1988; Hedreen, 1990).

It has only recently become evident that the matrix is not merely a homogeneous tissue surrounding striosomes, but itself contains discrete input and output zones – matrisomes – within it (Graybiel *et al.*, 1991). For instance, sensorimotor cortical fibre projections do not innervate all of the matrix, but only isolated zones within it (Malach and Graybiel, 1986; Flaherty and Graybiel, 1991). Thus the entire striatum, and not just the striosomal system, appears to have a modular organization. Such modularity is reminiscent of the layers and columns of the cerebral cortex.

In functional terms, this patchwork may allow individual inputs to the striatal matrix to be parcelled among different striatal subsystems. The degree of convergence and divergence of inputs of the striatum, and the degree to which they select different output modules influence information processing in the striatum.

Other inputs to the basal ganglia

DIRECT AND INDIRECT CORTICAL INPUTS

Two of the loop nuclei linked to the striatum and pallidum, the CM-PF complex of the thalamus and the subthalamic nucleus, receive inputs directly from the motor cortex. There are also projections from motor cortex to other sites in the basal ganglia circuit (e.g. to the tegmental pedunculopontine nucleus), but they are apparently not strong. The motor cortex projects to the CM nucleus, and the premotor cortex innervates the PF nucleus. CM and PF in turn project to the striatum, so the striatum receives indirect as well as direct information from the motor and premotor cortical areas. The fibre projection from the motor cortex to the subthalamic nucleus, which is dense and somatotopic, is accompanied by a weaker fibre projection from neighbouring cortical areas. The subthalamic nucleus projects to both segments of the pallidum and to the SNpr, thus providing a route by which signals from sensorimotor cortex can reach these nuclei without passing through the striatum. The subthalamic nucleus is now considered a pivotal modulator of basal ganglia circuitry (see below).

INPUTS FROM THE BRAINSTEM

Except for the well-known nigrostriatal pathway and a small nigropallidal pathway, direct brainstem inputs to the basal ganglia are sparse. Serotonin-containing fibres from the dorsal raphe nucleus reach the striatum, pallidum and the substantia nigra. The noradrenaline-containing locus coeruleus projects to the ventral striatum, but not strongly to the dorsal striatum or the pallidum. Besides these direct brainstem inputs, the pallidum and the striatum receive information indirectly, via the CM-PF complex, from the reticular formation (including the tegmental pedunculopontine region) and from the spinothalamic tracts. The brainstem inputs to the SNpc, discussed further below, include projections from parts of the subcortical limbic system, but the SNpr, like the pallidum, receive few non-striatal inputs. In general, nuclei in the basal ganglia circuit – except the striatum – receive most of their subcortical inputs from each other, not from other nuclei.

This limited access to the nuclei of the basal ganglia circuit, combined with the rich interconnections of these nuclei, is one of the best pieces of evidence that the basal ganglia circuit is a functional unit. Strong internal connectivity does not imply, however, that the extrinsic inputs to these nuclei are not important. For example, it may be that the input to the subthalamic nucleus from the motor cortex provides the main excitatory drive for this key nucleus, and limbic inputs to the SNpc may condition dopaminergic actions on the entire system.

PROJECTIONS FROM THE STRIATUM TO THE PALLIDUM AND THE SNpr

Compared to the cortex, the striatum is unusual in that most of its neurons are output neurons rather than interneurons. And nearly all of its outputs are directed towards the substantially smaller pallidum and substantia nigra (Tables 1.2 and 1.3). These two nuclei are thus, in a sense, bottle-necks in the primary basal ganglia circuit, a fact that may account for the devastating motor disturbances that damage to them can produce. Two subdivisions of these nuclei, the GPi and SNpr, play similar roles in relaying information from the striatum to thalamocortical circuits, and the GPi and SNpr share many other connections and neurochemical characteristics. Indeed, GPi and SNpr are in some ways more similar to each other than are GPe and GPi or SNpr and SNpc.

Striatal output neurons are classified as medium spiny neurons by their size and their abundance of dendritic spines. They release gamma-aminobutyric acid (GABA) as their neurotransmitter, and generally contain one or more neuropeptide co-transmitters as well. Because GABA hyperpolarizes active and resting neurons, when striatal neurons fire, they inhibit the normally high tonic activity of the pallidum and substantia nigra (Chevalier and Deniau, 1990). Striatal neurons

Table 1.2 Connections of the pallidum

EXTERNAL SEGMENT OF PALLIDUM (GPe)	
Inputs	*Outputs (GABA)*
From striatum: from matrix cell clusters: (GABA and encephalin)	To subthalamic nucleus
From subthalamic nucleus (glutamate)	To striatum
From thalamus: primarily from centre median nucleus	To GPi
From pedunculopontine nucleus	
From SNpc: sparse	
INTERNAL SEGMENT OF PALLIDUM (GPi)	
Inputs	*Outputs (GABA)*
From striatum: from matrix cell clusters (GABA and substance P)	To VA-VL
From subthalamic nucleus (glutamate)	To CM-PF
From thalamus: primarily from parafascicular nucleus	To pedunculopontine nucleus
	To lateral habenular nucleus
From pedunculopontine nucleus	To striatum
From SNpc: sparse	To GPe
VENTRAL PALLIDUM	
Inputs	*Outputs*
From ventral striatum	To mediodorsal nucleus of the thalamus
From amygdala	To hypothalamus
From dorsal raphe nucleus	To amygdala
From locus coeruleus	To lateral habenular nucleus
From SNpc and ventral tegmental area	

CM-PF = Centre median parafascicular nucleus; GABA = gamma-aminobutyric acid; SNPc = subthalamic nucleus pars compacta; VA-VI = ventral anterior–ventral lateral nucleus of the thalamus.

Table 1.3 Connections of the substantia nigra

SUBSTANTIA NIGRA PARS RETICULATA (SNpr)	
Inputs	*Outputs* (GABA)
From striatum: matrix in caudate nucleus and parts of putamen (GABA, neuropeptides)	To VA-VL thalamus
From subthalamic nucleus (glutamate)	To superior colliculus
From SNpc (dopamine)	To MD thalamus
From pedunculopontine nucleus	To pedunculopontine nucleus
SUBSTANTIA NIGRA, PARS COMPACTA (SNpc) AND VENTRAL TEGMENTAL AREA (VTA)	
Inputs	*Outputs (dopamine)*
From striatum (GABA, neuropeptides)	To striatum
From striosomes to SNpc	From cell group A8 and part of SNpc to matrix
From ventral striatum to ventral tegmental area	From part of SNpc to striosomes
From amygdala	From SN pars lateralis to both striosomes and matrix
From lateral preoptic hypothalamus	
From dorsal raphe nucleus	From cell group A10 to ventral striatum and amygdala
From frontal cortex	
From pallidum: sparse	To pallidum: sparse
From subthalamic nucleus: sparse	To subthalamic nucleus: sparse

GABA = Gamma-aminobutyric acid; MD = medial dorsal thalamic nucleus; SNpc = substantia nigra nucleus pars compacta; VA-VL = ventral anterior–ventral lateral nuclei of the thalamus.

probably also inhibit each other through their rich local axon collaterals. This may account for the characteristic very low firing rates of striatal neurons (Groves, 1983).

Despite occasional reports to the contrary, it is clear that both the caudate nucleus and the putamen project to all four striatal targets: GPe, GPi, SNpc and SNpr. The fibre bundles that form the striatopallidal and striatonigral pathways set up a roughly radial projection topography. The putamen – including the sensorimotor zone – projects more strongly to GPe and GPi, and less strongly to the SNpr, whereas the caudate nucleus – including the eye movement zone – projects more strongly to the SNpr. The SNpc apparently receives most of its striatal inputs from the ventral striatum and from striosomes, which are more abundant in the caudate nucleus than in the putamen. The ventral striatum also has its own projection target in the ventral pallidum, a region that lies below the anterior commissure within the substantia innominata, near the nucleus basalis of Meynert.

Until recently, it was believed that striatal outputs were all collaterals of each other. In the rat, single striatal neurons do indeed project to both segments of the pallidum and to the substantia nigra (Staines and Fibiger, 1984; Loopuijt and van der Kooy, 1985). But in higher mammals, neurons projecting to a given striatal target nucleus apparently send few collaterals to other target nuclei (Feger and Crossman, 1984; Beckstead and Cruz, 1986). This target restriction could provide a neural mechanism by which the striatum can control the activity of different parts of the pallidum and nigra independently. Selective output channelling is now thought to be of great importance for movement control.

Striatal neurons projecting to the GPe, GPi and substantia nigra differ neurochemically. Although each set of neurons contains GABA as a transmitter, they appear to have predominantly different co-transmitters: striatal fibres projecting to GPe contain encephalin, whereas those projecting to GPi and SNpr are more likely to contain substance P and dynorphin. This difference in co-transmitters suggests that pharmacological manipulations could target individual striatal output systems independently. However, pharmacological differences between the pathways are unlikely to be absolute. For instance, some neurons coexpress encephalin, dynorphin and substance P (Penny *et al.*, 1986; Besson *et al.*, 1990); and encephalin-containing projections are not entirely restricted to the GPe; the inner part of GPi also has considerable encephalin levels.

Striatal projection systems are segregated not only at the level of single neurons, but also at the level of macroscopic clusters of neurons. As mentioned above, the outputs to GPe, GPi and SNpr all arise primarily from the matrix, whereas striosomes project mainly to the SNpc or to the immediately surrounding SNpr. Within the matrix there appears to be distinct patches and bands of neurons projecting to GPe, GPi and SNpr (Desban *et al.*, 1989; Jiménez-Castellanos and Graybiel, 1989; Giménez-Amaya and Graybiel, 1990; Selemon and Goldman-Rakic, 1990), each set of clusters forming a branching three-dimensional network of matrisomes. The relationship between matrix input and output modules may be key to understanding basal ganglia processing. There is new evidence that all matrix regions receiving inputs from a body part representation in cortex send reconvergent inputs to pairs of sites in GPe and GPi (Flaherty and Graybiel 1993, 1994). This suggests that both segments may reintegrate striatal information about the body.

Despite the predominance of striatal output neurons, there are also several types of striatal interneurons. The cholinergic and somatostatin-containing interneurons have received the most attention recently. Cholinergic interneurons are large, aspiny cells that interact directly with medium spiny output neurons. Interactions between acetylcholine and dopamine have long been assumed because of the opposing effects dopaminergic and cholinergic drugs have on movement disorders, but ultrastructural studies show little direct dopaminergic input to the cholinergic interneurons. The striatal matrix, especially the sensorimotor part of the putamen, is richer in cholinergic cell bodies, neuropil and uptake sites than are striosomes. However, striosomes have denser muscarinic M1 binding than the matrix (Nastuk and Graybiel, 1988). Somatostatin-containing interneurons are medium-sized aspiny cells that, like the cholinergic neurons, are sprinkled through the striatum. Both cholinergic and somatostatin-containing neuropil are more dense in the matrix than in striosomes. In Huntington's disease, the somatostatin-containing and cholinergic interneurons are selectively spared (Nemeroff *et al.*, 1983; Ferrante *et al.*, 1987) – in dramatic contrast to the degeneration of nearby medium spiny projection neurons.

LOOP PATHWAYS OF THE BASAL GANGLIA

Inputs from the striatum to the pallidum and substantia nigra influence two sorts of pathways: those leading out of the basal ganglia, and loop pathways that project back to the basal ganglia. Output pathways will be discussed in the last section. The main loop pathways are the following:

1. Striatum → SNpc → striatum.
2. Pallidum → subthalamic nucleus → pallidum.
3. Striatum → GPi → CM-PF thalamus → striatum.

Mesostriatal pathways

Because the degeneration of nigrostriatal dopamine-containing fibres is pathognomonic of Parkinson's disease, this pathway has received much attention. Dopamine released in the striatum is made both in the cell bodies of SNpc neurons and in their striatal axon terminals. In the striatum, dopamine release is thought to be multiply controlled by the inputs and intrinsic circuitry of the SNpc, by autoreceptors for dopamine on the nigrostriatal axon terminals, and possibly by local circuits in the striatum itself.

The SNpc and striatum are often said to be reciprocally interconnected, but this may be true only for neurons in striosomes. Most striatonigral neurons are in the matrix, however, and project not to the SNpc but to the SNpr – which is not known to project back to the striatum. Nevertheless, the dendrites (and some cell bodies) of dopamine-containing neurons of the SNpc extend into SNpr. These may mediate interactions between the SNpc and SNpr.

Work to date suggests that there are four main groups of inputs to the SNpc (Table 1.3): (1) striatal input from striosomes and the ventral striatum; (2) limbic input from the central nucleus of the amygdala, the lateral preoptic area of the hypothalamus, and the dorsal raphe nucleus; (3) cortical input from the frontal cortex, including the supplementary motor cortex; and (4) some fibres from the pallidum and subthalamic nucleus. The SNpc thus provides a means for a number of nuclei – many of them related to the limbic system – to exert an influence on striatal activity. The diversity of inputs to the SNpc is in sharp contrast to the restricted inputs to the SNpr.

The striatum, besides receiving input from the SNpc, receives projections from the other major midbrain dopaminergic cell groups: the retrorubral region (cell group A8) and the ventral tegmental area (A10 cell group). Different dopaminergic cell groups project selectively to either striosomes or matrix in the dorsal striatum (Jiménez-Castellanos and Graybiel, 1987; Langer and Graybiel, 1989). The ventral tegmental area is the primary source of dopamine for the ventral striatum, prefrontal cortex and limbic targets, but some dopamine-containing fibres from the medial SNpc also innervate these regions. These specializations of striatal dopaminergic innervation have implications for disease. For instance, both in Parkinson's disease and following exposure to the neurotoxin 1-methyl-4-phenyl-1,2,3,6-tetrahydropyridine (MPTP), there is greater cell loss in the SNpc than in the ventral tegmental area (Langston *et al.*, 1984). Thus in parkinsonian disorders the limbic functions of the striatum could be spared relative to striatal sensorimotor functions. However, it is important to remember that dopaminergic neurons have a much less clear relation to movement than do neurons in the striatum and pallidum. Dopaminergic neurons on the SNpc do not fire in relation to movement or preparation for movement, but to stimuli that are behaviourally relevant (Schultz and Romo, 1990).

Dopamine-containing axon terminals synapse directly on striatal output neurons, as do the excitatory inputs from the cerebral cortex and thalamus. The arrangements of these synapses reflect dopamine's modulatory function. Many of the dopaminergic synapses on striatal neurons are on the necks of dendritic spines, whereas it is the heads of the spines that receive synaptic inputs from cortical fibres (Freund *et al.*, 1984). Dopamine-containing terminals are thus in a position to modulate transmission of cortical inputs selectively, at the level of individual spines, rather than to produce the non-selective modulation that they would produce were they near the axon hillock of the striatal neurons.

There has been a long debate over whether dopamine is excitatory or inhibitory: electrical stimulation of the substantia nigra causes a mixture of excitatory and inhibitory postsynaptic effects in striatal neurons, but application of dopamine directly into the striatum inhibits the already low basal firing rate of its neurons. Whether these effects are monosynaptic or not is not known. Recent evidence from whole-cell voltage clamp study of striatal neurons suggests that the effects of dopamine are mediated at least in part by potassium channels (Freedman and Weight, 1988), and appear to be voltage-dependent (Rutherford *et al.*, 1988; Kitai *et al.*, 1990). If they are voltage-dependent, the results of activity at a dopaminergic synapse will depend on the state of local activity in the recipient neuron. This conditional action fits well with the long-postulated notion that the monoaminergic pathways have a filtering effect on their target structures, enhancing the signal-to-noise ratio.

The nature of the postsynaptic dopamine receptor is, of course, crucial to its response to dopamine, and different dopamine receptors have different anatomical distributions in the basal ganglia. In the rat, dopamine D_2 receptors are found on encephalin neurons projecting to the globus pallidus (the rat homologue of the primate GPe), whereas D_1 receptors are found on substance P neurons projecting to the substantia nigra (Gerfen *et al.*, 1990). These differential effects set up the possibility, to be tested, that D_2-active drugs could target the encephalin-containing GPe pathway, and D_1 drugs target the substance P-containing GPi-SNpr pathway. Besides the D_1 and D_2 receptor subtypes, three new subtypes, the D_3, D_4 and D_5 receptors, have recently been cloned (Sokoloff *et al.*, 1990; Sunahara *et al.*, 1991; Van Tol *et al.*, 1991). Only the D_1 and D_2 subtypes have had their second-messenger effects characterized. D_1 receptors are positively coupled to adenylate cyclase (Stoof and

Kebabian, 1981) and to phosphatidyl inositol turnover (Mahan *et al.*, 1990), whereas D_2 receptors are negatively coupled to adenylate cyclase (Stoof and Kebabian, 1981) and to phosphatidyl inositol turnover (Pizzi *et al.*, 1988). It had long been postulated that D_2 receptors mediate the antipsychotic effects of neuroleptics such as haloperidol, but the discovery of the D_3 and D_4 receptors makes re-evaluation of this hypothesis necessary. In contrast with the D_1 and D_2 receptors, which are found in both the dorsal and ventral striatum, the D_3 receptor is concentrated especially in the striatum, and thus may have a special role in limbic or affective functions. Atypical neuroleptics, such as clozapine, have high affinity for D_4 receptors, and have fewer extrapyramidal side-effects than do the traditional neuroleptics, such as haloperidol, which tend to bind to D_2 receptors (Van Tol *et al.*, 1991). Neuroleptics such as haloperidol may also have effects through their binding to sigma sites, which are highly concentrated in the SNpc (Largent *et al.*, 1984; Gundlach *et al.*, 1986) – especially in the part of the SNpc that projects to striosomes (Graybiel *et al.*, 1989).

D_1 and D_2 receptors, along with nearly all other dopamine-related compounds, are differentially distributed with respect to striosomes and matrix. D_3, D_4 and D_5 receptors have not yet been evaluated for their compartmental affiliations. D_1 binding sites are denser in striosomes than in matrix (Besson *et al.*, 1990), whereas D_2 binding sites (and also high-affinity dopamine uptake sites) are denser in matrix than in striosomes (Joyce *et al.*, 1986; Graybiel and Moratalla, 1989). These differences, together with other neurochemical differences between the two compartments, make it possible for dopamine to have different effects on striosomal and matrix neurons. In fact, basal release of newly synthesized dopamine is higher in matrix-rich regions that in regions that contain many striosomes, and acetylcholine has different effects on that release in the two compartments (Kemel *et al.*, 1989).

Drugs that bind to dopamine receptors or change dopamine levels in the striatum change gene transcription in striatal neurons. For instance, they stimulate synthesis of encephalin in encephalin-containing neurons, most of which project to GPe. By contrast, they produce a decrease in the synthesis and content of substance P in substance P-containing neurons, most of which – at least in the matrix – project to GPi and SNpr (Gerfen *et al.*, 1990). Curiously, although the opioid peptide dynorphin coexists with substance P in striatal projection neurons, the effects of dopaminergic drugs on these two peptides are not the same. Because D_1 receptors are richer in the substance P- and dynorphin-rich striosomes, whereas D_2 sites are richer in the encephalin-rich matrix, D_1- and D_2-mediated effects on striatal output pathways could be significantly different.

The pallidum, although not a major target of the SNpc, is not devoid of dopamine-containing innervation. It is interesting that the two segments of the pallidum themselves, as well as their striatal control pathways, are distinguished by different types of dopamine receptor subtypes: ligands for D_1 receptors mainly bind to GPi, and ligands for D_2 receptors mainly bind to GPe (Richfield *et al.*, 1987; de Keyser *et al.*, 1988; Camps *et al.*, 1989). The GPi also receives a denser dopaminergic input than does the GPe (Parent and Smith, 1987; Besson *et al.*, 1990).

The effects of psychomotor stimulant dopamine agonists such as amphetamine and cocaine may be mediated in striatal neurons by expression of immediate-early genes such as c-*fos* (Graybiel *et al.*, 1990; Young *et al.*, 1991). Curiously, dopamine antagonists such as haloperidol also increase the expression of c-*fos*, but this effect seems to be mediated by D_2 rather than D_1 receptors (Dragunow *et al.*, 1990a; Miller, 1990). The products of these immediate-early genes are DNA-binding proteins that influence the transcription of other genes, including the gene for encephalin

(Sonnenberg *et al.*, 1989). It is possible that such immediate-early genes mediate such long-term behavioural effects of dopaminergic drugs as tardive dyskinesias and addictive syndromes. Determining the patterns within the basal ganglia of postsynaptic changes in gene transcription may help in understanding the pathological changes seen in Parkinson's disease and other basal ganglia disorders, and transcriptional regulation may be important in their treatment as well. For example, the effects of dopamine agonists on striatal c-*fos* can be duplicated in grafts derived from embryonic striatal tissue which have been implanted into damaged striatum (Cenci *et al.*, 1990; Dragunow *et al.*, 1990b; Liu *et al.*, 1991).

The GPe-subthalamic loop

The subthalamic nucleus is reciprocally interconnected with the pallidum (Table 1.4). GPe sends a massive projection to the subthalamic nucleus, which projects to GPi and SNpr, and also back to the GPe. The output neurons of the subthalamic nucleus are now thought to use glutamate as a neurotransmitter, and to be excitatory, not inhibitory as was long believed (Nakanishi *et al.*, 1987; Smith and Parent, 1988). This is a pivotal finding, because it helps explain how striatal activity can have remarkably different effects on basal ganglia output, depending on whether it excites neurons projecting to GPi and SNpr – the direct pathway, or neurons projecting to GPe – the indirect pathway (Fig. 1.2). GPi and SNpr both inhibit the VA-VL nuclei of the thalamus. The subthalamic loop, however, could modulate this inhibition. Striatal activity inhibits GPi's and SNpr's tonic inhibition of the thalamus, so cortical activation of striato-GPi and striatonigral neurons should increase thalamocortical activity. But striatal activity also inhibits GPe's inhibition of the subthalamic nucleus, permitting the subthalamic nucleus to excite GPi. GPi should then increase its inhibition of the thalamus and decrease thalamocortical activity (Albin *et al.*, 1989).

Until recently, it was thought that nearly all GPe output was directed towards the subthalamic nucleus; that is, that there was no direct way for the GPe to influence the output from GPi to the thalamus. There now is evidence, however, that GPe and GPi are reciprocally interconnected (Hazrati *et al.*, 1990; Kincaid *et al.*, 1990; Smith and Bolam, 1990). This resurrects the once-postulated notion of a step-by-step pathway from the striatum through GPe to GPi to the thalamus. The GPe-to-GPi pathway could have the same effects as the subthalamic loop: the striatum, by

Table 1.4 Connections of the subthalamic nucleus

Inputs	*Outputs*
From GPe: GABA	To GPi: glutamate
From cortex, especially motor cortex: glutamate	To GPe: glutamate
From pedunculopontine nucleus	To SNpr
	To ventral pallidum
	To VA-VL
	To striatum
	To pedunculopontine nucleus

GABA = Gamma-aminobutyric acid; GPe = external segment of the globus pallidus; GPi = internal segment of the globus pallidus; SNpr = subthalamic nucleus pars reticulata; VA-VL = ventral anterior-ventral lateral nucleus of the thalamus.

projecting to GPe, could disinhibit GPi neurons and increase inhibition of the thalamus, decreasing thalamocortical activity.

This simple circuit model has testable and practical implications. For instance, if the presence of the subthalamic loop dampens thalamocortical activity, removal of the loop should increase it, and increase motor activity. This result is seen in hemiballism, long known to follow subthalamic lesions. The effect of subthalamic lesions could have a therapeutic role in Parkinson's disease: in MPTP-treated parkinsonian monkeys, lesions of the subthalamic nucleus produce an immediate, dramatic alleviation of akinesia, tremor and rigidity (Bergman *et al.*, 1990). Such subthalamic lesions are thought to counteract a pathological increase in subthalamic activity in the parkinsonian monkey, an increase produced by a decrease of GPe activity relative to GPi activity (Miller and DeLong, 1987; Filion *et al.*, 1988).

Observations made on Huntington's disease brains suggest a pathological process in which GPe activity increases relative to GPi activity. In early-stage Huntington's disease, there is evidence that encephalin immunostaining in GPe selectively decreases, whereas substance P immunostaining in GPi is relatively spared (Reiner *et al.*, 1988; Albin *et al.*, 1990), although this has recently become controversial (Ferrante *et al.*, 1990). A specific deficit in GPe encephalin staining suggests that striatal neurons projecting to GPe are selectively damaged relative to those projecting to GPi. According to the model described above, this would decrease the striatum's inhibition of GPe and hence increase GPe's inhibition of the subthalamic nucleus. The resulting reduction of activity in GPi would decrease inhibition of the thalamus, ultimately leading to increased thalamocortical activity and chorea.

As this circuit model is further developed, several aspects of basal ganglia wiring will need to be added. Firstly, the motor cortex directly excites the subthalamic nucleus, and thus might bypass the cortex-to-striatum-to-GPe-to-subthalamic nucleus projection of the indirect pathway. Secondly, given the modular organization of inputs from cerebral cortex, and the modular organization of striatal output neurons projecting to GPe and GPi, it may be that different cortical commands are sent into the GPe and GPi pathways. Thirdly, striatal inputs may synapse only on certain pallidal output neurons; certainly not all neurons in the pallidum fire equally following striatal stimulation. Finally, the 'plus and minus sign' analysis of the basal ganglia circuit ignores the effects of the neuropeptides coexisting in the striatal pathways. Nevertheless, this model is appealing because of its simplicity and its success in predicting clinical findings. Now that the Huntington's disease gene has been cloned (Huntington's Disease Collaborative Research Group, 1993), information about its effects must be incorporated into the model.

The GPi–CM-PF–striatum loop

Outputs from GPi reach not only the VA and VL nuclei, but also the CM and PF nuclei (Table 1.5). As with the other basal ganglia paths, the ventral striatum has its own thalamic loop, involving the subparafascicular nucleus. The function of the CM-PF complex is a mystery – current theories of basal ganglia interactions have nothing substantive to say about it. Yet CM and PF are very large in the primate brain, and they project strongly to the striatum. CM and PF receive significant inputs from motor cortex (to CM), premotor cortex (to PF), and some inputs from the brainstem, and this brings extrinsic signals as well as feedback information to the striatum. Because both CM and PF project to discrete cell clusters within the striatal matrix, they may selectively target particular striatal output modules projecting to

Table 1.5 Connections of the basal ganglia-related thalamus

Inputs	*Outputs*
VENTRAL ANTERIOR (VA) AND VENTRAL LATERAL (VL) NUCLEI	
From GPi to VA and some VL	To frontal cortex
From SNpr to some VA	From VA to areas including supplementary motor area, frontal eye fields
From cerebellum to VL	From VL to areas including motor cortex
CENTRE MEDIAN (CM) AND PARAFASCICULAR (PF) NUCLEI	
Inputs	*Outputs*
From GPi	To striatum
From cortex	From CM to matrix in sensorimotor region of putamen
From motor cortex to CM	From PF to matrix in caudate nucleus and part of putamen
From premotor cortex to PF	From subparafascicular nucleus to ventral striatum
From amygdala to subparafascicular nucleus	To pallidum
From SNpr	From CM to GPe, some GPi
From superior colliculus	From PF to GPi, some GPe
From pedunculopontine nucleus	To cortex
From locus coeruleus	
From dorsal raphe nuclei	
From brainstem reticular formation	
From spinothalamic tracts	
MEDIODORSAL NUCLEUS	
Inputs	*Outputs*
From basolateral amygdala	To prefrontal cortex, also cingulate cortex and supplementary motor area
From hypothalamus	To basolateral amygdala
From olfactory bulb	
Fom ventral pallidum	
From SNpr	
Fron pontine reticular formation	

GPe = external segment of the globus pallidus; GPi = internal segment of the globus pallidus; SNpr = subthalamic nucleus pars reticulata.

GPe, GPi and SNpr. CM and PF are anatomically, and perhaps functionally, differentiated from each other in that CM projects primarily to the sensorimotor region of the putamen, whereas PF projects to the associative regions of both caudate nucleus and putamen (Sadikot *et al*., 1990). CM and PF both send fibres back to the pallidum: CM primarily to GPe, and PF primarily to GPi (Sadikot and Parent, 1989). They project sparsely to cerebral cortex and subcortical regions as well.

Other basal ganglia loops

The tegmental pedunculopontine nucleus is part of yet another basal ganglia loop. It receives input from the GPi, SNpr and motor cortex – inputs that suggest a motor rather than limbic role for the pedunculopontine nucleus. Most of the output of the pedunculopontine nucleus is sent back to the substantia nigra, especially to the SNpc, and also to the pallidum, subthalamic nucleus and CM-PF thalamus. But there are descending projections from the pedunculopontine nucleus as well. One such is to the reticular formation of the caudal brainstem and apparently includes the inhibitory area of Magoun, a region known to influence activity in the spinal cord. Neurons in the region of the pedunculopontine nucleus are cholinergic, and it is intriguing that they are selectively vulnerable in parkinsonian disorders, especially in progressive supranuclear palsy (Hirsch *et al.*, 1987; Zweig *et al.*, 1987). Cholinergic neurons in this region supply cholinergic input to the SNpc and the superior colliculus (Beninato and Spencer, 1986; Woolf and Butcher, 1986).

OUTPUTS OF THE BASAL GANGLIA

Compared to the tangled loops of interconnections among the basal ganglia and their allied nuclei, their outputs to other parts of the brain are few indeed. GPi and SNpr both send inhibitory input to the nuclei of the VA and VL thalamus, to the tegmental pedunculopontine nucleus, and to the lateral habenular nucleus. The SNpr, but apparently not GPi, also sends a fibre projection directly to the superior colliculus.

GPi and SNpr outputs to the thalamus

The fibre projections to the VA and VL nuclei are the best-known of the GPi and SNpr outputs, because they are by far the strongest outputs, and because VA and VL project to premotor and supplementary motor cortex. The deep cerebellar nuclei project to VL as well, and it was long thought that VL might be a site where the basal ganglia and cerebellum, the two classical extrapyramidal motor systems, could interact. More recent evidence suggests, however, that the basal ganglia and cerebellum project mainly to different subdivisions within the motor-related thalamus. For example, in the VLO subnucleus of VL, GPi projects to cell-dense islands, whereas the cerebellum projects to the cell-sparse regions in between them (Asanuma *et al.*, 1983). The cerebellum innervates other parts of VL, whereas the GPi predominantly innervates VA. SNpr also sends fibres to the adjacent mediodorsal thalamic nucleus.

The gross anatomical segregation of inputs to VA and VL does not rule out the possibility that cerebellar and basal ganglia systems have some interactions in the thalamus. The separation does, however, indicate that different regions of the cerebral cortex are most strongly influenced by the basal ganglia and cerebellum, because the different VA and VL input fields have outputs to distinct regions of cortex. The cerebellum-recipient region sends fibres primarily to motor cortex and some premotor cortex; the GPi-recipient region sends fibres to non-overlapping parts of premotor cortex and some motor cortex; and the SNpr-recipient regions of VL and the mediodorsal nucleus send fibres yet farther forward to the frontal lobes, including the frontal eye fields and prefrontal cortex (Asanuma *et al.*, 1983; Schell and Strick, 1984; Ilinsky *et al.*, 1985). Curiously the Vim subnucleus, which apparently does not receive inputs from the basal ganglia, is the thalamic nucleus in which lesions block parkinsonian tremor. Lesions in the VL nucleus relieve parkinsonian rigidity, but not tremor (Narabayashi, 1989).

Because the supplementary motor cortex is thought to play a role in premovement cortical activity, in contrast to a more immediate executive function for motor cortex, the influence of the basal ganglia's path to the cortex is also thought to be mainly at the level of movement planning. In contrast, the fibre projection from the cerebellum via VL to motor cortex is considered to have more influence on movement execution. The frontal regions to which SNpr projects may have a role in motor memory and working memory (Fuster, 1989). Such hypotheses, despite their vagueness, have been popular because certain aspects of basal ganglia motor disorders suggest disorders at the level of motor scheme or movement initiation rather than at the level of detailed movement execution. These include the difficulty that parkinsonian patients have in initiating and terminating movements, and the unwilled nature of choreic movements. Such functional distinctions are not absolute, however, and the anatomical distinctions are not either. For instance, there is recent evidence that basal ganglia-affiliated areas of the thalamus do project to certain areas of motor cortex (Holsapple *et al.*, 1991). Moreover, electrophysiological studies show that most basal ganglia neurons fire too late during the course of a movement to have much role in movement initiation (Mink and Thack, 1991a,b).

SNpr outputs to the superior colliculus

The oculomotor connections of the basal ganglia are unique in having a major tectal output in addition to their thalamic output. There is a strong GABAergic fibre projection from the SNpr to the superior colliculus. Fibres from SNpr innervate the middle layers of the superior colliculus, which contain many neurons that fire before saccadic eye movements. This pathway has been intensively studied, and, in the monkey, has been shown to influence whether saccadic eye movements occur or not. When saccadic eye movements are made, the tonic activity of SNpr neurons briefly decreases (Hikosaka and Wurtz, 1983). Because the output from the SNpr to the superior colliculus is inhibitory, this brief decrease allows a burst of spikes in the cells of the superior colliculus, and this, in turn, can trigger the initiation of saccades. Saccade-related bursts of activity have been recorded in the part of the caudate nucleus that projects to the SNpr. The path from striatum to SNpr to the superior colliculus, like the path from striatum to thalamus, is a doubly inhibitory one (Deniau and Chevalier, 1985). Injection of GABAergic agonists into SNpr, or of GABAergic antagonists into the superior colliculus, mimics the activity of this pathway and facilitates saccades (Hikosaka and Wurtz, 1985a,b). The path from SNpr to the thalamus may also infleunce eye movements, because the thalamic target of SNpr fibres projects in part to the frontal eye fields, but little is yet known about this cortically directed path.

Some of the eye movement neurons in the caudate nucleus and in the SNpr show behavioural state dependence (Hikosaka *et al.*, 1989). It may be that this dependence reflects the inputs from the frontal lobes to the caudate nucleus. The activity of some of these eye movement neurons is related to the remembered positions of targets. SNpr's projection to the superior colliculus, and also its projection via the thalamus to frontal cortex, may thus play some role in controlling behaviours contingent on stored as well as externally generated signals.

Other basal ganglia outputs

Hypotheses that explain the function of the basal ganglia exclusively in terms of basal ganglia effects on cortical mechanisms neglect not only the projections to the superior colliculus, but also those to the tegmental pedunculopontine nucleus, and the lateral habenular nucleus. The lateral habenular nucleus is interconnected with sites in the limbic system, tegmental motor region, and expecially the dorsal raphe nucleus. Because the dorsal raphe nucleus is, in turn, the major source of serotonergic inputs to several parts of basal ganglia circuitry, the lateral habenular nucleus, too, is to some extent part of a loop system of the basal ganglia. This is one of the many basal ganglia circuits remaining to be explored.

SUMMARY

Recent advances in research on the basal ganglia include: (1) a large increase in knowledge of the modular design of the striatum and its projections to GPe, GPi and SNpr; (2) a new view of the mechanisms by which increased or decreased activity in the subthalamic nucleus may lead to akinetic and choreic movement disorders respectively; (3) a new base of information about neurophysiological processing in basal ganglia circuitry, especially in relation to saccadic eye movement; and (4) indications that dopaminergic drugs can selectively interact with different basal ganglia circuits and can alter gene transcription within circuit nuclei.

References

Albin RL, Young AB, and Penney JB (1989) The functional anatomy of basal ganglia disorders. *Trends Neurosci*, **12**, 366–75

Albin RL, Young AB, Penney JB, Handelin B, Balfour R, Anderson KD *et al.* (1990) Abnormalities of striatal projection neurons and NMDA receptors in pre-symptomatic Huntington's disease. *N Engl J Med*, **322**, 1293–7

Alexander GE and DeLong MR (1985) Microstimulation of the primate neostriatum: II. Somatotopic organization of striatal microexcitable zones and their relation to neuronal response properties. *J Neurophysiol*, **53**, 1433–46

Alheid GF and Heimer L (1988) New perspectives in basal forebrain organization of special relevance for neuropsychiatric disorders: the striatopallidal, amygdaloid, and corticopetal components of the substantia innominata. *Neuroscience*, **27**, 1–39

Asanuma C, Thach WT, and Jones EG (1983) Distribution of cerebellar terminations and their relation to other afferent terminations in the ventral lateral thalamic region of the monkey. *Brain Res Rev*, **5**, 237–65

Beckstead RM and Cruz CJ (1986) Striatal axons to the globus pallidus, entopeduncular nucleus and substantia nigra come mainly from separate cell populations in cat. *Neuroscience*, **19**, 147–58

Beninato M and Spencer RF (1986) A cholinergic projection to the rat superior colliculus demonstrated by retrograde transport of horseradish peroxidase and choline acetyltransferase immunohistochemistry. *J Comp Neurol*, **253**, 525–38

Bergman H, Wichmann T, and DeLong MR (1990) Reversal of experimental parkinsonism by lesions of the subthalamic nucleus. *Science*, **249**, 436–8

Besson M-J, Graybiel AM, and Quinn B (1990) Coexpression of neuropeptides in the cat's striatum: an immunohistochemical study of substance P, dynorphin B and enkephalin. *Neuroscience*, **39**, 33–58

Bolam JP, Izzo PN, and Graybiel AM (1988) Cellular substrate of the histochemically-defined striosome/matrix system of the caudate nucleus: a combined Golgi and immunocytochemical study in cat and ferret. *Neuroscience*, **24**, 853–75

Camps M, Cortes R, Gueye B, Probst A, and Palacios JM (1989) Dopamine receptors in human brain: autoradiographic distribution of D2 sites. *Neuroscience*, **28**, 275–90

Carlsson M and Carlsson A (1990) Interactions between glutamatergic and monoaminergic systems within the basal ganglia – implications for schizophrenia and Parkinson's disease. *Trends Neurosci*, **13**, 272–6

Cenci MA, Mandel RJ, Kalen P, Wictorin K, and Björklund A (1990) C-*fos* induction in intrastriatal grafts of fetal nigral and striatal tissue: functional role of D1 dopamine receptors in graft–host interactions. *Soc Neurosci Abstr*, **16**, 469

Chevalier G and Deniau JM (1990). Disinhibition as a basic process in the expression of striatal functions. *Trends Neurosci*, **13**, 277–80

Crutcher MD and Alexander GE (1990) Movement-related neuronal activity selectively coding either direction or muscle pattern in three motor areas of the monkey. *J Neurophysiol*, **64**, 151–63

de Keyser J, Claeys A, de Backer JP, Ebinger G, Roels F, and Vauquelin G (1988) Autoradiographic localization of D1 and D2 dopamine receptors in the human brain. *Neurosci Lett*, **91**, 142–7

Deniau JM and Chevalier G (1985) Disinhibition as a basic process in the expression of striatal functions. II. The striato-nigral influence on thalamocortical cells of the ventromedial thalamic nucleus. *Brain Res*, **334**, 227–33

Desban M, Gauchy C, Kemel ML, Besson MJ, and Glowinski J (1989) Three-dimensional organization of the striosomal compartment and patchy distribution of striatonigral projections in the matrix of the cat caudate nucleus. *Neuroscience*, **29**, 551–66

DiFiglia M (1990) Excitotoxic injury of the neostriatum: a model for Huntington's disease. *Trends Neurosci*, **13**, 286–9

Dragunow M, Robertson GS, Faull RLM, Robertson HA, and Jansen K (1990a) D2 dopamine receptor antagonists induce *fos* and related proteins in rat striatal neurons. *Neuroscience*, **37**, 287–94

Dragunow M, Williams M, and Faull RLM (1990b) Haloperidol induces *Fos* and related molecules in intrastriatal grafts derived from fetal striatal primordia. *Brain Res*, **530**, 309–11

Dunnett SB and Iverson SD (1980) Regulatory impairments following selective kainic acid lesions of the neostriatum. *Behav Brain Res*, **1**, 497–506

Dunnett SB and Iverson SD (1982) Sensorimotor impairments following localized kainic acid and 6-hydroxydopamine lesions of the neostraitum. *Brain Res*, **248**, 121–7

Feger J and Crossman AR (1984) Identification of different subpopulations of neostriatal neurons projecting to globus pallidus or substantia nigra in the monkey: a retrograde fluorescence double-labelling study. *Neurosci Lett*, **49**, 7–12

Ferrante RJ and Kowall NW (1987) Tyrosine hydroxylase-like immunoreactivity is distributed in the matrix compartment of normal human and Huntington's disease striatum. *Brain Res*, **416**, 141–6

Ferrante RJ, Beal MF, Kowall NW, Richardson EP Jr, and Martin JB (1987) Sparing of acetylcholinesterase-containing striatal neurons in Huntington's disease. *Brain Res*, **411**, 162–6

Ferrante RJ, Kowall NW, Harrington K, and Richardson EP Jr (1990) Terminal striatal substance P- and met-enkephalin-projections in the globus pallidus are equally affected in Huntington's disease. *Soc Neurosci Abstr*, **16**, 1120

Filion M, Tremblay L, and Bédard PJ (1988) Abnormal influences of passive limb movement on the activity of globus pallidus neurons in parkinsonian monkeys. *Brain Res*, **444**, 165–76

Flaherty AW and Graybiel AM (1991) Corticostriatal transformations in the primate somatosensory system. Projections from physiologically mapped body-part representations. *J Neurophysiol*, **66**, 1249–63

Flaherty AW and Graybiel AM (1993) Output architecture of the primate putamen. *J Neurosci*, **13**, 3222–37

Flaherty AW and Graybiel AM (1994) Input–output modularity of the sensorimotor striatum in the squirrel monkey. *J Neurosci* (in press)

Fotuhi M, Koliatsos VE, Alexander GE, and DeLong MR (1989) Patterns of sensorimotor integration in the primate neostriatum: primary somatosensory cortex (SC) and motor cortex (MC) project to coextensive territories in the putamen. *Soc Neurosci Abstr*, **15**, 285

Freedman JE and Weight FF (1988) Single potassium channels activated by D2 dopamine receptors in acutely dissociated neurons from rat corpus striatum. *Proc Natl Acad Sci USA*, **85**, 3618–22

Freund TF, Powell JF, and Smith AD (1984) Tyrosine hydroxylase immunoreactive boutons in synaptic contact with identified striatonigral neurons, with particular reference to dendritic spines. *Neuroscience*, **13**, 1189–215

Fuster JM (1989) *The Prefrontal Cortex*. New York, Raven

Gerfen CR (1989) The neostriatal mosaic: striatal patch-matrix organization is related to cortical lamination. *Science*, **246**, 385–8

Gerfen CR, Engber TM, Mahan LC, Susel Z, Chase TN, Monsma FJ Jr *et al.* (1990) D1 and D2 dopamine receptor-regulated gene expression of striatonigral and striatopallidal neurons. *Science*, **250**, 1429–32

Giménez-Amaya J-M and Graybiel AM (1990) Compartmental origins of the striatopallidal projection in the primate. *Neuroscience*, **34**, 111–26

Graybiel AM (1984) Neurochemically specified subsystems in the basal ganglia. In Evered D and O'Connor M, eds, *Functions of the Basal Ganglia*. Ciba Foundation Symposium 107, *London*, Pitman Press 114–43

Graybiel AM (1990) Neurotransmitters and neuromodulators in the basal ganglia. *Trends Neurosci*, **13**, 244–54

Graybiel AM, Besson MJ, and Weber E (1989) Neuroleptic-sensitive binding sites in the nigrostriatal system: evidence for a differential distribution of sigma sites in the substantia nigra, pars compacta of the cat. *J Neurosci*, **9**, 326–38

Graybiel AM and Moratalla R (1989) Dopamine uptake sites in the striatum are distributed differentially in striosome and matrix compartments. *Proc Natl Acad Sci USA*, **86**, 9020–24

Graybiel AM, Moratalla R, and Robertson HA (1990) Amphetamine and cocaine induce drug-specific activation of the c-*fos* gene in striosome-matrix and limbic subdivisions of the striatum. *Proc Natl Acad Sci USA*, **87**, 6912–16

Graybiel AM, Flaherty AW, and Giménez-Amaya J-M (1991) Striosomes and matrisomes. In Bernard G, Carpenter MB, di Chiara G, Morelli M, and Stanzione P, eds, *The Basal Ganglia, III*, New York, Plenum Press, 3–12

Groves PM (1983) A theory of the functional organization of the neostriatum and the neostriatal control of voluntary movement. *Brain Res Rev*, **5**, 109–32

Gundlach AL, Largent BL, and Snyder SH (1986) Autoradiographic location of sigma receptor binding sites in guinea pig and rat central nervous system with (+)3H-3-(3-hydroxyphenyl)-N-(1-propyl)piperidine. *J Neurosci*, **6**, 1757–70

Hazrati L-N, Parent A, Mitchell S, and Haber SN (1990) Evidence for interconnections between the two segments of the globus pallidus in primates: a PHA-L anterograde tracing study. *Brain Res*, **533**, 171–5

Hedreen JC (1990) Pathological changes in early Huntington's disease. *Soc Neurosci Abstr*, **16**, 1121

Hikosaka O and Sakamoto M (1986) Cell activity in monkey caudate nucleus preceding saccadic eye movements. *Exp Brain Res*, **63**, 659–62

Hikosaka O and Wurtz RH (1983) Visual and oculomotor functions of monkey *Macaca mulatta* substantia nigra pars reticulata. 4. Relation of substantia nigra to superior colliculus. *J Neurophysiol*, **49**, 1285–301

Hikosaka O and Wurtz RH (1985a) Modification of saccadic eye movements by gamma aminobutyric-acid-related substances. I. Effect of muscimol and bicuculline in monkey *Macaca mulatta* superior colliculus. *J Neurophysiol*, **53**, 266–91

Hikosaka O and Wurtz RH (1985b) Modification of saccadic eye movements by gamma aminobutyric-acid-related substances. II. Effects of muscimol in monkey (*Macaca mulatta*) substantia nigra pars reticulata. *J. Neurophysiol*, **53**, 292–308

Hikosaka O, Sakamoto M, and Usui S (1989) Functional properties of monkey caudate neurons. III. Activities related to expectation of target and reward. *J Neurophysiol*, **61**, 814–32

Hirsch EC, Graybiel AM, Duyckaerts C, and Javoy-Agid F (1987) Neuronal loss in the pedunculopontine tegmental nucleus in Parkinson disease and in progressive supranuclear palsy. *Proc Natl Acad Sci USA*, **84**, 5976–80

Holsapple JW, Preston JB, and Strick PL (1991) The origin of thalamic inputs to the 'hand' representation in the primary motor cortex. *J Neurosci*, **11**, 2644–54

Huerta MF and Kaas JH (1990) Supplementary eye fields as defined by intracortical microstimulation: connections in macaques. *J Comp Neurol*, **293**, 299–330

Huntington's Disease Collaborative Research Group (1993) A novel gene containing a trinucleotide repeat that is expanded and unstable on Huntington's disease chromosomes. *Cell*, **72**, 971–83

Ilinsky IA, Jouandet ML, and Goldman-Rakic PS (1985) Organization of the nigrothalamocortical system in the rhesus monkey. *J Comp Neurol*, **236**, 315–30

Jiménez-Castellanos J and Graybiel AM (1987) Subdivisions of the dopamine-containing A8–A9–A10 complex identified by their differential mesostriatal innervation of striosomes and extrastriosomal matrix. *Neuroscience*, **23**, 223–42

Jiménez-Castellanos J and Graybiel AM (1989) Compartmental origins of striatal efferent projections in the cat. *Neuroscience*, **32**, 297–321

Jones EG, Coulter JD, Burton H, and Porter R (1977) Cells of origin and terminal distribution of corticostriatal fibers arising in the sensory-motor cortex of monkeys. *J Comp Neurol*, **173**, 53–80

Joyce JN, Sapp DW, and Marshall JF (1986) Human striatal dopamine receptors are organized in compartments. *Proc Natl Acad Sci USA*, **83**, 8002–6

Kawaguchi Y, Wilson CJ, and Emson PC (1990) Projection subtypes of rat neostriatal matrix cells revealed by intracellular injection of biocytin. *J Neurosci*, **10**, 3421–38

Kemel M-L, Desban M, Glowinski J, and Gauchy D (1989) Distinct presynaptic control of dopamine release in striosomal and matrix areas of the cat caudate nucleus. *Proc Natl Acad Sci USA*, **86**, 9006–10

Kennard C and Lueck CJ (1989) Oculomotor abnormalities in diseases of the basal ganglia. *Rev Neurol*, **145**, 587–95

Kincaid AE, Newman SW, Young AB, and Penney JB (1990) Evidence for a projection from the globus pallidus to the entopeduncular nucleus in the rat. *Soc Neurosci Abstr*, **16**, 427

Kish SJ, Shannak K, and Hornykiewicz O (1988) Uneven patterns of dopamine loss in the striatum of patients with idiopathic Parkinson's disease – pathophysiologic and clinical implications. *New Engl J Med*, **318**, 876–80

Kitai ST, Surmeier DJ, and Stefani A (1990) Dopaminergic modulation of voltage-dependent potassium conductances in rat neostriatal neurons. *Soc Neurosci Abstr*, **16**, 418

Künzle H (1975) Bilateral projections from precentral motor cortex to the putamen and other parts of the basal ganglia. An autoradiographic study in *Macaca fascicularis*. *Brain Res*, **88**, 195–209

Künzle H (1977) Projections from the primary somatosensory cortex to basal ganglia and thalamus in the monkey. *Exp Brain Res*, **30**, 481–92

Langer LF and Graybiel AM (1989) Distinct nigrostriatal projection systems innervate striosomes and matrix in the primate striatum. *Brain Res*, **498**, 344–50

Langston JW, Forno LS, Rebert CS, and Irwin I (1984) Selective nigral toxicity after systemic administration of 1-methyl-4-phenyl-1,2,3,6-tetrahydropyridine (MPTP) in the squirrel monkey. *Brain Res*, **292**, 390–4

Largent BL, Gundlach AL, and Snyder SH (1984) Psychotomimetic opiate receptors labeled and visualized with (+)[3H]3-(3-hydroxyphenyl)-N-(1-propyl)piperidine. *Proc Natl Acad Sci USA*, **81**, 4983–7

Liu F-C, Graybiel AM, Dunnett SB, and Robertson HA (1991) Intrastriatal grafts derived from fetal striatal primordia. III. Induction of modular patterns of *Fos*-like immunoreactivity by cocaine. *Exp Brain Res*, **85**, 501–6

Loopuijt LD and van der Kooy D (1985) Organization of the striatum: collateralization of its efferent axons. *Brain Res*, **348**, 86–99

Mahan LC, Burch RM, Monsma F J Jr, Sibley DR (1990) Expression of striatal D1 dopamine receptors coupled to inositol phosphate production and Ca^{2+} mobilization in *Xenopus* oocytes. *Proc Natl Acad Sci USA*, **87**, 2196–200

Malach R and Graybiel AM (1986) Mosaic architecture of the somatic sensory-recipient sector of the cat's striatum. *J Neurosci*, **6**, 3436–58

Miller JC (1990) Induction of c-*fos* mRNA expression in rat striatum by neuroleptic drugs. *J Neurochem*, **54**, 1453–5

Miller WC and DeLong MR (1987) Altered tonic activity of neurons in the globus pallidus and subthalamic nucleus in the primate MPTP model of parkinsonism. In Carpenter MB and Jayaraman, A (eds), *The Basal Ganglia: Structure and Function*, New York, Plenum Press, 415–29

Mink JW and Thach WT (1991a) Basal ganglia motor control. III. Pallidal ablation: normal reaction time, muscle cocontraction, and slow movement. *J Neurophysiol*, **65**, 330–51

Mink JW and Thach WT (1991b) Basal ganglia motor control. II. Late pallidal timing relative to movement onset and inconsistent pallidal coding of movement parameters. *J Neurophysiol*, **65**, 301–29

Nakanishi H, Kita H, and Kitai ST (1987) Intracellular study of rat substantia nigra pars reticulata neurons in an *in vitro* slice preparation: electrical membrane properties and response characteristics to subthalamic stimulation. *Brain Res*, **437**, 45–55

Narabayashi H (1989) Stereotaxic Vim thalamotomy for treatment of tremor. *Eur Neurol*, **29** (suppl 1), 29–32

Nastuk MA and Graybiel AM (1988) Autoradiographic localization and biochemical characteristics of M1 and M2 muscarinic binding sites in the striatum of the cat, monkey, and human. *J Neurosci*, **8**, 1052–62

Nemeroff CB, Youngblood WW, Manberg PJ, Prange AJ Jr, and Kizer JS (1983) Regional brain concentrations of neuropeptides in Huntington's chorea and schizophrenia. *Science*, **221**, 972–5

Parent A and Smith Y (1987) Differential dopaminergic innervation of the two pallidal segments in the squirrel monkey (*Saimiri sciureus*). *Brain Res*, **426**, 397–400

Parthasarathy HB, Schall JD, and Graybiel AM (1992) Distributed but convergent ordering of striatal projections: the frontal eye field and the supplementary eye field in the monkey. *J Neurosci*, **12**, 4468–88

Penny GR, Afsharpour S, and Kitai ST (1986) The glutamate decarboxylase-, leucine enkephalin-methionine enkephalin- and substance P-immunoreactive neurons in the neostriatum of the rat and cat: evidence for partial population overlap. *Neuroscience*, **17**, 1011–45

Penny GR, Wilson CJ, and Kitai ST (1988) Relationship of the axonal and dendritic geometry of spiny projection neurons to the compartmental organization of the neostriatum. *J Comp Neurol*, **269**, 275–89

Pizzi M, Da Prada M, Valerio A, Memo M, Spano PF, and Haefely WE (1988) Dopamine D_2 receptor stimulation inhibits inositol phosphate generating system in rat striatal slices. *Brain Res*, **456**, 235–40

Ragsdale CW and Graybiel AM (1990) A simple ordering of neocortical areas established by the compartmental organization of their striatal projections. *Proc Natl Acad Sci USA*, **87**, 6196–9

Reiner A, Albin RL, Anderson KD, D'Amato CJ, Penney JB, and Young AB (1988) Differential loss of striatal projection neurons in Huntington disease. *Proc Natl Acad Sci USA*, **85**, 5733–7

Richfield EK, Young AB, and Penney JB (1987) Comparative distribution of dopamine D-1 and D-2 receptors in the basal ganglia of turtles, pigeons, rats, cats, and monkeys. *J Comp Neurol*, **262**, 446–63

Rutherford A, Garcia-Munoz M, and Arbuthnott GW (1988) An afterhyperpolarization recorded in striatal cells *in vitro*: effect of dopamine administration. *Exp Brain Res*, **71**, 399–405

Sadikot AF and Parent A (1989) Differential projections of centre median and parafascicular nuclei in squirrel monkey. *Soc Neurosci Abstr*, **15**, 288

Sadikot AF, Parent A, and François C (1990) The centre median and parafascicular thalamic nuclei project respectively to the sensorimotor and associative-limbic striatal territories in the squirrel monkey. *Brain Res*, **510**, 161–5

Schell GR and Strick PL (1984) The origin of thalamic inputs to the arcuate premotor and supplementary motor areas. *J Neurosci*, **4**, 539–60

Schultz W and Romo R (1990) Dopamine neurons of the monkey midbrain: contingencies of responses to stimuli eliciting immediate behavioral reactions. *J Neurophysiol*, **63**, 607–24

Sedvall G (1990) PET imaging of dopamine receptors in human basal ganglia: relevance to mental illness. *Trends Neurosci*, **13**, 302–7

Selemon LD and Goldman-Rakic PS (1990) Topographical intermingling of striatonigral and striatopallidal neurons in the rhesus monkey. *J Comp Neurol*, **297**, 359–76

Seto-Ohshima A, Emson PC, Lawson E, Mountjoy CQ, and Carrasco LH (1988) Loss of matrix calcium-binding protein-containing neurons in Huntington's disease. *Lancet*, 1(8597), 1252–5

Smith Y and Bolam JP (1990) Convergence of pallidal and striatal inputs to neurones in the entopeduncular nucleus and substantia nigra of the rat: application of a new double anterograde labeling method at electron microscopic level. *Soc Neurosci Abstr*, **16**, 236

Smith Y and Parent A (1988) Neurons of the subthalamic nucleus in primates display glutamate but not GABA immunoreactivity. *Brain Res*, **453**, 353–6

Sokoloff P, Giros B, Martres M-P, Bouthenet M-L, and Schwartz J-C (1990) Molecular cloning and characterization of a novel dopamine receptor (D_3) as a target for neuroleptics. *Nature*, **347**, 146–51

Sonnenberg JL, Rauscher GJ III, Morgan JI, and Curran T (1989) Regulation of proenkephalin by *fos* and *jun*. *Science*, **246**, 1622–5

Staines WA and Fibiger HC (1984) Collateral projections of neurons of the rat globus pallidus to the striatum and substantia nigra. *Exp Brain Res*, **56**, 217–20

Stanton GB, Goldberg ME, and Bruce CJ (1988) Frontal eye field efferents in the macaque monkey: I. Subcortical pathways and topography of striatal and thalamic terminal fields. *J Comp Neurol*, **271**, 473–92

Stoof JC and Kebabian JW (1981) Opposing roles for D-1 and D-2 dopamine receptors in efflux of cyclic AMP from rat neostriatum. *Nature*, **294**, 366–8

Sunahara RK, Guan H-C, O'Dowd BF, Seeman P, Laurier LG, Ng G *et al.* (1991) Cloning of the gene for a human dopamine D_5 receptor with higher affinity for dopamine than D_1. *Nature*, **350**, 614–19

Turski L, Bressler K, Rettig K-J, Löschmann P-A, and Wachtel H (1991) Protection of substantia nigra from MPP^+ neurotoxicity by N-methyl-D-aspartate antagonsists. *Nature*, **349**, 414–18

Van Tol HHM, Bunzow JR, Guan H-C, Sunahara RK, Seeman P, Niznik HB *et al.* (1991) Cloning of the gene for a human dopamine D_4 receptor with high affinity for the antipsychotic clozapine. *Nature*, **350**, 610–14

Vonsattel J-P, Myers RH, Stevens TJ, Ferrante RJ, Bird ED, and Richardson EP Jr (1985) Neuropathological classification of Huntington's disease. *J Neuropath Exp Neurol*, **44**, 559–77

Woolf NJ and Butcher LL (1986) Cholinergic systems in the rat brain. III. Projection from the pontomesencephalic tegmentum to the thalamus, tectum, basal ganglia and basal forebrain. *Brain Res Bull*, **16**, 603–37

Young ST, Porrino LJ, and Iadarola MJ (1991) Cocaine induces striatal c-*Fos*-immunoreactive proteins via dopaminergic D1 receptors. *Proc Natl Acad Sci USA*, **88**, 1291–5

Zweig RM, Whitehouse PJ, Casanova MF, Walker LC, Jankel WR, and Price DL (1987) Loss of pedunculopontine neurons in progressive supranuclear palsy. *Ann Neurol*, **22**, 18–25

2
Experimental models of basal ganglia disease

M. A. Sambrook, A. R. Crossmann and I. J. Mitchell

Introduction

Diseases of the basal ganglia account for a very significant proportion of the total spectrum of disability arising from neurological disorders. Although Parkinson's disease and Huntington's chorea were clinically recognized well over 100 years ago, it is only during the last 2–3 decades that our understanding of the pathophysiological mechanisms causing them has started to assume a coherent form. These recent advances have to a large extent relied upon experimental research in animals.

Clinical research has until very recently been based upon careful documentation of the neurological features of movement disorders and associating them with the pathological findings at postmortem. By implication, the retrieval of information has been painstakingly slow. Recently, computed tomography and magnetic resonance imaging have improved the process of linking the clinical manifestations of movements disorders with changes in the structure of the basal ganglia. These developments, however, have simply highlighted the need for a better understanding of the functional importance of not only the individual components of the basal ganglia, but their overall role in the mediation of voluntary movements. Positron emission tomography is now starting to provide this type of information, but at the present time, particularly in basal ganglia-related diseases, its major deficit is one of definition.

These very considerable obstacles have created a need to try and reproduce the clinical disorders seen in humans with experimental models in animals. The sophistication of the motor system in the primate has dictated that such experiments are best performed in the monkey, although a vast amount of basic and supportive research has been possible in lower species of animals. Naturally, the authenticity of any model has to be carefully judged before extrapolating the experimental findings to the human disorder that it is supposed to represent and this has stimulated research into more precise methods of creating them. A brief examination of those methods is needed before examining their individual application.

Electrolytic coagulation was used in initial experiments and in retrospect might appear to have been a rather crude experimental technique. Ablative lesions do not respect anatomical boundaries and they bear little if any relevance to progressive degenerative disease, particularly if there is a selective loss of neurons within a structure. They have, however, played a very significant part in our understanding of basal ganglia function. Where disorders of movement are due to cerebral infarction their role is obvious and this is only too well-illustrated by the pioneering work of Whittier and Mettler in 1949 who investigated the mechanism of ballism with subthalamic lesions. A decade later Poirier and his colleagues used similar techniques to establish very important information about the separate mechanisms causing hypokinesia and tremor in parkinsonism.

As the neurochemical complexity of the basal ganglia has become apparent, the need to influence more specifically neuronal function has increased. The relatively specific dopaminergic neurotoxin, 6-hydroxydopamine, was extensively used in the rodent to cause degeneration of the nigrostriatal pathway by means of local intracerebral injection. It would probably have found much wider application in the monkey if 1-methyl-4-phenyl-1,2,3,6-tetrahydropyridine (MPTP) had not been accidently discovered in humans. When administered systemically, MPTP produced a parkinsonian syndrome in the monkey with focal degeneration of the substantia nigra and the locus coeruleus. This ideal research tool offered the opportunity of replicating Parkinson's disease with such remarkable accuracy that research has been stimulated into not only the neural mechanisms of the condition but also its aetiology.

The excitotoxins, kainic acid and quinolinic acid, cause localized cell death after intracerebral injection. They do not affect specific groups of neurons but fibres of passage at the site of injection are spared and they have therefore been used to create more selective ablative lesions. However, their lack of cell specificity is probably the explanation for the disappointing results obtained so far in replicating Huntington's disease by widespread injections of these agents into the caudate nucleus and putamen.

Localized intracerebral injections of neurotransmitter agonists and antagonists can be used temporarily to enhance or impede synaptic activity in a very specific manner. The advantage of such a technique relates to its transient effect with minimal tissue damage and the ability to repeat it. The method of administration does however demand considerable ingenuity since restraint has to be limited or, preferably, absent. By manipulating neurotransmission in both the medial and lateral pallidal segments and the subthalamic nucleus this methodology has led to the development of very authentic models of chorea and ballism and enabled detailed examination of the neural mechanisms causing them.

The application of these techniques for the creation of models of movement disorders will be further examined and their contribution towards our understanding of chorea, ballism, parkinsonism, drug-induced dyskinesia and dystonia will be analysed.

CHOREA AND BALLISM

Ablative lesions of the subthalamic nucleus

It is generally accepted that ballism is a severe form of chorea, an observation that was first made by Martin in 1927. He was not the first to describe the disorder, but his own experiences, combined with a review of the literature, resulted in the recognition of the syndrome of the body of Luys. The usual cause of damage to the subthalamic nucleus was infarction due to arteriosclerosis and hypertension. The term ballism stressed the involvement of the proximal limb musculature which results in wild throwing actions of the limbs.

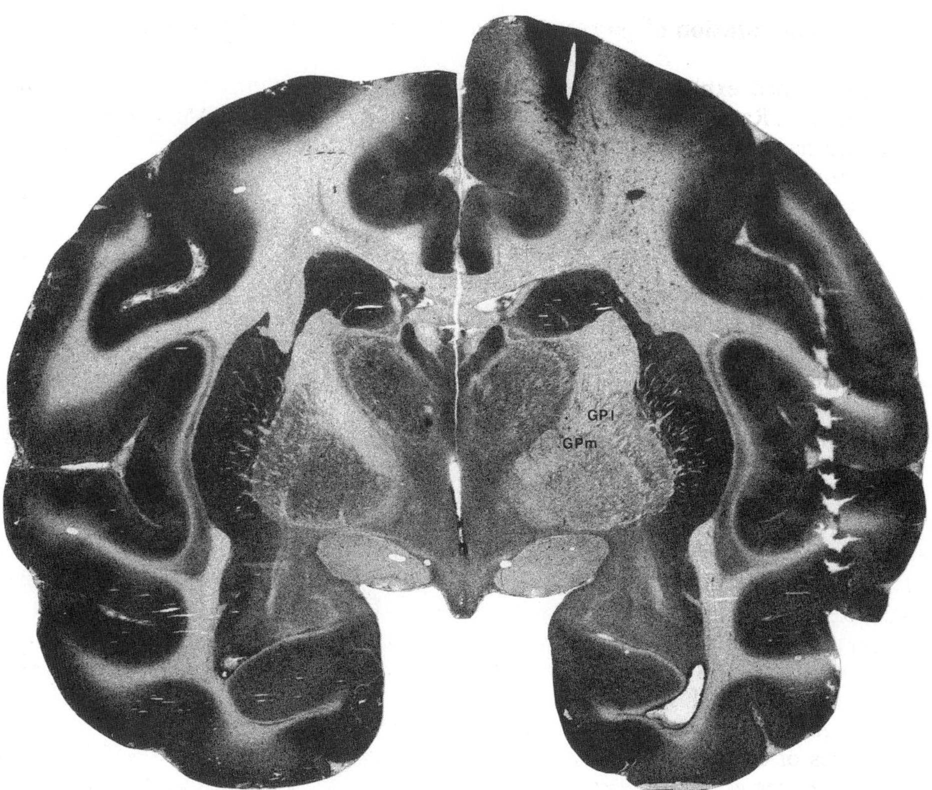

Figure 2.1 A direct reversal print of a 2-deoxyglucose autoradiograph from an animal which received an injection of bicuculline into the right subthalamic nucleus. This injection caused ballism in the contralateral limbs. 2-Deoxyglucose uptake is reduced in the medial (GPm) and lateral (GPl) pallidal segments ipsilateral to the injection.

The mode of onset of the disorder, its dramatic clinical features and its common association with the subthalamic nucleus understandably presented the ideal opportunity to recreate the condition in the primate using an ablative lesion. Whittier and Mettler (1949) and Carpenter *et al.* (1950) demonstrated that coagulation of the subthalamic nucleus resulted in a disorder for which they used the term choreoid hyperkinesia and which from their description ranged from mild chorea to the simian equivalent of ballism. It was necessary to destroy at least 20% of the nucleus, although hyperkinesia was observed with smaller lesions if there was associated damage to the subthalamopallidal pathway. The same workers utilized the model to investigate possible ways of alleviating the disorder and described beneficial results from secondary lesions in the medial pallidum.

Thus ballism came to be accepted as a 'release' phenomenon. The major efferent projections of the subthalamic nucleus were until recently considered to be inhibitory. They are directed to the globus pallidus and the substantia nigra pars reticulata, which in turn have major projections to the ventral-tier thalamic nuclei. Partial or complete loss of the inhibitory action of the subthalamic nucleus upon the medial pallidum appeared to offer the most logical explanation for the hyperkinesia.

Subthalamic infusion of gamma-aminobutyric acid (GABA) antagonists

The established explanation for ballism was attractive and clearly invited further investigation. Rather than destroying the subthalamic nucleus, it was considered that it should be possible to create the same effect by blocking the inhibitory action of the subthalamopallidal pathway in the medial pallidal segment. The available evidence supported GABA as the most likely neurotransmitter (Perkins and Stone, 1981; Rouzaire-Dubois *et al.*, 1983). A different type of experimental approach was required which would enable injections or infusions of very small volumes of neurotransmitter agonists and antagonists into the target area. Guide cannulae were stereotaxically implanted under general anaesthesia while the injections or infusions were by necessity administered to the unrestrained animal to permit immediate and detailed observation of their effect (Needham *et al.*, 1983).

The initial results were confusing and appeared completely to contradict established data. Using obliquely and vertically sited guide cannulae directed at the lentiform and subthalamic nuclei, hemiballism was seen after injections of GABA antagonists into the subthalamic nucleus but not the medial pallidal segment. The most precisely located injections in the subthalamic nucleus created the most severe form of hyperkinesia for 1–2 hours but only after a minimum latency of 6 minutes (Crossman *et al.*, 1984). During this initial period the animals remained unchanged. Similar injections directed at the periphery of the nucleus resulted in a milder form of dyskinesia resembling chorea but with a longer latency. The apparent conclusion to be drawn from this series of experiments was that ballism was associated with increased activity of subthalamic neurons, through blockade of the GABAergic pallidosubthalamic pathway (Vincent *et al.*, 1982).

A series of complementary studies eventually provided the explanation for these findings. Feger *et al.* (1989) injected the GABA antagonist bicuculline methiodide into the subthalamic nucleus of the rat and, using recording techniques, demonstrated an initial increase in neuronal discharge activity followed by prolonged arrest of spike formation. They concluded that the physiological action of bicuculline within the confined space of the subthalamic nucleus was quickly superseded by depolarization blockade and that this was in fact the most efficient way of temporarily halting subthalamic activity.

Metabolic mapping studies

Sokoloff *et al.* (1977) developed the technique of metabolic mapping to assess neuronal activity by using radioactively labelled 2-deoxyglucose (2-DG) as a measure of cell metabolism. The available evidence suggests that changes in the cerebral uptake of 2-DG reflect sodium pump activity associated with the production and release of neurotransmitters in nerve terminals rather than the generation of somatic spikes (Schwartz *et al.*, 1979).

2-DG was administered to animals with hemiballism produced by infusion of GABA antagonists into the subthalamic nucleus (Mitchell *et al.*, 1985a). Autoradiographic interpretation of the results using the uninjected side for comparison demonstrated that there was a 20% reduction in 2-DG uptake by the ipsilateral medial pallidal segment, thereby confirming that the activity of subthalamic neurons was decreased (Figure 2.1). Only a small reduction (6%) in 2-DG uptake was observed in the ipsilateral substantia nigra pars reticulata. This would suggest that the subthalamonigral pathway is of less importance in the mediation of the movement disorder than the projection to the globus pallidus and would coincide with previous reports that nigral lesions are ineffective for the alleviation of dyskinesia (Strominger and Carpenter, 1965).

Surprisingly, the above findings were associated with a 13–17% reduction in 2-DG uptake in the ventral anterior and the ventral lateral thalamic nuclei, suggesting a parallel reduction in the activity of the subthalamopallidal and the pallidothalamic pathways. This finding was not consistent with the former pathway being inhibitory. Using different experimental techniques, information from two sources provided important support for this conclusion. Firstly, Kitai and Kita (1987) demonstrated that stimulation of subthalamic neurons produced monosynaptic excitatory postsynaptic potentials in the rat substantia nigra. It is known that in the rat single subthalamic neurons project to both the substantia nigra and the entopeduncular nucleus, the equivalent of the medial pallidal segment in the primate. Secondly, Parent *et al.* (1989) demonstrated immunonistochemically that cell bodies in the subthalamic nucleus of the squirrel monkey do not show immunoreactivity for GABA but react strongly after incubation with an antiserum against glutamate.

Kynurenic acid infusion into the medial pallidum

If indeed the subthalamopallidal pathway was excitatory, then glutamate would seem the most likely candidate. To test the hypothesis, guide cannulae were implanted in the monkey and directed towards the medial pallidum. Infusions of the broad-spectrum glutamate antagonist kynurenic acid into this structure resulted in the appearance of dyskinesia ranging from mild contralateral hemichorea to hemiballism (Robertson *et al.*, 1989a). Infusions of GABA antagonists were again ineffective but very mild chorea was observed after injections of the GABA agonist muscimol.

GABA antagonism in the lateral pallidum

Huntington's chorea is characterized by degeneration of GABAergic striatal efferent neurons projecting upon the lateral and medial segments of the globus pallidus. Reiner *et al.* (1988) have demonstrated that the projection to the lateral pallidum is more severely affected initially. It has already been demonstrated that infusions of GABA antagonists into the medial pallidum are not associated with chorea. A further series of experiments were therefore performed to investigate the effect of GABA blockade in the lateral globus pallidus. Using the same methods as described above, bicuculline methiodide was infused into this structure and resulted in mild to moderate contralateral chorea (Crossman *et al.*, 1988). The abnormal movements were very characteristic of those seen in humans and exactly resembled the choreiform movements seen with some of the injections of bicuculline into the subthalamic nucleus and kynurenic acid into the medial pallidum described above.

2-DG studies were performed in the animals which developed chorea after bicuculline infusion into the lateral pallidum (Mitchell *et al.*, 1985b). 2-DG uptake was markedly increased in the subthalamic nucleus ipsilateral to the infused site. This was interpreted as an increase in the terminal activity of pallidosubthalamic neurons which were disinhibited as a result of GABA antagonism in the lateral pallidum. The change in 2-DG activity was most apparent in the dorsolateral part of the subthalamic nucleus which receives afferents from the ventral portion of the lateral pallidum, the site from which dyskinesia could be most easily elicited. This was confirmed with neuronal tracing studies using horseradish peroxidase. These changes in 2-DG activity in the subthalamic nucleus were associated with a decrease in isotope uptake in the ipsilateral medial pallidum and ventral anterior and ventral lateral thalamic nuclei, presumably due to the inhibition of subthalamopallidal and pallidothalamic neurons, as seen in ballism caused by primary lesions of the subthalamic nucleus.

Conclusions

It is possible to replicate both chorea and ballism in the monkey by the use of various techniques. The resulting dyskinesia is an accurate reproduction of the disorders seen in humans. A careful examination of the methods used together with complementary studies in both primates and subprimates permits the following conclusions to be drawn:

1. The neural mechanisms causing chorea and ballism are in many ways similar. Both disorders can be produced by decreasing the activity of the subthalamopallidal pathway, either by primary inhibition of subthalamic neurons or by blocking their terminal activity in the medial pallidum.
2. Chorea also occurs in association with GABA antagonism in the lateral pallidum. Here, disinhibition of pallidosubthalamic neurons causes inhibition of the subthalamic nucleus. The different clinical manifestations arising from acute infarction of the subthalamic nucleus and progressive degeneration of the striatum can be adequately explained by these conclusions. The latter, producing gradual destruction of the large topographically organized striatum, would through its lateral pallidal projection produce regional inhibition of subthalamic neurons and localized involuntary movements, whereas the former, depending on its extent, would produce either mild chorea or ballism.
3. The subthalamopallidal pathway is excitatory and mediated via glutamate.
4. In both of these hyperkinetic disorders the pallidothalamic pathway is also underactive. The neurons comprising this pathway are inhibitory and utilize GABA as the neurotransmitter. This would suggest that chorea and ballism are associated with an increase in thalamocortical activity, the movement disorder being mediated via the corticospinal and corticobulbar systems.
5. If motor programs are mediated primarily via the striatal projection to the medial pallidum and from there to the thalamus, then there is no reason to conclude from these results that the production of those programs in chorea and ballism is impaired. It would explain the tendency in these disorders for involuntary movements to interfere with the expression of voluntary actions. In Huntington's chorea it is suggested that GABAergic projection neurons from the striatum to the lateral pallidum are preferentially involved in the early stages of the disease. This situation is experimentally reproduced by GABA blockage in the lateral pallidum. As projection neurons to the medial pallidum become involved at a later stage, the ability to express motor programs is lost and hypokinesia develops.

PARKINSON'S DISEASE

The prevalence of Parkinson's disease in Europe and the North American continent is approximately 1 per 1000. The disorder can present in early and middle life and for these reasons it is a major cause of neurological disability. Levodopa therapy has revolutionized the management of Parkinson's disease, but in turn this form of treatment has become associated with severe and disabling side-effects which now present a challenge almost equal in magnitude to the untreated disorder.

In the light of these observations, authentic animal replicas of Parkinson's disease, particularly in the primate, have been avidly sought. Such replicas would permit many avenues of research into the aetiology, the neural mechanisms, the effect of new forms of treatment, the reasons for the side-effects of levodopa therapy and the possibility of slowing down the progression of the condition. The most exciting developments are of recent origin but a brief survey of the history of attempts to produce primate models of parkinsonism is informative.

Lesions of the ventromedial brainstem tegmentum in the primate

While ablative lesions of the ventromedial brainstem tegmentum have consistently failed to reproduce the complete clinical picture of Parkinson's disease, they have introduced important insight into the mechanism of the various components of the disorder. Unilateral lesions of the substantia nigra do not appear to produce any discernible effect upon movement or tone in the contralateral limbs, although administration of dopaminomimetic drugs may induce turning. Bilateral nigral lesions may induce a degree of hypokinesia (Carpenter and McMasters, 1964). Tremor, usually described as postural, has only occurred in association with hypokinesia after more extensive lesions involving the ventromedial part of the mesencephalic or upper pontine tegmentum (Ward *et al.*, 1948; Poirier, 1960). In these animals histological analysis has demonstrated that in addition to retrograde degeneration of the substantia nigra pars compacta, the lesions have destroyed the rubrospinal and rubrotegmental system and the brachium conjunctivum and resulted in a reduction of noradrenaline and 5-hydroxytryptamine, in addition to severe depletion of striatal dopamine (Poirier *et al.*, 1966). Alternatively, animals with lesions of the cerebellum or brainstem-related structures which did not primarily induce tremor developed tremor after administration of drugs such as harmaline, reserpine, α-methyl-*p*-tyrosine, phenothiazines and butyrophenones which are known to influence central monoaminergic systems. These findings implied that the development of hypokinesia and tremor required a combination of severe striatal dopamine depletion and involvement of the rubro-olivo-cerebello-rubral loop (Poirier *et al.*, 1975). Rigidity was rarely seen and, in fact, in the majority of reported experiments, limb tone was reduced.

6-Hydroxydopamine lesions

The neurotoxin 6-hydroxydopamine is reasonably selective for dopaminergic neurons but has only infrequently been used in primates. In studies performed in the marmoset, unilateral injection of the neurotoxin into the nigrostriatal pathway induced severe striatal dopamine depletion. The animals developed hypokinesia, torticollis and circling behaviour but no demonstrable tremor or rigidity. The hypokinesia disappeared and the torticollis and turning were reversed after the administration of apomorphine (Sambrook *et al.*, 1979). It is probable that further studies of the use of this neurotoxin in the primate have been largely abandoned due to the appearance of MPTP.

MPTP-induced parkinsonism in the primate

Parkinsonism is a well-recognized side-effect of the administration of neuroleptic drugs. The mechanism is through competitive inhibition for striatal dopamine receptors. Although the clinical features strongly resemble Parkinson's disease, there are no associated pathological changes.

In 1976, a chemistry student was admitted to hospital in Bethesda with what was intially considered to be acute schizophrenia. He failed to respond to electroconvulsive therapy and antipsychotic drugs and his catatonic state, mutism and rigidity were eventually diagnosed as acute parkinsonism. Further investigation revealed that the patient had been synthesizing narcotic drugs and that his symptoms had developed after self-administration of a specimen contaminated with MPTP. The case was reported by Davis *et al.* in 1979. The patient responded well to treatment with levodopa but commited suicide 18 months later. Severe degeneration of the substantia nigra pars compacta was demonstrated at autopsy.

Further cases were reported and all were related to the administration of meperidine-related compounds (Langston *et al.*, 1983). The clinical effect of MPTP and its mechanism of action were widely investigated in animals and led to a literature 'explosion' of the subject in the 1980s. Intravenous administration of MPTP to the rhesus monkey produced a disorder which was remarkably similar to idiopathic Parkinson's disease (Burns *et al.*, 1983). The animals developed akinesia, rigidity and a flexed posture with a variable degree of tremor. The tremor was more commonly postural in nature and primarily involved the head and occasionally the unsupported upper limbs. As in humans, pathological examination revealed severe degeneration of the substantia nigra pars compacta and marked striatal dopamine depletion.

Yet the similarity between MPTP-induced parkinsonism in the monkey and Parkinson's disease appeared even more remarkable with further evaluation. The clinical features could be reversed with levodopa therapy which, after a period of several weeks, became associated with peak-dose dyskinesia and rapid fluctuations in response to treatment (the on–off phenomenon). The dyskinesia had both choreiform and dystonic qualities, as typically seen in humans. These features were only seen in severely parkinsonian animals and appeared to increase in extent and duration with prolonged administration of levodopa (Clarke *et al.*, 1987).

It was initially reported that MPTP caused exclusive degeneration of the A8 and A9 nigrostriatal dopaminergic neurons in primates. However, Mitchell *et al.* (1986) reported degeneration of the ventral tegmental area and of the noradrenergic-containing cells of the locus coeruleus. In older animals these features were also accompanied by intraneuronal eosinophilic inclusions resembling Lewy bodies (Forno *et al.*, 1986). Neurochemical studies demonstrated that dopamine depletion was not confined to the striatum but extended into the nucleus accumbens and was associated with a moderate to profound loss of noradrenaline from both the nucleus accumbens and the cerebral cortex. The decrease in noradrenaline occurred irrespective of the presence of degeneration of the locus coeruleus but was most prominent in association with it. Dopamine D_2 receptor autoradiography using tritiated spiperone and sulpiride demonstrated an increase in specific binding in the caudate nucleus and putamen ranging from 40 to 180%, with the greatest increase in the ventrolateral putamen (Sambrook *et al.*, 1987).

Species specificity and mechanism of action of MPTP

The response of various species to MPTP administration is extremely variable. The rat is resistant and does not appear to develop any histological changes in the substantia nigra, although striatal dopamine depletion has been reported (Jarvis and Wagner, 1985). The mouse is more sensitive but much larger doses than those required to produce a comparable effect in the primate are needed (Heikkila *et al.*, 1984). Both histological and neurochemical changes are seen in the mouse, although the former have proved difficult to reproduce consistently and it is notable that recovery usually occurs after several months. Factors such as the mode of administration and the age and sex of the animal appear to introduce significant variables into the response to MPTP and eventual elucidation of these may well improve our understanding of the mechanism of action of the toxin and its possible relevance to Parkinson's disease (Langston and Irwin, 1986). The dog and the cat are moderately susceptible to the toxic effect of MPTP and nigral cell loss has been reported (Parisi and Burns, 1986; Schneider *et al.*, 1986).

The mechanism of action of MPTP has been extensively studied. It rapidly enters the brain after systemic administration and appears to be concentrated in glial cells and sites rich in monoamine oxidase B activity (Chiba *et al.*, 1984). This enzyme catalyses the oxidation of MPTP to the ion 1-methyl-4-phenylpyridinium (MPP^+), a highly toxic metabolite which inhibits mitochrondrial respiration (Nicklas *et al.*, 1985). It is, however, only the accumulation of this ion in certain parts of the brain which determines its eventual toxicity (Javitch and Snyder, 1985). This accumulation is facilitated by the catecholamine uptake system which concentrates MPP^+ in dopaminergic and noradrenergic neurons. It follows that the toxicity of MPTP can be blocked by the simultaneous administration of monoamine oxidase B or catecholamine uptake inhibitors (Heikkila *et al.*, 1985; Javitch and Snyder, 1985). The final concentration of MPP^+ in dopaminergic neurons appears to be the critical factor which determines its toxicity. In the primate the level of MPP^+ in the substantia nigra increases over 48–72 hours following MPTP administration, whereas it quickly decreases in other brain tissues after 24 hours (Irwin and Langston, 1985). In contrast, MPP^+ has a very short half-life in the rodent, which may well explain the reduced sensitivity of this animal to the toxic effect of MPTP (Markey *et al.*, 1984).

The selective vulnerability of certain neurons has been related to their neuromelanin content, a pigment which is absent in rodents and is present in highest concentrations in older primates. This might explain the increased susceptibility of these animals and humans to the toxic action of MPTP, the neuromelanin possibly potentiating its action by facilitating the accumulation of MPP^+ in nigral neurons (D'Amato *et al.*, 1986). Based on the 'toxic' theory of Parkinson's disease it has been suggested that the progression of this degenerative condition might be reduced by monoamine oxidase B inhibitors and the results of trials appear to support this hypothesis (Birkmayer *et al.*, 1985; Shoulson *et al.*, 1989; Tetrud and Langston, 1989).

In conclusion, the MPTP-induced model of parkinsonism in the monkey and in humans is most remarkable in its resemblance to idiopathic Parkinson's disease. It has created a new impetus of research into the disorder, several aspects of which will be examined below.

Neuronal metabolic studies in MPTP-induced parkinsonism

The demonstrated authenicity of the MPTP-induced model of parkinsonism in the monkey makes it an ideal subject for studies of neuronal activity using the well-established 2-DG technique developed by Sokoloff *et al.* (1977). Several groups of research workers have reported their results, based upon systemically treated monkeys and hemiparkinsonian animals which have received unilateral intracarotid infusions of MPTP (Schwartzman and Alexander, 1985; Porrino *et al.*, 1987 and Mitchell *et al.*, 1989). Despite variations in the findings, some of which appear to be based upon the effect of dopaminergic agents on the regional uptake of 2-DG, a consistent pattern of change in neuronal activity seems to emerge from these studies.

The disordered striatal activity arising from the loss of dopamine is most obviously demonstrated in the terminal fields of GABAergic projection neurons from the caudate nucleus and the putamen. The changes in the lateral pallidal segment are most obvious where a marked increase (24–27%) in 2-DG uptake is observed. This indicates increased terminal activity of these neurons, a conclusion supported by ligand-binding studies which have demonstrated downregulation of GABA receptors in this region (Griffiths, 1988; Robertson *et al.*, 1989b). The increased release of GABA results in inhibition of lateral pallidal neurons, the majority of which project to the subthalamic nucleus. Autoradiographic studies confirm that terminal activity in the subthalamic nucleus is decreased and since pallidosubthalamic neurons are again inhibitory and utilize GABA (Vincent *et al.*, 1982), this will be associated with an increase in subthalamic neuronal activity (Figure 2.2).

It now appears to have been convincingly demonstrated that subthalamopallidal neurons are excitatory using glutamate as the neurotransmitter (see page 32). The increased activity of these neurons in MPTP-induced parkinsonism should be associated with increased 2-DG uptake in both the medial and lateral pallidal segments to which they project. It is probable that the increased activity already referred to in the lateral pallidum is partly due to increased subthalamic neuronal terminal activity. There is, however, no clearly significant pattern of change in the medial pallidum, although the suggestion is of a slight increase. It has been hypothesized that the activity of striatal projection neurons to the medial and lateral pallidal segments is reversed in parkinsonism, the latter being increased, as reasoned above, and the former decreased (Penney and Young, 1986). This would certainly be consistent with the different neuronal projections to these two regions. In the striatal neuronal terminals of the lateral pallidum, GABA coexists with the neuromodulator encephalin, whereas terminals in the medial pallidum contain GABA and subtance P. Ligand-binding studies again provide supportive evidence in the form of increased [^{3}H]flunitrazepam binding in the medial pallidal segment in Parkinson's disease, suggesting decreased activity of striatal projection neurons to this region (Griffiths, 1988; Robertson *et al.*, 1989b). It could thus be concluded that the lack of any significant change in 2-DG uptake in the medial pallidum is due to the balance of converging neuronal activity from the putamen and subthalamic nucleus.

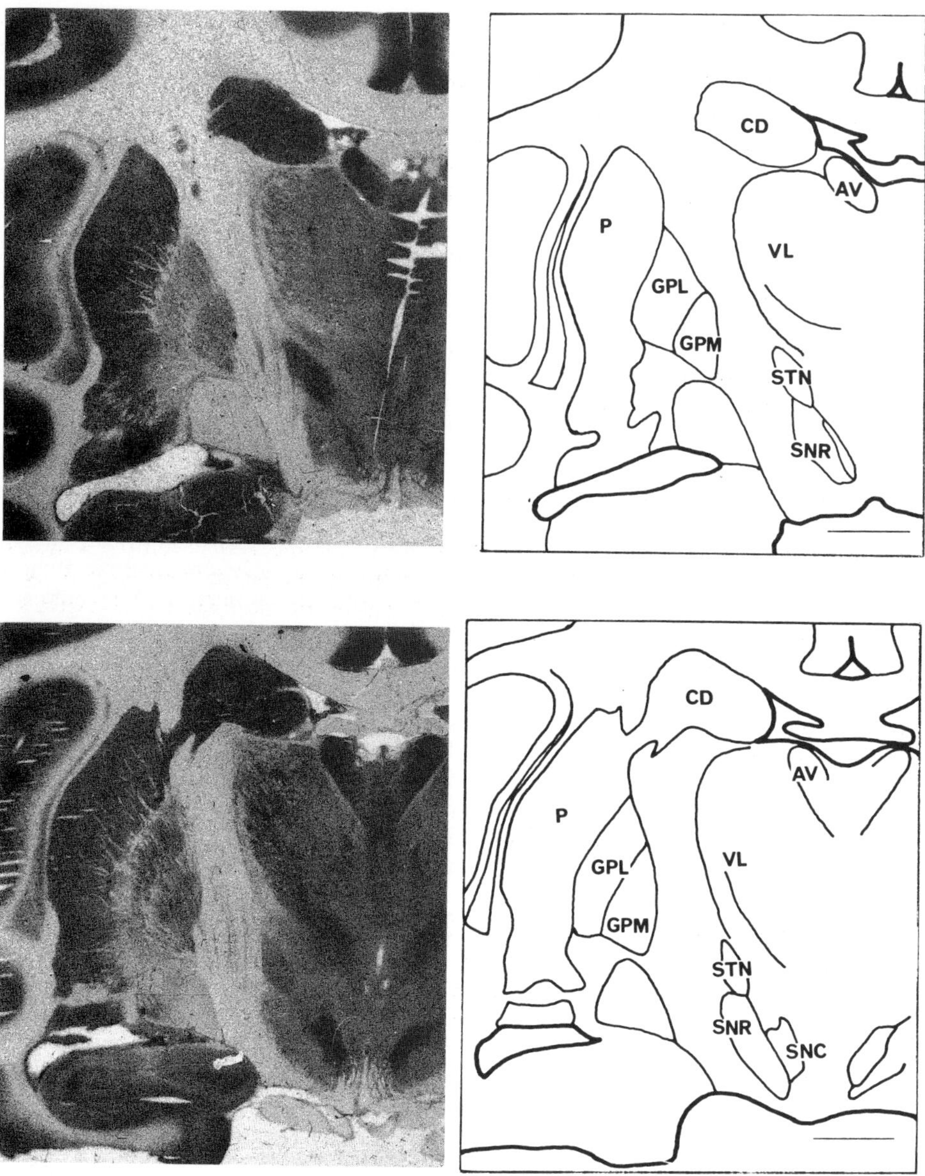

Figure 2.2 A direct reversal print of a 2-deoxyglucose autoradiograph from a control animal (above) and an animal with 1-methyl-4-phenyl-1,2,3,6-tetrahydropyridine (MPTP)-induced parkinsonism (below). Increased uptake of isotope can be seen in the medial (GPM) and lateral (GPL) pallidal segments and the ventrolateral thalamic nucleus (VL) of the parkinsonian animal. Uptake is reduced in the subthalamic nucleus (STN). The increased concentration of isotope in the substantia nigra, pars compacta (SNC) is associated with degenerative changes and microglial infiltration. AV = Anterior ventral nucleus; CD = caudate nucleus; P = putamen; SNR = substantia nigra pars reticulata.

The terminal projection fields of the medial pallidum in the thalamus and pedunculopontine nucleus are associated with increased 2-DG activity, suggesting that despite the lack of obvious change in isotope uptake in the medial pallidum itself, the activity of its projection neurons is increased. These neurons are inhibitory and utilize GABA. The neuronal recording studies of Miller and Delong (1987) and Filion *et al.* (1988) support this conclusion. These authors have demonstrated an unselective increase in medial pallidal activity and suggested that it inhibits the expression of normal motor patterns generated in the striatum. At the same time, the reduction in activity of projection neurons from the striatum to the medial pallidum, as argued above, will impede the transmission of these normal motor patterns and contribute to the disordered function. The attractiveness of these conclusions is enhanced when they are compared with the findings already reported in chorea and ballism, where the changes in 2-DG activity are a mirror image of those found in MPTP-induced parkinsonism.

Levodopa-induced choreiform dyskinesia and dystonia

The major problem encountered in the long-term treatment of Parkinson's disease is based upon the extreme difficulty in balancing levodopa therapy to provide a reversal of symptoms without producing side-effects. In the majority of patients a compromise is eventually established which provides for the relief of akinesia, rigidity and tremor for a significant part of the time but accepts mild to moderate dyskinesia as an inevitable consequence of this relief. In addition patients experience rapid and disabling changes in their mobility, known as the on–off effect. A way of preventing or ameliorating this aspect of treatment would present a major breakthrough in the management of the disorder.

The MPTP-induced model of parkinsonism faithfully replicates this aspect of Parkinson's disease. Chronic levodopa therapy is associated with the gradual appearance of peak-dose dyskinesia in the form of chorea and dystonia over a period of several weeks or months. In order of preference it most commonly affects the lower limbs, the upper limbs and even the spinal, tongue and facial muscles (Clarke *et al.*. 1987). As in Parkinson's disease, it is typically seen in those animals with the most severe form of the disorder. Furthermore, the most severely parkinsonian animals tend predominantly to develop dystonia whereas the less disabled experience mainly chorea. A mixture of both is not uncommonly seen. It is important to note that in the MPTP-induced model of parkinsonism these complications of treatment develop during regular levodopa therapy and without progressive nigral degeneration. This tends to support the hypothesis that peak-dose dyskinesia and the on–off effect are complications which are not only related to the severity of the disease but are induced by long-term treatment (Rajput *et al.*, 1984).

Neuronal metabolic studies performed in animals with peak-dose dyskinesia (Mitchell *et al.*, 1992) demonstrate only a partial reversal of the pattern of 2-DG uptake seen in parkinsonism. 2-DG activity is reduced in the lateral pallidum and increased in the subthalamic nucleus. This can be interpreted as a decrease in striatolateral pallidal activity and disinhibition of lateral pallidal neurons, which in turn results in increased inhibition of the subthalamic nucleus. These findings represent the converse of parkinsonism. The more surprising result is found in the medial pallidum where isotope uptake is increased and not decreased, as might be expected. The change in parkinsonism has been referred to above and represents the balance

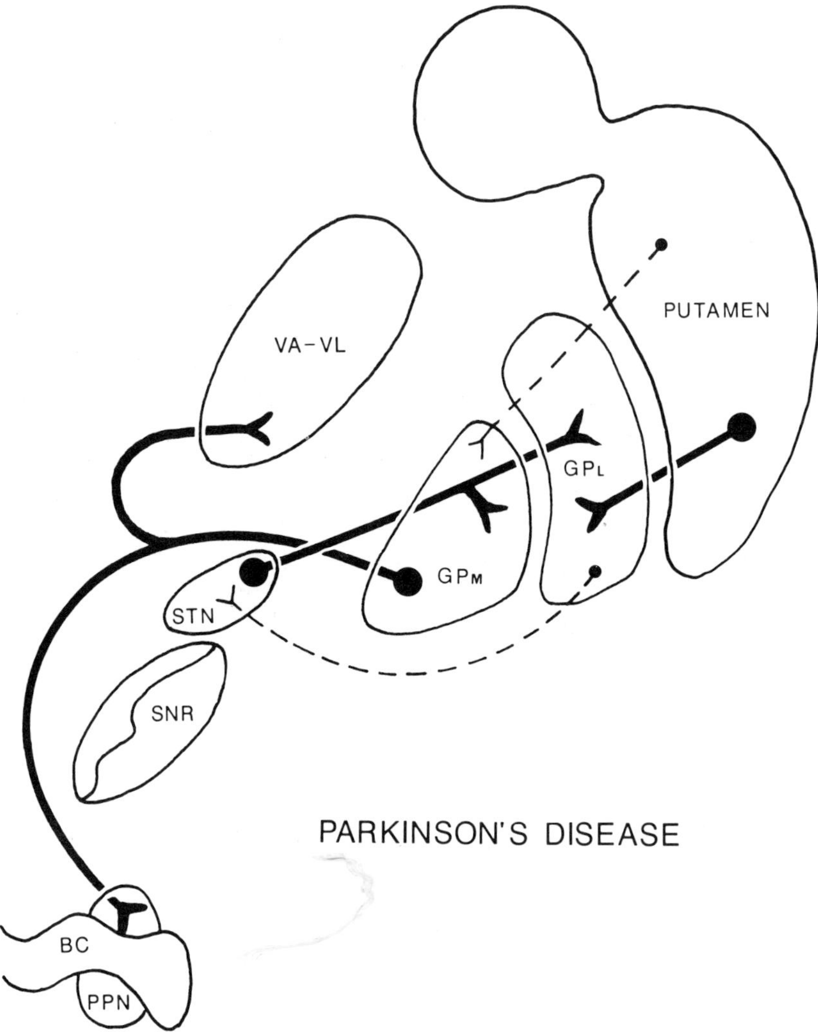

Figure 2.3 A summary of the changes in basal ganglia neuronal activity occurring in (a) 1-methyl-4-phenyl-1,2,3,6-tetrahydropyridine (MPTP)-induced parkinsonism and (b) levodopa-induced dyskinesia in the monkey, as deduced from neuronal metabolic studies using 2-deoxyglucose. BC = Brachium conjunctivum; GPL and GPM = lateral and medial globus pallidus; PPN = pedunculopontine nucleus; SNR = substantia nigra pars reticulata; STN = subthalamic nucleus; VA-VL = ventral anterior and ventral lateral thalamic nuclei.

of terminal activity of neurons projecting from the striatum and subthalamic nucleus, resulting in a slight increase in 2-DG activity. During peak-dose dyskinesia, isotope uptake in the medial pallidum is markedly increased. This can only be due to a very significant rise in striatomedial pallidal neuronal activity since the subthalamic nucleus is strongly inhibited. The lack of subthalamic excitation and the increase in striatal inhibition reduces the activity of medial pallidal neurons which project to the thalamus and pedunculopontine nucleus, as confirmed by the reduced 2-DG uptake in these areas (Figure 2.3).

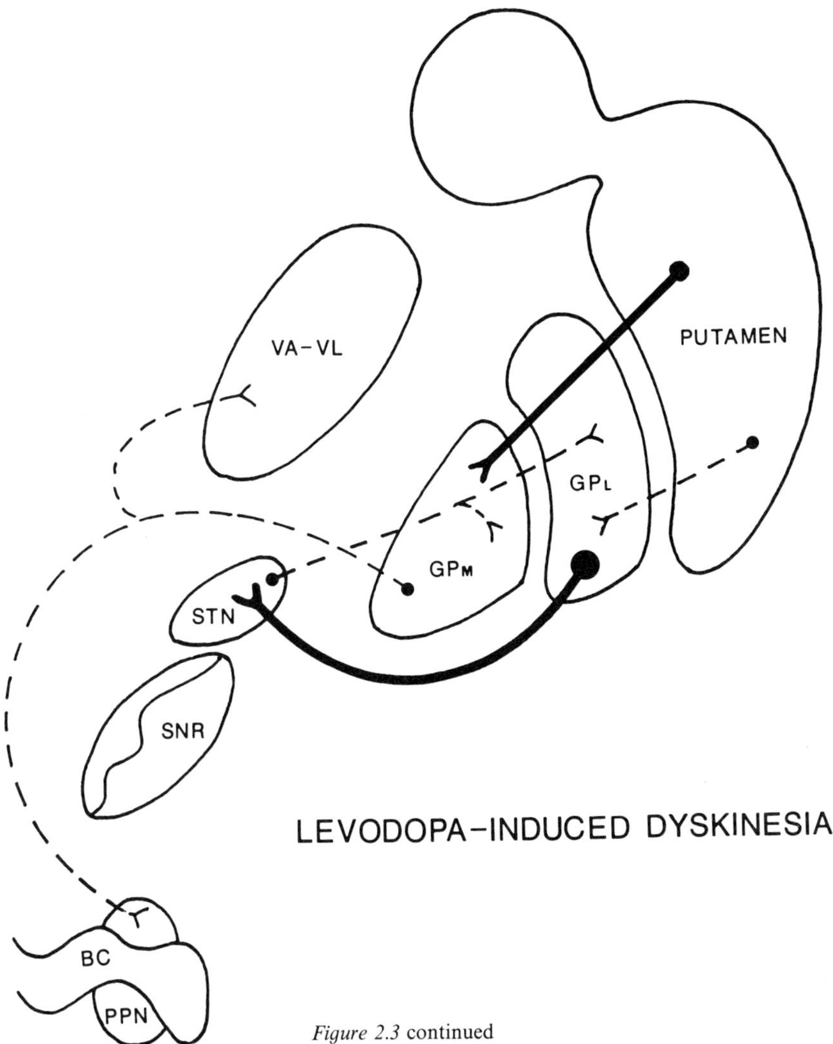

Figure 2.3 continued

These medial pallidal changes are present in peak-dose chorea but are most marked in peak-dose dystonia. This naturally invites a comparison of the mechanisms of chorea and dystonia. In both disorders the activity of the medial pallidum appears to be critical. This activity is in turn governed by two factors: subthalamic excitation and striatal inhibition. In classical chorea produced by GABA blockade in the lateral pallidum a reduction in subthalamic excitation appears to be the only change and is associated with a reduction in pallidothalamic activity. In the later stages of Huntington's disease, where there is degeneration of striatal neurons projecting to the medial pallidum as well, striatal inhibiton is decreased and it is suggested that this accounts for the appearance of hypokinesia. In peak-dose dystonia subthalamic excitation is reduced and striatal inhibition is increased, which in theory would reduce medial pallidal activity to a much more severe degree than in chorea. This suggests that the difference between the two disorders might be based on the degree of thalamic and possibly pedunculopontine disinhibition secondary to changes in medial pallidal activity.

Therapeutic implications from the MPTP-induced model of parkinsonism

The 2-DG findings in levodopa-induced dyskinesia present an opportunity to manipulate the disordered neuronal activity by means of a partially destructive lesion in the terminal projection field in the thalamus of medial pallidal neurons. Using the model of levodopa-induced dyskinesia in the MPTP-treated monkey, it has been possible by the technique of neuronal tracing (using horseradish peroxidase) to establish the precise area within the thalamus to which medial pallidal neurons project and thereby perform appropriate thalamotomies. With lesions in the ventral anterior and ventral lateral thalamus, peak-dose choreiform dyskinesia can be reduced or abolished without apparently increasing the severity of the parkinsonian symptoms. These findings have their equivalent in humans. Narabayashi *et al.* (1984) demonstrated that thalamotomies placed anterior to the midpoint of the AC–PC line (joining the anterior and posterior commissures) can alleviate levodopa-induced dyskinesia, as distinct from posteriorly placed lesions previously used for the treatment of tremor. In the light of these observations and with improved imaging techniques, the procedure of thalamotomy clearly needs re-evaluation.

Peak-dose dystonia, however, does not appear to be appreciably changed by thalamotomy. Two reasons can be considered to explain this. Since the mechanism of dystonia appears to be a progression of chorea with a greater reduction of medial pallidal activity, the ineffectiveness of the operation may simply be a factor of size which can be overcome by the use of larger lesions. Alternatively, the projection from the medial pallidum to the pedunculopontine nucleus may be important for the mediation of dystonia. There is no scientific evidence to support this statement but, none the less, it invites further investigation.

An increase in subthalamic neuronal activity is a prominent feature of the neural mechanisms of MPTP-induced parkinsonism. It is interesting to consider whether pharmacological or surgical manipulation of this activity might be beneficial in the treatment of Parkinson's disease. MPTP-induced parkinsonism in the marmoset can be temporarily reversed by injection of the glutamate antagonist, kynurenic acid, into the medial pallidum bilaterally (Graham *et al.*, 1990; Brotchie *et al.*, 1991). While glutamate antagonisn in the medial pallidum is open to consideration in Parkinson's disease, it seems unlikely that a localized effect could be achieved through the systemic administration of glutamate antagonists in view of the widespread distribution of glutamate receptors in the central nervous system and the probable downregulation of those in the medial pallidum. A therapeutic opening might appear if it was possible to demonstrate a specific characterization of these receptors.

Alternatively, lesioning of the subthalamic nucleus presents a direct approach which has a more immediate clinical application. Bergman *et al.* (1990) used ibotenic acid for this purpose and confirmed its potential for reversing experimentally induced parkinsonism. However, the traditional neurosurgical technique for producing brain lesions relies on radiofrequency thermocoagulation and it seemed appropriate to evaluate this in the MPTP model of Parkinson's disease.

Radiofrequency lesioning of the subthalamic nucleus has now been performed unilaterally and bilaterally using a 60° oblique approach to produce localized damage to the nucleus with minimal involvement of surrounding structures (Aziz *et al.*, 1991 and 1992). To an inherently critical investigator (MAS) the results have proved to be most exciting. In summary, a well-placed lesion which ablated 40–50% of the nucleus *unilaterally* produced very significant reversal of rigidity, tremor and hypokinesia with marked improvement in balance and mobility. A second contralateral lesion only produced further benefit if the first was not accurately targeted. Provided that lesion placement was correct and a significant proportion of the nucleus was destroyed, the effects were permanent. The inevitable concern that subthalamic nucleus lesions will produce spontaneous dyskinesia or exaggerate apomorphine-induced dyskinesia has not materialized experimentally.

It is interesting to reflect that subthalamotomy, as opposed to subthalamic nucleotomy, was first described as an effective lesion for the treatment of Parkinson's disease by Andy *et al.* in 1963. The area targeted primarily included the fields of Forel and ansa lenticularis since it was considered potentially dangerous to involve the subthalamic nucleus, as this might result in hemiballism.

In the light of these experimental findings it will be very interesting to watch for the inevitable neurosurgical development – subthalamotomy revisited. Subthalamic nucleotomy might just prove to be the most significant development in Parkinson's disease since the advent of levodopa.

References

Andy OJ, Jurko MF, and Sias FR (1963) Subthalamotomy in the treatment of parkinsonian tremor. *J Neurosurg*, **20**, 860–70

Aziz TZ, Peggs D, Sambrook MA, and Crossman AR (1991) Lesion of the subthalamic nucleus for the alleviation of MPTP-induced parkinsonism in the primate. *Movement Disorders*, **6**, 288–92

Aziz TZ, Peggs D, Agarwal E, Sambrook MA, and Crossman AR (1992) Subthalamic nucleotomy alleviates parkinsonism in the experimental primate. *Br J Neurosurg*, **6**, 575–582

Bergman H, Wichmann T, and DeLong MR (1990) Reversal of experimental parkinsonism by lesions of the subthalamic nucleus. *Science*, **249**, 1436–8

Birkmayer W, Knoll J, Riederer P, Youdim MBH, Hars V, and Marton J (1985) Increased life expectancy resulting from addition of L-deprenyl to Madopar treatment in Parkinson's disease: a longterm study. *J Neural Transm*, **64**, 113–27

Brotchie JH, Mitchell IJ, Sambrook MA, and Crossman AR (1991) Alleviation of parkinsonism by antagonism of excitatory amino acid transmission in the medial segment of the globus pallidus in rat and primate. *Movement Disorders*, **6**, 133–8

Burns RS, Chiueh CC, Markey SP, Ebert MH, Jacobowitz DM, and Kopin IJ (1983) A primate model of parkinsonism: selective destruction of dopaminergic neurons in the pars compacta of the substantia nigra by N-methyl-4-phenyl-1,2,3,6-tetrahydropyridine. *Proc Natl Acad Sci USA*, **80**, 4546–50

Carpenter MB and McMasters RE (1964) Lesions of the substantia nigra in the Rhesus monkey. Efferent fiber degeneration and behavioral observations. *Am J Anat*, **114**, 293–320

Carpenter MB, Whittier JR, and Mettler FA (1950) Analysis of choreoid hyperkinesia in the rhesus monkey. Surgical and pharmacological analysis of hyperkinesia resulting from lesions in the subthalamic nucleus of Luys. *J Comp Neuro*, **92**, 293–332

Chiba K, Trevor AJ, and Castagnoli N Jr (1984) Metabolism of the neurotoxic tertiary amine, MPTP, by brain monoamine oxidase. *Biochem Biophys Res Comm*, **120**, 574–8

Clarke CE, Sambrook MA, Mitchell IJ, and Crossman AR (1987) Levodopa-induced dyskinesia and response fluctuations in primates rendered parkinsonism with 1-methyl-4-phenyl-1,2,3,6-tetrahydropyridine (MPTP). *J Neurol Sci*, **78**, 273–80

Crossman AR, Sambrook MA, and Jackson A (1984) Experimental hemichorea/hemiballismus in the monkey. Studies on the intracerbral site of action in a drug-induced dyskinesia. *Brain*, **107**, 579–96

Crossman AR, Mitchell IJ, Sambrook MA, and Jackson A (1988) Chorea and myoclonus in the monkey induced by GABA-antagonism in the lentiform complex: the site of drug action and a hypothesis of the neural mechanisms of chorea. *Brain*, **111**, 1211–33

D'Amato RJ, Lipman ZP, and Snyder SH (1986) Selectivity of the parkinsonian neurotoxin MPTP: toxic metabolism MPP+ binds to neuromelanin. *Science*, **231**, 987–9

Davis GC, Williams AC, Markey SP, Ebert MH, Caine ED, Reichert CM *et al.* (1979) Chronic parkinsonism secondary to intravenous injection of meperidine analogues. *Psychiatry Res*, **1**, 249–54

Feger J, Vezole I, Renwart N, and Robledo P (1989) The rat subthalamic nucleus: electrophysiological and behavioural data. In Crossman AR and Sambrook MA, eds *Neural Mechanisms in Disorders of Movement*, London, John Libbey, 37–43

Filion M, Tremblay L, and Bedard PJ (1988) Abnormal influences of passive limb movement on the activity of globus pallidus neurons in parkinsonian monkeys. *Brain Res*, **444**, 165–76

Forno LS, Langston JW, DeLanney LE, and Ricaurte GA (1986) Locus coeruleus lesions and eosinophilic inclusions in MPTP-treated monkeys. *Ann Neurol*, **20**, 449–55

Graham WC, Robertson RG, Sambrook MA, and Crossman AR (1990) Injection of excitatory amino acid antagonists into the medial pallidal segment of the MPTP-treated primate reverses motor symptoms of parkinsonism. *Life Sci*, **47**, 91–7

Griffiths P (1988) Alterations in neurotransmitter receptors and iron content in Parkinson's disease and Alzheimer's disease. PhD Thesis, University of Manchester

Heikkila RE, Hess A, and Duvoisin RC (1984) Dopaminergic neurotoxicity of 1-methyl-4-phenyl-1,2,3,6-tetrahydropyridine in mice. *Science*, **224**, 1451–3

Heikkila RE, Manzino L, Cabbat FS, and Duvoisin RC (1985) Studies on the oxidation of the dopaminergic neurotoxin 1-methyl-4-phenyl-1,2,5,6-tetrahydropyirdine by monoamine oxidase B. *J Neurochem*, **45**, 1049–54

Irwin I and Langston JW (1985) Selective accumulation of MPP+ in the substantia nigra: a key to neurotoxicity? *Life Sci*, **36**, 207–12

Jarvis MF and Wagner GC (1985) Neurochemical and functional consequences following 1-methyl-4-phenyl-1,2,3,6-tetrahydropyridine (MPTP) and methamphetamine. *Life Sci*, **36**, 249–54

Javitch JA and Snyder SH (1985) Uptake of MPP+ by dopamine neurons explains selectivity of parkinsonism-inducing neurotoxin, MPTP. *Eur J Pharmacol*, **106**, 455–6

Kitai ST and Kita H (1987) Anatomy and physiology of the subthalamic nucleus: a driving force of the basal ganglia. In Carpenter MB and Jayaraman A, eds, *The Basal Ganglia II: Structure and Function–Current Concepts*, New York, Plenum Press, 357–73

Langston JW and Irwin I (1986) MPTP: current concepts and controversies. *Clin Neuropharmacol*, **9**, 485–507

Langston JW, Ballard P, Tetrud JW, and Irwin I (1983) Chronic parkinsonism in humans due to a product of meperidine analogue synthesis. *Science*, **219**, 979–80

Markey SP, Johannessen JN, Chiueh CC, Burns RS, and Herkenham MA (1984) Intraneuronal generation of a pyridinium metabolite may cause drug-induced parkinsonism. *Nature*, **311**, 464–7

Martin JP (1927) Hemichorea resulting from a local lesion of the brain. (The syndrome of the body of Luys.) *Brain*, **50**, 637–51

Miller WC and Delong MR (1987) Altered tonic activity of neurons in the globus pallidus and subthalamic nucleus in the primate MPTP model of parkinsonism. Carpenter MB and Jayaraman A, eds, *The Basal Ganglia II: Structure and Function–Current Concepts*, New York, Plenum Press, 395–403

Mitchell IJ, Sambrook MA, and Crossman AR (1985a) Subcortical changes in the regional uptake of [^{3}H]-2-deoxyglucose in the brain of the monkey during experimental choreiform dyskinesia elicited by injection of a gamma-aminobutyric acid antagonist into the subthalamic nucleus. *Brain*, **108**, 421–38

Mitchell IJ, Jackson A, Sambrook MA, and Crossman AR (1985b) Common neural mechanisms in experimental chorea and hemiballismus in the monkey. Evidence from 2-deoxyglucose autoradiography. *Brain Res*, **339**, 346–50

Mitchell IJ, Cross AJ, Sambrook MA, and Crossman AR (1986) MPTP-induced parkinsonism in the monkey: neurochemical pathology and regional brain metabolism. *J Neural Transm*, **(Suppl XX)**, 41–6

Mitchell IJ, Clarke CE, Boyce S, Robertson RG, Peggs D, Sambrook MA *et al.* (1989) Neural mechanisms underlying parkinsonian symptoms based upon regional uptake of 2-deoxyglucose in monkeys exposed to 1-methyl-4-phenyl-1,2,3,6-tetrahydropyridine. *Neuroscience*, **32**, 213–26

Mitchell IJ, Boyce S, Sambrook MA and Crossman AR (1992) A 2-DG study of the effects of dopamine agonists in the parkinsonian primate brain. *Brain*, **115**, 809–824

Narabayashi H, Yokochi F, and Nakajima Y (1984) Levodopa-induced dyskinesia and thalamotomy. *J Neurol Neurosurg Psychiatry*, **47**, 831–9

Needham GA, Soden PD, Sambrook MA, and Crossman AR (1983) A remotely operated pump for intracerebral micro-injection in the primate. *J Neurosci Methods*, **7**, 281–8

Nicklas WJ, Vyas I, and Heikkila RE (1985) Inhibiton of NADH-linked oxidation in brain mitochondria by 1-methyl-4-phenylpyridine, a metabolite of the neurotoxin 1-methyl-4-phenyl-1,2,3,6-tetrahydropyridine. *Life Sci*, **36**, 2503–8

Parent A, Hazrati LN, and Smith Y (1989) The subthalamic nucleus in primates. A neuroanatomical and immunohistochemical study. In Crossman AR and Sambrook MA, eds, *Neural Mechanisms in Disorders of Movement*, London, John Libbey, 29–35

Parisi JE and Burns RS (1986) MPTP-induced parkinsonism in man and experimental animals. *J Neuropathol Exp Neurol*, **44**, 325
Penney JB and Young AB (1986) Striatal inhomogeneities and basal ganglia function. *Movement Disorders*, **1**, 3–15
Perkins MN and Stone TW (1981) Iontophoretic studies on pallidal neurones and the projection from the subthalamic nucleus. *Q J Exp Physiol*, **66**, 225–36
Poirier LJ (1960) Experimental and histological study of midbrain dyskinesia. *J Neurophysiol*, **23**, 534–51
Poirier LJ, Sourkes TL, Bouvier G, Boucher R, and Carabin S (1966) Striatal amines, experimental tremor and the effect of harmaline in the monkey. *Brain*, **89**, 37–52
Poirier LJ, Pechadre JC, Larochelle L, Dankova J, and Boucher R (1975) Stereotaxis lesions and movement disorders in monkeys. In Meldrum BS and Marsden CD, eds, *Advances in Neurology, Vol 10, Primate Models of Neurological Disorders*, New York, Raven Press, 5–22
Porrino LJ, Burns RS, Crane AM, Palombo E, Kopin IJ, and Sokoloff L (1987) Changes in local cerebral glucose utilisation associated with Parkinson's syndrome induced by MPTP in the primate. *Life Sci*, **40**, 1656–64
Rajput AH, Stern W, and Laverty WH (1984) Chronic low-dose levodopa therapy in Parkinson's disease: an argument for delaying levodopa therapy. *Neurology*, **34**, 991–6
Reiner A, Albin RL, Anderson KD, D'Amato CJ, Penney JB, and Young AB (1988) Differential loss of striatal projection neurones in Huntington's disease. *Proc Natl Acad Sci* (*USA*), **85**, 5733–7
Robertson RG, Farmery SM, Sambrook MA, and Crossman AR (1989a) Dyskinesia in the primate following injection of an excitatory amino acid antagonist into the medial segment of the globus pallidus. *Brain Res*, **476**, 317–22
Robertson RG, Clarke CE, Boyce S, Sambrook MA, and Crossman AR (1989b) GABA/benzodiazepine receptors in the primate basal ganglia following treatment with MPTP: evidence for the differential regulation of striatal output by dopamine. In Crossman AR and Sambrook MA, eds, *Neural Mechanisms in Disorders of Movement*, London, John Libbey, 165–73
Rouzaire-Dubois B, Scarnati E, Hammond C, Crossman AR, and Shibazaki T (1983) Microiontophoretic studies on the nature of the neurotransmitter in the subthalamo-entopeduncular pathway of the rat. *Brain Res*, **271**, 11–20
Sambrook MA, Crossman AR, and Slater P (1979) Experimental torticollis in the marmoset produced by injection of 6-hydroxydopamine into the ascending nigrostriatal pathway. *Exp Neurol*, **63**, 583–93
Sambrook MA, Clarke CE, Robertson RG, Mitchell IJ, Boyce S, Graham WC *et al.* (1987) New parallels between Parkinson's disease and MPTP-induced parkinsonism in the monkey. In Carpenter MB and Jayaramen A, eds, *Basal Ganglia II: Structure and Function–Current Concepts*, New York, Plenum Press, 395–403
Schneider JS, Yuwiler A, and Markham CH (1986) Production of a parkinsonian-like syndrome in the cat with n-methyl-4-phenyl-1,2,3,6-tetrahydropyridine (MPTP): behavior, histology and biochemistry. *Exp Neurol*, **91**, 293–307
Schwartz WJ, Smith CB, Davidsen L, Savaki H, and Sokoloff L (1979) Metabolic mapping of functional activity in the hypothalamo-neurophypophysical system of the rat. *Science*, **205**, 723–5
Schwartzman RJ and Alexander GM (1985) Changes in the local cerebral metabolic rate for the MPTP primate model of Parkinson's disease. *Brain Res*, **358**, 137–43
Shouson I and Parkinson Study Group (1989) Effect of deprenyl on the progression of disability in early Parkinson's disease. *N Engl J Med*, **321**, 1364–71
Sokoloff L, Reivich M, Kennedy C, Des Rosiers MH, Patlack CS, Pettigrew KD *et al.* (1977) The [^{14}C] deoxyglucose method for the measurement of local cerebral glucose utilisation: theory, procedure and normal values in the conscious and anaesthetised albino rat. *J Neurochem*, **28**, 897–916
Strominger NL and Carpenter MB (1965) Effects of lesions in the substantia nigra upon subthalamic dyskinesia in the monkey. *Neurology*, **15**, 587–94
Tetrud JW and Langston JW (1989) The effect of deprenyl (selegiline) on the natural history of Parkinson's disease. *Science*, **245**, 519–22
Vincent SR, Kimura H, and McGeer EG (1982) A histochemical study of GABA-transaminase in the efferents of the pallidum. *Brain Res*, **241**, 162–5
Ward AA, McCulloch WS, and Magoun HW (1948) Production of an alternating tremor at rest in monkeys. *J Neurophysiol*, **11**, 317–30
Whittier JR and Mettler FA (1949) Studies on the subthalamus of the rhesus monkey. I. Anatomy and fiber connections of the subthalamic nucleus of Luys. *J Comp Neurol*, **90**, 281–317

3
Movement disorders: genetic aspects

A. E. Harding

This chapter will focus on inherited, or possibly inherited, movement disorders in which recent advances have been made, either in understanding their genetic basis or in applying molecular genetic techniques to clinical practice. This particularly applies to idiopathic torsion dystonia (ITD) and Huntington's disease (HD); genetic aspects of Parkinson's disease (PD) and neurocanthocytosis (NA) will also be discussed.

DYSTONIAS

The inheritance of idiopathic torsion dystonia

Idiopathic or primary torsion dystonia is a disorder characterized by involuntary sustained muscle contractions, frequently causing twisting and repetitive movements or abnormal postures (Fahn *et al.*, 1987) without other associated neurological features. It should be distinguished from symptomatic dystonia secondary to, for example, birth trauma, Wilson's disease, other degenerative disorders, encephalitis and neuroleptic drugs. The prevalence of ITD may be as high as 250 per million (Nutt *et al.*, 1988). A particularly high incidence of ITD has long been recognized in Ashkenazi Jews.

The clinical features of ITD are highly variable and severity is largely determined by age of onset, with most cases of generalized ITD developing before the age of 20 years; focal dystonias usually develop in adult life and segmental dystonia has a wide range of age of onset of symptoms (Marsden and Harrison, 1974). No consistent structural basis for ITD has been observed, but biochemical dysfunction of the basal ganglia or brainstem is suspected as these structures are frequently involved in symptomatic dystonia.

It has been clear for many years that ITD is often familial, but the precise genetic basis for these disorders has been controversial. Despite early studies providing good evidence that ITD was most commonly of autosomal dominant inheritance with reduced penetrance and variable expression in both Jewish and non-Jewish cases (Zeman *et al.*, 1959), Eldridge, in a study of 41 Jewish families in the USA, proposed that this disorder was usually of autosomal recessive inheritance and later estimated a heterozygote frequency of 1 in 65 in this racial group (Eldridge, 1970; Eldridge and Gottlieb, 1976).

Eldridge did not analyse this data statistically, and his studies were clearly biased in favour of familial cases. Three points emerged which do not favour the hypothesis that juvenile-onset generalized dystonia among Jews is nearly always caused by an autosomal recessive gene. In families containing index cases who had normal parents, the proportion of affected sibs was significantly lower than 25% if the data are corrected for ascertainment bias (Korczyn *et al.*, 1981). The parental consanguinity rate was only about 1.5%, and the incidence of dystonia amongst cousins and other second- or third-degree relatives of index cases was higher than would be expected for the proposed gene frequency.

Jewish patients with affected children or parents have been reported on numerous occasions, including in the first description of inherited dystonia by Schwalbe (Truong and Fahn, 1988), and they are clinically indistinguishable from those suggested to exhibit autosomal recessive inheritance. Eldridge felt that these were due to pseudodominance, that is the result of heterozygote–homozygote mating (Eldridge and Koerber, 1979; Eldridge, 1981). Again, the observed incidence of this occurrence is much too high for the quoted gene frequency and parental consanguinity rate.

A study of primary torsion dystonia in Israel confirmed the relatively high incidence of this disease amongst Ashkenazi Jews originating from eastern Europe (Korczyn *et al.*, 1980; Zilber *et al.*, 1984). Ascertainment was virtually complete. The genetic data did not meet predictions based on an autosomal recessive model and the authors concluded that the disorder could result from an autosomal dominant gene with low penetrance. The same conclusions were drawn from a recent study of dystonia developing before the age of 28 years in Ashkenazi Jews in the USA; penetrance was estimated at about 30% (Bressman *et al.*, 1989). Thirty-eight of the 43 probands in this study had generalized or multifocal dystonia. There was some evidence that isolated cases in Israel, as in the UK, result from fresh dominant mutation, as paternal age was increased (Bundey *et al.*, 1975; Zilber *et al.*, 1984), although this was not observed in the USA (Risch *et al.*, 1990). A recent detailed statistical analysis of the data reported by Eldridge (1970) suggests that they fit best with autosomal dominant inheritance with, again, approximately 30% penetrance (Pauls and Korczyn, 1990). Thus it has to be concluded that the hypothesis of autosomal recessive inheritance explaining the majority of Ashkenzai Jewish cases of dystonia is no longer tenable.

Large dominant pedigrees of dystonics, with variable expression but complete penetrance, have been well-documented in both Jewish and non-Jewish kindreds (Zeman *et al.*, 1959, Johnson *et al.*, 1962; Eldridge, 1970). The latter have often contained patients very similar to those with the severe juvenile-onset dystonia commonly seen amongst the Jewish population. The clinical distinction between dystonia in Jews and non-Jewish families has thus been disputed (Burke *et al.*, 1986). Furthermore, complex segregation analysis of the pedigrees reported by Eldridge (1970) showed no differences between Jewish and non-Jewish kindreds (Pauls and Korczyn, 1990).

Until recently there had been few genetic studies of unselected cases of ITD in populations which do not contain a substantial number of Ashkenazi Jews (Bundey *et al.*, 1975). Fletcher and colleagues (1990) studied 107 index cases with generalized, multifocal or segmental ITD from 100 British kindreds, ascertained independently of whether or not there was a positive family history. A total of 260 relatives was examined; 37 of these were affected on examination, of whom 18 were asymptomatic. In 45 families there were affected individuals in more than one generation, and in

17 kindreds members of three or more generations were affected. In six families cases were confined to a single generation (affected sibs in five kindreds and affected cousins in the sixth).

The disorder varied considerably within families, ranging from immobility before the age of 10 years to asymptomatic focal dystonia (e.g. writer's cramp or blepharospasm) in elderly subjects. Postural tremor alone occurred in six secondary cases. Analysis of the data resulting from this study provided evidence against multifactorial inheritance or a high proportion of autosomal recessive cases. The parental consanguinity rate was 1%. An increased incidence of ITD in Ashkenazi Jews was confirmed; 11 index cases were of Jewish origin but these were indistinguishable, both clinically and in terms of pedigree analysis, from the other patients. The conclusion of this study was that about 85% of cases of ITD in the UK are caused by a dominant gene or genes with reduced (approximately 40%) penetrance. There was no evidence for the existence of either X-linked or autosomal recessive forms of ITD, or genetic heterogeneity within dominant pedigrees or racial groups. About 14% of singleton cases probably represent fresh dominant mutation; the finding of Bundey *et al.* (1975), that mean paternal age is increased in this group of patients, was confirmed. The remaining 16% are likely to be non-genetic phenocopies, although these are not distinguishable from familial cases.

For genetic counselling purposes it was estimated from this study that the *a priori* risk of sibs or children of patients with familial ITD being similarly affected was 21%. The risk to offspring of single cases is 14%, and sibs 8%. These risks to healthy relatives fall with age, by 50, 75 and 90% at the ages of 15, 30 and 50 years respectively. These figures are only applicable to generalized, multifocal and segmental dystonia in the population studied; recurrence risks to relatives of Jewish patients in the USA and Israel can be derived from data reported in the relevant family studies (Zilber *et al.*, 1984; Bressman *et al.*, 1989; Risch *et al.*, 1990).

The genetic contribution to adult-onset focal dystonias is not as yet clearly established. These disorders are likely to be aetiologically more heterogeneous, despite the existence of cases of focal dystonia in large families containing other members with generalized ITD. Waddy and colleagues (1991) undertook a genetic study of idiopathic focal dystonias by examining 153 first-degree relatives of 40 index cases with torticollis (14), orofacial dystonias (16) and writer's cramp (10). Nine affected relatives were identified in six families; 8 of these had symptoms such as clumsiness or tremor, but none was aware that they had dystonia. A further 4 relatives were affected by history. Overall, 25% of index cases had relatives with dystonia. The results of segregation analysis suggested the presence of an autosomal dominant gene or genes with reduced penetrance as a common cause for focal dystonia.

If an autosomal dominant gene is responsible for some cases of focal dystonia, one major issue which arises is whether this is the same gene which causes generalized dystonia. None of the index cases studied by Waddy *et al.* (1991) had relatives with generalized dystonia, and there was a tendency for affected relatives to have the same type of dystonia as the index case. The presence of different genes causing different types of focal dystonia cannot be excluded, but four lines of evidence are compatible with the hypothesis that most cases of inherited dystonia, focal or generalized, are caused by a common mutation. Firstly, families containing cases of generalized dystonia would be expected to be ascertained through the most severely affected member, and thus would not have been included in this study. Second, focal dystonias are numerically nine times more common than generalized dystonia (Nutt *et al.*, 1988), so the incidence of generalized disease amongst secondary cases should be correspondingly low. Third, the segregation ratios for dystonia in sibs and parents were not significantly different from that reported in our genetic study of segmental and generalized dystonia in the UK (Fletcher *et al.*, 1990), although they were consistently lower. There may be more non-genetic phenocopies amongst the index cases with focal dystonia. Finally, a high proportion of secondary cases ascertained through probands with more severe disease has focal dystonia indistinguishable from that observed in index cases studied by Waddy and colleagues (Bressman *et al.*, 1989; Fletcher *et al.*, 1990). The only feature of this study of focal dystonias in favour of genetic heterogeneity is the absence of Ashkenazi Jews amongst the index cases, compared to 10.3% of probands with generalized or segmental dystonia in the UK (Fletcher *et al.*, 1990).

One question which frequently arises in genetic studies of ITD is the nature of the relationship between postural tremor and dystonia. Tremor often occurs in patients with dystonia (Marsden and Harrison, 1974) and has been observed alone in the relatives of dystonic patients in virtually every family study undertaken (Eldridge, 1970; Bundey *et al.*, 1975; Zilber *et al.*, 1984; Fletcher *et al.*, 1990). Whether this indicates that tremor may be the sole manifestation of the dominant ITD gene, or merely represents a coincidental occurrence of essential tremor in these families, requires study of a control population. The results of a case-control study of 72 patients with generalized and segmental ITD, examining the incidence of genetic and environmental factors possibly relevant to dystonia, are in favour of the former hypothesis. The only variables significantly more frequent in the patient group were a family history of tremor or stuttering (Fletcher *et al.*, 1991a); the latter has also been suggested to be a minor manifestation of ITD (Zeman *et al.*, 1960).

The variable severity and penetrance of ITD are currently unexplained. Intrafamilial correlation for both age of onset of symptoms and severity is low, suggesting environmental, rather than genetic, modification of the phenotype (Fletcher *et al.*, 1990). There is a growing body of evidence which incriminates peripheral trauma in the pathogenesis of dystonia (Koller *et al.*, 1989). Of the 104 patients with generalized and segmental ITD studied by Fletcher and colleagues (1990), 17 (16.4%) gave a history of trauma exacerbating dystonia within 2 months, or preceding the onset of dystonia in the same part of the body within 1 year. Eight of these 17 patients had affected relatives (Fletcher *et al.*, 1991b). It is possible that trauma can precipitate dystonic movements in individuals who are at risk of developing autosomal dominant ITD by virtue of being gene carriers.

An autosomal recessive form of dystonia has been proposed in four families from the Spanish gypsy population (Gimenez-Roldan *et al.*, 1988), based on observations of affected sibs with consanguineous parents in three of the kindreds. However, the consanguinity rate amongst Spanish gypsies is very high. Onset was before the age of 20 in three families, and all these patients had severe generalized dystonia. The fourth kindred was rather different, with onset of severe cranial dystonia, accompanied by dystonia and myoclonus in the upper limbs, in the third and fourth decades of life. The diagnosis of ITD is not absolutely certain in these patients; the results of detailed modern imaging studies and lysosomal enzyme assays were not reported.

An X-linked recessive dystonic syndrome appears to be particularly frequent on the Philippine island of Panay (Lee *et al.*, 1976; Fahn and Moskowitz, 1988). A recent study of 36 patients reported an age of onset between 12 and 52 years; the first symptom was usually focal dystonia but this became generalized within about 7 years (Kupke *et al.*, 1990a). Parkinsonism is common in this disorder, and may precede dystonia; this is not responsive to L-dopa. A further possible X-linked syndrome of generalized dystonia and deafness has been described in one kindred (Scribanu and Kennedy, 1976).

Genetic linkage studies in ITD

It is unlikely that the aetiology of ITD will be completely resolved until there are specific metabolic or genetic markers available for these conditions. The approach of reverse genetics is particularly appealing in dystonias, given the current lack of biochemical or pathological clues. Although genetic linkage studies of the dystonias are hampered by the possibility of disease heterogeneity which may not be clinically evident, as well as incomplete or absent expression of the disorder in some gene carriers, substantial progress has been made in the last few years. Genetic linkage analysis in one unusually large non-Jewish family with autosomal dominant ITD (Johnson *et al.*, 1962) has localized the defective gene to the end of the long arm of chromosome 9 (Ozelius *et al.*, 1989). Tight linkage between the dystonia locus and that encoding gelsolin, an actin-binding protein, at band 9q32–34 was demonstrated. Further studies in Jewish kindreds in the USA showed evidence for linkage between the loci for dystonia and argininosuccinate synthetase (ASS), which also maps to 9q32–34 (Kramer *et al.*, 1990). Thus it is probable (although not certain) that the gene or genes causing dystonia in these two populations are at the same locus (allelic). The authors suggested that one explanation for the higher penetrance in the non-Jewish family could be that different, but allelic, mutations produce susceptibility to dystonia in Jewish and non-Jewish families.

This ITD locus (DYT1) has subsequently been mapped to a 6 cM interval between ASS and AK1, with significant linkage disequilibrium between an extended ASS/ABL haplotype and ITD in both familial and sporadic Jewish cases (Kwiatkowski *et al.*, 1991; Ozelius *et al.*, 1992). This means that carrier detection and prenatal diagnosis are possible in Jewish ITD families in the USA, with a high degree of accuracy.

Genetic heterogeneity in autosomal dominant ITD has been demonstrated in families in Europe and Australia. Linkage studies with ASS in 27 small European families (3 Jewish and 24 non-Jewish) yielded a total lod score of −6.7 at a recombination fraction of 0.01. However, tight linkage to this marker could be excluded in three non-Jewish families; when these were excluded the maximum total lod score was 3.4. This suggests that there is a locus on chromosome 9q for this disorder in both non-Jewish and Jewish kindreds in the UK, but that one or more ITD loci map elsewhere. The ASS12/ABL4 haplotype observed in Jewish ITD families in the USA was significantly more frequent in Jewish, but not non-Jewish, kindreds in this study (Warner *et al.*, 1993). We have also studied a large Australian pedigree containing patients with ITD presenting in the second decade, often with prominent laryngeal involvement (Parker, 1985). Linkage to distal 9q loci was excluded (Ahmad *et al.*, 1993). It is also clear that the gene for essential tremor is not allelic to that on chromosome 9 causing ITD (Conway *et al.*, 1993). The X-linked dystonia–parkinsonism syndrome described in the Philippines has been mapped to the pericentromeric region of the X chromosome (Wilhelmsen *et al.*, 1990; Kupke *et al.*, 1990b, 1992).

Dopa-responsive dystonia

One type of dystonia which is clinically distinct from ITD is dopa-responsive dystonia (DRD) or Segawa's disease (Nygaard *et al.*, 1988). This syndrome usually comprises dystonia, often combined with parkinsonism, with onset in the first two decades of life, which responds dramatically and persistently to small doses of L-dopa. DRD is probably under-recognized, partly because it has a variable presentation including spastic diplegia; misdiagnosis as cerebral palsy has been reported (Boyd and Patterson, 1989). Inheritance is also autosomal dominant, probably with incomplete penetrance. It has been suggested that this disorder is due to abnormal activity of the enzyme tyrosine hydroxylase (TH), which converts tyrosine to dopa. Linkage studies in three families with DRD using a complementary DNA TH probe and other chromosome 11 markers have excluded TH as the disease locus (Fletcher *et al.*, 1989). The DRD locus has also been excluded from the region of chromosome 9 containing the American/Jewish ITD locus in one large kindred (Kwiatkowski *et al.*, 1990).

HUNTINGTON'S DISEASE

Gene mapping

The HD locus was mapped to the short arm of chromosome 4 (4p) in 1983 (Gusella *et al.*, 1983), and the clinical application of linked markers in this disease started around 1986 (see below). Critical to this is the assumption that there is only one HD locus, or that locus heterogeneity can be recognized. The use of chromosome 4 DNA markers for genetic prediction in a family exhibiting the HD phenotype but caused by a defective gene elsewhere in the genome would be grossly misleading. Conneally and colleagues (1989) examined a total of 63 families from a wide range of racial backgrounds (Caucasian, black American and Japanese) for evidence of linkage between the HD and G8 (D4S10) loci. The combined maximum lod score was 87.7 at a recombination fraction of 0.04. Only five small families generated mildly negative lod scores. There was no evidence of locus heterogeneity, that is, one linked and one unlinked locus, among these families, although a second rare locus could not be ruled out with certainty. In two disorders which may be confused clinically with HD, benign hereditary chorea and dentatorubropallidoluysian atrophy, linkage between the disease loci and distal chromosome 4p markers has been excluded (Quarrell *et al.*, 1988; Kondo *et al.*, 1990).

Linkage disequilibrium between some 4p markers, D4S98 and D4S95 (Fig. 3.1), has been described in HD families of mixed ancestry in Canada (Theilmann *et al.*, 1989) and others from the UK, 47% of whom were Welsh (Snell *et al.*, 1989). As well as suggesting that these two markers are particularly close to the HD locus, these studies were thought to indicate, as has been long suspected, that there may only be a few HD mutations which have spread around the world by means of immigration. However, this assumption is in question as an extensive recent analysis of linkage disequilibrium showed that many different haplotypes are associated with chromosomes carrying the HD mutation (MacDonald *et al.*, 1992).

After intensive effort since 1983, the HD gene has eventually been identified (MacDonald *et al.*, 1993). Progressing from the establishment of genetic linkage to isolating the mutant gene in any disease is a formidable task, as even closely linked DNA polymorphisms are usually more than a million bp (1 Mb) away from the disease gene. These difficulties were enhanced in HD by the position of the gene, in the terminal cytogenetic sub-band of chromosome 4, 4p16.3, between D4S10 and the telomere (Gilliam *et al.*, 1987). Many polymorphic loci distal to D4S10 have been identified. By using these for linkage analysis in reference and HD pedigrees (Whaley *et al.*, 1988; MacDonald *et al.*, 1989), and also by cloning large segments of DNA

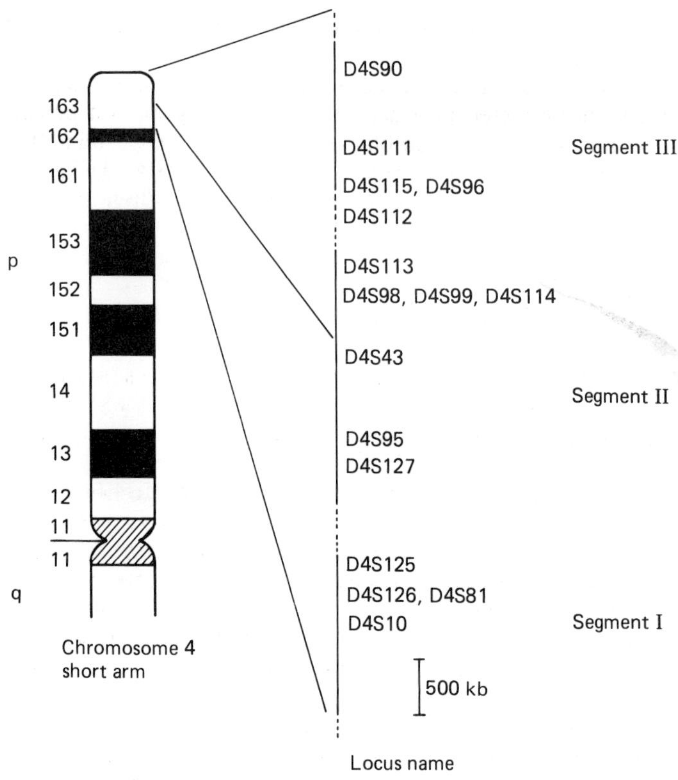

Figure 3.1 Physical map of chromosome 4p16.3, the region containing the Huntington's disease gene, as of 1989. This can be divided into three segments, which together contain about 5 million bp. Loci which are overlapping, or present within contiguous cloned sequences, are separated by commas. From MacDonald *et al.* (1989a), with permission from Cell Press.

using pulsed field electrophoresis to produce a physical map of 4p16.3 (Bucan *et al.*, 1990), three clusters of loci were defined (Fig. 3.1). Studies of recombination events in HD families initially suggested two possible locations for the HD gene, one telomeric and one more proximal (Fig. 3.1). The latter location became increasingly likely on the basis of observed recombination events and linkage disequilibrium data (MacDonald *et al.*, 1991, 1992; Bates *et al.*, 1992).

Work then focused on identifying genes within this 500 kb region, and analysing them for mutations. Eventually, an expressed sequence termed IT15 was identified. This gene contains a sequence of tandemly repeated trinucleotides (CAG) at one end. This repeat sequence varied in length in normal subjects (between 11 and 34 trinucleotides), but was longer in patients with HD, ranging from 42 to more than 100 repeats. It is not as yet clear whether there is any overlap between HD patients and controls in terms of repeat length. Preliminary data suggest an inverse correlation between repeat length and age of onset (MacDonald *et al.*, 1993). This is of particular interest as three other neurological diseases, myotonic dystrophy, X-linked bulbospinal neuronopathy and the fragile X syndrome, have been shown to be caused by an intragenic unstable trinucleotide repeat, the size of which is correlated with severity of phenotype (Suthers *et al.*, 1992).

The messenger RNA for the HD gene is about 11 kb in length and appears to be widely expressed. Its predicted product, termed Huntingtin, is a protein 348 kD in molecular mass, and bears no resemblance to any known protein. It is not as yet known whether the trinucleotide repeat sequence is translated. The next phase of unravelling the molecular pathogenesis of HD, determining function and malfunction of Huntingtin, is underway.

Determination of the HD phenotype

The discovery of DNA markers linked to the HD locus made it possible to identify individuals who are very likely to be homozygous for the mutant gene amongst the offspring of two affected parents, and this was confirmed by mutation analysis (MacDonald *et al.*, 1993). Such patients have been described from Venezuela and the USA (Wexler *et al.*, 1987; Myers *et al.*, 1989), and they do not appear to be more severely affected than heterozygotes. These observations suggest that the genetic defect in HD is unlikely to cause loss of function, such as an enzyme deficiency, as this would be expected to exhibit a dosage effect. An alteration in site or quantity of expression is more probable.

It has long been recognized that patients with particularly early-onset HD usually have affected fathers. Conversely, most late-onset cases inherit the gene from their mothers (Myers *et al.*, 1983). A detailed study of age at onset of symptoms in 3160 patients with HD showed that there was little difference between affected mothers and their offspring, but the distribution for age at onset in the offspring of affected fathers fell into two groups: a large one similar to that of the fathers and a smaller one which was, on average, 24 years younger than that of the fathers. Analysis of the grandparental origin of the HD gene suggested that the propensity for very early onset originates at the time of differentiation of the germ line of a male who inherits the HD gene from his mother, but that this propensity could be transmitted through the male line for a number of generations before the appearance of a juvenile-onset case (Ridley *et al.*, 1988).

It has been suggested that these observations are explicable on the basis of genomic imprinting (Reik, 1988; Ridley *et al.*, 1988), in which genes are labelled as being of maternal or paternal origin by means of a variable degree of methylation. Methylation can alter gene activation, inactivation and expression. Genes in ova and sperm differ in their degree of methylation, the latter tending to be relatively undermethylated. After conception, these methylation states persist except in cells which form the germline; genes in germline cells are remethylated as being of maternal or paternal origin, depending on the sex of the embryo. It is argued that the propensity for males with HD to have severely affected offspring arises when a HD allele is transmitted from a female to a male and remethylation of the allele (as being of paternal origin) is defective and leads to early or high-level expression of the harmful gene product. In contrast, genomic imprinting of HD alleles of maternal origin modifies the gene in favour of delayed or reduced expression and later onset of the disease in children of affected mothers. It is not clear whether methylation is relevant to expansion of trinucleotide repeats, but there is a parental sex effect in determining disease severity in myotonic dystrophy and the fragile X syndrome; in both cases repeat amplification is preferentially associated with female transmission.

Presymptomatic testing in HD

Since the identification of DNA markers linked to the HD locus, the potential problems of their clinical application in presymptomatic and prenatal diagnosis have been debated at length. These can broadly be divided into practical difficulties and ethical issues. Most of the former have been resolved by the identification of the HD mutation, but the latter largely persist.

An obvious, but sometimes overlooked prerequisite to predictive testing is that the diagnosis of HD in relatives is secure. This is particularly a problem in isolated cases without a family history (see below). The incidence of misdiagnosis of HD is as high as 15% (Folstein *et al.*, 1986), and this is particularly likely in isolated cases. It is incumbent on all centres undertaking testing to ensure that the diagnosis is correct by obtaining medical records, reviewing living patients if necessary, obtaining autopsy data if possible, and analysing DNA for the HD mutation in an affected relative. Even if there is clear evidence of a dominantly inherited syndrome of a movement disorder and dementia, the diagnosis of HD may be in doubt (Shiwach *et al.*, 1990). Alternative diagnoses include dentatorubropallidoluysian atrophy, olivopontocerebellar atrophy, familial Alzheimer's disease, and Gerstmann–Straussler syndrome.

A major practical limitation in presymptomatic testing was that imposed by pedigree structure. In order to determine which marker allele is segregating with the HD gene in a given family, it was preferable to test two generations containing affected individuals. For practical purposes this meant that for genetic prediction in an adult at risk (i.e. with an affected parent), there should be at least one parent and grandparent (affected or unaffected) available for testing. These restrictions meant that only between 15 and 75 per cent of adults at risk (the proportion depending on the population studied) could have a predictive test before the HD mutation was identified (Harper and Sarfarazi, 1985; Misra *et al.*, 1988; Farrer *et al.*, 1988; Brock *et al.*, 1989). The other major problem of testing using linked markers was that it was only possible to determine whether the subject had a low (minimum 2%) or high (maximum 98%) risk of carrying the HD gene, because of the possibility of recombination between the marker and disease loci. These two problems have now been resolved, assuming that all families with HD have the same type of mutation. Confirmation of the presence of the expanded repeat in an affected relative is desirable, but the need for extended family studies has gone. The method of mutation analysis described by MacDonald *et al.* (1993) is technically difficult, but an improved method should be suitable for service use (Goldberg *et al.*, 1993).

The uptake of predictive testing amongst those at risk has varied from 15% to those invited to participate to 75–85% of individuals who spontaneously request testing (Brock *et al.*, 1989; Craufurd *et al.*, 1989). Many of the latter who change their minds have not thought through the implications of testing in detail. Those proceeding with the test are more likely than not to be female, married, and to have children already. The commonest motive for being tested is resolution of uncertainty and increased ease in planning for the future, together with concern about the possible risk of existing children; surprisingly few (20–25%) indicate that they want testing in order to make reproductive decisions (Bloch *et al.*, 1989; Craufurd *et al.*, 1989).

Over 1500 presymptomatic tests for HD have been performed worldwide (Morris 1990; Tyler *et al.*, 1992; World Federation of Neurology Research Group on Huntington's Disease, 1993). The problems encountered have more commonly involved counselling and clinical aspects than the laboratory ones discussed above.

Both expected and unanticipated ethical and legal issues have arisen (Morris *et al.*, 1989; Huggins *et al.*, 1990; Shiwach *et al.*, 1990). International guidelines for the application of presymptomatic and prenatal testing have been published in an attempt to deal with these (World Federation of Neurology Research Group on Huntington's Disease, 1989).

It is important that individuals wishing to be tested understand the variable manifestations and natural history of HD. It is essential that the implications of a positive result are discussed in detail, in relation to emotional reactions in the immediate post-test period and the longer term, life insurance, employment and lifestyle in general, and effects on partners, parents, children, and other relatives. Subjects should understand that a positive result does not currently give accurate information on age of onset of symptoms, or their severity, but this situation may change when further data are obtained from studies of repeat length and phenotype.

The counselling required to transmit the above and ensure that the subject has sufficient information on which to base a decision to be tested usually takes at least three sessions, supplemented by written information. Most centres insist on a 'cooling off' period of at least three months, before consent is given and proceeding with the test, unless there are exceptional circumstances. It is best not to take blood from the subject at risk until that time, and the result should be given in person as soon as is feasible. Support for the subject must be available after the test. Those undergoing testing are encouraged to select a partner to accompany them at all stages of counselling related to the test (Tyler *et al.*, 1992).

Inappropriate use of the test may be requested by physicians, family members, or others such as insurance companies, employers, or adoption agencies. The decision to take the test is the sole choice of the individual concerned. It is generally thought that testing should not be performed on subjects under the age of majority but that they should be allowed to make an informed decision about testing after this age. Most parents appreciate this after discussion; the main motive for seeking testing of young children by parents is the hope that there will be a low risk result and their view is that HD need not be discussed with the children if this is the case. Early marriage or reproduction may provide exceptions to this recommendation. Requests for pre-adoption testing have been refused (Morris *et al.*, 1989).

Subjects with a past or current history of major psychiatric illness are usually asked to postpone testing. There was some controversy as to whether testing using linked markers should be undertaken in those showing equivocal clinical signs of HD. This is not uncommon; about 10% of those requesting presymptomatic tests are either definitely or possibly affected at the time of referral (Brock *et al.*, 1989; Morris *et al.*, 1989; Morris, 1990). It now seems reasonable to undertake mutation analysis in such subjects, but it is important to assess whether minor symptoms or signs can be attributed to HD with certainty in these circumstances.

Other ethical problems which have arisen in presymptomatic testing, which may persist with mutation analyses, include refusal to give blood samples by key relatives, unintentional risk alteration in family members, requests from one monozygous twin for testing when the other does not want it, and the need to confirm the suspicion of the applicant that a relative has HD when the latter has no desire to be assessed neurologically (Morris *et al.*, 1989; Huggins *et al.*, 1990). It is generally held that a family member's right to confidentiality supersedes the applicant's right to be tested.

In subjects given high risk results no persistent adverse consequences have been observed so far, although transient depression, of varying degree, is common (Wiggins, 1989; Meissen *et al.*, 1988; Brandt *et al.*, 1989; Craufurd *et al.*, 1989). Post-test suicide has not been reported. Some individuals given low risk results have described hostility from untested or affected siblings, and transient depression for a 'survivor effect' is common in such subjects.

Prenatal testing for HD

Prenatal tests for HD gene carrier status can be divided into two types: a direct mutation test, or what is referred to as prenatal exclusion testing. The former is possible when one prospective parent has HD or has had predictive testing. The latter was introduced for prospective parents at risk who did not have the appropriate pedigree structure for linkage-based presymptomatic testing in themselves, or who did not wish to undergo testing but wanted to avoid transmitting the HD gene to their children. This may still be the preferred option for some couples, although it does raise ethical difficulties. In either case, DNA is ideally analysed from chorionic villus samples obtained at 8–10 weeks' gestation and results are thus available in time for a first-trimester abortion. It is advisable to assess informativeness before conception, although human nature dictates that this is not always practical. Testing should not be undertaken unless the couple concerned is committed to terminating high-risk pregnancies.

Prenatal exclusion testing is done by determining which distal part of chromosome 4p has been inherited by the fetus from the parent at risk, using linked markers. This can be done if the affected parent of the prospective parent is dead, as long as the patient's spouse is alive. Take, for example, a fetus with a mother whose father has HD. The fetus will inherit the relevant part of chromosome 4 from either its maternal grandmother or its maternal grandfather. The former implies a 2% risk of the fetus carrying the HD gene, and the latter a near 50% risk, the same as that of the parent at risk. It should be stressed that a near 50% risk does not alter the risk of the prospective parent. The uptake of prenatal exclusion testing is relatively low, presumably reflecting attitudes towards terminating pregnancies which have a 50% chance of being unaffected (Craufurd *et al.*, 1989; Tyler *et al.*, 1990). Between 35 and 50% of couples counselled with a view to prenatal exclusion testing choose not to follow this option.

The ethical problems which arise in prenatal testing are similar to those discussed above in relation to presymptomatic testing. Continuation of pregnancies shown to be at high risk raises the possibility of the child having had an unsolicited presymptomatic test should the parent at risk have HD. This situation should be avoided by adequate prepregnancy counselling. All prenatal tests are potentially harmful to the pregnancy, and should not be undertaken unless the result will be acted on.

The problem of isolated cases of HD

The differential diagnosis of dominantly inherited chorea and dementia is small. Substantial diagnostic problems arise when a patient presents with the clinical features of HD but there is no family history of affected relatives. It is not clear what proportion of such patients has HD, and this creates difficulties in genetic counselling for their families. There are four possible explanations for isolated cases of what looks like HD: (1) they have a different disease; (2) the existence of relatives with HD is hidden by early death, exceptionally late onset of the disease in antecedents, or denial by the family; (3) non-paternity; and (4) fresh mutation. The second and third categories probably account for the majority of isolated cases. This issue should be resolved soon when such patients have been investigated for the presence of HD mutation.

Dominantly inherited disorders mimicking HD have been discussed earlier; an important and often overlooked condition which is often misdiagnosed as HD is neuroacanthocytosis (NA) (see below). Other potential causes of understandable diagnostic confusion include cerebrovascular disease, and tardive dyskinesia with psychiatric dysfunction (Folstein *et al.*, 1986). Quarrell *et al.* (1986) investigated 22 patients thought to have HD on clinical grounds apart from the absence of a definite family history. At least one parent of 7 of these had died before the age of 60 years, 1 was thought to be illegitimate, and the parent of another had died in a psychiatric hospital. Autopsies had been performed on 7 patients, and the diagnosis of HD was confirmed in 6; the seventh was thought to have cerebrovascular disease, although a later study suggested that this patient too had HD (Bateman *et al.*, 1992). These authors reviewed 49 patients in whom a diagnosis of HD seemed possible on clinical grounds, but who gave no history of definitely affected relatives. In 32 with progressive chorea and dementia, postural instability, and abnormal initiation of saccadic eye movements, the diagnosis was confirmed in all 7 patients who had had autopsies, affected relatives were found in 5 others, and HD remained probable in a further 13 who were re-examined. In the 17 with a less typical clinical picture, a diagnosis of HD appeared likely in 2. Other diagnoses such as cerebrovascular disease, NA, recrudescence of Sydenham's chorea, and drug-induced tardive dyskinesia could have explained the remainder. It was concluded that the likelihood of HD in a patient with the typical clinical features of this disorder but no family history is at least 75%, which for practical purposes implies a risk to their children hardly less than in familial HD (Bateman *et al.* 1992). The most plausible explanations for seemingly sporadic cases of HD are non-paternity and mild, late-onset disease which may be overlooked.

Fresh mutation has been thought to be exceptionally rare in HD, as might be expected from the effects of a late-onset disorder on biological fitness; this is probably slightly increased rather than decreased. Prior to the possibility of mutation analysis, the criteria for accepting a patient as representing a fresh mutation were: typical clinical features, preferably with pathological confirmation of HD; transmission to offspring; both parents confirmed as healthy over the age of about 65 years; and proof of paternity. Not surprisingly, no such case has been reported. Wolff *et al.* (1989) provided good evidence for the existence of a fresh mutation in a patient who had 15 healthy siblings. The parents had died in their 80s, free of neurological disease. Extensive serological testing showed no evidence of non-paternity. DNA analysis indicated that several of the patient's unaffected siblings shared one or both of her haplotypes for RFLPs linked to the HD locus. The study of MacDonald and colleagues (1993) showed direct evidence of fresh mutation in two patients with HD. Of interest is the observation that the parental allele which expanded sufficiently to produce the HD phenotype contained a trinucleotide repeat at the upper limit of normal. A similar phenomenon, of 'premutation', is seen in the fragile X syndrome (Suthers *et al.*, 1992).

NEUROCANTHOCYTOSIS

NA or chorea-acanthocytosis can be distinguished from the other main disorder causing neurological impairment and acanthocytosis, abetalipoproteinaemia, by the characteristic clinical features and lipid abnormalities of the latter (Hardie, 1989). NA is a disorder characterized by a variable, and often mixed, movement disorder, usually including chorea, acanthocytosis, normal serum lipid concentrations, and other neurological dysfunction such as areflexia which usually reflects the presence of an axonal neuropathy. The condition is probably underdiagnosed and, as noted above, often confused with HD. Approximately 50 cases have been reported in the English literature, and a similar number in Japanese papers (Hardie, 1989).

Hardie and colleagues (1990) described 19 cases; 12 of these were members of three families and the rest were sporadic. The age of onset of symptoms ranged from 8 to 62 (mean 32) years and the clinical features were very variable. Cognitive impairment and personality change occurred in more than 50%. Chorea was seen in nearly all symptomatic cases but dystonia, tics, involuntary vocalizations and an akinetic rigid syndrome were also observed. The last is particularly frequent in the late stages of the disease. One-third of patients had had seizures. Orofacial involuntary movements and orolingual dystonia were sometimes severe, occasionally with biting of the lips and tongue. Thirteen patients had depressed or absent tendon reflexes, but only 3 had distal muscle weakness.

Evidence of an axonal neuropathy was present in 7 of 14 patients investigated neurophysiologically. Sural nerve biopsies showed evidence of a chronic axonal neuropathy with prominent regenerative activity, predominantly affecting the large diameter myelinated fibres. Computed tomography (CT) scans usually showed cerebral atrophy, and occasionally caudate atrophy. Non-specific focal and symmetrical signal abnormalities from the caudate or lentiform nuclei were seen by magnetic resonance imaging (MRI) in 3 of 4 cases. Serum creatinine kinase activity was increased in 11 patients.

Postmortem examination in one case showed extensive neuronal loss and gliosis affecting the corpus striatum, pallidum, and substantia nigra, particularly the pars reticulata. The cerebral cortex was spared and there was no evidence of anterior horn cell loss in the spinal cord. Other reported autopsies have shown similar findings, except that previously no abnormalities have been found in the substantia nigra, and there may be loss of anterior horn cells (de Yebenes *et al.*, 1988).

The diagnosis of NA is often missed because of failure to examine at least three fresh blood films; films reported as showing crenation or anisopoikilocytosis are suspicious in this context. Ideally, phase contrast microscopy can be used to distinguish the appearance of true acanthocytes from the spherical regular crenation of echinocytes seen in a mumber of systemic diseases. Scanning electron microscopy of fresh red cells can also be useful in this context.

The genetics of NA are unclear. Both autosomal dominant and autosomal recessive inheritance have been proposed. In favour of the former is parent–child transmission in a small number of families (Levine *et al.*, 1968; Kito *et al.*, 1980; Sotanieni, 1983), but familial cases confined to a single generation or less certain pedigrees are more common. Isolated cases are almost certainly under-reported. Vance *et al.* (1987) concluded that NA is most likely to be an autosomal recessive disorder and this is supported by parental consanguinity which has been described in five families (e.g. Sotanieni, 1983; Hardie *et al.*, 1990). However, the existence of families containing affected members in more than one generation requires either a different mode of inheritance or the possibility of genetic heterogeneity. Published pedigrees have included only one example of male-to-male transmission, in which an affected male had a brother and a paternal uncle with seizures and 'mental symptoms', and a son with acanthocytosis alone but no neurological impairment (Kito *et al.*, 1980). Of all familial cases reported in the English literature, 31 were male and 18 female, and in sporadic cases the sex ratio was 9 male:4 female (overall 40 male, 22 female).

These data suggest the possibility of an X-linked dominant gene causing NA. In favour of this is the combination of NA and the McLeod phenotype reported in one family (Hardie *et al.*, 1990). The McLeod phenotype, comprising acanthocytosis associated with abnormal expression of Kell blood antigens, usually with raised serum creatinine kinase (CK) concentrations and subclinical myopathy, is caused by a mutant gene on the short arm of the X chromosome (Bertelson *et al.*, 1988). In relation to this it is of interest that many patients with NA have elevated serum CK activity, and that involuntary movements have been noted in some males with the McLeod phenotype (Marsh, 1983). It will be of interest to test the hypothesis of X-linked inheritance in NA using genetic linkage analysis.

PARKINSON'S DISEASE

The role of genetic factors in the aetiology of PD has been controversial for many years; family studies were hampered by variable diagnostic criteria and the difficulties of assessing the significance of such a common disorder occurring in more than one member of a family (Duvoisin, 1986). The genetic hypothesis was discarded by many when a twin study showed similar concordance rates between monozygotic and dizygotic twins (Ward *et al.*, 1983), but the controversy has re-emerged. There are four main reasons for this. First is the recent publication of a large Italian kindred with PD (Golbe *et al.*, 1990). As many as 41 members spanning four generations were affected. Atypical features included early age of onset (mean 46.5 years), an aggressive course (death within a mean of 7 years), and a low incidence of tremor. Nevertheless, patients were L-dopa-responsive, and postmortem examination showed Lewy bodies and a typical distribution of neuronal degeneration in both autopsied subjects. The authors ascribed their findings to autosomal dominant inheritance with incomplete penetrance. Degl'Innocenti *et al.* (1989) have also reported a large kindred of what appears to be familial, but otherwise clinically typical, PD.

Second, mitochondrial complex I deficiency has been reported in both substantia nigra (Schapira *et al.*, 1990a; Mann *et al.*, 1992a) and platelets (Parker *et al.*, 1989) of patients with PD. Some subunits of this complex are encoded by mitochondrial DNA (mtDNA), which is exclusively maternally inherited. The mitochondrial genetic hypothesis is the only one which can entirely account for previous observations on PD in twins, with uneven distribution of defective mitochondrial genes within oocytes explaining the lack of concordance between monozygotic twin pairs. Third, genetic susceptibility to PD is indicated by an increased incidence of alleles associated with poor metabolism of debrisoquine in PD compared to controls (Armstrong *et al.*, 1992; Smith *et al.*, 1992). Finally, Duvoisin and colleagues have recently reappraised their twin study, and now conclude that it neither proves nor disproves the genetic hypothesis (Johnson *et al.*, 1990). F^{18} fluorodopa positron emission tomography (PET) scanning in asymptomatic co-monozygous twins of PD patients suggests that concordance is higher if subclinical disease is taken into account, although this was also true, but to a lesser extent, for dizygous twins (Burn *et al.*, 1992).

The clinical and genetic features of familial PD in the UK were investigated by examining the families of 20 probands who were selected on the basis of having clinically typical PD and at least one affected relative (Maraganore *et al.*, 1991). Forty-nine secondary cases were identified. These subjects were clinically indistinguishable from sporadic cases of idiopathic PD. Non-random ascertainment of probands did not permit comparison of the observed incidence of secondary PD cases to that expected from population data, and the question as to whether familial clustering of PD is genetic, coincidental, or due to shared environmental factors remains unanswered. If it is assumed that familial PD has a genetic component, the similar incidence of the disease in the parents and sibs of index cases suggested that an autosomal dominant gene or genes with reduced penetrance is the most likely explaination for this. The data did not support the possibilities of either polygenic or mitochondrial inheritance; there was a slight excess of paternal transmission.

The mitochondrial hypothesis has been explored further by analysing mtDNA in the brain of patients dying with PD. Schapira *et al.* (1990b) and Lestienne *et al.* (1990) analysed restriction fragments of mtDNA in substantia nigra and cerebral cortex from PD brains. There was no significant polymorphism common to the PD group, nor evidence of a significant proportion of mtDNA with large deletions. Ikebe and colleagues (1990), however, found a proportion of mtDNA with the 4.9 kb 'common deletion' in PD brain (including striatum) using the polymerase chain reaction. Quantification of deleted mtDNA in a 73-year-old PD patient initially suggested that these were increased 17-fold (Ozawa *et al.*, 1990), but recent evidence indicates that this is merely an age-related phenomenon (Lestienne *et al.*, 1991; Mann *et al.*, 1992b). Furthermore, a proportion of mutated mtDNA which is only detectable using the polymerase chain reaction is hardly likely to be the cause of any biochemical defect. It has also been proposed that point mutations of mtDNA may be relevant to the pathogenesis of PD (Ikebe *et al.*, 1992), but it can be questioned whether such mutations are of any pathological significance whatsoever. The mitochondrial genone is highly polymorphic, making it difficult to argue pathogenicity for mutations unless they are heteroplasmic and occur in more than one unrelated disease subject and not in a large number of normal controls. Such evidence has not been provided in PD (Ikebe *et al.*, 1992).

It is clear that the genetic hypothesis of PD should be explored further. An obvious approach is genetic linkage studies in large kindreds containing sufficient affected members. Leaving genetic hypotheses aside, familial clustering of PD could be explained by a shared environmental insult. Calne and colleagues (1987) felt that their observation of correlation between family members for calendar year of onset (as opposed to age) supported this hypothesis. However, this was only reported in six kindreds, and the data of Maraganore *et al.* (1991) showed insignificant correlation for year of onset, with only slightly positive coefficients for both parents and sibs. Some such correlation would be expected as a result of ascertainment bias.

References

Ahmad F, Davis MB, Waddy HM, Oley CA, Marsden CD and Harding AE (1993) Evidence for locus heterogeneity in autosomal dominant torsion dystonia. *Genomics*, **15**, 9

Armstrong M, Daly AK, Cholerton S, Bateman CN, and Idle JR (1992) Mutant debrisoquine hydroxylation genes in Parkinson's disease. *Lancet*, **339**, 1017–18

Bateman D, Boughey AM, Scaravilli, F, Marsden CD, and Harding AE (1992) A follow up study of isolated cases of suspected Huntington's disease. *Ann Neurol*, **31**, 293–8

Bates GP, Valdes J, Hummerich H, Baxendale S, Le Paslier DL, Monaco AP *et al.* (1992) Characterization of a yeast artificial chromosome contig spanning the Huntington's disease gene candidate region. *Nature Genet*, **1**, 180–7

Bertelson CJ, Pogo AP, Chaudhuri A, Marsh WL, Redman CM, Banerjee D *et al.* (1988) Localization of the McLeod locus (XK) within Xp21 by deletion analysis. *Am J Hum Genet*, **42**, 703–11

Bloch M, Fahy M, Fox S, and Hayden MR (1989) Predictive testing for Huntington disease: II. Demographic characteristics, life-style patterns, attitudes, and psychosocial assessments of the first fifty-one candidates. *Am J Med Genet*, **32**, 217–24

Boyd K and Patterson V (1989) Dopa responsive dystonia; a treatable condition misdiagnosed as cerebral palsy. *B Med J*, **298**, 1019–20

Brandt J, Quaid KA, Folstein SE, Garber P, Maestri NE, Abbott MH *et al.* (1989) Presymptomatic diagnosis of delayed-onset disease with linked DNA markers. The experience in Huntington's disease. *JAMA*, **261**, 3108–14

Bressman SB, de Leon D, Brin MF, Risch N, Burke RE, Greene PE *et al.* (1989) Idiopathic dystonia among Ashkenzai Jews: evidence for autosomal dominant inheritance. *Ann Neurol*, **26**, 612–20

Brock DJ, Mennie M, Curtis A, Millan F, Baron, L, Raeburn JA *et al.* (1989) Predictive testing for Huntington's disease with linked DNA markers. *Lancet*, **ii**, 463–6

Bucan M, Zimmer M, Whaley WL, Poustka A, Youngman S, Allitto BA *et al.* (1990) Physical maps of 4p16.3, the area expected to contain the Huntington disease mutation. *Genomics*, **6**, 1–15

Bundey S, Harrison MJG, and Marsden CD (1975) A genetic study of torsion dystonia. *J Med Genet*, **12**, 12–19

Burke RE, Brin MF, Fahn S, Bressman SB, and Moskowitz C (1986) Analysis of the clinical course of non-Jewish, autosomal dominant torsion dystonia. *Movement Disorders*, **1**, 163–78

Burn DJ, Mark MH, Playford ED, Maraganore DM, Zimmerman TR, Duvoisin RC *et al.* (1992) Parkinson's disease in twins studied with ^{18}F-DOPA and positron emission tomography. *Neurology*, **42**, 1894–1900

Calne S, Schoenberg B, Martin W, Uitti RJ, Spencer P, and Calne DB (1987) Familial Parkinson's disease: possible role of environmental factors. *Can J Neurol Sci*, **14**, 303–5

Conneally PM, Haines JL, Tanzi RE, Wexler NS, Penchaszadeh GK, Harper PS *et al.* (1989) Huntington disease: no evidence for locus heterogeneity. *Genomics*, **5**, 304–8

Conway D, Bain PG, Warner TT, Davis MB, Findley LJ, Thompson PD, Marsden CD and Harding AE (1993) Linkage analysis with chromosome 9 markers in hereditary essential tremor. *Movement Disorders*, **8**, 374

Craufurd D, Dodge A, Kerzin-Storrar L, and Harris R (1989) Uptake of presymptomatic predictive testing for Huntington's disease. *Lancet*, **ii**, 603–5

Degl'Innocenti F, Maurello MT, and Marini P (1989) A parkinsonian kindred. *Ital J Neuro Sci*, **10**, 307–10

de Yebenes JG, Brin MF, Mena MA, de Felipe C, del Rio RM, Bazan E *et al.* (1988) Neurochemical findings in neuroacanthocytosis. *Movement Disorders*, **3**, 300–12

Duvoisin R (1986) Genetics of Parkinson's disease. *Adv Neurol*, **45**, 307–12

Eldridge R (1970) The torsion dystonias: literature review and genetic and clinical studies. *Neurology*, **20** (suppl), 1–78

Eldridge R (1981) Inheritance of torsion dystonia in Jews. *Ann Neurol*, **10**, 203–4

Eldridge R and Gottlieb R (1976) The primary hereditary dystonias: genetic classification of 768 families and revised estimate of gene frequency, autosomal recessive form, and selective bibliography. *Adv Neurol*, **14**, 457–74

Eldridge R and Koerber T (1979) Torsion dystonia: autosomal recessive form. In Goodman RM, Motulsky SG, eds, *Genetic Disorders among Ashkenazi Jews*, New York, Raven Press, 213–51

Fahn S and Moskowitz C (1988) X-linked recessive dystonia and Parkinsonism in Filipino males. *Ann Neurol*, **24**, 179

Fahn S, Marsden CD, and Calne DB (1987) Classification and investigation of dystonia. In Marsden CD, Fahn S, eds, *Movement Disorders 2*, London, Butterworths, 332–58

Farrer LA, Myers RH, Cupples LA, and Connneally PM (1988) Considerations in using linkage analysis as a presymptomatic test for Huntington's disease. *J Med. Genet*, **25**, 577–88

Fletcher NA, Holt IJ, Harding AE, Nygaard TG, Mallet J, and Marsden CD (1989) Tyrosine hydroxylase and L-dopa responsive dystonia. *J Neurol Neurosurg Psychiatry*, **52**, 112–14

Fletcher NA, Harding AE, and Marsden CD (1990) A genetic study of idiopathic torsion dystonia in the United Kingdom. *Brain*, **113**, 379–96

Fletcher NA, Harding AE, and Marsden CD (1991a) A case control study of idiopathic torsion dystonia. *Movement Disorders*, **6**, 304–9

Fletcher NA, Harding AE, and Marsden CD (1991b) The relationship between trauma and idiopathic torsion dystonia. *J Neurol Neurosurg Psychiatry*, **54**, 713–17

Folstein SE, Leigh RJ, Parhad IM, and Folstein MF (1986) The diagnosis of Huntington's diseases. *Neurology*, **36**, 1279–83

Gilliam TC, Tanzi RD, Haines JL, Bonner TI, Faryniarz AG, Hobbs WJ *et al.* (1987) Localization of the Huntington's disease gene to a small segment of chromosome 4 flanked by D4S10 and the telomere. *Cell*, **50**, 565–71

Giminez-Roldan S, Delgado G, Marin M, Villanueva JA, and Mateo D (1988) Hereditary torsion dystonia in gypsies. *Adv Neurol*, **50**, 73–81

Golbe LI, Di Iorio G, Bonavita V, Miller DC, and Duvosin RC (1990) A large kindred with autosomal dominant Parkinson's disease. *Ann Neurol*, **27**, 276–82

Goldberg YP, Andrew SE, Clarke LA, Hayden MR (1993) A PCR method for accurate assessment of trinucleotide repeat expansion in Huntington disease, *Human Molecular Genetics*, **6**, 635–636

Gusella JF, Wexler NS, Conneally PM, Naylor SL, Anderson MA, Tanzi Re *et al.* (1983) A polymorphic DNA marker genetically linked to Huntington's disease. *Nature*, **306**, 234–8

Hardie RJ (1989) Acanthocytosis and neurological impairment – a review. *Q J Med*, **71**, 291–306

Hardie RJ, Pullon HWH, Harding AE, Owen JS, Pires M, Daniels GL *et al.* (1990) Neuroacanthocytosis. A clinical, haematological and pathological study of 19 cases. *Brain*, **114**, 13–49

Harper PS and Sarfarazi M (1985) Genetic prediction and family structure in Huntington'c chorea. *Br Med J*, **290**, 1929–31

Huggins M, Bloch M, Kanani S, Quarrell OWJ, Theilman J, Hedrick A *et al.* (1990) Ethical and legal dilemmas arising during predictive testing for adult-onset disease; the experience of Huntington disease. *Am J Hum Genet*, **47**, 4–12

Ikebe S, Tanaka M, Ohno K, Sato W, Hattori K, Kondo T, Mizuno Y, and Ozawa T (1990) Increase of deleted mitochondrial DNA in the striatum in Parkinson's disease and senescence. *Biochem Biophys Res Commun*, **170**, 1044–8

Ikebe S, Hattori N, Mizuno Y, Ranaka M, and Ozawa T (1992) Point mutations of mitochondrial DNA in Parkinson's disease. *Movement Disorders*, **7** (suppl 1), 71

Johnson W, Schwartz G, and Barbeau A (1962) Studies on dystonia musculorum deformans. *Arch Neurol*, **7**, 301–13

Johnson WG, Hodge SE, and Duvoisin R (1990) Twin studies and the genetics of Parkinson's disease – a reappraisal. *Movement Disorders*, **5**, 187–94

Kito S, Itoga E, Hiroshige Y, Matsumoto N, and Miwa S (1980) A predigree of amyotrophic chorea with acanthocytosis. *Aerch Neurol*, **37**, 514–17

Koller WC, Wong GF, and Lang A (1989) Post-traumatic movement disorders: a review. *Movement Disorders*, **4**, 20–36

Kondo I, Ohta H, Yazaki M, Ideda JE, Gusella JF, and Kanazawa I (1990) Exclusion mapping of the hereditary dentatorubropallidoluysian atrophy gene from the Huntington's disease locus. *J Med Genet*, **27**, 105–8

Korczyn AD, Kahana E, Zilber N, Streifler M, Carasso R, and Alter M (1980) Torsion dystonia in Israel. *Ann Neurol*, **8**, 387–91

Korczyn AD, Zilber N, Kahana E, and Alter M (1981) Inheritance of torsion dystonia in Jews. *Ann Neurol*, **10**, 204–5

Kramer PL, de Leon D, Ozelius L, Risch N, Bressman SB, Brin MF *et al.* (1990) Dystonia gene in Ashkenazi Jewish population is located on chromosome 9q32–34. *Ann Neurol*, **27**, 114–20

Kupke KG, Lee LV, Viterbo GH, Arancillo J, Donlon T, and Muller U (1990a) X-linked recessive torsion dystonia in the Philippines. *Am J Med Genet*, **36**, 1–6

Kupke KG, Lee LV, and Muller U (1990b) Assignment of the X-linked torsion dystonia gene to Xq21 by linkage analysis. *Neurology*, **40**, 1438–42

Kupke KG, Graeber MB, and Muller U (1992) Dystonia-Parkinsonism syndrome (XDP) locus: flanking markers in Xq12-q21.1 *Am J Hum Genet*, **50**, 808–15

Kwiatkowski DJ, Nygaard TG, Schuback DE, Perman S, Trugman JM, Bressman SB *et al.* (1990) Identification of a highly polymorphic microsatellite VNTR within the argininosucinnate synthetase locus: exclusion of the dystonia gene on 9q32–34 as the cause of dopa-responsisive dystonia in a large kindred. *Am J Hum Genet*, **48**, 121–8

Kwiatkowski DJ, Ozelius L, Kramer PL, Perman S, Schuback DE, Gusella JF *et al.* (1991) Torsion dystonia genes in two populations confined to a small region on chromosome 9q32–34. *Am J Human Genet*, **49**, 366–71

Lee LV, Pascasio FM, Fuentes FD, and Viterbo GH (1976) Torsion dystonia in Panay, Philippines. *Adv Neurol*, **14**, 137–51

Lestienne P, Nelson J, Riederer P, Jellinger K, and Reichmann H (1990) Normal mitochondrial genome in brain from patients with Parkinson's disease and complex I defect. *J Neurochem*, **55**, 1810–12

Lestienne P, Riederer P, and Jellinger K (1991) Mitochondrial DNA in postmortem brain from patients with Parkinson's disease. *J Neurochem*, **56**, 1819

Levine IM, Estes JW, and Looney JM (1968) Hereditary neurological disease with acanthocytosis. *Arch Neurol*, **19**, 403–9

MacDonald ME, Haines JL, Zimmer M, Cheng SV, Youngman S, Whaley WL *et al.* (1989) Recombination events suggest potential sites for the Huntington's disease gene. *Neuron*, **3**, 183–90

MacDonald ME, Lin C, Srinidi L, Bates G, Altherr M, Whaley WL *et al.* (1991) Complex patterns of linkage disequilibrium in the Huntington disease region. *Am J Hum Genet*, **49**, 723–34

MacDonald ME, Novolletto A, Lin C, Tagle D, Barnes G, Bates G *et al.* (1992) The Huntington's disease candidate region exhibits many different haplotypes. *Nature Genet*, **1**, 99–103

MacDonald ME, Ambrose CM, Duyao MP, Myer RH, Lin C, Srinidhi L *et al.* (1993) A novel gene containing a trinucleotide repeat that is expanded and unstable on Huntington's disease chromosomes. *Cell*, **72**, 971–83

Mann VM, Cooper JM, Krige D, Caniel SE, Schapira AHV, and Marsden CD (1992) Brain skeletal muscle and platelet mitochondrial function in Parkinson's disease. *Brain*, **115**, 333–42

Maraganore DM, Harding AE, and Marsden CD (1991) A clinical and genetic study of familial Parkinson's disease. *Movement Disorders*, **6**, 205–11

Marsden CD and Harrison MJG (1974) Idiopathic torsion dystonia (dystonia musculorum deformans): a review of forty-two patients. *Brain*, **97**, 793–810

Marsh WL (1983) Deleted antigens of the Rhesus and Kell blood groups: association with cell membrane defects. In Garratty, ed, *Blood Group Antigens and Disease*, Arlington, American Association of Blood Banks, 165–85

Misra VP, Baraitser M, and Harding AE (1988) Genetic prediction in Huntington's disease: what are the limitations imposed by pedigree structure? *Movement Disorders*, **3**, 233–6

Morris MJ (1990) Huntington's disease: presymptomatic testing. *Curr Opin Neurol Neurosurg*, **3**, 337–41

Morris MJ, Tyler A, Lazarou L, Meredith L, and Harper PS (1989) Problems in genetic prediction for Huntington's disease. *Lancet*, **ii**, 601–3

Myers RH, Goldman D, Bird ED, Sax DS, Merril CR, Schoenfield M *et al.* (1983) Maternal transmission in Huntington's disease. *Lancet*, **i**, 208–10

Myers RH, Leavitt J, Farrer LA, Jagadeesh J, McFarlene H, Mostromauro CA *et al.* (1989) Homozygote for Huntington disease. *Am J Hum Genet*, **45**, 615–18

Nutt JG, Muenter MD, Aronson A, Kurland LT, and Melton LJ (1988) Epidemiology of focal and generalized dystonia in Rochester, Minnesota. *Movement Disorders*, **3**, 188–94

Nygaard TG, Marsden CD, and Duvoisin RC (1988) Dopa responsive dystonia. *Adv Neurol*, **50**, 377–84

Ozawa T, Tanaka M, Ikebe S, Ohno K, Kondo T, and Mizuno Y (1990) Quantitative determination of deleted mitochondrial DNA relative to normal DNA in parkinsonism striatum by a kinetic PCR analysis. *Biochem Biophys Res Commun*, **172**, 483–9

Ozelius L, Kramer PL, Moskowitz CB, Kwiatkowski DJ, Brin MF, Bressman SB *et al.* (1989) Human gene for torsion dystonia located on chromosome 9q32–34. *Neuron*, **2**, 1427–34

Ozelius LJ, Kramer PL, de Leon D, Risch N, Bressman SB, Schuback DE *et al.* (1992) Strong allelic association between torsion dystonia gene (DYT1) and loci on chromosome 9q34 in Ashkenazi Jews. *Am J Hum Genet*, **50**, 619–28

Parker N (1985) Hereditary whispering dysphonia. *J Neurol Neurosurg Psychiatry*, **48**, 218–24

Parker WD, Boyson SJ, and Parks JK (1989) Abnormalities of the electron transport chain in idiopathic Parkinson's disease. *Ann Neurol*, **26**, 719–23

Pauls DL and Korczyn AD (1990) Complex segregation analysis of dystonia pedigrees suggests autosomal dominant inheritance. *Neurology*, **40**, 1107–10

Quarrell OWJ, Tyler A, Cole G, and Harper PS (1986) The problem of isolated cases of Huntington's disease in South Wales 1974–1984. *Clin Genet*, **30**, 433–9

Quarrell OWJ, Youngman S, Sarfarazi M, and Harper PS (1988) Absence of close linkage between benign hereditary chorea and the locus D4S10 (probe G8). *J Med Genet*, **25**, 191–4

Reik W (1988) Genomic imprinting: a possible mechanism for the parental origin effect in Huntington's disease. *J Med Genet*, **25**, 805–8

Ridley RM, Frith CD, Crow TJ, and Conneally PM (1988) Anticipation in Huntington's disease is inherited through the male line but may originate in the female. *J Med Genet*, **25**, 589–95

Risch NJ, Bressman SB, de Leon D, Brin MF, Burke RE, Greene PE *et al.* (1990) Segregation analysis of idiopathic torsion dystonia in Ashkenazi Jews suggests autosomal dominant inheritance. *Am J Hum Genet*, **46**, 533–8

Schapira AHV, Mann VM, Cooper JM, Dexter D, Daniel SE, Jenner P *et al.* (1990a) Anatomic and disease specificity of NADH CoQ reductase (complex I) deficiency in Parkinson's disease. *J Neurochem*, **55**, 2142–5

Schapira AHV, Holt IJ, Sweeney M, Harding AE, Jenner PG, and Marsden CD (1990b) Mitochondrial DNA analysis in Parkinson's disease. *Movement Disorders*, **5**, 294–7

Scribanu N and Kennedy C (1976) Familial syndrome with dystonia, neural deafness, and possible intellectual impairment: clinical course and pathological findings. *Adv Neurol*, **14**, 235–43

Shiwach RS, Lindenbaum RH, and Miciak A (1990) Predicting Huntington's disease. *Lancet*, **i**, 230

Smith CAD, Gough AC, Leigh PN, Summers BA, Harding AE, Maraganore DM *et al.* (1992) Association between the CYP2D6-debrisoquine hydroxylase polymorphism and susceptibility to Parkinson's disease. *Lancet*, **339**, 1375–7

Snell RG, Lazarou LP, Youngman S, Quarrell OWJ, Wasmuth JJ, Shaw DJ *et al.* (1989) Linkage disequilibrium in Huntington's disease: an improved localisation for the gene. *J Med Genet*, **26**, 673–5

Sotaniemi KA (1983) Chorea-acanthocytosis: neurological disease with acanthocytosis. *Acta Neurol Scand*, **68**, 53–6

Suthers GK, Huson SM, and Davies KE (1992) Instability versus predictability: the molecular diagnosis of myotonic dystrophy. *J Med Genet* **29**, 761–5

Theilmann J, Kanani S, Shiang R, Robbins C, Quarrell O, Huggins M *et al.* (1989) Non-random association between alleles detected at D4S95 and D4S98 and the Huntington's disease gene. *J Med Genet*, **26**, 676–81

Truong DD and Fahn S (1988) A early description of dystonia: translation of Schwalbe's thesis and information on his life. *Adv Neurol*, **50**, 651–64

Tyler A, Ball D, Craufurd D (1992) Presymptomatic testing for Huntington's disease in the United Kingdom, *British Medical Journal*, **304**, 1593–1596

Tyler A, Quarrell OWJ, Lazarou LP, Meredith AL, and Harper PS (1990) Exclusion testing in pregnancy for Huntington's disease. *J Med Genet*, **27**, 488–95

Tyler A, Quarrell OWJ, Lazarou LP, Meredith AL, and Harper PS (1990) Exclusion testing in pregnancy for Huntington's disease. *J Med Genet*, **27**, 488–95

Vance JM, Pericak-Vance MA, Bowman MH, Payne CS, Fredane L, Siddique T *et al.* (1987) Chorea-acanthocytosis: a report of three new families and implications for genetic counseling. *Am J Med Genet*, **28**, 403–10

Waddy HM, Fletcher NA, Harding AE, and Marsden CD (1991) A genetic study of idiopathic focal dystonias. *Ann Neurol*, **29**, 320–4

Ward CD, Duvoisin RC, Ince SE, Nutt JD, Eldridge R, and Calne DB (1983) Parkinson's disease in 65 pairs of twins and in a set of quadruplets. *Neurology*, **33**, 815–24

Warner TT, Fletcher NA, Davis MB, Ahmad F, Conway D, Feve A, Rondot P, Marsden CD and Harding AE (1993) Linkage analysis in British and French families with idiopathic torsion dystonia. *Brain*, **116**, 739

Wexler NS, Young AB, Tanzi RE, Travers H, Starosta-Rubinstein S, Penney JB *et al.* (1987) Homozygotes for Huntington's disease. *Nature*, **326**, 194–7

Whaley WL, Michiels F, MacDonald ME, Romano D, Zimmer M, Smith B *et al.* (1988) Mapping of D4S98/S114/S113 confines the Huntington's defect to a reduced physical region at the telomere of chromosome 4. *Nuclei Acids Res*, **16**, 11769–80

Wiggins S (1989) Early follow-up of persons participating in the Canadian National Collaborative study of predictive testing for Huntington's disease. *Am J Hum Genet*, **45**, A282

Wilhelmsen KC, Weeks DE, Nygaard TG, Mowkowitz CB, Rosales RL, dela Paz DC *et al.* (1991) Genetic mapping of "LUBAG" (X-linked dystonia-parkinsonism) in a Filipino kindred to the pericentromeric region of the X chromosome. *Ann Neurol*, **29**, 124–31

Wolff G, Deuschl G, Wienker TF, Hummel K, Bender K, Lucking CH *et al.* (1989) New mutation of Huntington's disease. *J Med Genet*, **26**, 18–27

World Federation of Neurology Research Group on Huntington's Disease (1989) Ethical issues policy statement on Huntington's disease molecular genetics predictive test. *J Neurol Sci*, **94**, 327–32

World Federation of Neurology Research Group on Huntington's Disease (1993) Presymptomatic testing for Huntington's disease. A world-wide survey. *J Med Genet*, in press

Zeman W, Kaelbling R, and Pasamanick B (1959) Dystonia musculorum deformans I. The hereditary pattern. *Am J Hum Genet*, **11**, 188–202

Zeman W, Kaelbling R, and Pasamanick B (1960) Idiopathic dystonia musculorum deformans II. The formes frustes. *Neurology*, **10**, 1068–75

Zilber N, Korczyn AD, Kahana E, Fried K, and Alter M (1984) Inheritance of idiopathic torsion dystonia among Jews. *J Med Genet*, **21**, 13–26

4
Functional imaging of movement disorders

David J. Brooks

INTRODUCTION

Structural imaging (computed tomography (CT)) and magnetic resonance imaging (MRI) are frequently unrewarding in movement disorders. When degenerative syndromes are examined structural changes are often only evident by the time the disease is far advanced. No abnormalities are seen in idiopathic dystonia or tremor. Functional imaging provides a more sensitive means for detecting and characterizing the effects of movement disorders. To date most reports have concerned positron emission tomography (PET) rather than single photon emission tomography (SPECT), and so this chapter will concentrate on the former technique. Where relevant, SPECT findings will be compared with those of PET.

There are three basic approaches to examining the changes in cerebral function associated with movement disorders. Firstly, abnormalities in resting levels of regional cerebral metabolism and blood flow can be examined. Secondly, abnormal cortical and subcortical activity associated with involuntary movements (dystonia/tremor) can be detected. Additionally, patients with movement disorders can be asked to perform motor tasks with a view to demonstrating aberrations in their pattern of cerebral activation. Thirdly, dysfunction of neurotransmitter systems can be revealed. The pre- and postsynaptic dopaminergic system has been most extensively studied, and this chapter will concentrate on the association between changes in this system and movement disorders.

PET measurements are performed by administering a tracer tagged with a short-lived positron-emitting isotope. These isotopes are usually generated by a cyclotron, and include ^{15}O ($t_{1/2}$ 2.03 minutes), ^{11}C ($t_{1/2}$ 20.4 minutes), ^{18}F ($t_{1/2}$ 110 minutes), and ^{76}Br ($t_{1/2}$ 16 hours). The subject is then scanned, and axial tomographic maps of regional cerebral tracer uptake are obtained. By comparing the kinetics of tracer accumulation in different brain regions with that in arterial plasma, regional cerebral tracer uptake can be quantitatively related to metabolism, blood flow, integrity of nerve terminal function, or receptor density. SPECT tracers are longer lived, and are usually labelled with either ^{123}I or ^{99m}Tc. SPECT measurements are currently semiquantitative. Commonly used PET and SPECT tracers, and their biological applications, are detailed in Table 4.1. In this chapter functional imaging in movement disorders has been divided into two main sections: the akinetic–rigid syndromes and involuntary movements disorders.

Table 4.1 Positron emission tomography (PET) and single photon emission tomography (SPECT) tracers in common use for studying movement disorders

Biological application	*Tracer*
Blood flow	$C^{15}O_2$, $H_2{}^{15}O$, $CH_3{}^{18}F$, $^{13}NH_3$ ^{99m}Tc-HMPAO, ^{133}Xe
Oxygen metabolism	$^{15}O_2$
Glucose metabolism	^{18}F-2-fluoro-2-deoxyglucose (^{18}FDG)
Dopamine storage	^{18}F-6-fluorodopa (^{18}F-dopa)
Dopamine reuptake sites	^{11}C-nomifensine (^{11}C-NMF)
Dopamine D_1 sites	^{11}C-SCH 23390/39166
Dopamine $D_{2/3}$ sites	^{11}C-raclopride (RAC) ^{123}I-iodobenzamide (IBZM) ^{11}C-methylspiperone (MSP) ^{18}F-fluorospiperone (FSP) ^{18}F-fluoroethylspiperone (FESP) ^{76}Br-bromospiperone (BSP)
Monoamine oxidase B activity	^{11}C-deprenyl

THE AKINETIC–RIGID SYNDROMES

Parkinson's disease

Parkinson's disease (PD) is ultimately a pathological diagnosis, being characterized by Lewy body degeneration of the pigmented and other brainstem nuclei, the ventrolateral substantia nigra compacta projections to putamen in particular being targeted (Spokes *et al.*, 1979; German *et al.*, 1989; Fearnley and Lees, 1991). In a recent pathological series all PD patients examined were found to have occasional cortical, as well as brainstem, Lewy bodies (Hughes *et al.*, 1992). When cortical involvement becomes extensive the condition is usually termed diffuse Lewy body disease (DLBD), rather than PD, but currently it remains unclear whether DLBD and PD are simply part of a spectrum. Most cases of DLBD present as levodopa-responsive akinetic–rigid syndromes, but this condition can manifest as isolated dementia indistinguishable from Alzheimer's disease (Byrne *et al.*, 1989).

Few PET studies on PD patients have been pathologically validated; the diagnosis is generally based on clinical criteria such as initial unilateral onset of rest tremor, rigidity, and bradykinesia, progressing to bilateral involvement over a few years with a good therapeutic response to L-dopa. Hypomimia, postural instability, and reduced arm swing are taken as supportive features. Atypical features are conventionally taken to be a poor L-dopa response, the presence of supranuclear gaze problems, cerebellar ataxia, or early autonomic failure. Cases of proven Lewy-body PD have been reported, however, that had a poor response to L-dopa (Hughes *et al.*, 1992) or supranuclear gaze problems (Lewis and Gawell, 1990; Fearnley *et al.*, 1991). A number of patients with atypical parkinsonian syndromes are also known to retain a reasonable L-dopa response throughout their illness (Fearnley and Lees, 1990). As a consequence the

PET findings presented below for patients clinically diagnosed as having PD should be treated with a degree of caution until pathological validation becomes available.

Metabolic and activation studies

PET measurements of regional cerebral oxygen and glucose metabolism with $^{15}O_2$ and ^{18}FDG primarily reflect the metabolism of nerve terminal synaptic vesicles. Consequently levels of metabolism in the basal ganglia reflect the metabolic activity of afferent projections to those nuclei, and of interneurons, rather than that of basal ganglia efferent projections. Primates can be made hemiparkinsonian by administering a unilateral carotid injection of 1-methyl-4-phenyl-1,2,3,6-tetrahydropyridine (MPTP). This destroys all ipsilateral substantia nigra compacta–striatal dopaminergic projections. In primates destruction of the nigra compacta results in an increase in lateral, but not medial, pallidal glucose utilization (Crossman, 1990). Striatopallidal fibres are principally gabaminergic and inhibitory in action. Increased lateral pallidal metabolism following nigral destruction suggests that the nigrostriatal dopaminergic system has an inhibitory action on striatolateral pallidal projections.

Using PET, increased oxygen and glucose metabolism can be demonstrated in the lentiform nucleus contralateral to the affected limbs in hemiparkinsonian patients (Wolfson *et al.*, 1985; Miletich *et al.*, 1988). Unfortunately the current resolution of PET is not sufficient to separate putamen and pallidal activity. When subjects with bilateral PD are studied, metabolism of the lentiform nucleus is normal or mildly reduced. This finding suggests that the increased lentiform metabolism seen in early asymmetrical PD is either only a transient adaptive mechanism, or that chronic L-dopa treatment returns function in this pathway to normal in time. Acutely, L-dopa therapy appears to have little effect on striatal metabolism (Leenders *et al.*, 1985a). This is not entirely surprising as nigrostriatal projections account for only a small percentage of the total striatal synaptic activity, and have both inhibitory and excitatory actions. As a consequence, large changes in activity of the dopaminergic system after administration of exogenous dopa may lead to only small overall changes in the total striatal activity.

Hemiparkinsonian patients, early into their disease, show small but significant decreases in frontal blood flow and metabolism contralateral to their affected limbs (Perlmutter and Raichle, 1985; Wolfson *et al.*, 1985). Bilaterally affected PD patients show more diffuse cortical hypometabolism; their levels of glucose utilization correlate with their psychometric performance (Kuhl *et al.*, 1984a; Peppard *et al.*, 1988). ^{18}FDG scans of frankly demented PD patients show an Alzheimer pattern of impaired brain glucose utilization, posterior parietal and temporal association areas being most affected, while non-demented patients have normal cortical function or mild frontal hypometabolism (Kuhl *et al.*, 1984b, 1985; Wolfson *et al.*, 1985; Otsuka *et al.*, 1991). Only 1 demented PD patient has had pathological findings correlated with ^{18}FDG PET and no Alzheimer cortical changes were evident (Schapiro *et al.*, 1990). Currently it remains unclear whether the pattern of glucose hypometabolism in demented PD patients reflects coincidental Alzheimer's disease, cortical Lewy body disease, loss of cholinergic projections, or some other degenerative process. As lesions of the nucleus basalis of Meynert in primates result in transient diffuse cortical hypometabolism (Kiyosawa *et al.*, 1989), loss of cholinergic projections is unlikely to be responsible for the Alzheimer pattern of reduced ^{18}FDG uptake found in demented PD patients.

In normal subjects stereotyped movements of a joystick in a forward direction with the right hand result in contralateral regional cerebral blood flow (rCBF) increases in the lentiform nucleus and sensorimotor cortex (SMC), and bilateral increases in caudal anterior cingulate, supplementary motor area (SMA), and lateral premotor cortex (PMC) (Playford *et al.*, 1992a). Joystick movements in freely selected directions result in additional bilateral activation of rostral anterior cingulate, SMA, PMC, parietal association areas, and dorsolateral prefrontal cortex (DLPFC). When PD patients, scanned after cessation of treatment for 12 hours, perform the same joystick tasks, normal activation of SMC, PMC and lateral parietal association areas occurs, but there is selectively impaired activation of the contralateral lentiform nucleus, and of the anterior cingulate, SMA, and DLPFC; that is, those cortical areas that receive their main input from the basal ganglia.

It is thought that the SMA and DLPFC play a crucial role in generating volitional motor programmes while parietal association and lateral premotor cortex are responsible for generating motor responses to external cues (Goldberg, 1985; Goldman-Rakic, 1987; Thaler and Passinghau, 1989; Mushiake *et al.*, 1990). An inability to activate SMA and DLPFC in PD could explain the difficulty these patients experience in initiating motor actions. Jenkins *et al.* (1992) have demonstrated that when apomorphine, a combined D_1 and D_2 agonist, is given subcutaneously to PD patients, resolution of their akinesia is associated with a significant increase in SMA blood flow, providing further evidence for the role of this structure in the generation of motor programs. Similar findings have been reported using ^{133}Xe SPECT (Rascol *et al.*, 1992).

The presynaptic dopaminergic system

After its intravenous administration, ^{18}F-dopa is taken up by the terminals of the nigrostriatal dopaminergic projections and stored as ^{18}F-dopamine and its metabolites (Firnau *et al.*, 1987). The rate of striatal ^{18}F accumulation reflects both transport of ^{18}F-dopa into striatum, and its subsequent decarboxylation by dopa decarboxylase. ^{11}C-Nomifensine binds reversibly to striatal dopamine reuptake sites, and so also provides a measure of integrity of nigrostriatal projections (Tedroff *et al.*, 1988, 1990). In MPTP-lesioned primates striatal uptake of both ^{18}F-dopa and ^{11}C-nomifensine are severely diminished (Chieuh *et al.*, 1986; Leenders *et al.*, 1988a).

Garnett *et al.* (1984) and Nahmias *et al.* (1985) published the first reports on striatal ^{18}F-dopa uptake in PD. Their subjects had hemiparkinsonism, and were early into their disease. PET showed normal caudate, but bilaterally reduced putamen tracer uptake, activity being most depressed in the putamen contralateral to the affected limbs. These studies were the first demonstration that subclinical involvement of dopaminergic projections to the putamen contralateral to clinically unaffected limbs in PD could be detected. Subsequently a number of groups have confirmed these observations (Leenders *et al.*, 1986a,b; Martin *et al.*, 1986; Brooks *et al.*, 1990a). Two studies have reported a significant correlation between depression in striatal ^{18}F-dopa uptake of PD patients, and their degree of locomotor disability (Leenders *et al.*, 1986a; Brooks *et al.*, 1990a). Patients with a sustained response to L-dopa therapy show greater striatial ^{18}F-dopa accumulation than those with a fluctuating response (Leenders *et al.*, 1986b).

On average PD patients show a 50% loss of specific putamen ^{18}F-dopa uptake (Brooks *et al.*, 1990a) compared to a 60–80% loss of ventrolateral nigra compacta cells at postmortem (Rinne *et al.*, 1989; Fearnley and Lees, 1991). Putamen dopamine levels are reduced by over 90% in PD (Bernheimer *et al.*, 1973; Kish *et al.*, 1988) and so striatal ^{18}F-dopa uptake is likely to reflect the terminal density of the nigrostriatal projections rather than the levels of endogenous striatal dopamine present. Specific putamen uptake of the active (+) enantiomer of ^{11}C-nomifensine is also reduced to around 50% of normal levels in PD, while caudate ^{11}C-NMF uptake is relatively preserved (Leenders *et al.*, 1990; Salmon *et al.*, 1990). In individual PD patients putamen ^{11}C-NMF uptake correlates with locomotor status, and also with ^{18}F-dopa uptake, confirming that both these tracers are markers of integrity of the nigrostriatal dopaminergic terminals.

It has been estimated that patients do not develop symptoms of parkinsonism until they have lost 40–50% of their nigra compacta cells, and 80% of their putamen dopamine. PET should, therefore, provide a means of detecting subclinical nigral dysfunction in at-risk subjects. Using ^{18}F-dopa PET, Calne *et al.* (1985) studied 4 asymptomatic subjects who had been exposed to MPTP. These workers were able to demonstrate subnormal striatal tracer uptake in 2 of these 4 subjects. Sawle *et al.* (1992a) have examined striatal ^{18}F-dopa uptake in a family where 4 out of 10 siblings developed dopa-responsive parkinsonism in their fourth decade. The 4 affected siblings all showed severely reduced striatal tracer accumulation. A fifth, asymptomatic, sibling also had impaired putamen ^{18}F-dopa uptake and 1 year later went on to develop akinesia and 'inner tremulousness'. Subclinical nigral dysfunction has also been demonstrated in asymptomatic co-twins of PD patients (Burn *et al.*, 1992). Six out of 17 co-twins had putamen ^{18}F-dopa uptake reduced more than 2 s.d. below the normal mean. One of these 6 co-twins had developed clinical PD when reviewed 2 years after PET. It seems clear, therefore, that ^{18}F-dopa PET is capable of detecting subclinical PD in at-risk subjects. Whether such subjects should receive a neuroprotective agent if their scans are abnormal remains uncertain.

It has been suggested that Parkinson's disease may be initiated by a subclinical toxic or infective insult in early life, but only becomes clinically evident when additional cell loss from the nigra due to a normal ageing process causes the cell population to fall below 50% (Calne *et al.*, 1986). In order to test this hypothesis two groups have studied the relationship between age and specific striatal ^{18}F-dopa uptake in normal subjects over an age range of 20–80 years. Results were conflicting, one group finding no age effect on striatal tracer uptake (Sawle *et al.*, 1990a), while the other group found a significant decline of ^{18}F-dopa uptake with age (Martin *et al.*, 1989).

Bhatt *et al.* (1991a) serially measured striatal ^{18}F-dopa uptake over 3.3–3.9 years in groups of 9 PD and 7 normal subjects. Both the PD and normal groups showed similar 5% falls in mean striatal : cerebellar ^{18}F-dopa uptake ratios. These workers concluded that the decline in nigral function in PD is slow and similar to that associated with natural ageing. As, however, the mean striatal : cerebellar ^{18}F-dopa uptake ratio of their PD patients was only 18% lower than the mean value for their controls, a mean 5% fall in striatal : cerebral ^{18}F-dopa uptake ratio could represent a significant nigral cell loss. Sawle *et al.* (1992b) have recently reported a mean 48% fall in specific putamen ^{18}F-dopa uptake over 3 years in a group of 5 PD patients, suggestive of an on-going degenerative rather than an ageing process. Currently the role of ageing in PD remains uncertain. Recent pathological studies suggest the pattern of nigral cell and striatal dopamine loss due to natural ageing is different from that in PD (Fearnley and Lees, 1991; Kish *et al.*, 1992). As there is evidence of reactive microglia in the nigra in PD patients at autopsy, indicative of an active inflammatory process, it is unlikely that ageing alone is responsible for the onset of symptoms in PD (McGeer *et al.*, 1988).

Recently PD has been treated with striatal implants of either autologous adrenal medullary tissue, or fetal mesencephalic grafts. PET provides a means of examining graft function post transplantation. Guttman *et al.* (1989) PET scanned 6 PD patients following adrenal transplantation. ^{68}Ga-EDTA scans showed the continuing presence of blood–brain barrier (BBB) disruption at 6 weeks and 6 months following surgery. Graft ^{18}F-dopa uptake was inconsistently increased at 6 weeks following surgery, and the authors felt that any increase in tracer uptake could probably be explained by the presence of BBB disruption. Sawle *et al.* (1992c) performed ^{18}F-dopa PET on 2 PD patients before, and serially for 13 months after, fetal engraftment into the putamen contralateral to the more affected limbs. Patency of the blood–graft barrier was established at 6 months in 1 of these subjects using Gd-enhanced MRI. Both of these patients maintained a sustained clinical improvement of the limbs contralateral to the putamen engrafted. Figure 4.1 shows serial PET images of striatal ^{18}F-dopa uptake in the first patient before and after surgery. It can be seen that there is a progressive increase in tracer uptake by the grafted left putamen over 13 months. The second patient showed a similar progressive increase in ^{18}F-dopa uptake into the grafted right putamen. Interestingly, while graft ^{18}F-dopa uptake increased progressively over 1 year in both patients, clinical improvement reached a plateau by 6 months. The reason for this dissociation between graft function and clinical response is unclear, but may reflect the localized site of action of the graft.

The postsynaptic striatal dopamine system

At least five different subtypes of dopamine receptors have now been described but broadly they fall into D_1-type (D_1, D_5) which are adenyl cyclase-dependent, and D_2-type (D_2–D_4), which are not. The locomotor functions mediated by the dopaminergic system are thought primarily to involve striatal D_2 receptors. Only one PET study on striatal D_1 receptors status in PD has been reported to date: in untreated hemiparkinsonian patients, later shown to be levodopa-responsive, no side-to-side difference in striatal ^{11}C-SCH23390 was evident (Rinne *et al.*, 1990a). This finding suggests that in spite of the presence of striatal deafferentiation there is no compensatory upregulation of D_1 sites in PD.

Table 4.1 shows that there are a number of suitable PET tracers for studying striatal D_2 receptor density. These tracers are antagonists which bind either irreversibly (^{11}C-methylspiperone, ^{18}F-fluorethylspiperone) or reversibly (^{76}Br-bromospiperone, ^{11}C-raclopride). The advantage of reversible antagonists is that their uptake at equilibrium is independent of cerebral perfusion and that they can be displaced by cold tracer to provide measurements of both receptor density (B_{max}) and affinity (K_d). Their affinity for D_2 sites, however, is weaker than that of the irreversibly bound antagonists, and they are less able to distinguish absolute changes in D_2 site density from changes in D_2 site occupancy by endogenous dopamine. The cerebellum and cortex are relatively devoid of D_2 receptors and equilibrium levels of tracer binding in these regions are frequently taken to reflect non-specific striatal binding in PET studies.

Leenders *et al.* (1985b) reported normal striatal uptake of ^{11}C-MSP in 4 untreated PD patients. Brücke *et al.* (1991) and Schwarz *et al.* (1992) have also noted normal striatum : frontal uptake ratios of IBZM in *de novo* PD patients who were responsive

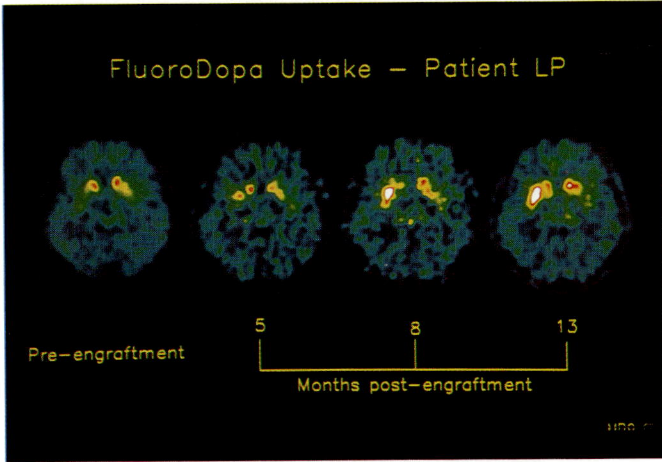

Figure 4.1 Positron emission tomography images of striatal ^{18}F-dopa uptake in a Parkinson's disease patient 1 year before, and 5, 8 and 13 months after engraftment of the left putamen with fetal mesencephalic tissue. Courtesy of Dr S. V. Sawle.

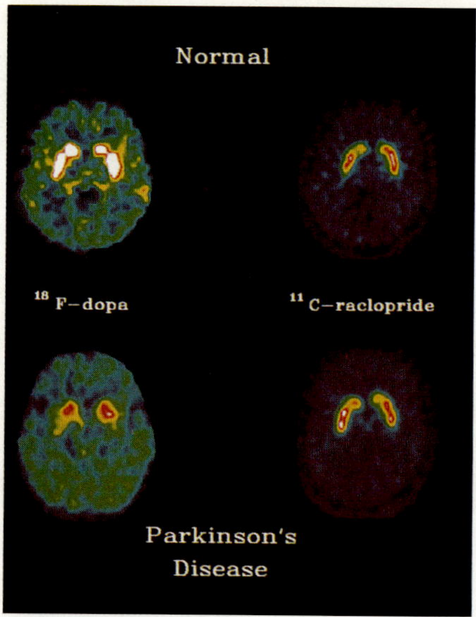

Figure 4.2 Positron emission tomography scans of striatal ^{18}F-dopa and ^{11}C-raclopride in a normal subject and untreated patients with hemiparkinsonism affecting the left limbs. The PD patients show reduced ^{18}F-dopa and normal ^{11}C-raclopride uptake. Courtesy of Dr D. J. Burn.

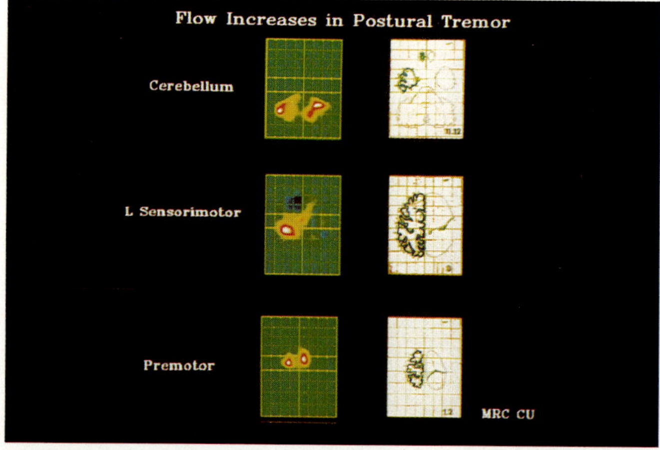

Figure 4.3 A map showing the cerebral regions where statistically significant (white areas) blood flow increases occurred in association with postural tremor of the right arm. Unilateral arm tremor led to significant bilateral cerebellar and premotor cortex, and contralateral sensorimotor cortex, activation. Courtesy of Dr J. G. Colebatch.

to dopaminergic agents. Brooks *et al.* (1992a) studied 6 untreated PD cases with ^{11}C-raclopride. Four had normal and 2 had significantly elevated (124 and 138% of normal) equilibrium putamen : cerebellum tracer uptake ratios while all 6 had normal caudate uptake ratios. Mean putamen ^{11}C-raclopride uptake for the group was increased by 11%. Leenders *et al.* (1991) have recently reported a mean 20% increase in putamen ^{11}C-raclopride binding in 18 untreated PD cases. Two groups have examined side-to-side striatal ^{11}C-raclopride uptake in untreated PD patients with asymmetrical disease (Rinne *et al.*, 1990b; Sawle *et al.*, 1990b). In these studies mean tracer uptake by the striatum or putamen contralateral to the more affected limbs was 10–15% higher than in the ipsilateral putamen. On balance, PET findings suggest that in untreated PD, putamen D_2 sites are either normal or mildly upregulated. Caudate D_2 sites appear to remain at normal levels. Where putamen ^{18}F-dopa and ^{11}C-raclopride uptake have both been measured in individual untreated PD patients, an inverse correlation between the binding of the two tracers has been found (Fig. 4.2).

Using ^{11}C-MSP, Leenders *et al.* (1985b) reported a mean 20% decrease in striatal tracer uptake in 5 PD patients chronically treated with levodopa. Hagglund *et al.* (1987) and Shinotoh *et al.* (1990), however, found normal levels of striatal ^{11}C-MSP uptake in their treated PD patients. Wienhard *et al.* (1990) reported an 18% decrease in mean caudate ^{18}F-FESP binding in 7 treated PD cases. Leenders *et al.* (1991) studied 9 PD cases after treatment with L-dopa for 3 months and found normal levels of putamen ^{11}C-raclopride binding while Brooks *et al.* (1992a) noted a 30% fall in putamen and caudate ^{11}C-raclopride binding in 5 chronically treated PD patients who had developed fluctuating responses to levodopa. Brücke *et al.* (1991) reported a 17% decrease of striatal : frontal uptake ratio of IBZM in their medicated PD patients. On balance, functional imaging suggests that treated PD patients have normal or reduced levels of striatal D_2 sites, reduced levels occurring particularly in chronically treated PD cases who have developed a fluctuating response to therapy.

MULTIPLE SYSTEM ATROPHY

This condition, occasionally known as Shy–Drager syndrome, includes striatonigral degeneration (SND), olivopontocerebellar atropy (OPCA), and progressive autonomic failure (PAF) in its spectrum. About 10% of cases initially diagnosed as Parkinson's disease are found to have this condition at autopsy (Quinn, 1989). The pathology of MSA is distinct from PD, and consists of neuronal loss from the basal ganglia, brainstem nuclei, cerebellar nuclei and intermediolateral columns of the cord, without neuronal inclusion body formation. In its early stages MSA may be clinically difficult to distinguish from PD, as it can present as an akinetic–rigid syndrome which is initially L-dopa-responsive (Fearnley and Lees, 1990). With time cerebellar ataxia and severe autonomic failure tend to become evident, and response to L-dopa diminishes. As with PD, most PET studies on MSA and SND cases lack pathological validation. Reported findings in SND usually refer to patients with L-dopa-resistant parkinsonism without supranuclear gaze problems or cortical dysfunction.

Metabolic studies

De Volder *et al.* (1989) have studied regional cerebral glucose utilization with ^{18}FDG in 7 cases of probable striatonigral degeneration. Two cases also had autonomic failure and cerebellar ataxia. There was a general 20% decrease in grey matter glucose utilization in the SND group, but putamen and caudate were particularly affected with 46 and 36% reductions in glucose metabolism respectively. Frontal cortex was more severely affected than other cortical areas, and cerebellar metabolism was reduced in the 2 patients with ataxia. Otsuka *et al.* (1991) have also reported significantly reduced striatal glucose metabolism in 8 cases of probable SND. These findings contrast with PD where striatal metabolism is preserved.

Fulham *et al.* (1991) examined ^{18}FDG uptake in 7 OPCA patients with autonomic failure, and in 8 PAF patients. They found significantly reduced cerebellar and frontal but normal striatal glucose utilization in the OPCA patients, and normal levels of rCMRGlc (regional cerebral glucose metabolism) in PAF. These findings suggest that PET provides a potential means of determining whether patients presenting with isolated autonomic failure have PAF or MSA. Glucose utilization has been examined in cases of sporadic and familial OPCA without autonomic failure of rigidity (Rosenthal *et al.*, 1988). These patients had reduced cerebellar and brainstem glucose metabolism; the individual levels correlated inversely with the level of ataxia present.

The dopaminergic system

As in PD, specific putamen ^{18}F-dopa and ^{11}C-nomifensine uptake is reduced to around 50% of normal levels in SND and individual levels of putamen ^{18}F-dopa uptake correlate with locomotor function (Brooks *et al.*, 1990a,b; Salmon *et al.*, 1990). Caudate ^{18}F-dopa and ^{11}C-nomifensine uptake are significantly more depressed in SND compared with PD (Brooks *et al.*, 1990b; Otsuka *et al.*, 1991). The ventrolateral nigra sends dopamine projections to the putamen, while the medial nigra projects to caudate. The above PET findings suggest that medial nigra is more severely involved in MSA than PD. Pathological studies corroborate this conclusion: some MSA patients show similar selective ventrolateral nigral cell to that seen in PD while others show extensive nigral involvement (Spokes *et al.*, 1979; Goto *et al.*, 1989; Fearnley and Lees, 1990). Why the ventrolateral nigra is targeted in PD and MSA remains unclear. One suggestion is that these nigral cells are the least melanized, and if melanin provides a protection against free radical damage, hypomelanized cells will be more susceptible to toxic damage (Gibb *et al.*, 1990).

^{18}F-dopa uptake has also been studied in patients with pure autonomic failure (Brooks *et al.*, 1990b). Those few PAF patients who have come to pathology have shown degeneration of the intermediolateral columns of the spinal cord similar to that seen in MSA, but also Lewy bodies in the nigra and sympathetic ganglia similar to that seen in PD patients (Vanderhaegen *et al.*, 1970). In contrast to PD, however, the PAF patients showed little nigral cell loss. Striatal ^{18}F-dopa uptake was normal in 5 out of 7 PAF patients, suggesting that their dysautonomia was not associated with underlying nigral dysfunction. Two subjects, however, showed reduced putamen ^{18}F-dopa uptake and one of these subsequently developed a pseudobulbar palsy typical of MSA.

It has been suggested that OPCA, SND and PAF all represent extremes of an MSA spectrum. Against this hypothesis are the reports of normal striatal ^{18}F-dopa uptake in sporadic OPCA with autonomic failure (Brooks, 1992) and PAF (Brooks *et al.*, 1990b), normal striatal glucose metabolism in OPCA (Fulham *et al.*, 1991) and normal cerebellar glucose metabolism in SND (De Volder *et al.*, 1989). These PET findings suggest that OPCA, SND and PAF may all exist as separate conditions.

Brooks *et al.* (1992) studied striatal dopamine D_2 receptor density in SND with ^{11}C-raclopride and found significant mean 10 and 11% reductions in equilibrium caudate and putamen : cerebellum tracer uptake ratios, respectively, equivalent to a mean 14 and 15% loss of caudate and putamen D_2 sites. Only 2 of their 10 SND patients, however, had significantly reduced caudate or putamen ^{11}C-raclopride uptake. Shinotoh *et al.* (1990) have also reported a reduction in mean striatal ^{11}C-MSP binding in 4 SND cases but again the SND and normal ranges of tracer uptake overlapped. Schwarz *et al.* (1992) studied striatal IBZM uptake in *de novo* parkinsonian patients with a negative apomorphine response. Eight had reduced, and 4 normal tracer uptake. On balance, functional imaging suggests that a moderate loss of striatal D_2 sites occurs in SND, but that a number of these parkinsonian patients who fail to respond to dopaminergic agents have normal levels of striatal D_2 receptors. It is likely, therefore, that degeneration of brainstem and pallidal rather than dopaminergic projections is responsible for their poorly L-dopa-responsive rigidity.

PROGRESSIVE SUPRANUCLEAR PALSY (PSP)

This condition is generally taken to refer to Steele–Richardson–Olszewski syndrome, and is characterized pathologically by neurofibrillary tangle formation and neuronal loss in the basal ganglia, superior colliculi, brainstem nuclei and the periaqueductal grey matter (Steele *et al.*, 1964). There are, however, a number of other degenerative causes of supranuclear gaze problems. PSP is fully manifested as L-dopa-resistant akinetic–rigid syndrome, in association with a supranuclear downgaze palsy, a bulbar palsy and dementia of frontal type. In the early stages of the disease, however, the patient may present as a partially L-dopa-responsive akinetic–rigid syndrome with mild supranuclear gaze difficulties, making a clear distinction from other parkinsonian disorders difficult (Jackson *et al.*, 1983; Maher and Lees, 1986).

Metabolic studies

There have been several reports of regional cerebral glucose and oxygen metabolism in patients with probable PSP, some of whom have later had the diagnosis confirmed at autopsy (D'Antona *et al.*, 1985; Foster *et al.*, 1988; Leenders *et al.*, 1988b; Goffinet *et al.*, 1989; Blin *et al.*, 1990a). Cortical metabolism tends to be globally depressed in this condition, the motor and prefrontal areas being particularly affected. Frontal levels of metabolism have been shown to correlate with performance on psychometric tests of frontal function (Blin *et al.*, 1990a). Hypofrontality is not specific for PSP and can be seen in SND, Pick's disease, and Huntington's disease. Striatal metabolism is also depressed in PSP and cerebellar and thalamic metabolism may also be affected. ^{18}FDG scans, therefore, cannot be reliably used to distinguish PSP from MSA or SND, though the preservation of striatal metabolism in PD helps to distinguish this condition from the multiple system degenerations.

The dopaminergic system

Two studies (Leenders *et al.*, 1988b; Bhatt *et al.*, 1991b) have reported that striatal ^{18}F-dopa uptake in PSP is significantly reduced, and that individual levels of uptake correlate inversely with disease duration. The resolution of the scanners used in these studies was unfortunately too low to separate caudate and putamen signals. Brooks *et al.* (1990a) measured putamen and caudate ^{18}F-dopa influx constants in PSP and found putamen and caudate tracer uptake to be similarly reduced (37 and 48% of normal, respectively). These PET findings suggest that the nigra is uniformly involved in PSP and this is in agreement with pathological reports (Jellinger *et al.*, 1980; Kish *et al.*, 1985). In contrast, a group of PD patients with a similar degree of locomotor disability showed significant sparing of caudate ^{18}F-dopa uptake (putamen 48% and caudate 84% of normal). Nine out of 10 PSP patients had significantly reduced caudate ^{18}F-dopa uptake compared to only 4 out of 16 PD cases. There was no correlation between putamen or caudate ^{18}F-dopa uptake in the PSP patients and their level of locomotor function. Unlike PD and SND, where locomotor disability appears to result primarily from loss of dopaminergic fibres, loss of mobility in PSP is probably a consequence of degeneration of pallidal and brainstem projections.

Striatal dopamine D_2 receptor density in PSP has been studied with PET in a number of centres. Baron *et al.* (1986) scanned 7 PSP patients with the reversible D_2 antagonist ^{76}Br-bromospiperone (BSP) and reported a 24% fall in the mean equilibrium striatum : cerebellum tracer uptake ratio. Two of their 7 patients, however, had striatal BSP uptake within the normal range and only 3 showed a significant fall in striatal tracer binding. Wienhard *et al.* (1990) found a 17% fall in caudate ^{18}F-fluoroethylspiperone binding potential in their two PSP patients. Brooks *et al.* (1992a) studied 9 PSP patients with ^{11}C-raclopride. They found mean 24 and 9% falls in equilibrium caudate and putamen : cerebellum ^{11}C-raclopride uptake ratios, equivalent to a 32 and 12% loss of caudate and putamen D_2 sites, respectively. Four of these 9 PSP patients, however, had striatal tracer uptake that fell within the normal range. In view of these PET findings it is likely that in PSP, as in SND, degeneration of pallidal and brainstem projections is responsible for the poor L-dopa-response of this akinetic–rigid syndrome rather than a primary loss of dopamine receptors.

CORTICOBASAL DEGENERATION (CBD)

This syndrome, also known as corticodentatonigral degeneration with neuronal achromasia, has characteristic clinical features (Riley *et al.*, 1990). Patients present with an akinetic–rigid limb which becomes dyspraxic or exhibits alien behaviour. Cortical sensory loss, dysphasia, myoclonus, supranuclear gaze problems and bulbar dysfunction may also be evident. Intellect is spared until late. Eventually all four limbs become involved and the condition is invariably poorly L-dopa-responsive. The pathology consists of collections of swollen, achromatic Pick cells, without argyrophilic inclusion bodies, concentrated in the posterior frontal, inferior parietal, and superior temporal lobes, and in the dentate nuclei and substantia nigra (Gibb *et al.*, 1989).

There have been three reports of PET studies on patients with the clinical syndrome of CBD. Sawle *et al.* (1991a) studied 6 patients with ^{18}F-dopa and $^{15}O_2$. Striatal ^{18}F-dopa uptake was strikingly asymmetrical, being most depressed contralateral to the more affected limbs. Caudate and putamen tracer uptake were equally severely depressed in CBD, in contrast to PD. Mesial frontal ^{18}F-dopa uptake was also significantly depressed. As might be predicted from the distribution of the pathology, cortical oxygen metabolism ($rCMRO_2$) was most significantly reduced in posterior

Table 4.2 Positron emission tomography findings in akinetic–rigid syndromes

	PD	*PD (demented)*	*SND*	*PSP*	*CBD*
Glucose metabolism	Normal	Low parietal/ temporal	Low striatal/ frontal	Low striatal/ frontal	Low striatal/ inferior parietal
F-dopa uptake	Putamen <caudate	Putamen <caudate	Putamen $\leqslant$caudate	Putamen =caudate	Putamen =caudate
Striatal D_2 sites	Normal or raised if untreated Normal or low if treated		Normal or low	Normal or low	?

CBD = Corticobasal degeneration; PD = Parkinson's disease; PSP = progressive supranuclear palsy; SND = striatonigral degeneration.

frontal, inferior parietal and superior temporal regions. Again these $rCMRO_2$ reductions were strikingly asymmetrical, being most severe contralateral to the more affected limbs. The authors felt that these PET findings distinguished CBD from Alzheimer's and Pick's disease, where posterial parietal and inferior frontal hypometabolism predominate respectively, and from PSP, where frontal and striatal metabolism are more symmetrically reduced.

Eidelberg *et al.* (1991) have studied 5 CBD patients with PET. The found that inferior parietal, hippocampal, and thalamic glucose metabolism and striatal ^{18}F-dopa uptake were significantly depressed contralateral to the more affected limbs compared to ipsilateral function. This contrasted with PD patients who had symmetrical levels of regional cerebral glucose metabolism. Blin *et al.* (1990b) have reported similar asymmetrical reductions in inferior parietal and thalamic FDG uptake in CBD. To date, no PET studies on the integrity of dopaminergic receptors in this condition are available.

Table 4.2 summarizes PET findings in parkinsonian syndromes.

THE INVOLUNTARY MOVEMENT DISORDERS

Dystonia

Idiopathic torsion dystonia (ITD) is now thought to be a dominantly inherited condition with about a 40% penetrance (Fletcher *et al.*, 1990). It has been linked to a genetic locus on chromosome 9 in both caucasian and Jewish kindreds (Ozelius *et al.*, 1989; Kramer *et al.*, 1990). Dopa-responsive dystonia (DRD) is also familial, but appears to have a different gene locus to ITD. Pathological studies have failed to identify consistent structural or neurotransmitter abnormalities in ITD, though depressed levels of brainstem and basal ganglia monoamines were reported in 2 cases (Hornykiewicz *et al.*, 1986). Patients with acquired hemidystonia tend to have lesions of the caudate, lentiform nucleus, or ventral thalamus (Marsden *et al.*, 1985), and so ITD may well be associated with dysfunction of connections between these structures and the motor cortical association areas.

A problem with PET studies on dystonia to date has been the heterogeneity of the cohorts of patients examined. Familial, sporadic and acquired dystonics have been grouped together, and hemi- and focal dystonics have often been selected in order to provide side-to-side comparisons of basal ganglia function. As a consequence, the relevance of some of the PET findings in dystonia to familial ITD remains unclear.

METABOLIC AND ACTIVATION STUDIES

Chase *et al.* (1988) studied 6 sporadic cases of idiopathic dystonia with ^{18}FDG. Three of their patients had generalized, 1 focal, 1 segmental, and 1 multifocal dystonia, and all had normal CT or MRI brain scans. Three of the 6 dystonics had increased lenticular, and 2 of these 3 increased caudate, glucose utilization contralateral to the more affected limbs. After thalamotomy 1 of these 3 patients showed partial resolution of the lentiform nucleus hypermetabolism. Eidelberg *et al.* (1990) have also reported increased lentiform nucleus glucose metabolism contralateral to the affected limbs in 2 cases of idiopathic hemidystonia with normal MRI. One of his cases was familal and the other sporadic. As ^{18}FDG uptake primarily reflects synaptic activity, increased lentiform glucose metabolism in ITD could be due to abnormally raised cortical input into putamen, putamen input into pallidum, or interneuronal activity.

In contrast to the above two studies. Gilman *et al.* (1988) were unable to find any consistent pattern of abnormal ^{18}FDG uptake in their 5 patients with sporadic asymmetrical ITD; 1 showed contralateral caudate hypermetabolism. Stoessl *et al.* (1986) also failed to find any consistent changes in rCMRGlc in 16 patients with torticollis, 4 of whom had additional focal limb dystonia. These authors, however, noted an abnormally poor covariance between striatal and thalamic glucose metabolism in their torticollis patients, and postulated that striatal–thalamic connections were functionally disturbed.

Temple and Perlmutter (1990) examined the integrity of central sensory connections in a group of 11 subjects with idiopathic hemi- or focal dystonia, generally writer's cramp. They used vibrotactile stimulation to activate the SMC, and measured the resultant increase in blood flow. The dystonic subjects had a 20% attenuation of their SMC blood flow response to tactile stimulation compared with normal controls, and the authors suggested that this reduced SMC activation was a consequence of abnormal function of basal ganglia–thalamic–SMC projections. Their dystonic patients were on average 25 years older than their controls, however, and so it remains uncertain whether their attenuated SMC blood flow response to activation was due to pathology, or simply age artefact.

Playford *et al.* (1992b) have recently performed PET activation studies on 6 familial ITD patients, measuring rCBF while they performed joystick movements. Although the ITD patients were bradykinetic compared to age-matched controls, they showed significantly higher levels of left putamen and supplementary motor area activation. The authors concluded that dystonia is associated with inappropriate overactivity of basal ganglia–SMA projections.

THE DOPAMINERGIC SYSTEM

Leenders *et al.* (1988c) reported striatal ^{18}F-dopa uptake in 4 patients with sporadic hemidystonia and 2 patients with torticollis. Three of these hemidystonic patients had background rigidity, however, and so strictly had acquired dystonia–parkinsonism rather than ITD. One of these 3 also had a calcified lesion in the midbrain tegmentum. The 6 subjects all had abnormal striatal ^{18}F-dopa uptake, and in the 4 hemidystonics this was most depressed in the striatum contralateral to the affected limbs. The 4 hemidystonic patients also had striatal D_2 receptor integrity assessed with ^{11}C-methylspiperone. In three the striatal ^{11}C-MSP binding was normal, while the patient with the midbrain lesion showed increased striatal ^{11}C-MSP uptake. This patient was thought to have striatal D_2 receptor upregulation secondary to the deafferentiation resulting from loss of nigrostriatal dopaminergic projections.

Martin *et al.* (1988) measured striatal ^{18}F-dopa uptake in 4 dystonic subjects. One of these had dopa-responsive dystonia and his striatal ^{18}F-dopa uptake was normal. The other 3 had sporadic ITD; 2 of these had impaired striatal tracer uptake. Playford *et al.* (1991) studied a cohort of 11 familial ITD cases with ^{18}F-dopa PET. Eight of these patients had normal studies while the other 3 showed mild impairment of putamen ^{18}F-dopa uptake. It was concluded that nigral dysfunction had low penetrance in ITD and its presence was probably unrelated to disease symptomatology. Two asymptomatic obligate gene carriers that were studied both had normal striatal ^{18}F-dopa uptake.

Two centres have reported ^{18}F-dopa PET findings in DRD. Sawle *et al.* (1991b) studied 6 subjects with clinically typical disease and found normal striatal tracer uptake in 4 of the 6. The group as a whole showed a uniform 25% fall in mean caudate and putamen tracer uptake. The authors speculated that this mild reduction in striatal ^{18}F-dopa uptake could reflect either pathology of the nigrostriatal terminals as a consequence of the disease, or downregulation of dopa decarboxylase activity due to chronic exposure to L-dopa therapy. Snow *et al.* (1992) studied 4 DRD patients and found normal striatal ^{18}F-dopa uptake in all of these cases.

In conclusion, PET findings in dystonia have been inconsistent, in part due to the heterogeneity of the patient groups studied. When abnormalities have been found in ITD, they have consisted of resting lentiform or caudate hypermetabolism contralateral to the more affected limbs and reduced striatal ^{18}F-dopa uptake. The majority of DRD patients have normal striatal ^{18}F-dopa uptake. Activation studies on ITD patients suggest that the lentiform nucleus and supplementary motor areas may be inappropriately overactive when these patients perform motor tasks.

Tremor

PET scans to date on tremor patients have fallen into two main categories: studies to determine the abnormal regional cerebral metabolic and blood flow changes associated with the presence of involuntary tremor, and studies to determine the types of tremor that are associated with nigral dysfunction, as evidenced by reduced striatal ^{18}F-dopa binding.

METABOLIC AND ACTIVATION STUDIES

Dubinsky and Hallett (1987) first reported that postural tremor was associated with abnormally high medullary glucose metabolism, probably arising from the inferior olive, and suggested that essential tremor (ET) is associated with hyperactivity of olivocerebellar connections. Colebatch *et al.* (1990) studied rCBF in 4 ET patients under three different conditions: when relaxed and tremor-free; with their right arm extended, resulting in an involuntary tremor; and when relaxed with the examiner imposing a passive oscillation on the patient's wrist. Results were compared with 4 normal controls under three different conditions: when relaxed; when holding their right arms in an extended posture; and when initiating a postural tremor by voluntarily oscillating their right wrists.

In the 4 ET patients the presence of an involuntary postural tremor of the right arm was associated with significant bilateral cerebellar, bilateral premotor cortex, and contralateral SMC increases in blood flow. Figure 4.3 is a map of statistical significance, and shows the areas that were significantly activated in the group of 4 ET patients. When controls extended their right arms without tremor, and when relaxed tremor-free ET patients had an oscillation passively imposed on their wrist, there was no significant cerebellar activation. This finding suggests that it was the involuntary tremor in ET patients that was specifically associated with cerebellar activation. When controls imitated a postural tremor with their right arms, ipsilateral cerebellar activation occurred, and there was additional activation of the supplementary motor area compared with involuntary tremor. The authors agreed with Dubinsky and Hallett (1987) that ET is likely to be associated with overactivity of olivary–cerebellar connections.

Colebatch *et al.*'s study (1990) has now been extended (Brooks *et al.*, 1992b). It has become apparent with greater numbers that even at rest, without tremor, ET patients have abnormally raised cerebellar blood flow compared to controls. The same group has also studied patients with neuropathic postural tremor. These patients also showed bilaterally raised levels of cerebrellar blood flow at rest and in the presence of tremor. This finding is against the hypothesis that neuropathic tremor (NT) arises simply as a consequence of mismatch of afferent and efferent traffic in peripheral nerves and suggests that both ET and NT have a central origin. Parker *et al.* (1992) have recently reported PET rCBF findings in 7 patients with unilateral parkinsonian rest tremor. These patients had an electrode stereotactically placed in the contralateral ventral thalamus. Electrical stimulation abolished the tremor and led to a bilateral fall in cerebellar blood flow. It is becomining apparent that overactivity of cerebellar connections may underlie all forms of tremor, whether the tremor is essential, neuropathic, or parkinsonian in character.

THE DOPAMINERGIC SYSTEM

Uncertainty exists over the relationship between isolated rest tremor and PD. Patients occasionally present with a 3–5 Hz rest tremor indistinguishable from that seen in PD, but without significant bradykinesia or rigidity when postures are adopted that abolish the tremor. There have been no pathological reports on such cases, and it is unclear whether they have a *forme fruste* of PD with Lewy body brainstem disease, or an alternative condition. Brooks *et al.* (1992c) have examined striatal ^{18}F-dopa uptake in 11 patients with isolated 3–5 Hz rest tremor. In 4 cases tremor was first evident in the legs. All 11 rest tremor patients had reduced putamen ^{18}F-dopa uptake contralateral to the more affected limbs. Mean putamen and caudate tracer uptake were 50 and 80% of normal, similar to that found in PD. The authors concluded that isolated rest or foot tremor probably represents a phenotype of PD. It remains uncertain whether these patients will eventually develop the full clinical syndrome of PD; 2 of the 11 patients scanned have had tremor for 14 and 20 years without progression.

While rest tremor is a characteristic of PD, postural tremor indistinguishable from ET occurs just as frequently and can be a presenting feature (Lance *et al.*, 1963; Findley *et al.*, 1981; Jankovic and Frost, 1981). Patients with a large-amplitude postural tremor may have a low-amplitude break-through rest component (Marsden *et al.*, 1983), and frequently have cogwheel rigidity on synkinesis and reduced arm swing, particularly if they are elderly (Critchley, 1956; Salisachs and Findlay, 1984). As these signs are also features of PD, this has led to occasional difficulties in clinically distinguishing ET from PD. In four retrospective series, 10–25% of patients initially diagnosed as PD were later reclassified as having essential tremor (Marshall, 1962; Critchley, 1972; Rautakorpi, 1978; Larsen and Calne, 1983). Clinical surveys are divided over the relationship between ET and PD; some have reported no relationship (Cleeves *et al.*, 1988) while others have found that up to 19% of ET cases later convert to PD (Geraghty *et al.*, 1985). One survey has reported an increased 20% prevalence of ET in relatives of PD patients (Lang *et al.*, 1986). Fourteen ET cases have come to autopsy to date. These have all shown non-specific histopathological changes, arguing against a relationship between ET and PD (Rajput *et al.*, 1991). These autopsy findings, however, do not rule out postural tremor as a presenting feature of PD.

Brooks *et al.* (1992) have examined the relationship between essential tremor and nigral integrity by performing ^{18}F-dopa PET on 8 patients with familial ET and 12 patients with sporadic postural tremor. The 8 familial ET cases all had putamen and caudate ^{18}F-dopa uptake within the normal range, arguing against an association of ET and PD. Putamen ^{18}F-dopa uptake was normal in 10, and reduced in 2 of the sporadic postural tremor cases. One of these patients had putamen tracer uptake in the PD range. His postural arm tremor had been present for 2 years and over the following 18 months he developed typical PD with bradykinesia and rest tremor. The authors concluded that, while there was no evidence for an association between familial ET and PD, postural tremor could represent an isolated manifestation of PD. 'Soft' signs of parkinsonism, such as the presence of low-amplitude tremor when seated relaxed, reduced arm swing on walking, and the presence of sustained cogwheel rigidity on synkinesis, proved to be unreliable predictors of the presence of nigral dysfunction in postural tremor patients.

Chorea and tardive dyskinesia

The pathology of Huntington's disease (HD) involves loss of spiny neurons from the striatal and dentate nuclei. Those patients with predominant chorea show selective loss of striatolateral pallidal projections, while those with akinetic–rigid syndromes show additional severe loss of striatomedial pallidal fibres (Albin *et al.*, 1990). The condition is dominantly inherited, and associated with an abnormally raised number of repeats on the short arm of chromosome 4. The degenerative disorders neuroacanthocytosis (NA) and dentatorubropallidoluysian atrophy are also associated with chorea, as are benign familial chorea and the inflammatory diseases systemic lupus erythematosus and Sydenham's chorea. Patients with tardive dyskinesia exhibit chorea, though stereotypies are usually also evident. The pathology of tardive dyskinesia is uncertain; neurochemical studies on a primate tardive dyskinesia model have reported severe depletion of subthalamic levels of gamma-aminobutyric acid (Gunne *et al.*, 1984) while postmortem studies on human tardive dyskinesia cases have found low subthalamic glutamate decarboxylase activity (Andersson *et al.*, 1989).

METABOLIC STUDIES

Several centres have established that affected HD patients have severely reduced caudate, and more moderately reduced lentiform nucleus, glucose and oxygen metabolism, and that this is present in early disease when CT and MRI are generally normal (Kuhl *et al.*, 1982; Hayden *et al.*, 1986; Leenders *et al.*, 1986c). Levels of striatal glucose metabolism correlate with the locomotor function of these patients (Young *et al.*, 1986). In early disease cortical metabolism is preserved in HD, but subsequently declines as dementia becomes prominent, the frontal cortex being targeted (Kuhl *et al.*, 1984a; Kuwert *et al.*, 1990a). While caudate hypometabolism is a characteristic of HD, its presence is not specific for this condition. Caudate glucose utilization is also reduced in neuroacanthocytosis and dentatorubropallidoluysian atrophy (Hosokawa *et al.*, 1987; Dubinsky *et al.*, 1989) and may be normal or reduced in benign familial chorea (Suchowersky *et al.*, 1986; Kuwert *et al.*, 1990b). In contrast to the degenerative causes of chorea, striatal glucose metabolism has been reported to be elevated in chorea secondary to systemic lupus erythematosus (Guttman *et al.*, 1987), Sydenham's chorea (KL Leenders, personal communication) and tardive dyskinesia (Pahl *et al.*, 1987). PET, therefore, provides a potential means of distinguishing the degenerative choreas from those associated with inflammatory disorders or neuroleptic treatment.

The sensitivity and specificity of PET for the detection of subclinical caudate hypometabolism in subjects at risk for HD are still controversial. Grafton *et al.* (1990) have performed ^{18}FDG PET on 54 at-risk subjects for HD and found low caudate metabolism in 12 cases. Nine of the 12 patients identified as high-risk from either DNA linkage studies or their subsequent development of the disease had low caudate metabolism – a concordance of 75%. One of 8 low-risk cases also had abnormal caudate function. Five out of the 6 at-risk subjects with 'soft' signs of HD had low caudate metabolism. The authors concluded that PET provides a sensitive means of detecting caudate dysfunction in subjects at risk for HD. Results from other centres have been less striking. Young *et al.* (1987) found no abnormalities of caudate metabolism in 29 at-risk subjects while Hayden *et al.* (1987) reported reduced caudate glucose utilization in 3 out of 8 high-risk, and 1 out of 5 low-risk subjects. Present evidence suggests that if ^{18}FDG PET is abnormal in subjects at risk for HD they are likely to develop chorea, but a normal study does not exclude this disorder.

THE DOPAMINERGIC SYSTEM

Using the tracer ^{11}C-MSP, Wong *et al.* (1985) have studied striatal dopamine D_2 receptor integrity in 13 affected patients with HD and 9 at-risk relatives. They found a significant reduction in the mean caudate : cerebellar tracer uptake ratio of the affected group and individual uptake ratios correlated inversely with clinical disease duration. The at-risk subjects all had normal striatal ^{11}C-MSP uptake. Subsequently two other centres have confirmed reduced striatal ^{11}C-MSP binding in single patients with HD (Leenders *et al.*, 1986c; Hagglund *et al.*, 1987). Reduced caudate ^{18}F-FESP uptake has also been reported in 2 HD cases (Wienhard *et al.*, 1990) and reduced striatal IBZM binding in 10 cases (Brücke *et al.*, 1991). There has been one published case report on striatal ^{18}F-dopa uptake in HD (Leenders *et al.*, 1986c). This was normal within the 1.7 cm resolution of the PET camera used.

The finding of reduced striatal D_2 site binding potential, like that of reduced caudate metabolism, is not specific for HD. Brooks *et al.* (1991) have reported a mean 70% reduction of striatal ^{11}C-raclopride binding in 3 NA patients. These workers also examined ^{18}F-dopa uptake in 6 NA subjects. Caudate and anterior putamen tracer uptake was normal but posterior putamen tracer uptake was selectively reduced by 60%. Similar findings were obtained for a patient with akinetic–rigid HD (unpublished observations). The parallel PET findings in HD and NA are not surprising as the striatal pathology of these two conditions is similar (Bird *et al.*, 1978; de Yebenes *et al.*, 1988; Hardie *et al.*, 1991). The selective abnormality of posterior putamen ^{18}F-dopa uptake in NA and HD suggests the presence of focal pathology in the ventrolateral nigra. This has indeed been noted in NA (Hardie *et al.*, 1991).

While striatal D_2 receptor density is severely reduced in degenerative causes of chorea, two PET studies have established, using the tracers ^{76}Br-BSP and ^{11}C-MSP, that D_2 density is preserved in tardive dyskinesia (Blin *et al.*, 1989; Andersson *et al.*, 1990). This finding argues against the hypothesis that tardive dyskinesia results from striatal D_2 receptor upregulation following prolonged exposure to neurolepsis. To date only one study on D_2 receptor status has been reported in an inflammatory cause of chorea (Turkanski *et al.*, 1993). Striatal D_2 binding was normal in a case of SLE chorea, suggesting that measurement of striatal D_2 density as well as glucose metabolism will provide a means of distinguishing the degenerative choreas from other causes.

THE FUTURE

This chapter has reviewed the way that functional imaging has been used to date to demonstrate and distinguish the characteristic patterns of derangement of regional cerebral metabolism and the dopaminergic system in the akinetic–rigid syndromes and involuntary movement disorders. More excitingly, PET is able to detect subclinical functional abnormalities, and so identify subjects at risk for degenerative disorders such as PD and HD. In the future PET will provide a means of monitoring the therapeutic effects of engraftment or stereotactic lesioning in movement disorders, and may help to establish the role of nerve growth factors and neuroprotective agents in the treatment of degenerative disease.

The use of PET for studying abnormalities in patterns of cerebral activation in PD, dystonia and tremor has also been reviewed. These studies are still in their infancy, and provide a potential means of learning about the networks associated with generation of involuntary movements, and of detecting the effects of selective basal ganglia pathology on activation of cortical areas.

Finally the majority of pharmacological studies on movement disorders with PET and SPECT have involved the dopaminergic system, though tracers to study the serotonin, benzodiazepine, cholinergic and opiate systems are also available. The hunt continues for suitable tracers to study glutamatergic and peptidergic systems. If suitable reversible antagonist tracers become available it should in theory become possible to examine changes in receptor occupancy by endogenous transmitters when activation paradigms are performed. Suitable agonist tracers may allow high- and low-affinity receptor subclasses to be distinguished. While functional imaging is unlikely ever to reveal the cause of a movement disorder, its potential for demonstrating the functional consequences of these diseases remains unparalleled.

References

Albin RL, Reiner A, Anderson KD, Penney JB, and Young AB (1990) Striatal and nigral neuron subpopulations in rigid Huntington's disease: implications for the functional anatomy of chorea and rigidity-akinesia. *Ann Neurol*, **27**, 357–65

Andersson U, Haggstrom J-E, Levin ED, Bondesson U, Valverius M, and Gunne, LM (1989) Reduced glutamate decarboxylase activity in the subthalamic nucleus of patients with tardive dyskinesia. *Movement Disorders*, **4**, 37–46

Andersson U, Eckernas SA, Hartvig P, Ulin J, Langstrom B, and Haggstrom JE (1990) Striatal binding of ^{11}C-NMSP studied with positron emission tomography in patients with persistent tardive dyskinesia: no evidence for altered dopamine receptor binding. *J Neural Transm*, **79**, 215–26

Baron JC, Maziere B, Loc'h, C *et al.* (1986) Loss of striatal (76Br)bromospiperone binding sites demonstrated by positron tomography in progressive supranuclear palsy. *J Cereb Blood Flow Metab*, **6**, 131–6

Bernheimer H, Birkmayer W, Hornykiewicz O, Jellinger K, and Seitelberger F (1973) Brain dopamine and the syndromes of Parkinson and Huntington–clinical, morphological and neurochemical correlations. *J Neurol Sci*, **29**, 415–55

Bhatt MH, Snow BJ, Martin WRW, Pate BD, Ruth TJ, and Calne DB (1991a) Positron emission tomography suggests that the rate of progression of idiopathic parkinsonism is slow. *Ann Neurol*, **29**, 674–7

Bhatt MH, Snow BJ, Martin WRW, Peppard R, and Calne DB (1991b) Positron emission tomography in progressive supranuclear palsy. *Arch Neurol*, **48**, 389–91

Bird TD, Cedarbaum S, Valpey RW, and Stahl WL (1978) Familial degeneration of the basal ganglia with acanthocytosis: a clinical, pathological, and neurochemical study. *Ann Neurol*, **3**, 747–52

Blin J, Baron JC, Cambon H *et al.* (1989) Striatal dopamine D_2 receptors in tardive dyskinesia: PET study. *J Neurol Neurosurg Psychiatry*, **52**, 1248–52

Blin J, Baron JC, Dubois P *et al.* (1990a) Positron emission tomography study in progressive supranuclear palsy. *Arch Neurol*, **47**, 747–52

Blin J, Vidhailhet M, Bonnet AM *et al.* (1990b) PET study in corticobasal degeneration. *Movement Disorders*, **5** (suppl 1), 19

Brooks DJ (1992) PET in autonomic failure. In Bannister R, Mathias CJ, eds, *Autonomic Failure*, 3rd edn, Oxford, Oxford University Press

Brooks DJ, Ibañez V, Sawle GV *et al.* (1990a) Differing patterns of striatal 18F-dopa-uptake in Parkinson's disease, multiple system atrophy and progressive supranuclear palsy. *Ann Neurol*, **28**, 547–55

Brooks DJ, Salmon EP, Mathias CJ *et al.* (1990b) The relationship between locomotor disability, autonomic dysfunction, and the integrity of the striatal dopaminergic system, in patients with multiple system atrophy, pure autonomic failure, and Parkinson's disease, studied with PET. *Brain*, **113**, 1539–52

Brooks DJ, Ibanez V, Playford ED *et al.* (1991) Presynaptic and postsynaptic striatal dopaminergic function in neuroacanthocytosis: a positron emission tomographic study. *Ann Neurol*, **30**, 166–71

Brooks DJ, Ibanez V, Sawle GV *et al.* (1992a) Striatal D_2 receptor status in Parkinson's disease, striatonigral degeneration, and progressive supranuclear palsy, measured with ^{11}C-raclopride and PET. *Ann Neurol*, **31**, 184–92

Brooks DJ, Jenkins IH, Baines P, Thompson PD, Findley LJ, and Marsden CD (1992b) A comparison of the abnormal patterns of cerebral activation associated with neuropathic and essential tremor. *Neurology*, **42**, Supp 3, 373

Brooks DJ, Playford ED, Ibanez V *et al.* (1992c) Isolated tremor and disruption of the nigrostriatal dopaminergic system: an ^{18}F-dopa PET study. *Neurology*, **42**, 1554–60

Brücke T, Podreka I, Angelberger P *et al.* (1991) Dopamine D2 receptor imaging with SPECT: studies in different neuropsychiatric disorders. *J Cereb Blood Flow Metab* **11**, 220–8

Burn DJ, Mark MH, Playford ED *et al.* (1992) Parkinson's disease in twins studied with ^{18}F-dopa and positron emission tomography. *Neurology*, **42**, 1894–1900

Byrne E, Lennox G, Lowe J, and Godwin-Austin RB (1989) Diffuse Lewy body disease: clinical features in 15 cases. *J Neurol Neurosurg Pshchiatry*, **52**, 709–17

Calne CB, Langston JW, Martin WR *et al.* (1985) Positron emission tomography after MPTP: observations relating to the cause of Parkinson's disease. *Nature*, **317**, 246–8

Calne DB, Eisen A, McGeer EG, and Spencer P (1986) Alzheimer's disease, Parkinson's disease and motoneurone disease: a biotrophic interaction between aging and environment. *Lancet*, **1**, 1067–70

Chase T, Tamminga CA, and Burrows H (1988) Positron emission studies of regional cerebral glucose metabolism in idiopathic dystonia. *Adv Neurol*, **50**, 237–41

Chieuh CC, Burns RS, Kopin IJ *et al.* (1986) 6-18F-Dopa/positron emission tomography visualized degree of damage to brain dopamine in basal ganglia of monkeys with MPTP-induced parkinsonism. In Markey SP, Castagnoli N, Trevor AJ, and Kopin IJ, eds, *MPTP: A Neurotoxin Producing a Parkinsonian Syndrome*, Orlando, Academic Press, 327–38

Cleeves L, Findley LJ, and Koller W (1988) Lack of association between essential tremor and Parkinson's disease. *Ann Neurol*, **24**, 23–6

Colebatch JG, Findley LJ, Frackowiak RSJ, Marsden CD, and Brooks DJ (1990) Preliminary report: activation of the cerebellum in essential tremor. *Lancet*, **336**, 1028–30

Critchley M (1956) Neurological changes in the aged. *J Chronic Dis*, **3**, 459–77

Critchley E (1972) Clinical manifestations of essential tremor. *J Neurol Neurosurg Psychiatry*, **35**, 365–72

Crossman AR (1990) A hypothesis on the pathophysiological mechanisms that underlie levodopa- or dopamine agonist-induced dyskinesia in Parkinson's disease: implications for future strategies in treatment. *Movement Disorders*, **5**, 100–8

D'Antona R, Baron JC, Samson Y *et al.* (1985) Subcortical dementia: frontal cortex hypometabolism detected by positron tomography in patients with progressive supranuclear palsy. *Brain*, **108**, 785–800

De Volder AG, Francard J, Laterre C *et al.* (1989) Decreased glucose utilisation in the striatum and frontal lobe in probable striatonigral degeneration. *Ann Neurol*, **26**, 239–47

de Yebenes JG, Brin MF, Mena MA *et al.* (1988) Neurochemical findings in neuroacanthocytosis. *Movement Disorders*, **3**, 302–12

Dubinsky R and Hallett M (1987) Glucose hypermetabolism of the inferior olive in patients with essential tremor. *Ann Neurol*, **22**, 118

Dubinsky RM, Hallett M, Levey R, and Di Chiro G (1989) Regional brain glucose metabolism in neuroacanthocytosis. *Neurology*, **39**, 1253–5

Eidelberg D, Dhawan V, Cedarbaum J, Greene P, and Fahn S (1990) Contralateral basal ganglia hypermetabolism in primary unilateral limb dystonia, *Neurology*, **40** (suppl 1), 399

Eidelberg D, Dhawan V, Moeller JR *et al.* (1991) The metabolic landscape of cortico-basal ganglionic degeneration: regional asymmetries studied with positron emission tomography. *J Neurol Neurosurg Psychiatry*, **54**, 856–62

Fearnley JM and Lees AJ (1990) Striatonigral degeneration: a clinicopathological study. *Brain*, **113**, 1823–42

Fearnley JM and Lees AJ (1991) Ageing and Parkinson's disease: substantia nigra regional selectivity. *Brain*, **114**, 2283–301

Fearnley JM, Revesz T, Brooks DJ, Frackowiak RSJ, and Lees AJ (1991) Diffuse Lewy body disease presenting with a supranuclear downgaze palsy. *J Neurol Neurosurg Psychiatry*, **54**, 159–61

Findley LJ, Gresty MA, and Halmagyi GM (1981) Tremor, the cogwheel phenomenon and clonus in Parkinson's disease. *J Neurol Neurosurg Psychiatry*, **44**, 534–46

Firnau G, Sood S, Chirakal R, Nahmias C, and Garnett ES (1987) Cerebral metabolism of 6-[18F]fluoro-L-3,4-dihydroxyphenylalanine in the primate. *J Neurochem*, **48**, 1077–82

Fletcher NA, Harding AE, and Marsden CD (1990) A genetic study of idiopathic torsion dystonia in the United Kingdom. *Brain*, **113**, 379–95

Foster NL, Gilman S, Berent S, Morin EM, Brown MB, and Koeppe RA (1988) Cerebral hypometabolism in progressive supranuclear palsy studied with positron emission tomography. *Ann Neurol*, **24**, 399–406

Fulham MJ, Dubinsky RM, Polinsky RJ *et al.* (1991) Computed tomography, magnetic resonance imaging and positron emission tomography with [^{18}F]fluorodeoxyglucose in multiple system atrophy and pure autonomic failure. *Clin Autonomic Res*, **1**, 27–36

Garnett ES, Nahmias C, and Firnau G (1984) Central dopaminergic pathways in hemiparkinsonism examined by positron emission tomography. *Can J Neurol Sci*, **11**, 174–9

Geraghty JJ, Jankovic J, and Zetusky WJ (1985) Association between essential tremor and Parkinson's disease. *Ann Neurol*, **17**, 329–33

German DC, Manaye K, Smith WK, Woodward DJ, and Saper CB (1989) Midbrain dopaminergic cell loss in Parkinson's disease: computer visualaization. *Ann Neurol*, **26**, 507–14

Gibb WRG, Luthert P, and Marsden CD (1989) Corticobasal degeneration. *Brain* **112**, 1171–92

Gibb WRG, Fearnley JM, and Lees AJ (1990) The anatomy and pigmentation of the human substantia nigra in relation to selective neuronal vulnerability. *Adv Neurol*, **53**, 31–4

Gilman S, Junck L, Young AB *et al.* (1988) Cerebral metabolic activity in idiopathic dystonia studied with positron emission tomography. *Adv Neurol*, **50**, 231–6

Goffinet AM, De Volder AG, Gillain C *et al.* (1989) Positron tomography demonstrates frontal lobe hypometabolism in progressive supranuclear palsy. *Ann Neurol*, **25**, 131–9

Goldberg G (1985) Supplementary motor area structure and function: review and hypotheses. *Behavior Brain Sci*, **8**, 567–616

Goldman-Rakic PS (1987) Circuitry of primate prefrontal cortex and regulation of behaviour by representation memory. In Plum F, ed, *The Nervous System: Higher Functions of the Brain*, Bethesda: Americal Physiology Society, 373–417

Goto S, Hirano A, and Matsumoto S (1989) Subdivisional involvement of nigrostriatal loop in idiopathic Parkinson's disease and striatonigral degeneration. *Neuroscience*, **26**, 766–70

Grafton ST, Mazziotta JC, Pahl JJ *et al.* (1990) A comparison of neurological, metabolic, structural, and genetic evaluation in persons at risk for Huntington's disease. *Ann Neurol*, **28**, 614–21

Gunne LM, Haggstrom J-E, and Sjoquist B (1984) Association with persistent neuroleptic-induced dyskinesia of regional changes in brain GABA synthesis. *Nature*, **309**, 347–9

Guttman M, Lang AE, Garnett ES *et al.* (1987) Regional cerebral glucose metabolism in SLE chorea: further evidence that striatal hypometabolism is not a correlate of chorea. *Movement Disorders*, **2**, 201–10

Guttman M, Burns RS, Martin WR *et al.* (1989) PET studies of Parkinsonian patients treated with autologous adrenal implants. *Can J Neurol Sci*, **16**, 305–9

Hagglund J, Aquilonius SM, Eckernas SA *et al.* (1989) Dopamine receptor properties in Parkinson's disease and Huntington's chorea evaluated by positron emission tomography using 11C-N-methyl-spiperone. *Acta Neurol Scand*, **75**, 87–94

Hardie RJ, Pullon HWH, Harding AE *et al.* (1991) Neuroacanthocytosis. A clinical, haematological, and pathological study of 19 cases. *Brain*, **114**, 13–50

Hayden MR, Martin WRW, Stoessl AJ *et al.* (1986) Positron emission tomography in the early diagnosis of Huntington's disease. *Neurology*, **36**, 888–94

Hayden MR, Hewitt J, Martin WRW, Clark C, and Amman A (1987) Studies in persons at risk for Huntington's disease. *N Engl J Med*, **317**, 382–3

Hornykiewicz O, Kish SJ, Becker LE, Farley I, and Shannnak K (1986) Brain neurotransmitters in dystonia musculorum deformans. *N Engl J Med*, **315**, 347–52

Hosokawa S, Ichiya Y, Kuwabara Y *et al.* (1987) Positron emission tomography in cases of chorea with different underlying diseases. *J Neurol Neurosurg Psychiatry*, **50**, 1284–7

Hughes AJ, Daniel SE, Kilford L, and Lees AJ (1992) The accuracy of the clinical diagnosis of Parkinson's disease: a clinicopathological study of 100 cases. *J Neurol Neursurg Psychiatry*, **55**, 181–4

Jackson JA, Jankovic J, and Ford J (1983) Progressive supranuclear palsy: clinical features and response to treatment in 16 patients. *Ann Neurol*, **13**, 273–8

Jankovic J, and Frost JD (1981) Quantitative assessment of parkinsonian and essential tremor: clinical application of triaxial accelerometry. *Neurology*, **31**, 1235–40

Jellinger K, Riederer P, and Tomananga M (1980) Progressive supranuclear palsy: clinico-pathological and biochemical studies. *J Neural Transm* (suppl 16), 111–28

Jenkins, IH, Fernandez W, Playford ED *et al.* (1992) Akinesia and Parkinson's disease: impaired activation of the supplementary motor area is reversed by apomorphine. *Ann Neurol*, **32**, 749–57

Kish SJ, Chang LJ, Mirchandani LJ, Shannak K, and Hornykiewicz O (1985) Progressive supranuclear palsy: relationship between extrapyramidal disturbances, dementia, and brain neurotransmitter markers. *Ann Neurol*, **18**, 530–6

Kish SJ, Shannak K, and Hornykiewicz O (1988) Uneven pattern of dopamine loss in the striatum of patients with idiopathic Parkinson's disease. *N Engl J Med*, **318**, 876–80

Kish SJ, Shannak K, Rajput A, Deck JHN, and Hornykiewicz O (1992) Aging produces a specific pattern of striatal dopamine loss: implications for the etiology of idiopathic Parkinson's disease. *J Neurochem*, **58**, 642–8

Kiyosawa M, Baron JC, Hamel E *et al.* (1989) Time course of effects of unilateral lesions of the nucleus basalis of Meynert on glucose utilisation by the cerebral cortex. Positron emission tomography in baboons. *Brain*, **112**, 435–55

Kramer PL, De Leon D, Ozelius L *et al.* (1990) Dystonia gene in Ashkenazi Jewish population is located on chromosome 9q32–34. *Ann Neurol*, **27**, 114–20

Kuhl DE, Phelps ME, Markham CH, Metter EJ, Riege WH, and Winter EJ (1982) Cerebral metabolism and atrophy in Huntington's disease determined by 18FDG and computed tomographic scans. *Ann Neurol*, **12**, 425–34

Kuhl DE, Metter EJ, Riege WH, and Markham CH (1984a) Patterns of cerebral glucose utilisation in Parkinson's disease and Huntington's disease. *Ann Neurol*, **15** (suppl) S119–25

Kuhl DE, Metter EJ, and Riege WH (1984b) Patterns of local cerebral glucose utilisation determined in Parkinson's disease by the 18F-fluorodeoxyglucose method. *Ann Neurol*, **15**, 419–24

Kuhl DE, Metter EJ, Benson DF *et al.* (1985) Similarities of cerebral glucose metabolism in Alzheimer's and Parkinsonian dementia. *J Cereb Blood Flow Metab*, **5**, S169–70

Kuwert T, Lange HW, Langen KJ, Herzog H, Aulich A, and Feinendegen LE (1990a) Cortical and subcortical glucose consumptions measured by PET in patients with Huntington's disease. *Brain*, **113**, 1405–23

Kuwert T, Lange HW, Langen KJ *et al.* (1990b) Normal striatal glucose consumption in two patients with benign hereditary chorea as measured by positron emission tomography. *J Neurol*, **237**, 80–4

Lance JW, Schwab RS, and Peterson EA (1963) Action tremor and the cogwheel phenomenon in Parkinson's disease. *Brain*, **86**, 95–110

Lang AE, Kierens C, and Blair RDG (1986) Family history of tremor in Parkinson's disease. *Adv Neurol*, **45**, 313–16

Larsen TA and Calne DB (1983) Essential tremor. *Clin Neuropharmacol*, **6**, 185–206

Leenders KL, Wolfson L, Gibbs JM *et al.* (1985a) The effects of L-DOPA on regional cerebral blood flow and oxygen metabolism in patients with Parkinson's disease. *Brain*, **108**, 171–91

Leenders KL, Herold S, Palmer AJ *et al.* (1985b) Human cerebral dopamine system measured *in vivo* using PET. *J Cereb Blood Flow Metab*, **5** (suppl) S157–8

Leenders KL, Palmer A, Turton S *et al.* (1986a) DOPA uptake and dopamine receptor binding visualized in the human brain *in vivo*. In Fahn S, Marsden CD, Jenner P, and Teychenne P, eds, *Recent Developments in Parkinson's disease*, New York, Raven Press, 103–13

Leenders KL, Palmer AJ, Quinn N *et al.* (1986b) Brain dopamine metabolism in patients with Parkinson's disease measured with positron emission tomography. *J Neurol Neurosurg Psychiatry*, **49**, 853–60

Leenders KL, Frackowiak RSI, Quinn N, and Marsden CD (1986c) Brain energy metabolism and dopaminergic function in Huntington's disease measured *in vivo* using positron emission tomography. *Movement Disorders*, **1**, 69–77

Leenders KL, Aquilonius SM, Bergstrom K *et al.* (1988a) Unilateral MPTP lesion in a rhesus monkey: effects on the striatal dopaminergic system measured *in vivo* with PET using various novel tracers. *Brain Res*, **445**, 61–7

Leenders KL, Frackowiak RS, and Lees AJ (1988b) Steele-Richardson-Olszewski syndrome. Brain energy metabolism, blood flow and fluorodopa uptake measured by positron emission tomography. *Brain*, **111**, 615–30

Leenders KL, Quinn N, Frackowiak RSJ, and Marsden CD (1988c) Brain dopaminergic system studied in patients with dystonia using positron emission tomography. *Adv Neurol*, **50**, 243–7

Leenders KL, Salmon EP, Tyrrell P *et al.* (1990) The nigrostriatal dopaminergic system assessed *in vivo* by positron emission tomography in healthy volunteer subjects and patients with Parkinson's disease. *Arch Neurol*, **47**, 1290–8

Leenders KL, Antonini A, Schwarz J, Oertel W, and Hess K (1991) Dopamine D_2 receptors measured *in vivo* in patients with Parkinson's disease. In Narabayashi H, ed, *10th International Symposium on Parkinson's Disease*, Tokyo, 121

Lewis AJ and Gawell MJ (1990) Diffuse Lewy body disease with dementia and oculomotor dysfunction. *Movement Disorders*, **5**, 143–7

McGeer PL, Itagaki S, Akiyama H, and McFeer EG (1988) Rate of cell death in Parkinsonism indicates active neuropathological process. *Ann Neurol*, **24**, 574–6

Maher ER and Lees AJ (1986) The clinical features and natural history of the Steele-Richardson-Olszewski syndrome (progressive supranuclear palsy). *Neurology*, **36**, 1005–8

Marsden CD, Obeso JA, and Rothwell JC (1983) Benign essential tremor is not a single entity. In Yahr MD, ed, *Current Concepts of Parkinson's Disease and Related Disorders*, Amsterdam, Excerpta Medica, 31–46

Marsden CD, Obeso JA, Zarranz JJ, and Lang AE (1985) The anatomical basis of the symptomic hemidystonias. *Brain*, **108**, 463–83

Marshall J (1962) Observations on essential tremor. *J Neurol Neurosurg Psychiatry*, **25**, 122–5

Martin WRW, Stoessl AJ, Adam MJ *et al.* (1986) Positron emission tomography in Parkinson's disease: glucose and dopa metabolism. *Adv Neurol*, **45**, 95–8

Martin WRW, Stoessl AJ, Palmer M *et al.* (1988) PET scanning in dystonia. *Adv Neurol*, **50**, 223–9

Martin WRW, Palmer MR, Patlak CS, and Calne DB (1989) Nigrostriatal function in humans studied with positron emission tomography. *Ann Neurol*, **26**, 535–42

Miletich RS, Chan T, Gillespie M, Di Chiro G, and Stein S (1988) Contralateral basal ganglia metabolism is abnormal in hemiparkinsonian patients. An FDG-PET study. *Neurology*, **28**, S260

Mushiake H, Inase M, and Tanji J (1990) Selective coding of motor sequence in the supplementary motor area of the monkey cerebral cortex. *Exp Brain Res*, **82**, 208–10

Nahmias C, Garnett ES, Firnau G, and Lang A (1985) Striatal dopamine distribution in Parkinsonian patients during life. *J Neurol Sci*, **69**, 223–30

Otsuka M, Ichiya Y, Hosokawa S *et al.* (1991) Striatal blood flow, glucose metabolism, and ^{18}F-dopa uptake: difference in Parkinson's disease and atypical parkinsonism. *J Neurol Neurosurg Psychiatry*, **54**, 898–904

Ozelius L, Kramer PL, Moskowitz CB *et al.* (1989) Human gene for torsion dystonia located on chromosome 9q32–34. *Neuron*, **2**, 427–34

Pahl JJ, Mazziotta JC, Cummings J *et al.* (1987) Positron emission tomography in tardive dyskinesia and Huntington's disease. *J Cereb Blood Flow Metab*, **7**, 1253–5

Parker F, Tzourio N, Blond S, Petit H, and Mazoyer B (1992) Evidence for a common network of brain structures involved in parkinsonian tremor and voluntary repetitive movement. *Brain Res*, **584**, 11–17

Peppard RF, Martin WRW, Guttman M *et al.* (1988) The relationship of cerebral glucose metabolism to cognitive deficits in Parkinson's disease. *Neurology*, **38** (suppl 1), 364

Perlmutter JS and Raichle ME (1985) Regional blood flow in hemiparkinsonism. *Neurology*, **35**, 1127–34

Playford ED, Sawle GV, Fletcher NA, Marsden CD, and Brooks DJ (1991) Familial torsion dystonia: an ^{18}F-dopa PET study. *J Cereb Blood Flow Metab*, **11** (suppl 2), S816

Playford ED, Jenkins IH, Passingham RE, Nutt J, Frackowiak RSJ, and Brooks DJ (1992a) Impaired mesial frontal and putamen activation in Parkinson's disease: a PET study. *Ann Neurol*, **32**, 151–61

Playford ED, Passingham RE, Marsden CD, and Brooks DJ (1992b) Abnormal activation of striatum and supplementary motor area in dystonia. *Movement Disorders*, **7**, suppl 144

Quinn N (1989) Multiple system atrophy – the nature of the beast. *J Neurol Neurosurg Psychiatry*, **52**, 78–89
Rajput AH, Rozdilsky B, Ang L, and Rajput A (1991) Clinicopathologic observations in essential tremor: report of six cases. *Neurology*, **41**, 422–4
Rascol O, Sabatini U, Chollet F *et al.* (1992) Supplementary and primary sensory motor area activity in Parkinson's disease. Regional cerebral blood flow changes during finger movements and effects of apomorphine. *Arch Neurol*, **49**, 144–8
Rautakorpi I (1978) Essential tremor. An epidemiological, clinical, and genetic study. Thesis. University of Turku, Finland
Riley DE, Lang AE, Lewis A *et al.* (1990) Cortical-basal ganglionic degeneration, *Neurology*, **40**, 1203–12
Rinne JO, Rummukainen J, Lic M, Paljarvi L, and Rinne UK (1989) Dementia in Parkinson's disease is related to neuronal loss in the medial substantia nigra. *Ann Neurol*, **26**, 47–50
Rinne JO, Laihinen A, Nagren K *et al.* (1990a) PET demonstrates different behaviour of striatal dopamine D1 and D2 receptors in early Parkinson's disease. *J Neurosci Res*, **27**, 494–9
Rinne UK, Laihinen A, Rinne JO, Nagren K, Bergman J, and Ruotsalainen U (1990b) Positron emission tomography demonstrates dopamine D2 receptor supersensitity in the striatum of patients with early Parkinson's disease. *Movement Disorders*, **5**, 55–9
Rosenthal G, Gilman S, Koeppe RA *et al.* (1988) Motor dysfunction in olivopontocerebellar atrophy is related to cerebral metabolic rate studied with positron emission tomography. *Ann Neurol*, **24**, 414–19
Salisachs P and Findley LJ (1984) Problems in the differential diagnosis of essential tremor. In Findley LJ, Capildeo R, eds, *Movement Disorders: Tremor*, London, MacMillan Press, 219–24
Salmon EP, Brooks DJ, Leenders KL *et al.* (1990) A two-compartment description and kinetic procedure for measuring regional cerebral [11C]nomifensine uptake using positron emission tomography. *J Cereb Blood Flow Metab*, **10**, 307–16
Sawle GV, Colebatch JG, Shah A, Brooks DJ, Marsden CD, and Frackowiak RS (1990a) Striatal functin in normal aging: implications for Parkinson's disease. *Ann Neurol*, **28**, 799–804
Sawle GV, Brooks DJ, Ibañez V, and Frackowiak RSJ (1990b) Striatal D2 receptor density is inversely proportional to dopa uptake in untreated hemi-Parkinson's disease. *J Neurol Neurosurg Psychiatry*, **53**, 177–70
Sawle GV, Brooks DJ, Marsden CD, and Frackowiak RSJ (1991a) Corticobasal dgeneration: a unique pattern of regional cortical oxygen metabolism and striatal fluorodopa uptake demonstrated by positron emission tomography. *Brain*, **114**, 541–56
Sawle GV, Leenders KL, Brooks DJ *et al.* (1991b) Dopa-responsive dystonia: [18F]dopa positron emission tomography. *Ann Neurol*, **30**, 24–30
Sawle GV, Wroe SJ, Lees AJ, Brooks DJ, and Frackowiak RSJ (1992a) The identification of presymptomatic parkinsonism: clinical and [^{18}F]dopa PET studies in an Irish kindred. *Ann Neurol*, **32**, 609–17
Sawle GV, Turjanski N, Brooks DJ, and Frackowiak RSJ (1992b) The rate of disease progression in Parkinson's disease: PET findings in patients receiving medical treatment or following foetal mesencephalic transplantation. *Neurology*, **42**, supp 3, 295
Sawle GV, Bloomfield PM, Bjorklund A *et al.* (1992c) Transplantation of fetal dopamine neurons in Parkinson's disease: PET [^{18}F]-6-L-fluorodopa studies in two patients with putaminal implants. *Ann Neurol*, **31**, 166–73
Schapiro MB, Grady C, Ball MJ, DeCarli C, and Rapoport SI (1990) Reductions in parietal/temporal cerebral glucose metabolism are not specific for Alzheimer's disease. *Neurology*, **40** (suppl 1), 152
Schwarz J, Tatsch K, Arnold G *et al.* (1992) I-iodobenzamide-SPECT predicts dopaminergic responsiveness in patients with de-novo parkinsonism. *Neurology*, **42**, 556–61
Shinotoh H, Aotsuka A, Yonezawa H *et al.* (1990) Striatal dopamine D_2 receptors in Parkinson's disease and striato-nigral degeneration determined by positron emission tomography. In Nagatsu T *et al.*, eds, *Basic, Clinical, and Therapeutic Advances of Alzheimer's and Parkinson's Diseases*, vol 2, New York, Plenum Press, 107–10
Snow B, Okada A, Martin WRW, Duvoisin RC, and Calne DB (1992) PET scanning in dopa-responsive dystonia, parkinsonism-dystonia, and young-onset parkinsonism. In Segawa M, ed, *Hereditary Progressive Dystonia*, Carnforth, New York, Parthenon Publishing, 181–88
Spokes EGS, Bannister R, and Oppenheimer DR (1979) Multiple system atrophy with autonomic failure. Clinical, hostological, and neurochemical observations on four cases. *J Neurol Sci*, **43**, 59–62
Steele JC, Richardson JC, and Olszewski J (1964) Progressive supranuclear palsy. A heterogeneous degeneration involving the brain stem, basal ganglia, and cerebellum, with vertical gaze and pseudobulbar palsy. *Arch Neurol*, **10**, 333–59
Stoessl AJ, Martin WRW, Clark C *et al.* (1986) PET studies of cerebral glucose metabolism in idiopathic torticollis. *Neurology*, **36**, 653–7

Suchowersky O, Hayden MR, Martin WRW, Stoessl AJ, Hildebrand AM, and Pate BD (1986) Cerebral metabolism of glucose in bening hereditary chorea. *Movement Disorders*, **1**, 33–45

Tedroff J, Aquilonius S-M, Hartvig P *et al.* (1988) Monoamine re-uptake sites in the human brain evaluated *in vivo* by means of 11C-nomifensine and positron emission tomography: the effects of age and Parkinson's disease. *Acta Neurol Scand*, **77**, 192–201

Tedroff J, Aquilonius S-M, Laihinen A *et al.* (1990) Striatial kinetics of [11C]-(+)-nomifensine and 6-[18F]fluoro-L-dopa in Parkinson's disease measured with positron emission tomography. *Acta Neurol Scand*, **81**, 24–30

Temple LW and Perlmutter JS (1990) Abnormal vibration-induced cerebral blood flow responses in idiopathic dystonia. *Brain*, **113**, 691–707

Thaler DE and Passingham RE (1989) The supplementary motor cortex and internally directed movement. In Crossman AR, Sambrook M, eds, *Neural Mechanisms in Disorders of Movement*, London, Libby, 175–81

Turjanski N, Burn DJ, Lammertsma AA, Dolan R, Harding AE, Quinn N, Kennard C, and Brooks DJ (1993) PET studies on D_1 and D_2 receptor status in chorea. *Neurology*, **43**, sipp 2, A333

Vanderhaegen JJ, Perier O, and Sternon JE (1970) Pathological findings in idiopathic orthostatic hypotension: its relationship with Parkinson's disease. *Arch Neurol*, **22**, 207–14

Wienhard K, Coenen HH, Pawkik G *et al.* (1990) PET studies of dopamine receptor distribution using [18F]fluoroethylspiperone: findings in disorders related to the dopaminergic system. *J Neural Transm*, **81**, 195–213

Wolfson LI, Leenders KL, Brown LL, and Jones T (1985) Alterations of regional cerebral blood flow and oxygen metabolism in Parkinson's disease. *Neurology*, **35**, 1399–405

Wong DF, Links JM, Wagner HN Jr *et al.* (1985) Dopamine and serotonin receptors measured in-vivo in Huntington's disease with C-11 N-methylspiperone PET imaging. *J Nucl Med*, **26**, P107

Young AB, Penney JB, Starosta-Rubinstein S *et al.* (1986) PET scan investigations of Huntington's disease: cerebral metabolic correlates of neurological features and functional decline. *Ann Neurol*, **20**, 296–303

Young AB, Penney JB, Starosta-Rubinstein S *et al.* (1987) Normal caudate glucose metabolism in persons at-risk for Huntington's disease. *Ann Neurol*, **44**, 254–7

5
Eye movement abnormalities in extrapyramidal diseases

Rick Stell and Adolfo M. Bronstein

The movements of the eyes conform to well-defined functional subtypes, namely saccades, smooth pursuit, vestibular, optokinetic and vergence eye movements, each with relatively independent anatomical pathways. Such organization provides selective vulnerability to pathological processes so that clinical descriptions simply stating that a certain motor disorder has 'abnormal eye movements' are outdated and imprecise; some diseases can severely affect one type of eye movement and spare others. Ocular movements can be easily recorded and are simpler to interpret than limb movements and, in fact, fine analysis of eye movements in extrapyramidal diseases can contribute to a better understanding of the abnormal motor mechanisms operating in a certain condition. Of more general interest, examination of eye movements plays an important part in the clinical diagnosis of patients with movement disorders since oculomotor abnormalities are frequent and sometimes severe in these patients.

In this chapter we will firstly review some basic anatomofunctional aspects of the various oculomotor subsystems and the evidence for the basal ganglia being involved in the control of eye movements. Finally, we will discuss the oculomotor abnormalities present in some diseases of the basal ganglia and attempt a clinical summary.

BASIC ANATOMY, PHYSIOLOGY AND CLINICAL EXAMINATION OF THE OCULOMOTOR SYSTEM

Conjugate eye movements belong to two basic types, slow or fast. The former comprise the slow phase of vestibular and optokinetic reflexes and smooth pursuit ('following') movements; essentially, slow eye movements tend to stabilize the eyes on a visual target. Fast eye movements basically tend to shift the eyes from one target to another and comprise saccades and quick components ('beats') of vestibular and optokinetic nystagmus. A comprehensive review on the function, mechanisms and structures involved in eye movements has appeared (Carpenter, 1988). More clinical aspects can be found in Rudge (1983), Leigh and Zee (1983) and Baloh and Honrubia (1990). Kennard and Lueck (1989) and Lang and Marsden (1983) have published reviews on oculomotor function in basal ganglia diseases.

Saccades

These are rapid eye movements whose peak velocities are directly related to the amplitude of the saccade; in the case of the largest saccades velocities up to 700°/s are attained. Saccades, particularly those made without an accompanying head movement, are a relatively late acquisition in evolution. Their purpose is to bring targets of interest on to the fovea and can be tested at the bedside by asking the subject rapidly to refixate between two targets, usually the examiner's fingers. The clinician can examine various subtypes of saccadic movements by asking the subject to look right–left, up–down; (1) at command (without targets); (2) at the patient's own pace (self-paced) between two fixed targets; or (3) at a sudden presentation of a novel visual target, reinforced verbally or not (Fig. 5.1). Clinical observation suggests a somewhat hierarchic organization of saccadic movements. Incipient neurological disease affecting the cerebral hemispheres will initially involve saccades made at command or spontaneous repetitive refixations between two fixed targets; later on, saccades elicited by visual targets and, finally, fast phases of optokinetic nystagmus may be involved, signalling a progression from a more voluntary, higher-order type of motor control to a more reflexive one. Quick components of vestibular and optokinetic nystagmus are grouped together with saccades because they have the same amplitude/velocity profile and they share the same neural generators.

Saccades are characterized in terms of their velocity, latency and accuracy; recordings are useful but not imperative. The presence of slow saccades usually indicates dysfunction of the pontine (paramedian pontine reticular formation; PPRF) or mesencephalic saccidic generators which are involved in the production of horizontal and vertical saccades respectively. It must be remembered, however, that more peripheral lesions, from the oculomotor nuclei down to the extraocular muscles, can also produce saccadic slowing, particularly in diffuse degenerative processes. Saccades usually consist of one or two refixation steps. If three or more saccades are required to achieve a target they are considered to be hypometric. Whilst hypometric saccades may occur in normal fatigued subjects, they are considered pathological if they predominante in one direction or occur in more than 50% of large refixations. Hypometric saccades tend to occur as a result of lesions involving supranuclear oculomotor pathways anywhere from the cerebral cortex to the superior colliculi, and are often found in disease of the basal ganglia (Troost *et al.*, 1974; Spector and Troost, 1981). Hypermetric saccades are less common than hypometric saccades and are due to cerebellar disease (Fig. 5.2).

There are at least two parallel pathways by which the cortex can generate saccades (Schiller *et al.*, 1980; Leichnetz, 1981). The first originates in the frontal eye fields (Broadman area 8), which receives visual information from the primary visual cortex and the posterior parietal cortex. This pathway projects directly and indirectly, via the ipsilateral superior colliculus, to the reticular saccade generators in the midbrain and pons; some of these indirect projections are now known to reach the colliculus via basal ganglia structures (Fig. 5.3), as will be discussed in more detail in the next section (Hikosaka and Wurtz, 1983). Secondly, there are projections from the posterior parietal cortex to the superior colliculus and paramedian reticular formation. The more anterior, frontocollicular projection is thought to be predominantly concerned with the production of higher-order saccades such as voluntary and predictive saccades and saccades made to remembered targets (Collin *et al.*, 1982; Deng *et al.*, 1986). Parietocollicular projections, on the other hand, are more concerned with the production of reflexive saccades to novel visual stimuli (Tusa *et*

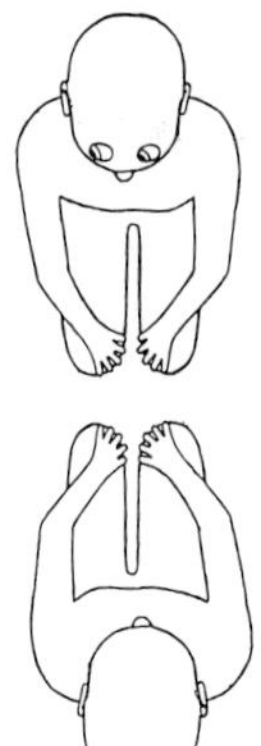

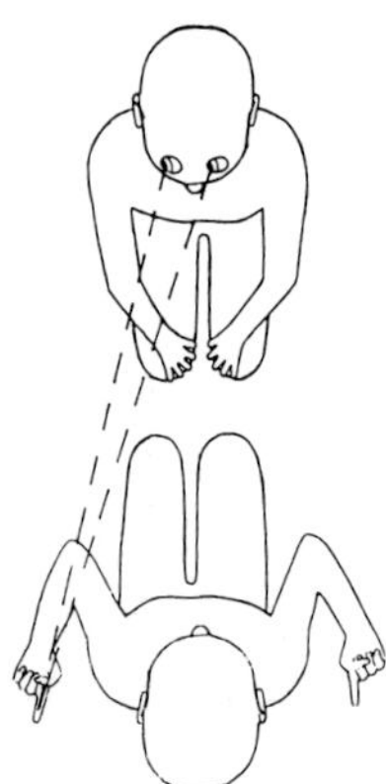

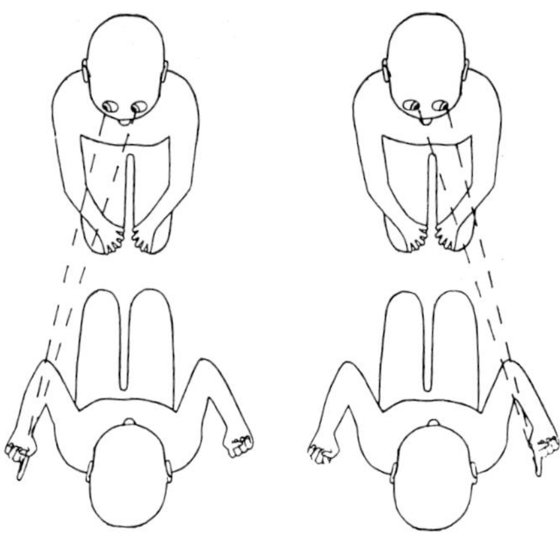

Figure 5.1 Clinical examination of saccades. On command: the examiner is seated facing the patient and, without suggesting any target, asks the patient to look right, pauses, then left, and so on. Self-paced: the examiner's fingers are presented as continuous targets to the right and left of the patient, who is asked to look alternately between them, at his or her own pace, as many times as he or she can. Visually elicited: the examiner shows clenched fists and asks the patient to look at the finger whenever this is clocked up (or when the whole hand opens up, in order to present a large target capable of attracting the patient's attention). The production of visually elicited saccades can be facilitated by simultaneous verbal reinforcement, saying 'right' or 'left' appropriately in the direction in which the patient should look. Incipient cortical or basal ganglia disease predominantly affects saccades on command, self-paced, or other types of voluntary saccades. As disease progresses, or in cerebellar–brainstem lesions, all types of saccades will be more evenly involved.

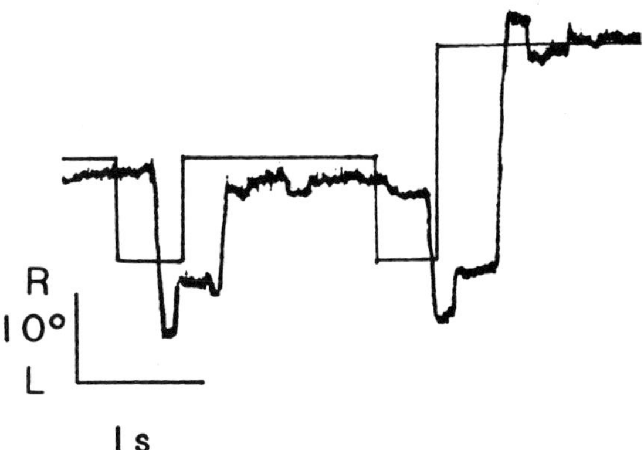

Figure 5.2 Saccadic dysmetria in a patient with cerebellar ectopia. Target trajectory is superimposed upon the electro-oculogram record to facilitate the identification of hypermetric saccades. In contrast to hypometria, which is a less specific finding, hypermetria indicates cerebellar disease.

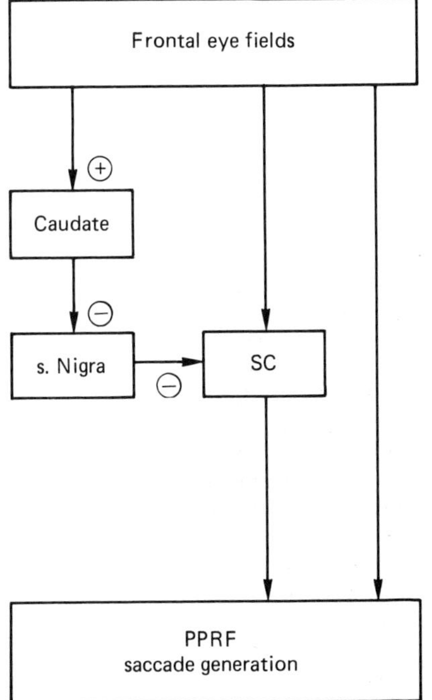

Figure 5.3 Schematic diagram of the anatomical connections from the frontal eye fields to the pontine saccade generators (paramedian pontine recticular formation; PPRF). Although a direct frontal–PPRF pathway exists, most saccades are thought to be mediated via the superior colliculus (SC). Activation of the frontocaudate-nigrocollicular pathway effectively leads to collicular disinhibition, thereby facilitating or triggering saccades. Descending pathways from the posterior parietal cortex (not shown here) also generate saccades via the SC.

al., 1986). All these areas, from the cortex to the reticular formation, are, by definition, supranuclear gaze structures. Saccades are generated by the contralateral cerebral cortex and the ipsilateral PPRF (i.e. a rightward saccade depends on the left hemisphere and the right pons).

Smooth pursuit

Smooth pursuit eye movements are slow eye movements whose purpose is to maintain foveation of slowly moving targets. The gain of the smooth pursuit system refers to the ratio of the peak slow eye movement velocity to the peak target velocity. If pursuit eye velocity fails to match target velocity (i.e. pursuit gain is less than unity), a series of corrective saccades compensate and produce the characteristic 'cogwheel' or broken pursuit pattern. Smooth pursuit may be tested at the bedside by asking the subject carefully to follow a slowly moving target which the patient must be able to see clearly. Smooth pursuit normally exhibits 'catch-up' saccades if target motion excedes a velocity of 30–40°/s or a frequency of 0.5 Hz; therefore, the examiner must be familiar with the normal appearance of visual following. Smooth pursuit gain falls with age, fatigue, drugs and alcohol, but if these are excluded as a cause, a reduced gain is a sensitive, though non-specific sign of central nervous system disease. During clinical or oculographic investigation of smooth pursuit it is crucial to elicit the patient's attention and cooperation; in fact, many 'broken pursuits' become normal with appropriate encouragement and attractive targets.

The pathways involved in smooth pursuit are not well-known and involve widespread cortical, brainstem and cerebellar areas (see Lisberger *et al.*, for review). Crucial structures are the parietal cortex and the cerebellar flocculus; the dorsal lateral pontine nucleus, the pretectal accessory optic system, the dorsal cerebellar vermis and the vestibular nuclei seem to be participate as well. Smooth pursuit is controlled by the ipsilateral cerebral and cerebellar cortex, i.e. 'broken' pursuit to the right may be due to a right parietal or cerebellar lesion.

Vestibulo-ocular reflex (VOR)

Vestibular eye movements are slow-phase eye movements produced in response to head movement, to which they are equal in amplitude and opposite in direction. They maintain images of the surroundings stationary upon the retina during head movements and thus prevent visual blurring. VOR gain refers to the ratio of the peak eye velocity to the peak head velocity; in the light this ratio is normally unity over a large range of frequencies and velocities of head rotation. Hypoactive or hyperactive gains produce a sensation of target movement or blurring during head movement, termed oscillopsia (Bender, 1965; Gresty *et al.*, 1977; Bronstein and Hood, 1987). The VOR is examined clinically at the bedside by having the patient fixate upon the examiner's nose whilst the patient's head is either passively or actively turned (doll's head manoeuvre). If there is any impediment to turn the head upon the shoulders (e.g. neck pain or rigidity), the patient may be oscillated *en bloc* on an ordinary swivel chair (Fig. 5.4). If VOR gain is unity, eye movements will appear smooth to the examiner, without the presence of corrective saccades. In the case of marked hypoactivity of the VOR, careful observation of the patient's eyes whilst

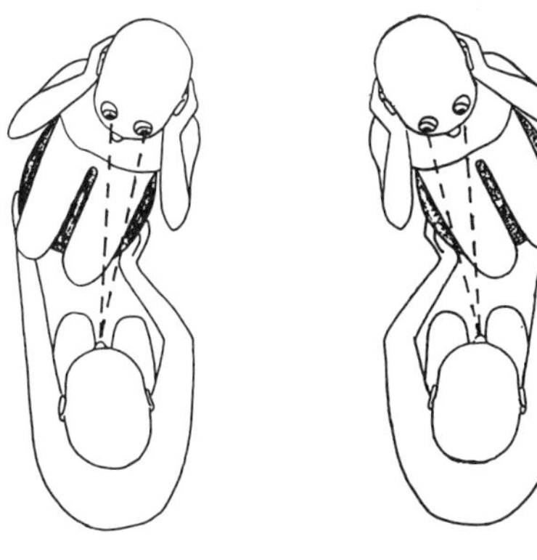

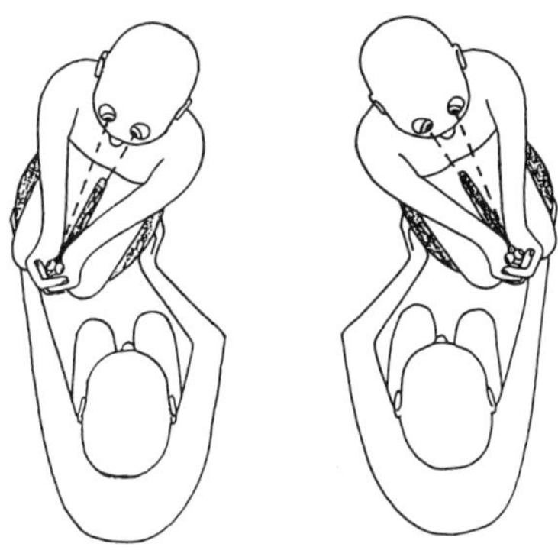

Figure 5.4 Clinical procedure to assess the vestibulo-ocular reflex (VOR) and VOR suppression. The patient is seated on a swivel chair which is oscillated manually by the examiner. During VOR the patient is instructed (and reminded frequently!) to keep fixation on the examiner's nose. In order to avoid spurious head movements during chair oscillation the patient may be asked to hold his or her head with his or her hands. In cooperative patients with good neck mobility, the conventional doll's head manoeuvre achieved by turning the patient's head on his or her shoulders is equally satisfactory. In either case, the examiner looks for improvement in the range of eye excursion in cases of gaze palsy, which would suggest a supranuclear origin, and for small saccades interspersed with the slow-phase VOR, which might indicate abnormal vestibular function. During VOR suppression the patient is asked to fixate his or her own thumbs while keeping the hands clasped in front. The presence of significant nystagmus during low-frequency (<0.3 Hz) oscillation indicates abnormal VOR suppression, a finding usually correlated with the presence of diminished ('broken up') pursuit.

turning will reveal small 'catch-up' saccades in the same direction as the slow-phase eye movement.

An alternative method of examination of the VOR is to oscillate the head whilst viewing the optic fundus with an ophthalmoscope (Zee, 1978). If the gain of the VOR is unity, the fundus will remain stationary; if it is hypoactive it will appear to move in the direction of the head rotation and in the opposite direction if the VOR is hyperactive; corrective saccades will also be evident and in general are easier to detect than the slow retinal drift. If reduced vestibular function is clinically suspected, formal rotational or caloric testing should be carried out. This need not involve complex or expensive equipment since the original caloric technique of Fitzgerald and Hallpike (1942), perhaps complemented with Frenzel's glasses, is perfectly adequate. In some patients with clinically diagnosed multiple system atrophy or cerebellar degenerations, absent vestibular function may not be suspected, yet may contribute to their unsteadiness. Occasionally, in some patients with downward gaze palsy, in whom accompanying neck rigidity does not permit an adequate doll's head manoeuvre, bilateral stimultaneous irrigation of the auditory external meati with cold water (20°C) for about 1 minute is needed in order to overcome the gaze limitation, thus confirming the supranuclear origin of the gaze paresis.

There are many parallel VOR pathways and this may explain the resilience of the VOR to central nervous system disease. The most basic is the disynaptic pathway from the vestibular end-organ to the vestibular nuclei within the brainstem and from there to the third, fourth and sixth nerve nuclei (for review see Precht, 1977, and Wilson and Melvill Jones, 1979). Low gain of the VOR usually signifies bilateral labyrinthine or eighth nerve disease and, more rarely, severe metabolic depression, or structural lesions disrupting intra-brainstem transmission. High VOR gain can occur in cerebellar disease, especially of the vestibulocerebellum (flocculus, nodulus, uvula and paraflocculus) and is thought to depend on loss of tonic inhibition of the cerebellum upon the vestibular nuclei (Baloh *et al.*, 1975; Gresty *et al.*, 1977).

The VOR at times must be suppressed, so that head and eye tracking of moving targets is possible, as it occurs in spectators watching the ball in a tennis match. VOR suppression can be tested clinically by oscillating subjects in a chair whilst they fixate upon the thumbs of their interlaced hands, with arms outstretched (Fig. 5.4). If VOR suppression is impaired the observer will note nystagmic beats in the direction of head motion during rotation, whereas the eyes remain stationary on the target if the VOR is effectively suppressed. VOR suppression is thought for the most part to be mediated through smooth pursuit mechanisms (Barnes, 1988); abnormalities of the two usually occur together (Halmagyi and Gresty, 1979) and in the same direction (i.e. broken pursuit to the right is usually accompanied by abnormal VOR suppression during rightwards rotation).

Optokinetic eye movements

Optokinetic slow-phase eye movements are produced in response to motion of large areas of the visual field. Their function is to aid the VOR to stabilize images on the retina during constant-velocity rotation or during very low-frequency head motion, at which times the VOR does not respond optimally. Frequently, the slow eye movement is interrupted by quick components of nystagmus which reset the eyes close to primary gaze (optokinetic nystagmus, OKN); in fact, the quick components normally take the eyes beyond primary gaze, in the direction of the oncoming visual stimuli (Hood and Leech, 1974). Clinically they can be tested by rotating a striped or dotted drum held in front of the subject. Alternatively, and frequently more effective than the hand-held drum, oscillating a newspaper or magazine in front of the patient's eyes generates good slow-phase eye movements. If one is interested in eliciting nystagmus, however, the patient frequently needs to be instructed simply to glance

Figure 5.5 (a) Optokinetic nystagmus responses in a patient with progressive supranuclear palsy (PSP), illustrating the characteristic deviation of the eyes in the direction of the slow component of nystagmus. The phenomenon is usually best detected during sudden reversal of drum rotation (right side of the figure) because at this point the eyes of normal subjects 'flick' in the direction of the quick component of nystagmus (arrow), whereas the patient's eyes drift slowly in the direction of drum rotation (dotted arrow). Electro-oculographic recordings; top trace indicates motion of a full field drum, each spike corresponding to a 20° interval. (b) Left beating vestibular nystagmus elicited by stopping rightwards whole-body rotation in the same patient as in Figure 5.5a. The nystagmus in the patient is less brisk than in the normal subject and the eyes deviate tonically in the orbit in the direction of the slow component of the nystagmus.

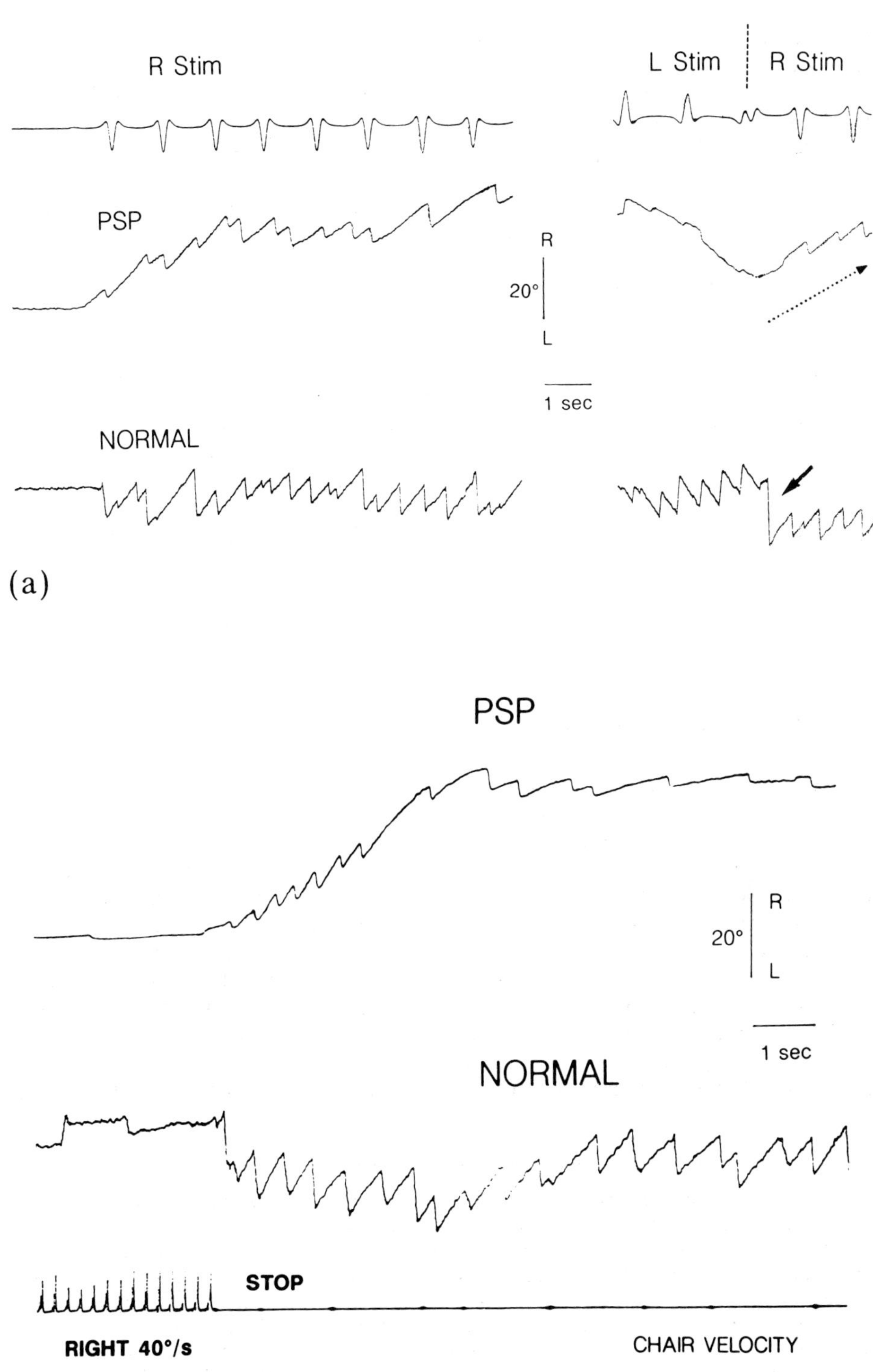
R Stim
L Stim
R Stim
PSP
R
20°
L
1 sec
NORMAL
(a)
PSP
R
20°
L
1 sec
NORMAL
STOP
RIGHT 40°/s
CHAIR VELOCITY
(b)

at what is in front of him/her rather than try to follow a particular word or feature in the page shown.

Optokinetic pathways are widespread in the central nervous system but not known in detail. The parietal and cerebellar (floccular) cortices are important in generating ipsilaterally directed slow-phase optokinetic eye movements (Baloh *et al.*, 1980; Zee *et al.*, 1981; Precht, 1982). Impairment of OKN usually correlates well with impaired smooth pursuit and in general has the same clinical significance, though the two may be affected separately (Barratt *et al.*, 1985). Parietal, brainstem/cerebellar lesions or diffuse central nervous system involvement produces low-velocity, deranged OKN. Unilateral hemispheric lesions may have a twofold effect on OKN by affecting the ipsilateral slow phase and the contralaterally directed quick phase; this usually results in a significant directional preponderance of the nystagmus (defined by the direction of the quick phase) ipsilateral to the lesion. A frequent sign in extrapyramidal disorders, detected during clinical or oculographic examination, is that during optokinetic stimulation the eyes deviate tonically in the direction of the slow component of the nystagmus (Dix *et al.*, 1971), opposite to what occurs in normal individuals, as described above (Fig. 5.5a). Although striking, the finding probably does not reflect a primary optokinetic abnormality but rather defective quick components of nystagmus secondary to a saccadic disorder; this abnormal ocular deviation in the direction of the slow phase in these patients can also be seen during vestibular nystagmus (Fig. 5.5b). This sign is found most frequently and with a greater severity in Steele–Richardson–Olszewski syndrome, but it is not specific of this condition and can be present in other frontal or basal ganglia disorders, in particular those with a supranuclear gaze palsy, whatever its cause.

Vergence eye movements

Vergence eye movements are disjunctive movements which ensure binocular foveal fixation of an object of interest and stereosopic vision. The major stimuli for vergence are retinal blur (accommodative vergence) and a disparity between the position of images on the two retinas, producing diplopia (fusional vergence). In demented or unmotivated patients, one should use the patient's own thumb or nose as a target before establishing that convergence is affected. Failure of convergence (and some limitation of upgaze), however, is common in the elderly, so it is not a very useful sign in patients above the age of 60 years. Within the oculomotor nucleus are neurons which discharge exclusively for vergence (Keller and Robinson, 1972; Mays, 1984; Mays *et al.*, 1986). Premotor neurons involved in vergence are found in the mesencephalic reticular formation dorsolateral to the oculomotor nucleus (Mays, 1984; Judge and Cumming, 1986).

THE ROLE OF THE BASAL GANGLIA IN EYE MOVEMENT CONTROL – A PHYSIOLOGICAL UPDATE

The basal ganglia themselves do not directly control eye movements and have no direct connections with the immediate premotor centres in the brainstem (PPRF), but receive afferents from the frontal eye fields which project to the caudate nucleus (Webster, 1965). The caudate nucleus in turn projects to the substantia nigra reticulata (SNr) and from this structure efferents project to intermediate and deep layers of the superior colliculus (Graybiel, 1978), thus gaining access to a saccadic pathway (Fig. 5.3). Both the caudate–SNr and the SNr–collicular pathways are mediated by gamma-aminobutyric acid (GABA)ergic inhibitory synapses (Vincent *et al.*, 1978). Using single cell recording techniques in primates, Hikosaka and Wurtz (1983) localized subgroups of reticulata saccade-related cells which decreased their firing rate in response to either visual or auditory targets but not both. Visually responsive cells were found to be task-specific: fixation-related cells responded to fixation of a stimulus and also to removal of the visual stimulus, whereas other cells decreased their firing rate only prior to saccades made to a remembered target position. Injections of the GABA agonist muscimol into the SNr of primates disinhibited the superior colliculus, leaving animals unable to maintain fixation and with frequent unwanted saccades which shifted the eyes off the target of interest (Hikosaka and Wurtz, 1985a). Injection of muscimol into the superior colliculus, on the other hand, produced slow hypometric saccades with long latencies, particularly to remembered saccades (Hikosaka and Wurtz, 1985b). The SNr therefore seems tonically to inhibit the superior colliculus and it is thought that the reduction of this tonic inhibition allows saccades to be generated. More recently, it has been demonstrated that cells within the caudate nucleus have saccade-related activity during tasks requiring a memory of target position (Hikosaka *et al.*, 1989). Thus, the experimental evidence suggests that the basal ganglia participate in the generation of saccades made in the context of specific behavioural tasks, especially those requiring visual memory of target position. The role of the basal ganglia in the generation of other types of eye movements is at present unknown, though minor abnormalities in other subtypes of saccades, smooth pursuit and the VOR are found in basal ganglia disease. However, since basal ganglia diseases rarely have pathology confined to these nuclei, it is likely that the more widespread ocular motor involvement in some of these conditions depends on associated pathological changes elsewhere.

EYE MOVEMENTS IN EXTRAPYRAMIDAL DISEASES

Parkinson's disease

A great deal has been written about eye movements in idiopathic Parkinson's disease (PD), in spite of the fact that clinical examination of ocular motility is usually unremarkable.

OCULOGRAPHIC STUDIES

There has been considerable disagreement as to the extent and nature of oculomotor abnormalities in Parkinson's disease. This may have in part resulted from a failure to account for the effect of medications on the eye movements (Shimizu *et al.*, 1977), a lack of age-matched normal controls (Shibasaki *et al.*, 1979) and/or from the inclusion of patients with severe disease and additional central nervous system lesions (White *et al.*, 1983a,b). One of the first quantitative studies of eye movements in PD (Corin, Elizan and Bender, 1972) suggested saccadic dysfunction; saccades made to random visual targets were found to be hypometric but of normal latency and with normal peak velocities. Subsequent studies (Shibasaki *et al.*, 1979; White *et al.*, 1983b), by contrast, reported prolonged latencies and saccadic slowing. Gibson *et al.* (1987) analysed eye movements in mildly affected untreated patients and found saccadic hypometria with normal saccadic velocities and latencies, though the latter showed a greater scatter than in normals. In addition, they found that the saccadic deficit improved in those patients whose other motor skills responded to L-dopa, a finding also noted by Highstein *et al.* (1969) and Rascol *et al.* (1989).

Another possible cause for conflicting results in the study of eye movements in PD may relate to the nature of the experimental conditions used. Using random non-predictive target displacements, few if any abnormalities were found (Bronstein and Kennard, 1985; Gibson *et al.*, 1987), whilst those studies assessing self-paced (Melvill Jones and de Jong, 1971) or predictive saccades (Bronstein and Kennard, 1985) have shown hypometric or delayed saccades (Fig. 5.6). This discrepancy is thought to relate to the different supranuclear pathways subserving saccades, as discussed in the preceding section; the more direct descending projections to the PPRF from the parietal or frontal cortices might mediate the generation of 'reflex' saccades and those via the basal ganglia to the superior colliculus might mediate 'voluntary' saccades. Hypometric saccades in PD may result from increased inhibition of the superior colliculus by the substantia nigra as a consequence of reduced caudate (GABAergic) inhibition of the substantia nigra.

It has long been held that parkinsonian patients have limited upgaze and convergence, though until recently this was based on the study of very few patients. Tanyeri *et al.* (1989) found that mild to moderately affected patients had normal horizontal and vertical saccades to a 'reflex' target, and only one patient had limitation of upgaze when compared to age-matched controls. This is in agreement with the clinical impression that limitation of upgaze in Parkinson's disease represents, in the main, an age-related phenomenon. The presence of a significant limitation of upgaze and slowing of vertical saccades, especially if present early in the course of the disease, should suggest an alternative diagnosis such as progressive supranuclear palsy.

Smooth pursuit in PD has frequently been reported to be of reduced gain (Melvill Jones and Mandl, 1976; White *et al.*, 1983b), but the abnormality described is only mild and pursuit has been found within normal limits in other studies (Bronstein and Kennard, 1985). There does however seem to be a correlation between limb bradykinesia and smooth pursuit abnormalities, suggesting that the basal ganglia may be implicated more directly in this ocular motor function (Gibson and Kennard 1986; Gibson *et al.*, 1987). The VOR in PD has been found to have a low gain in

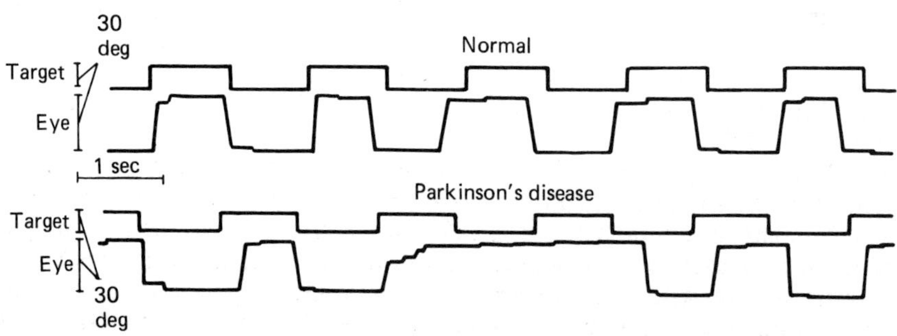

Figure 5.6 Saccadic eye movements in a patient with idiopathic Parkinson's disease and in an age-matched normal subject, during regular (predictive) motion of a target. The patient does not anticipate target motion regularly and on one occasion 'freezes' and produces a multiple-step hypometric saccade. Infrared recording; upward deflection indicates rightward motion. From Bronstein and Kennard (1985), with permission.

patients with advanced disease (White *et al.*, 1983a), though this is not a consistent finding (Teravainen and Calne, 1980). Hypoactive caloric responses have also been found, particularly in patients with postural instability (Reichert *et al.*, 1982). However, a cautious interpretation of results from vestibulo-ocular tests in the more severely affected patients is needed since vestibular nystagmus is profoundly affected by the level of alertness, a factor which is difficult to control when testing severely affected patients in the dark. An abnormal interaction between foveal and peripheral retinal visual information during pursuit and VOR suppression has been reported in parkinsonian patients (Hood and Waniewski, 1984). OKN has been found to be variably hypoactive or normal in PD, sometimes with deviation of the eyes in the direction of the slow component (Shibasaki *et al.*, 1979; Hood and Waniewski, 1984).

In addition to the above, a number of higher-order oculomotor abnormalities have been found in patients with PD. Flowers and Downing (1978) found that parkinsonian patients made hand-tracking errors of a moving target, especially when a predictive motor strategy was required, but failed to demonstrate a predictive deficiency in an ocular motor tracking task. They concluded that only the limbs show a predictive abnormality in PD. This issue was taken up by Bronstein and Kennard (1985), who confirmed that PD patients were able to make adequate predictive smooth pursuit eye movements, but demonstrated abnormal delay in the generation of saccades made to targets moving in a predictive manner. Patients were able to reduce their saccadic latencies during 'hidden' predictive sequences, but were not able to do so any further when instructed that the target would move in a predictive manner from the outset. Dejong and Melvill Jones (1971) found that parkinsonian patients were also unable to make regular self-paced saccades between two stationary visual targets, the saccades becoming increasingly hypometric and the eyes remaining longer than normal on each target before being able to make a refixation. Studies have also reported abnormalities of saccades when these were specifically made to remembered targets (Crawford *et al.*, 1989; Lueck *et al.*, 1990). These observations may be explained by reduced caudate inhibition of the SNr, producing increased inhibition of the superior colliculus, or by the presence of abnormal fronto-basalganglia interaction in PD.

CLINICAL OVERVIEW

From the best-controlled clinical studies it would seem that in the vast majority of patients with PD abnormalities of ocular movements are confined to specific higher-order types of saccades, such as self-paced, predictive and remembered saccades; more reflexive visually elicited saccades and other subsystems of eye movements are normal or only mildly involved. These findings would agree with what single cell studies in animals suggest as a possible role of the basal ganglia in oculomotor control.

The profusion of experimental literature to date has served to confuse rather than clarify the clinical problem of knowing how abnormal eye movements can be in a patient with a parkinsonian syndrome, before an alternative diagnosis to idiopathic PD should be contemplated. We believe that during clinical examination there usually is very little wrong with eye movements in a moderately affected PD patient, particularly if one keeps in mind that a mild degree of hypometria during saccades, 'broken up' pursuit, convergence and upgaze limitation are common findings in the normal elderly population. Some severely affected PD patients may show degrees of saccadic hypometria or broken pursuit, together with some deviation in the direction of the slow component during OKN, which clinically seems outside the normal range for their age. However, clinically significant slowing of saccades and limitations of gaze in any plane, apart from some moderate upgaze deficit, should evoke alternative diagnoses such as Steele–Richardson–Olszewski or multiple system atrophy. It must be admitted, however, that these clinical conclusions are hampered by the lack of personal or published experience correlating detailed oculomotor examinations with pathological studies in large numbers of patients with Parkinson's symptoms.

Huntington's disease

Huntington's disease (HD) is an inherited autosomal dominant disorder in which there is degeneration in the caudate, substantia nigra pars reticulata and frontal lobes with normal or raised levels of striatal dopamine. It is therefore an ideal condition with which to compare the eye movements of PD. From the first studies of Starr (1967), a predilection for involvement of the saccadic system with relative preservation of smooth pursuit was found, and was later confirmed by Petit and Milbled (1973). Patients with HD were found to have great difficulty initiating voluntary saccades without the use of head thrusts and/or frequent eye blinks, similar to those seen in congenital ocular motor apraxia (Leigh *et al.*, 1983). Saccadic latencies were prolonged and saccades were hypometric and occasionally slow. Vertical saccades were more severely affected than horizontal saccades in all respects (Petit and Milbled, 1973).

Clinical observation had suggested that patients with an earlier age of onset tended to have more severe ocular motor abnormalities than patients with late-onset disease. This was supported by a study of Lasker *et al.* (1988) who found that patients with onset of disease before the age of 30 had a high incidence of saccadic slowing but the velocity was normal in those in whom the disease began after the age of 30. Older-onset patients on the other hand had prolonged latencies. In addition, Huntingtonian patients were noted to have difficulty suppressing spontaneous saccades and saccades made to novel visual stimuli. Prominent square wave jerks were seen to intrude upon smooth pursuit and other forms of eye movement. Patients had great difficulty maintaining fixation upon any specific target and were unable to inhibit saccades to novel visual stimuli in the periphery of vision (Avanzini *et al.*, 1979). In addition patients were unable to make saccades in a direction opposite to a novel visual stimulus (antisaccades).

Dysfunction of the basal ganglia and frontal lobes is thought to be responsible for the combination of ocular motor disturbances seen in HD. The prominent fixational instability is thought to be due either to loss of frontal inhibition of the superior colliculi or to a reduction of GABAergic inhibition of the substantia nigra reticulata upon the superior colliculi. Inability to suppress saccades and saccadic distractibility have been found in humans following frontal lobe lesions (Guitton *et al.*, 1982). The cause of saccadic slowing in HD is not known; slow saccades usually indicate dysfunction of the reticular generators, though pathological studies of the midbrain and pons have failed to demonstrate abnormalities in HD (Leigh *et al.*, 1985).

Steele–Richardson–Olszewski syndrome

This condition, also known as progressive supranuclear palsy, was first described in 1964 by Steele, Richardson and Olszewski. The typical ocular motor abnormality initially involves vertical saccades which first become hypometric and then slow;

downgaze being affected relatively early (David *et al.*, 1968). Involvement of upgaze and convergence usually follow before horizontal saccades become affected. Smooth pursuit eye movements are relatively preserved but may become severely affected in the late stages of the disease (Troost and Daroff, 1977; Chu *et al.*, 1979). Eye movements induced by the oculocephalic manoeuvre are intact even when there is virtual absence of other voluntary eye movements, and it is this characteristic that makes the disorder supranuclear. An early though non-specific finding is the presence of gaze instability with frequent square wave jerks (involuntary saccades with a normal intersaccadic interval) which take the eyes off the target of interest and intrude upon smooth pursuit (Troost and Daroff, 1977). The VOR (Troost and Daroff, 1977) and OKN have variably been found to be of low gain. As the main abnormality remains within the saccadic system, OKN, rotational and caloric stimuli typically produce a tonic drift of the eyes in the direction of the slow phase (Dix *et al.*, 1971), as shown in Figure 5.5. With time patients may develop internuclear and nuclear involvement (Mastaglia and Grainger, 1975), with loss of the oculocephalic responses and of Bell's phenomenon.

Although the above ocular motor abnormalities are the hallmark of the condition, there are, however, pathologically proven cases of Steele–Richardson–Olszewski syndrome with normal eye movements (Dubas *et al.*, 1983) and cases where they only developed late in the course of the illness (Perkin *et al.*, 1978). Furthermore, the oculomotor disturbances are not specific and should be taken in the context of the clinical picture as a whole. Focal lesions and animal studies point to the rostral mesencephalic reticular formation in the prerubral fields (the rostral interstitial nucleus of the medial longitudinal fasciculus) as the site responsible for selective downgaze palsy (Kompf *et al.*, 1979; Buttner-Ennever *et al.*, 1989); whilst the impairment of downward saccades in progressive supranuclear palsy probably reflects involvement of such areas, pathologically the degenerative changes are too widespread to ascribe any particular ocular motor abnormality to the basal ganglia *per se*.

Wilson's disease

Most reviews suggest that eye movement disturbances are not prominent in Wilson's disease (Walshe, 1976; Sternlieb *et al.*, 1987). Various ocular motor abnormalities have been described however and include "jerky oscillations of the eye movements", involuntary upgaze, paresis of upgaze and slowed saccades with relative preservation of smooth pursuit and vestibular responses (Kirkham and Kamin, 1974). Goldberg and Van Noorden (1966) have in addition described an accommodative paresis. Gaze distractibility, noted by Wilson himself in his original description (Wilson, 1954), has been confirmed by Lennox and Jones (1989), who suggested that this was due more to frontal lobe dysfunction than to the basal ganglia. Smooth pursuit can also be moderately affected, as shown in Figure 5.7 from a patient with Wilson's disease with cerebellar signs. The saccadic abnormalities may respond to treatment with penicillamine (Kirkham and Kamin, 1974; Harbour *et al.*, 1988).

Niemann–Pick's disease type C (juvenile dystonic lipidosis)

This autosomal recessive condition presents with early jaundice and a failure to thrive, followed by a progressive ataxia, dystonia, dementia and a vertical

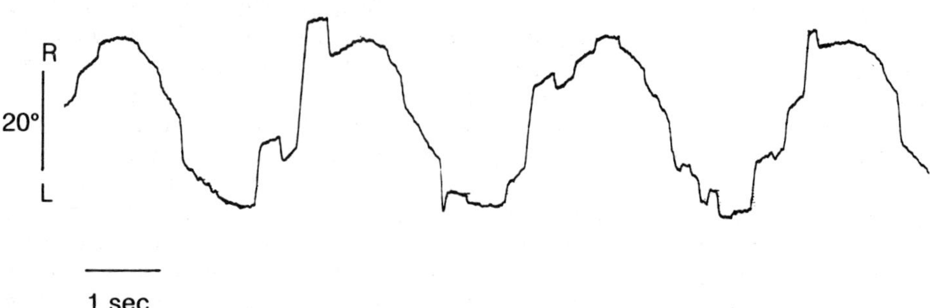

Figure 5.7 Eye movements (electro-oculogram) in a patient with Wilson's disease, including prominent cerebellar signs whilst following a target moving sinusoidally at 0.3 Hz. Slow-phase eye movement velocity is not adequate to match target velocity and is 'intruded' upon by square wave jerks and saccades.

supranuclear ophthalmoplegia (Norman *et al.*, 1967; Neville *et al.*, 1973). The exact classification and pathophysiologic characteristics are still controversial. In this variant, as opposed to Niemann–Pick types A and B, there are normal or only slightly reduced levels of sphyngomyelinase activity with only moderate neuronal sphyngomyelin accumulation. Niemann–Pick type C is a clinically heterogeneous disease with a wide variation of phenotypes from a neonatal rapidly fatal form to an adult form. One particular phenotype, reported by Cogan *et al.* (1981), consists of the triad of a downgaze paralysis, ataxia and athetosis and foam cells in the spleen liver and bone marrow (DAF syndrome). A supranuclear downgaze paresis is the most distinctive feature of the condition and may be one of the earliest signs of the disorder, though eventually, upgaze and horizontal eye movements become affected in addition.

Gilles de la Tourette syndrome

Gilles de la Tourette syndrome is characterized by multiple motor and vocal tics, and a variety of behavioural disturbances (Lees, 1985). The disorder is inherited through a sex-influenced autosomal dominant mode inheritance with variable expressivity. Pathological examinations of three brains have not revealed any specific abnormalities (reviewed in Lees 1985).

Blepharospasm and forced gaze deviation have been described in this syndrome and it is these findings which, in part, have prompted suggestions that the condition may be due to dysfunction of the basal ganglia (Frankel and Cummings, 1984). Despite the above, Bollen *et al.* (1988) were not able to find any abnormalities of saccades, smooth pursuit or fixation in 28 children with Tourette syndrome although remembered and predictive saccades were not studied.

Corticobasal degeneration

This condition was first described by Rebeiz *et al.* (1967) in 3 patients with a progressive movement disorder showing frontoparietal atrophy with cortical cell loss, Pick cells without Pick bodies and degeneration and gliosis in the thalamus and basal ganglia. The illness began in late adult life with either focal dystonia, myoclonus, and pain involving one arm which often moved involuntarily (alien limb), or alternatively as an akinetic–rigid parkinsonian syndrome. Eye movement abnormalities have been described in this condition (Gibb *et al.*, 1989; Riley *et al.*, 1990), but no quantitative studies have been reported. The abnormalities described are of a vertical and horizontal supranuclear gaze palsy, often with prominent eye blinks to facilitate saccade generation but no head thrusting. In patients studied by the authors (without pathology) there was difficulty in generating saccades to command, particularly without a target, and with marked hypometricity of the saccade that were able to be generated. These findings are more marked in the direction of the more severely affected limbs. Eye blinks and head thrusts were not utilized. Reflex saccades were relatively well-preserved. Smooth pursuit was of low gain, in some patients particularly whilst following the target in a direction opposite to that of the more involved limbs. This crossed disorder of pursuit and saccades found in some of these patients is explained by the fact that one cerebral hemisphere controls contralateral saccades and ipsilateral pursuit. Whilst similar oculomotor picture could be produced by a variety of unilateral hemispheric lesions (e.g. vascular, tumours); however, in the clinical context of a progressive movement disorder, this pattern of eye movement is quite typical of corticobasal degeneration.

Multiple system atrophy

Under the name multiple system atrophy, three progressive, non-familial neurological syndromes, with an apparently similar neuropathological picture, have been described. These patients may present with an akinetic–rigid syndrome with autonomic features (Shy–Drager-type), an akinetic–dystonic syndrome (striatonigral degeneration-type) or as a complex cerebellar degeneration (olivopontocerebellar atrophy or OPCA-type), although in the later stages these clinical syndromes tend to merge. Cell loss and gliosis occur in a number of sites, the emphasis depending on the phenotypic variant, but include the basal ganglia, inferior olives, pontine nuclei, cerebellar Purkinje cells, intermediolateral columns of the spinal cord and Onuf's nucleus. Though once thought to be rare, it has been estimated to make up approximately 10% of cases of parkinsonism in the UK (Quinn, 1989).

Oculomotor abnormalities are prominent in this condition (Berciano, 1982) but to date no detailed eye movement studies have appeared in the literature; no doubt the difficulty in ascertaining the diagnosis in the absence of pathological confirmation has delayed such a study. With this proviso our personal experience in cases with suspected multiple system atrophy includes the finding of supranuclear palsies in the form of mild limitations of gaze overcome by the doll's head manoeuvre, moderate saccadic slowing and hypometria. This disorder of gaze may occur in any direction i.e. without preference for downgaze, unlike Steele–Richardson–Olszewski syndrome, although this statement may reflect some reluctance of the authors to label supranuclear palsies which look typical of Steele–Richardson–Olszewski syndrome as multiple system atrophy and vice versa. Once again the issue awaits pathological verification. Features which help to distinguish between multiple system atrophy and other extrapyramidal disorders with supranuclear palsy are the presence of disproportionate impairment of slow-phase eye movements (smooth pursuit, optokinetic and vestibulo-ocular suppression) and the presence of gaze paretic or down-beating nystagmus – all signs indicating the concomitant involvement of cerebellar structures in multiple system atrophy, particularly of the OPCA type. It is of note, however, that in a recent series of 10 patients with pathologically proven striatonigral degeneration, in whom cerebellar signs were not conspicuous, eye movements were not reported either as abnormal or useful in distinguishing between this condition and idiopathic Parkinson's disease (Fearnley and Lees, 1990). Some patients with clinical diagnosis of multiple system atrophy show absent vestibular responses to caloric and rotational stimuli (Bronstein *et al*., 1991).

Neuroacanthocytosis

Neuroacanthocytosis is a disorder characterized by a progressive neurological illness associated with acanthocytes in the peripheral blood and a normal lipoprotein profile. In most patients the illness begins in the fourth and fifth decades. Prominent chorea, dystonia and tics with a particular involvement of orofacial structures are characteristic (Hardie, 1989). The pattern of inheritance has not yet been clearly defined but several families have been reported in which two or more members are affected (Levine *et al*., 1968; Vance *et al*., 1987). The eye movements in neuroacanthocytosis have not been characterized but in 2 cases examined personally by the authors the major findings were gaze distractibility and difficulty in generating saccades to command, similar to the findings in HD. In addition, episodic forced gaze deviations of the eyes were noted in 1 of the patients.

Primary dystonia

There have not been systematic studies of eye movements in idiopathic generalized dystonia, probably because they appear to be normal during routine clinical examination. Some forms of focal dystonia described below (torticollis and blepharospasm) and dystonia as part of more general motor disorders have received more attention.

SPASMODIC TORTICOLLIS (ST)

Idiopathic spasmodic torticollis is the most common form of focal primary dystonia. As with other forms of primary dystonia the pathology is unknown, but is assumed to involve the basal ganglia, as it may be produced by lesions and disorders affecting these structures (Rothwell and Obeso, 1987). No gross abnormality of eye movements is found on clinical examination. Occasionally a patient may have a first-degree, low-amplitude nystagmus contralateral to the torticollis, i.e. a patient with chin rotated to the right may have nystagmus on left gazes and with electrooculography in the dark this is not an uncommon finding (Bronstein and Rudge, 1986). Smooth pursuit is essentially normal; OKN is occasionally of higher region contralateral to the torticollis. Saccadic function, including remembered, predictive and self-paced saccades, is normal (Stell *et al*., 1990).

A possible link between the vestibular system and spasmodic torticullis has been suggested for over 70 years (Barre, 1929), based on clinical observations of isolated cases of 'otogenic' spasmodic torticollis and supported by lesion/stimulation studies of the vestibular pathways producing abnormal head postures (see Bronstein and Rudge, 1988, for review). Also suggestive is that the degree of torticollis can frequently be modified by body and head tilt and by turning when walking (Denny-Brown, 1968; Bronstein *et al.*, 1987). Subtle abnormalities of vestibular function had been noted in the past (Svien and Cody, 1969), usually consisting of spontaneous nystagmus in the dark and asymmetries of the caloric responses, but these were not usually emphasized (Matthews *et al.*, 1978). During caloric test, approximately one-third of patients in the light and two-thirds in the absence of fixation show an asymmetry of induced vestibular nystagmus with a preponderance in a direction opposite to that of the torticollis (Bronstein and Rudge, 1986); similar percentages were found during rotational tests. Stell *et al.* (1989) confirmed the above findings and demonstrated that the asymmetry of vestibular function was not simply the result of the abnormal head position as it persisted after correction of the head posture with botulinum toxin. Other studies in normal subjects (Bronstein and Hood, 1986) and in patients (Bronstein and Rudge, 1988; Stell *et al.*, 1991) demonstrated that an asymmetry of the cervical input to the balance centres could not explain the vestibular asymmetry, suggesting that the abnormalities found in spasmodic torticollis probably reflected a primary central bias of the mechanisms controlling head and eye position. At the present time it is felt that the vestibular asymmetry in spasmodic torticollis results from dysfunction of the basal ganglia or mesencephalic nuclei with which they communicate and which are important for the coordination of eye and head movement, such as the interstitial nucleus of Cajal. Lesions of this structure in animals have been noted to produce abnormal head and eye postures (Hassler and Hess, 1954; Fukushima *et al.*, 1985; Fukushima-Kudo *et al.*, 1987).

BLEPHAROSPASM

Blepharospasm can occur in structural lesions of the basal ganglia and brainstem, in 1-methyl-4-phenyl-1,2,3,6-tetrahydropyridine (MPTP)-induced human parkinsonism or as an isolated finding, in which case it is grouped as an idiopathic focal dystonia (Jankovic and Ford, 1983; Keane and Young, 1985; Kulisevski *et al.*, 1988). Clinical examination of ocular movements in idiopathic blepharospasm is unremarkable. There are obvious technical difficulties and possible artefacts when recording eye movements in essential blepharospasm. In a study in which the magnetic search eye coil technique was used to investigate visually elicited saccades, reduced accuracy of horizontal saccades, reduced peak velocity of large downward saccades and a general prolongation in latencies were found (Lueck *et al.*, 1990). In another study, using a video-based Purkinje image tracking system, visually elicited and remembered horizontal saccades were measured (Hotson and Boman, 1991); both types of saccades were equally found to have increased latencies and incresed variability in latencies but normal accuracy and peak velocities. The general conclusion from these studies was that the findings would be compatible with basal ganglia dysfunction, but probably not involving the substantia nigra pars reticulata, which is thought to be particularly involved in remembered saccades. It was argued that, although several patients had received botulinum toxin treatment, this was not the cause of the abnormal findings because the toxin would have induced saccadic slowing, rather than increased latency.

Ataxia telangiectasia

Ataxia telangiectasia (AT) is an autosomal recessive disorder characterized by cutaneous and conjunctival telangiectasia and a progressive neurological syndrome comprising choreoathetosis, myoclonus, cerebellar ataxia, peripheral neuropathy and abnormal eye movements (Louis-Bar, 1941; Sedgwick and Boder, 1972). Some 10–20% of patients develop malignancy, and survival beyond the third decade is unusual. Ataxia telangiectasia is clinically heterogeneous, with several of the above features being absent in any one patient, including the telangiectasia.

The eye movements in AT are severely impaired; the abnormality consisting of the combination of an impairment in the production of saccades and cerebellar ocular motor disturbances (Boder and Sedgwick, 1958; Smith and Cogan, 1959; Balon *et al.*, 1978; Stell *et al.*, 1989). All patients studied by the authors had extreme difficulty in generating saccades with the head fixed, so that head thrusts were often used. Those saccades which were produced were of increased latency and extremely hypometric but with normal peak velocities. Reflex saccades were equally impaired during optokinetic and vestibular stimulation, the eyes drifting in the direction of the slow phase of the induced nystagmus. This abnormality is similar to that present in congenital oculomotor apraxia (Cogan, 1952), although the head thrusts are not so pronounced. Congenital oculomotor apraxia affects only horizontal saccades whereas in ataxia telangiectasia both vertical and horizontal saccades are impaired. More importantly, patients with ataxia telangiectasia show, in addition to the above, typical cerebellar eye movement abnormalities: gaze evoked, rebound and down-beating nystagmus, impaired smooth pursuit, OKN and VOR suppression. A finding not previously noted, but present in 2 of our 4 patients, was periodic alternating nystagmus, a rare form of cerebellar nystagmus which alternates in direction in a regular fashion with cycles of between 120 and 720 seconds (Stell *et al.*, 1989). The combination of ocular motor abnormalities described is highly characteristic of ataxia telangiectasia and its presence should suggest the diagnosis even in the absence of other typical features of the disease.

AN ATTEMPTED CLINICAL SUMMARY

It may be useful to try to group the ocular motor signs encountered in patients with movement disorders into a few basic syndromes, namely supranuclear, apraxic, cerebellar, vestibular and pontomesencephalic. These syndromes may overlap with each other according to the structures impaired by each particular disease; for instance, in a 'pure' cerebellar degeneration the ocular motor findings would be relatively straightforward, whereas if in addition to cerebellar eye signs a supranuclear palsy and slow horizontal saccades were detected, a diagnosis of OPCA or multiple system atrophy should be considered. The following guidelines could be of some use as a general operational scheme:

1. The syndrome of *supranuclear gaze palsy* needs some clarification. The first point is to restrict the term to saccadic deficits only, i.e. by definition broken or even absent pursuit should not be considered gaze palsy. Secondly, it must be remembered that the term supranuclear palsy has a particularly vague connotation in the oculomotor system, since there are a number of parallel and serial structures involved in the generation of saccades above the level of the oculomotor nuclei.

This is in contrast to the somatomotor system where palsies can only be of the lower or upper motoneuron type. Accordingly, there is considerable variation as to how supranuclear lesions manifest themselves since lesions are not necessarily discrete but frequently involve several structures, from the cerebral cortex down to the brainstem reticular generators. Regarded in this way, a supranuclear gaze paresis would include, schematically listed in order of increasing severity: hypometric 'multiple-step' saccades, difficulties in initiating saccades, slowing of saccades, tonic deviation of the eyes in the direction of the slow component of nystagmus during OKN and, finally, limitations of gaze – improved somewhat by pursuit and OKN and significantly by the doll's head manoeuvre. Clinical use of the term supranuclear gaze palsy, however, is usually reserved for this latter stage and as such it tends to neglect the existing continuum preceding it. Such a continuum is not only due to progression of the pathological process but can also be seen as a reversible functional situation, as exemplified in patients with idiopathic PD who can develop a transient supranuclear gaze palsy during an intercurrent infection (Guiloff *et al.*, 1980). Although the palsy may show a preference for a certain direction of gaze (i.e. downward gaze in Steele–Richardson–Olszewski syndrome), as a general rule, all directions will become involved, in varying degrees, as disease progressses.

The following conditions may show features of a supranuclear palsy: progressive supranuclear palsy (Steele–Richardson–Olszewski), multiple system atrophy (OPCA type, Shy–Drager, striatonigral degeneration), adult Niemann–Pick disease, Diffuse Lewy body disease (Lewis and Gawel, 1990; Fearnley *et al.*, 1991) and less often in Wilson's disease, severe PD, corticobasal degeneration and the choreas (HD and neuroacanthocytosis).

2. *Apraxic syndrome*, in which subjects manifest difficulty in initiating saccades. As in other apraxias, the deficit is greater when the movement to be executed is self or internally initiated rather than reflexive, as with self-paced saccades, for saccades generated under these conditions are hypometric. If there is adequate neck mobility, head thrust may be used as this frequently improves gaze transference. Blinks are also used to release fixation, frequently at the beginning of a head thrust. Reflexive 'non-voluntary' saccades, as well as quick components of nystagmus, are relatively spared. There may be associated difficulty in inhibiting spontaneous saccade which will appear as gaze impersistence or gaze distractibility. Although frontal (premotor) or fronto-basal ganglia connections are thought to be involved in acquired oculomotor apraxia (Pierrot-Deseilligny *et al.*, 1988) the lesion responsible for the pure syndrome of congenital oculomotor apraxia in children is not established (Fielder *et al.*, 1986). Head thrusts with oculomotor apraxia can be found in ataxia telangiectasia (with saccades of normal speed and a florid cerebellar ocular motor syndrome) and in HD (frequently with slow saccades). Many extrapyramidal disorders, particularly in the early stages, show apraxic features in the oculomotor system without compensatory head thrusts. Selective difficulty in generating saccades to command, to remembered targets, and with self-paced and anticipatory saccades, implies a high-order deficit akin to apraxia in the broad sense of the term. In this sense, the subtle oculomotor disorder in PD and the earliest stage of most supranuclear palsies, as in Steele–Richardson–Olszewski syndrome, multiple system atrophy, corticobasal degeneration, can be considered apraxic.
3. *Pontomesencephalic syndrome*, in which, either as a result of a generalized atrophic process or secondary to selective reticular degeneration, the saccadic generators for

horizontal saccades (pons), vertical saccades (midbrain), or both are involved, resulting in a significant slowing of saccades. Combined degeneration of various structures, e.g. nigrocollicular-pontine, and direct nuclear or muscular involvement may also result in slowed saccades (Mizutani *et al.*, 1988). Slow saccades can be seen in later stages of disorders with supranuclear palsies, such as Steele–Richardson–Olszewski syndrome, Wilson's disease, multiple system atrophy and HD. In some forms of hereditary type of spinocerebellar degeneration, such as that described by Wadia and Swami (1971), the slowing is extreme (Zee *et al.*, 1976).

4. *Cerebellar eye syndrome*: typically, this syndrome affects slow-phase eye movements and eccentric gaze-holding mechanisms: deranged smooth pursuit, OKN, VOR suppression and gaze paretic nystagmus and down-beat nystagmus can occur. These signs are thought to depend on flocculonodular (archicerebellum, vestibulocerebellum) involvement. Saccadic dysmetria may also occur; hypermetric saccades being a specific sign of a cerebellar (dorsal vermis) lesion (Fig. 5.2), though less common than the slow-phase abnormalities. Square wave jerks may have a cerebellar origin and are almost always present in cases with ocular dysmetria; the opposite does not hold true, in that square waves can be seen in the absence of cerebellar disease or ocular dysmetria. Cerebellar eye signs in varying degrees can occur in a variety of sporadic or hereditary cerebellar degenerations, multiple system atrophy (particularly in OPCA type), Wilson's disease (not severe) and ataxia telangiectasia.
5. *Asymmetry of the VOR* can be frequently detected in patients with spasmodic torticollis by rotational or caloric tests, usually with the fast phases of nystagmus more active in the direction of occipital deviation. Occasionally, in cases with marked vestibular asymmetry, a low-amplitude nystagmus can be seen when the patient looks in the direction opposite to the chin deviation; in such cases OKN can be slightly more active in the direction of the occipital deviation.

   Absent nystagmic responses to caloric and rotational stimuli can occur in clinically diagnosed cases of multiple system atrophy and in familial cerebellar degenerations. This may be suspected clinically by careful inspection of the eye during the doll's head manoeuvre, when small catch-up saccades in the opposite direction of head motion interrupt the slow-phase eye movement.

CONCLUSION

Whilst it is clear that eye movements are disturbed in many basal ganglia disorders, in most conditions pathological changes extend outside the basal ganglia so that interpretation of the oculomotor findings in relation to the function of the basal ganglia is limited. Two possible exceptions are PD and, to some extent, HD, in which there are relatively circumscribed pathological changes within the basal ganglia. The study of these two clinically contrasting conditions, supported by experimental work in animals, strongly suggests that the basal ganglia are important for the production of saccades contingent upon specific experimental conditions. It is apparent that tasks requiring memory of previous target positions (remembered and predictive saccades) are dependent on basal ganglia integrity via fronto-caudato-nigro-collicular projections. In addition the basal ganglia are important, at least in part, for the suppression of unwanted saccades to novel visual stimuli.

It might be appropriate to conclude by reminding ourselves that there are fundamental anatomical and physiological differences between the somatomotor and the oculomotor systems and that such differences are likely to underly the often impressive differential involvement of one or the other by disease. Whilst patients can be devastated by parkinsonian or dystonic symptoms, the oculomotor physiologist often has to resort to the 'magnifying glass' of sophisticated recording techniques and complicated experimental paradigms in the search for eye signs in such diseases. The positive side of this approach is that such studies have provided some insight into the function of these structures and has aided in the clearer definition of several of the disorders.

Acknowledgements

We are grateful to the Dystonia Foundation for financial support for Dr Stell, to our colleagues at the National Hospital for referring their patients for examination, and to Prof. C. D. Marsden, Dr S. S. Mossman and Dr T. Anderson for useful comments on the manuscript. Special thanks to Miss Teresa Metcalfe for drawing Figures 5.1 and 5.4.

References

Avanzini G, Girotti F, Caraceni T, and Spreafico R (1979) Oculomotor disorders in Huntington's chorea. *J Neurol Neurosurg Psychiatry*, **42**, 581–9

Baloh RW and Honrubia V (1990) *Clinical Neurophysiology of the Vestibular System*, Philadelphia, F.A. Davis

Baloh, RW, Konrad HR, and Honrubia V (1975) Vestibulo-ocular function in patients with cerebellar atrophy. *Neurology*, **25**, 160–8

Baloh RW, Yee RD, and Boder E (1978) Eye movements in ataxia-telangiectasia. *Neurology*, **28**, 1099–104

Baloh RW, Yee SD, and Honrubia V (1980) Optokinetic nystagmus and parietal lobe lesions. *Ann Neurol*, **7**, 269–76

Barnes GR (1988) Head–eye co-ordination: visual and nonvisual mechanisms of VOR slow-phase modification. *Prog Brain Res*, **76**, 319–28

Barratt H, Gresty MA, and Page NGR (1985) Neurological evidence for dissociation of pursuit and optokinetic systems. *Acta Otolaryngol* (*Stockh*), **100**, 89–97

Barre JA (1929) Le torticollis spasmodique. *Rev Neurol* (*Paris*), **I**, 984–1013

Bender MB (1965) Oscillopsia. *Arch Nerol*, **13**, 204–13

Berciano J (1982) Olivopontocerebellar atrophy – a review of 117 cases. *J Neurol Sci*, **53**, 253–72

Boder E and Sedgwick RP (1958) Ataxia telangiectasia: a familial syndrome of progressive cerebellar ataxia, oculocutaneous telangiectasia and frequent pulmonary infection. *Paediatrics*, **21**, 526–54

Bollen EL, Roos RAC, Cohen AP, Minderra RB, Reulen JPH, Van De Wetering BJM *et al.* (1988) Oculomotor control in Gilles de la Tourette syndrome. *J Neurol Neurosurg Psychiatry*, **51**, 1981–3

Bronstein AM and Hood JD (1986) The cervico-ocular reflex in normal subjects and patients with absent vestibular function. *Brain Res*, **373**, 399–408

Bronstein AM and Hood JD (1987) Oscillopsia of peripheral vestibular origin. Central and cervical compensatory mechanisms, *Acta Otolaryngol* (*Stockh*), **104**, 307–14

Bronstein AM and Kennard C (1985) Predictive ocular motor control in Parkinson's disease. *Brain*, **108**, 925–40

Bronstein AM and Rudge P (1986) Vestibular involvement in spasmodic torticollis. *J Neurol Neurosurg Psychiatry*, **49**, 290–5

Bronstein AM and Rudge P (1988) The vestibular system in abnormal head postures and in spasmodic torticollis. In Fahn S, Marsden CD, Calne DB, eds, *Advances in Neurology*, New York, Raven Press, 493–500

Bronstein AM, Rudge P, and Beechey AH (1987) Spasmodic torticollis following unilateral VIII nerve lesions: neck EMG modulation in response to vestibular stimuli. *J Neurol Neurosurg Psychiatry*, **50**, 580–6

Bronstein AM, Mossman SS, and Luxon LM (1991) The neck–eye reflex in patients with reduced vestibular and optokinetic function. *Brain* (in press)

Buttner-Ennever JA, Acheson JF, Buttner U, Graham EM, Leonard TJK, and Ross Russel R (1989) Ptosis and supranuclear downgaze palsy. *Neurology*, **39**, 385–9

Carpenter RHS (1988) *Movement of the Eyes*, London, Pion

Chu FC, Reingold DB, Cogan DG, and Williams AC (1979) The eye movement disorders of progressive supranuclear palsy. *Ophthalmology*, **86**, 422–8

Cogan DG (1952) A type of congenital ocular motor apraxia presenting jerky head movements. *Trans Am Acad Ophthalmol Otolaryngol*, **56**, 853–62

Cogan DG, Chu FC, Bachman DM, and Barranger A (1981) The DAF syndrome. *Neuro-Ophthalmology*, **2**, 7–16

Collin NG, Cowey A, Latto R, and Marzi C (1982) The role of frontal eye-fields and superior colliculi in visual search and non-visual search in Rhesus monkeys. *Behav Brain Res*, **4**, 177–93

Corin MS, Elizan TS, and Bender MB (1972) Oculomotor function in patients with Parkinson's disease. *J Neurol Sci*, **15**, 251–65

Crawford TJ, Goodrich S, Henderson L, and Kennard C (1989) Predictive responses in Parkinson's disease: manual keypresses and saccadic eye movements to regular stimulus event. *J Neurol Neurosurg Psychiatry*, **52**, 1033–42

David NJ, Mackey EA, and Smith JL (1968) Further observations in progressive supranuclear palsy. *Neurology*, **18**, 349

Dejong JD and Melvill Jones G (1971) Akinesia, hypokinesia, and bradykinesia in the oculomotor system of patients with Parkinson's disease. *Exp Neurol*, **32**, 58–68

Deng SY, Goldberg ME, Segraves MA, Ungerleider LG, and Mishkin M (1986) The effect of unilateral ablation of the frontal eye fields on saccadic performance in the monkey. In Keller EL and Zee DS, eds, *Adaptive Processes in Visual and Oculomotor Systems. Advances in the Biosciences*, vol 57, Oxford, Pergamon Press, 201–8

Denny-Brown D (1968) Clinical symptomatology of diseases of the basal ganglia. In Vinken PJ and Bruyn GW, eds, *Handbook of Clinical Neurology*, vol 6, Amsterdam, North Holland, 133–72

Dix MR, Harrison MJG, and Lewis PD (1971) Progressive supranuclear palsy (the Steele–Richardson–Olszewski syndrome). A report of 9 cases with particular reference to the mechanism of the oculomotor disorder. *J Neurol Sci*, **13**, 237–56

Dubas F, Gray F, and Escourolle R (1983) Maladie de Steele–Richardson–Olszewski sans ophthalmoplegie. *Rev Neurol (Paris)*, **139**, 407–16

Fearnley JM and Lees AJ (1990) Striatonigral degeneration. A clinicopathological study. *Brain*, **113**, 1823–42

Fearnley JM, Revesz T, Brooks DJ, Frackowiak RSJ, and Lees AJ (1991) Diffuse Lewy body disease presenting with a supranuclear gaze palsy. *J Neurol Neurosurg Psychiatry*, **54**, 159–61

Fielder AR, Gresty MA, Dodd KL, Mellor DH and Levenne MI (1986). Congenital ocular motor apraxia. *Trans Ophthalmol Soc UK*, **105**, 589–98

Fitzgerald G and Hallpike CS (1942) Studies in human vestibular function: I. Observations on the directional preponderance of caloric nystagmus resulting from cerebral lesions. *Brain*, **65**, 115–80

Flowers KA and Downing AC (1978) Predictive control of eye movements in Parkinson's disease. *Ann Neurol*, **4**, 63–6

Frankel M and Cummings JL (1984) Neuro-ophthalmic abnormalities in Tourette's syndrome: functional and anatomical implications. *Neurology*, **34**, 359–61

Fukushima K, Takahashi K, and Kato M (1985) Interstitial vestibular interaction in the control of head posture. *Exp Brain Res*, **57**, 264–70

Fukushima-Kudo J, Fukushima K, and Tashiro K (1987) Rigidity and dorsiflexion of the neck in progressive supranuclear palsy and the interstitial nucleus of Cajal. *J Neurol Neurosurg Psychiatry*, **50**, 1197–203

Gibb WRG, Luthert PJ, and Marsden CD (1989) Corticobasal degeneration. *Brain*, **112**, 1171–92

Gibson JM and Kennard C (1986) A quantitative study of on-off fluctuations in the oculomotor system in Parkinson's disease. In Yahr M and Bergmann J, eds, *Advances in Neurology*, New York, Raven, 329–34

Gibson JM, Pimlott R, and Kennard C (1987) Ocular motor and manual tracking in Parkinson's disease and the effect of treatment. *J Neurol Neurosurg Psychiatry*, **50**, 853–60

Goldberg MF and von Noorden GK (1966) Ophthalmic findings in Wilson's hepatolenticular degeneration with emphasis on ocular motility. *Arch Ophthalmol*, **75**, 162–70

Graybiel AM (1978) Organization of the nigrotectal connection: an experimental tracer study in the cat. *Brain Res*, **143**, 339–48

Gresty MA, Hess K, and Leech J (1977) Disorders of the vestibulo-ocular reflex producing oscillopsia and mechanisms compensating for loss of labyrinthine function. *Brain*, **100**, 693–716

Guiloff RJ, George RJ, and Marsden CD (1980) Reversible supranuclear ophthalmoplegia associated with Parkinsonism. *J Neurol Neurosurg Psychiatry*, **43**, 552–4

Guitton D, Buchtel HA, and Douglas RM (1982) Disturbances of voluntary saccadic eye movement following discrete unilateral frontal lobe removals. In Lennerstrand G, Zee DS, and Keller EL, eds, *Functional Basis of Ocular Motility Disorders*, Oxford, Pergamon, 497–506

Halmagyi GM and Gresty MA (1979) Clinical signs of visual vestibular interaction. *J Neurol Neurosurg Psychiatry*, **42**, 934–9

Harbour RC, Sethi K, and DeChicchis A (1988) Eye movement abnormalities in Wilson's disease. In *Seventh International Neuro-Ophthalmology Congress Abstracts*, Vancouver, Canada

Hardie RJ (1989) Acanthocytosis and neurological impairment – a review. *Q J Med*, **71**, 264, 291–306

Hassler R and Hess WR (1954) Experimentelle und anatomische Befunde uber die Drehbewegungen und ihre nervosen Apparate. *Arch Psychiatr Nervenkr*, **192**, 488–526

Highstein S, Cohen B, and Mones R (1969) Changes in saccadic eye movements of patients with Parkinson's disease before and after L-Dopa. *Trans Am Neurol Assoc*, **97**, 277–9

Hikosaka O and Wurtz RH (1983) Visual and oculomotor functions of monkey substantia nigra pars reticulata. III. Memory-contingent visual and saccadic responses. *J Neurophysiol*, **49**, 1268–84

Hikosaka O and Wurtz RH (1985a) Modification of saccadic eye movements by GABA-related substances. II. Effect of muscimol in monkey substantia nigra pars reticulata. *J Neurophysiol*, **53**, 292–308

Hikosaka O and Wurtz RH (1985b) Modification of saccadic eye movements by GABA-related substances. I. Effect of muscimol and bicucculine in monkey superior colliculus. *J Neurophysiol*, **53**, 266–91

Hikosaka O, Sakamoto M, and Ushi S (1989) Functional property of monkey caudate neurons. III. Activities related to expectation of target and reward. *J Neurophysiol*, **61**, 814–32

Hood JD and Leech J (1974) The significance of peripheral vision in the perception of movement. *Acta Oto-Laryngol (Stockh)*, **77**, 72–9

Hood JD and Waniewski E (1984) Influence of peripheral vision upon vestibulo-ocular reflex suppression. *J Neurol Sci*, **63**, 27–44

Hotson JR and Boman DR (1991) Memory-contingent saccades and the SNpr postulate of essential blepharospasm. *Brain*, **114**, 295–307

Jankovic J and Ford J (1983) Blepharospasm and orofacial-cervical dystonia: clinical and pharmacological findings in 100 patients. *Ann Neurol*, **13**, 402–11

Judge SJ and Cumming BG (1986) Neurons in the monkey midbrain with activity related to vergence eye movement and accommodation. *J Neurophysiol*, **55**, 915–30

Keane JR and Young JA (1985) Blepharospasm with bilateral basal ganglia infarction. *Arch Neurol*, **52**, 1206–8

Keller EL and Robinson DA (1972) Abducens unit behaviour in the monkey during vergence movements. *Vision Res*, **12**, 369–82

Kennard C and Lueck CJ (1989) Oculomotor abnormalities in diseases of the basal ganglia. *Rev Neurol (Paris)*, **145**, 587–95

Kirkham TH and Kamin DF (1974) Slow saccadic eye movements in Wilson's disease. *J Neurol Neurosurg Psychiatry*, **37**, 191–4

Kompf D, Pasik T, Pasik P, and Bender MB (1979) Downward gaze in monkeys. Stimulation and lesion studies. *Brain*, **102**, 527–58

Kulisevski J, Marti MJ, Ferrer I, and Tolosa E (1988) Meige syndrome: neuropathology of a case. *Movement Disorders*, **3**, 170–5

Lang AE and Marsden CD (1983) Eye movement disorders in basal ganglia disease. In Clifford Rose F, ed, *The Eye in General Medicine*, London, Chapman and Hall

Lasker AG, Zee DS, Hain TC, Folstein SE, and Singer HS (1988) Saccades in Huntington's disease: slowing and dysmetria. *Neurology*, **38**, 427–31

Lees AJ (1985) *Tics and Related Disorders*, Edinburgh, Churchill Livingstone

Leigh RJ and Zee DS (1983) *The Neurology of Eye Movements*, Philadelphia, F.A. Davis

Leigh RJ, Newman SA, Folstein SE, Lasker AG, and Jensen BA (1983) Abnormal ocular motor control in Huntington's disease. *Neurology*, **33**, 1268–75

Leigh RJ, Parhad IM, Clark AW, Buttner-Ennever JA, and Folstein SE (1985) Brainstem findings in Huntington's disease: possible mechanisms for slow vertical saccades. *J Neurol Sci*, **71**, 247–56

Lennox G and Jones R (1989) Gaze distractibility in Wilson's disease. *Ann Neurol*, **25**, 415–17

Levine IM, Esles JW, and Looney JM (1968) Hereditary neurological disease with acanthocytes. *Arch Neurol*, **19**, 403–10

Lewis AJ and Gawel MJ (1990) Diffuse Lewy body disease with dementia and oculomotor dysfunction. *Movement Disorders*, **5**, 143–7

Leichnetz GR (1981) The prefrontal cortico-oculomotor trajectories in the Rhesus monkey. *J Neurol Sci*, **49**, 387–96

Lisberger SG, Morris EJ, and Tychsen L (1987) Visual motion processing and sensory-motor integration for smooth pursuit eye movements. *Annu Rev Neurosci*, **10**, 97–129

Louis-Bar D (1941) Sur un syndrome progressif comprenant des relangiectasies capillaires, cutanee et

conjectivales symetriques a disposition naevoide et des troubles cerebelleux. *Confin Neurol (Basel)*, **4**, 32–42
Lueck CJ, Tanyeri S, Crawford TJ, Henderson L, and Kennard C (1990) Antisaccades and remembered saccades in Parkinson's disease. *J Neurol Neurosurg Psychiatry*, **53**, 284–8
Mastaglia FL and Grainger KMR (1975) Internuclear ophthalmoplegia in progressive supranuclear palsy. *J Neurol Sci*, **25**, 303–8
Matthews WB, Beasley P, Parry-Jones W, and Garland G (1978) Spasmodic torticollis: a combined clinical study. *J Neurol Neurosurg Psychiatry*, **41**, 485–92
Mays LE (1984) Neural control of vergence eye movements: convergence and divergence neurons in midbrain. *J Neurophysiol*, **51**, 1091–108
Mays LE, Porter JD, Gamlin PDR, and Tello CA (1986) Neural control of vergence eye movements: neurons encoding vergence velocity. *J Neurophysiol*, **56**, 1007–21
Melvill Jones G and de Jong JD (1971) Dynamic characteristics of saccadic eye movements in Parkinson's disease. *Exp Neurol*, **31**, 17–31
Mizutani T, Satoh J, and Morimatsu Y (1988) Neuropathological background of oculomotor disturbances in olivopontocerebellar atrophy with special reference to slow saccade. *Clin Neuropathol*, **7**, 53–61
Neville BGR, Lake BD, Stephens R *et al.* (1973) A neurovisceral storage disease with vertical cupranuclear ophthalmoplegia and its relationship to Niemann–Pick disease. *Brain*, **96**, 97–120
Norman RM, Forrester RM, Tingey, AH (1967) The juvenile form of Niemann–Pick disease. *Arch Dis Child*, **42**, 91–6
Perkin GD, Lees AJ, Stern GM and Kocen RS (1978) Problems in the diagnosis of progressive supranuclear palsy (Steele–Richardson–Olszewski syndrome). *Can J Neurol Sci*, **5**, 167–73
Petit H and Milbled G (1973) Anomalies of conjugate ocular movements in Huntington's chorea: application to early detection. In Barbeau A, Chase TN, and Paulson GW, eds, *Advances in Neurology*, New York, Raven Press, 287–94
Pierrot-Deseilligny C, Gautier J-C, and Loron P (1988) Acquired ocular motor apraxia due to bilateral frontoparietal infarcts. *Ann Neurol*, **23**, 199–202
Precht W (1977) The functional synaptology of brainstem oculomotor pathways. In Baker R and Berthoz A, eds, *Control of Gaze by Brainstem Neurons, Development in Neuroscience*, vol 1, Amsterdam, Elsevier, 131–41
Precht W (1982) Anatomical and functional organization of optokinetic pathways. In Lennerstrand, G, Zee DS, Keller E, eds, *Functional Basis of Ocular Motility Disorders*, Oxford, Pegamon Press, 291–302
Quinn N (1989) Multiple system atrophy – the nature of the beast. *J Neurol Neurosurg Psychiatry*, (suppl), 78–89
Rascol O, Clanet M, Montastruc JL, Simonetta M, Soulier-Esteve MJ, Doyon B *et al.* (1989) Abnormal ocular movements in Parkinson's disease. Evidence of involvement of dopaminergic systems. *Brain*, **112**, 1193–214
Rebeiz JJ, Kolodny EH, and Richardson EP (1967) Corticodentatonigral degeneration with neuronal achromasia: a progressive disorder of late adult life. *Trans Am Neurol Assoc*, **92**, 23–6
Reichert WH, Doolittle J, and McDowell FH (1982) Vestibular dysfunction in Parkinson's disease. *Neurology*, **32**, 1133–8
Riley DE, Lang AE, Lewis A, Resch L, Ashby P, Hornykiewica O *et al.* (1990) Cortical-basal ganglionic degeneration. *Neurology*, **40**, 1203–12
Rothwell JC and Obeso JA (1987) The anatomical and physiological basis of torsion dystonia. In Marsden CD and Fahn S, eds, *Movement Disorders*, vol 2, London, Butterworths, 313–31
Rudge P (1983) *Clinical Neuro-otology*, Edinburgh, Churchill Livingstone
Schiller PH, True SD, and Conway JL (1980) Deficits in eye movements following frontal eye field and superior colliculus ablations. *J Neurophysiol*, **44**, 1175–89
Sedgwick RP and Boder B (1972) Ataxia-telangiectasia. In Vinken PJ, Bruyn GW, eds, *Handbook of Clinical Neurology*, vol 14, Amsterdam, North Holland, 267–339
Shibasaki H, Tsuji S and Kuroiwa Y (1979) Oculomotor abnormalities in Parkinson's disease. *Arch Neurol*, **36**, 360–4
Shimizu N, Coen B, Bala SP, Meridoza M, and Yar MD (1977) Ocular dyskinesias in patients with Parkinson's disease treated with levadopa. *Ann Neurol*, **1**, 167–71
Smith JL and Cogan DG (1959) Ataxia telangiectasia,. *Neurology*, **28**, 1099–104
Spector R and Troost BT (1981) The ocular motor system. *Ann Neurol*, **9**, 517–25
Starr A (1967) A disorder of rapid eye movements in Huntington's chorea. *Brain*, **90**, 545–64
Steele JC, Richardson JC, and Olszewski J (1964) Progressive supranuclear palsy. *Arch Neurol*, **10**, 333–59
Stell R, Bronstein AM and Marsden CD (1989a) Vestibulo-ocular abnormalities in spasmodic torticollis before and after botulinum toxin injections. *J Neurol Neurosurg Psychiatry*, **52**, 57–62
Stell R, Bronstein AM, Plant GT, and Harding AE (1989b) Ataxia telangiectasia: a reappraisal of the ocular motor features and their value in the diagnosis of atypical cases. *Movement Disorders*, **4**, 320–9

Stell R, Bronstein AM, Gresty M, Buckwell D, and Marsden CD (1990) Saccadic function in spasmodic torticollis. *J Neurol Neurosurg Psychiatry*, **49**, 290–5

Stell R, Gresty MA, Metcalfe T, and Bronstein AM (1991) Cervico-ocular function in patients with spasmodic torticollis. *J Neurol Neurosurg Psychiatry*, **54**, 39–41

Sternlieb I, Giblin DR, and Scienberg IH (1987) Wilson's disease. In Marsden CD and Fahn S, eds, *Movement Disorders 2*, Oxford, Butterworth-Heinemann, 288–302

Svien HJ and Cody DTR (1969) Treatment of spasmodic torticollis by suppression of labyrinthine activity. Report of a case. *Mayo Clin Proc* **44**, 825–7

Tanyeri S, Leuck CJ, Crawford TJ, and Kennard C (1989) Vertical and horizontal saccadic eye movements in Parkinson's disease. *Neuro-ophthalmology*, **9**, 165–77

Teravainen H and Calne DB (1980) Studies of Parkinsonian movement: 2. Initiation of fast voluntary eye movement during postural disturbance. *Acta Neurol Scand*, **62**, 149–57

Troost BT and Daroff RB (1977) The ocular motor defects in progressive supranuclear palsy. *Ann Neurol*, **2**, 397–403

Troost BT, Webber MD and Daroff RB (1974) Hypometric saccades. *Am J Ophthalmol*, **78**, 1002–5

Tusa RJ, Zee DS, and Herdman SJ (1986) Recovery of oculomotor function in monkeys with large unilateral cortical lesions. In Keller EL and Zee DS, eds, *Adaptive Processes in Visual and Oculomotor Systems, Advances in the Biosciences*, vol 57, Oxford, Pergamon Press, 209–16

Vance JM, Pericak-Vance MA, Bowman M, Payne CS, Fredane L, and Siddique T (1987) Chorea-acanthocytosis: a report of 3 new families and implications for genetic counselling. *Am J Med Genet*, **28**, 403–10

Vincent SR, Hattori T, and McGreer EG (1978) The nigrotectal projection: a biochemical and ultrastructural characterization. *Brain Res*, **151**, 159–64

Wadia NH and Swami RK (1971) A new form of heredo-familial spinocerebellar degeneration with slow eye movements (nine families). *Brain*, **94**, 359–74

Walshe JM (1976) Wilson's disease (hepatolenticular degeneration). In Vinken PJ, Bruyn GW, Klawans L, eds, *Handbook of Clinical Neurology*, Amsterdam, Elsevier, 379–414

Webster KE (1965) Cortico-striatal projections in the cat. *J Anat*, **99**, 329–37

White OB, Saint-Cyr JA, and Sharpe JA (1983a) Ocular motor deficits in Parkinson's disease. I. The horizontal vestibulo-ocular reflex and its regulation. *Brain*, **106**, 555–70

White OB, Saint-Cyr JA, Tomlinson RD, and Sharpe JA (1983b) Ocular motor deficits in Parkinson's disease. II. Control of the saccadic and smoot pursuit systems. *Brain*, **106**, 571–87

Wilson K (1954) *Neurology* 2nd edn, Ninian Bruce A, ed, Butterworth and Co Ltd 941–67

Wilson VJ, Melvill Jones G (1979) *Mammalian Vestibular Physiology*, New York, Plenum

Zee DS (1978) Ophthalmoscopy in examination of patients with vestibular disorders. *Ann Neurol*, **3**, 373–4

Zee DS, Optican LM, Cook JD, Robinson DA, and King Engel W (1976) Slow saccades in spino-cerebellar degeneration. *Arch Neurol*, **33**, 243–51

Zee DS, Yamazaki A, Butler PH, and Gucer G (1981) Effects of ablation of flocculus and paraflocculus on eye movements in primate. *J Neurophysiol*, **46**, 878–99

Part II

Akinetic–rigid syndromes

6
Problems in Parkinson's disease and other akinetic–rigid syndromes

C. David Marsden and Stanley Fahn

INTRODUCTION

Since we last wrote on this topic in 1987 in *Movement Disorders 2*, much has happened. This is reflected in our selection of new chapters in *Movement Disorders 3*. The initial emphasis is on the cause of Parkinson's disease. In *Movement Disorders 1*, published in 1982, Roger Duvoisin speculated upon the role of heredity and viruses. He concluded then that: 'Their near identity of dizygotic and monozygotic concordances effectively excludes genetic factors from consideration in the aetiology of Parkinson's disease'. However, he has now reappraised this conclusion (Duvoisin, 1993), to generate new interest in hereditary contributions to susceptibility to this illness, a point to which we will return. Because of the originally negative impact of twin studies, however, attention focused upon environmental factors. In 1982, the full impact of 1-methyl-4-phenyl-1,2,3,6-tetrahydropyridine (MPTP) had not struck and only smoking had emerged as an interesting topic, apart from the long-standing debate about a viral cause. By 1987, the saga of MPTP held the stage and Bill Langston provided a major review of its significance in *Movement Disorders 2*. Since then, it has been determined that its toxic effect is directed at complex I of mitochondria, specifically affecting the activity of NADH CoQ reductase. The full force of epidemiology is now being applied in an attempt to tease out some environmental agent causing Parkinson's disease, an area reviewed in Chapter 7.

A search for aetiological clues by measuring neurochemical changes in brain proceeds at a rapid pace, with much emphasis on mitochondrial dysfunction, particularly in complex I. There are several reports of reduced activity of NADH CoQ reductase in substantia nigra, other areas of brain, platelets and muscle in patients with Parkinson's disease; not all of these have been replicated. Conflicting findings make it difficult to understand the full value of these reports. We refer the reader to the latest review on mitochondrial function in Parkinson's disease by Schapira and his colleagues (1992). The meaning and specificity of complex I alterations in Parkinson's disease remain to be elucidated. Is this a primary defect or secondary to other factors, including environmental toxins, endogenous oxidative stress or genetic factors?

Oxidative stress has emerged as a leading hypothesis in the pathogenesis of Parkinson's disease, but the evidence is not yet available to prove this concept. In fact, Calne (1992) has raised a number of points against this hypothesis. On the other hand, recent reviews (Fahn and Cohen, 1992; Jenner *et al.*, 1992) summarize the evidence in favour of it. In a novel approach, Jenner and colleagues (1992) carried out biochemical analyses on brains of presumed presymptomatic Parkinson's disease, namely those with incidental Lewy bodies in the substantia nigra. These investigators measured levels of iron, ferritin, zinc, complex I activity and reduced glutathione. The only one found to be statistically significantly altered was a decrease of reduced glutathione concentration in the substantia nigra. This finding is interpreted as a sign of oxidative stress, and therefore strongly supports the oxidative stress hypothesis in the pathogenesis of Parkinson's disease.

Pathology has always been held to hold clues to the aetiology of the illness. In 1982, Lysia Forno reviewed the topic; in 1987 Kurt Jellinger provided his extensive experience. In Chapter 8 Bill Gibb and Andrew Lees review their detailed work on selective vulnerability of nigral zones, the effect of ageing and other issues, based upon classical neuropathology.

In 1987, we wrote on the possible role of deprenyl in slowing the rate of progression of Parkinson's disease, concluding that 'what is now required, urgently, is the appropriate randomized "blind" study to prove or disprove this hypothesis'. DATATOP has been exactly that, and represents a triumph of organization and execution (Parkinson Study Group, 1989). Its impact deserves the contribution of Ira Shoulson on neuroprotective therapy. Since Chapter 9 was written, the final report of deprenyl in DATATOP has been published (Parkinson Study Group, 1993), showing that deprenyl has prolonged symptomatic effects, based on clinical worsening after withdrawal of medication. Moreover, the benefit in delaying the need for levodopa therapy becomes less effective over time. On the other hand, the symptomatic effect of deprenyl may not entirely explain the delay in the need for levodopa, and some protective effect by deprenyl is possible. This seems reasonable because 2 months after washout from experimental medications, subjects who had been receiving deprenyl were less severely affected with Parkinson's disease than those who had been receiving placebo. The lack of a clear-cut interpretation leaves open the question of the role of monoamine oxidase inhibitors and other antioxidants in the early stage of Parkinson's disease.

The problems of levodopa therapy have been with us for many years, and the cause and management of fluctuations were topics of debate in 1982 and 1987. Fred Wooten's contribution on levodopa pharmacokinetics in 1987 covered existing knowledge then, but many new studies have since been published. Maral Mouradian and Tom Chase deal with the vexed issue of improving dopaminergic therapy in Chapter 10.

A novel topic since the last issue has been the development of neural transplantation. This is still an experimental field, not yet ripe for widespread clinical application. However, its implications are far-reaching, not only for Parkinson's disease, but potentially for many other neurological conditions. Kathy Sleece-Collier and John Sladek review basic studies in the field in Chapter 11, while Olle Lindvall (Chapter 12) gives a measured overview of the clinical position. Since these chapters were written, three recent articles have appeared, demonstrating mild to substantial benefit in patients with Parkinson's disease and with MPTP-induced parkinsonism (Freed *et al.*, 1992; Spencer *et al.*, 1992; Widner *et al.*, 1992). We can anticipate more studies on embryonic dopaminergic cell implants in patients with Parkinson's disease to determine the true value of this approach.

Another neurosurgical technique has been revived, namely pallidotomy. A report by Laitenen *et al.* (1992) suggests that a lesion in the posteroventrolateral part of the internal segment of the globus pallidus can reduce bradykinesia and tremor. Since this site appears to be the target of subthalamopallidal afferents, Laitinen's result can be matched with the reports by Bergmann *et al.* (1990) and Aziz *et al.* (1991), in which they report successful improvement of experimental parkinsonism in primates by lesioning the subthalamic nucleus, which is overactive in Parkinson's disease. There is also a report of disappearance of parkinsonian signs in a patient who suffered a subthalamic haematoma (Sellal *et al.*, 1992), lending support to the concept of the role of the subthalamic nucleus in Parkinson's disease.

For every 10 patients with Parkinson's disease, there is another with one of the parkinson-plus syndromes. In previous volumes we have attempted to cover these in sequence: in 1982 we discussed multiple system atrophy and autonomic failure (Roger Bannister and David Oppenheimer); in 1987, olivopontocerebellar atrophy (Roger Duvoisin), Steele–Richardson–Olszewski syndrome (Andrew Lees) and Wilson's disease (Irmin Sternlieb and Herb Scheinberg). We return to multiple system atrophy, for it probably represents one of the commonest other akinetic–rigid syndromes and causes great distress and difficulty in management; Niall Quinn provides his extensive knowledge of the topic in Chapter 13. Finally, this time round we invited Ray Watts, S. S. Mirra and E. P. Richardson to review corticobasal degeneration, which has grown in recognition in recent years (Chapter 14).

MANAGEMENT OF THE NEWLY DIAGNOSED CASE OF PARKINSON'S DISEASE

Since we wrote on this topic in 1987, matters have changed. Then, the major issue was when to start dopamine replacement therapy, and whether to use a levodopa preparation or a directly acting dopamine agonist. Now there are issues over immediate neuroprotective therapy.

As mentioned above, the DATATOP study, along with smaller controlled investigations (Tetrud and Langston, 1989; Myllyla *et al.*, 1992) have highlighted the possible capacity of deprenyl (selegiline) to slow the rate of progression of Parkinson's disease (see Chapter 9). How should this evidence influence our advice to patients just known to have Parkinson's disease and without any functional disability?

Firstly, it should be made clear that deprenyl does not stop or reverse Parkinson's disease. The evidence is that it delays the need to start dopamine replacement therapy, and this evidence is compelling. However, the issue of whether this is due, in part, to true neuroprotection from the cause or mechanisms responsible for the illness, or whether it is due entirely to a mild symptomatic effect of deprenyl is not yet conclusive. Although deprenyl withdrawal did lead to worsening (Parkinson Study Group, 1993), indicating prolonged symptomatic effects, this does not disprove an additional neuroprotective effect from deprenyl. In any case, delay of need for dopamine replacement treatment also means delay in the long-term problems known to occur during such therapy.

To us, this means that we recommend deprenyl treatment (5 mg morning and lunchtime) in all patients just diagnosed as having Parkinson's disease. We are reassured in this view by the lack (as yet) of any long-term unexpected side-effects of chronic deprenyl treatment. We also strongly support carefully controlled, placebo-designed studies testing other potentially neuroprotective drugs in early Parkinson's disease in the absence of any symptomatic drug, including deprenyl, because there is no conclusive evidence that deprenyl is actually protective. A note of caution should be made about introducing this dosage of deprenyl in patients already on levodopa therapy. The DATATOP study did not evaluate the role of deprenyl in such patients, only those on no therapy. Practical experience has shown that the addition of deprenyl on those taking levodopa can augment the dopaminergic response and induce psychosis or confusion, particularly on those who are already on maximally tolerated doses of levodopa. If patients are already on levodopa, and insist on trying deprenyl in addition, we start with a small dose of deprenyl – 2.5 mg at breakfast – and increase the dose only if the drug is well-tolerated.

If deprenyl may be good for Parkinson's disease, what about other akinetic–rigid syndromes? There is no evidence, one way or the other, as to whether deprenyl has any effect on multiple system atrophy, Steele–Richardson–Olszewski syndrome, corticobasal degeneration, etc. Nor are there data to suggest that, theoretically, deprenyl might have any useful effect in these conditions. However, nothing else is known to be of neuroprotective benefit. In the face of ignorance, deprenyl can be given to these patients or, preferably, we recommend entering them into a clinical trial of such treatment.

Deprenyl is not the only antioxidative drug that was evaluated in DATATOP. Tocopherol (vitamin E) with and without deprenyl was tested as well. The results, however, showed no benefit from vitamin E at a dosage of 2000 u/day (Parkinson Study Group, 1993). Whether other antioxidants, such as ascorbate, would be beneficial would need to be determined by a similar controlled trial. It should be pointed out that the failure of tocopherol to provide protection does not invalidate the oxidant stress hypothesis. There could be many reasons why tocopherol failed to provide benefit, including inadequate dose, failure to enter the brain in sufficient concentration, and tocopherol's site of action.

PRESYMPTOMATIC DIAGNOSIS OF PARKINSON'S DISEASE

The possibility of slowing the rate of progression of the underlying pathology of Parkinson's disease by drug therapy has highlighted the need for early diagnosis. Current theory suggests the progressive pathology in the brain may begin many years before clinical evidence of the disease appears. How long is not known, but estimates suggest as long as 20–30 years! If an effective neuroprotective treatment is developed, it should be started before, rather than after symptoms appear. The treatment of symptomless hypertension has had a considerable effect upon the incidence of stroke. Techniques for presymptomatic diagnosis are therefore being sought. Positron emission tomography (PET) using [^{18}F]fluorodopa can detect about a 30% decrease in striatal dopamine synthesis and storage (see Chapter 4), and may be used as the 'gold standard'. More sensitive, specific and cost-effective ideas need to be explored.

WHAT TO DO WHEN DISABILITY WARRANTS FURTHER TREATMENT OF PARKINSON'S DISEASE

Despite deprenyl (selegiline), symptoms and disability will increase, at a variable rate, in most patients with Parkinson's disease. At some stage, disability will reach a point requiring further treatment. The level at which this occurs depends upon individual circumstances (work, family, age and philosophy all play a part). When this decision is reached, the problem is which drug to employ. The options are conventional levodopa preparations (Sinemet or, in Europe, Madopar), longer-acting forms of levodopa (Sinemet CR or Madopar CR) or directly acting dopamine agonists (bromocriptine, lisuride or pergolide). The objective is to employ a strategy that will give the longest period of stable smooth benefit without side-effects (mainly dyskinesias, fluctuations and psychiatric complications). There is some evidence to suggest that directly acting dopamine agonists are associated with a lower risk of the emergence of fluctuations in response and dyskinesias. However, fewer patients gain adequate therapeutic benefit from dopamine agonists compared to levodopa, which will improve the vast majority of patients. This dilemma has led to wide debate as to the best strategy for treatment at this critical time (Kurlan, 1988).

Some have taken the view that a combination of levodopa and a directly acting dopamine agonist may be the best insurance for long-term success (Rinne, 1985). Support for this approach has been obtained from open comparative studies (Rinne, 1985, 1987), although a recent small randomized trial of combined bromocriptine and levodopa versus levodopa alone was less convincing (Weiner *et al.*, 1993). Indeed, Weiner *et al.*, who provide a careful critique of previous studies, conclude that 'the usefulness of early combination therapy remains, at best, questionable'.

Two other issues are relevant. Firstly, some have raised the question as to whether treatment with a directly acting dopamine agonist at the time of diagnosis may be as effective as deprenyl (selegiline) in delaying the need for levodopa. The hypothesis is that such agents, by reducing endogenous dopamine synthesis, might provide neuroprotection against dopamine-derived oxidative stress, or at least delay the need for levodopa. Secondly, some have advocated the use of delayed-release levodopa preparations (Sinemet CR or Madopar CR) when the need for such treatment arises. The hypothesis behind this idea is that smooth delivery of levodopa, rather than the pulsatile peaks and troughs produced by conventional Sinemet or Madopar, might also delay the emergence of fluctuations and dyskinesias. However, neither of these concepts has been verified by rigorous long-term comparative trials.

Against this background it is clear that the best advice to patients with Parkinson's disease at this critical point in their illness is fraught with uncertainty. Indeed, opinions outweigh facts. The patient's views must carry weight, but in the final analysis where doubt exists, the best opinion is to suggest enrolment in well-designed clinical trials to answer the questions raised. Some such trials are in progress, but more should be started.

Meanwhile, what do we do? Both of us take the view that when disability warrants further therapy, the best option is to start a delayed-release levodopa preparation (Sinemet CR or Madopar CR). Most patients, in our experience, gain adequate relief with relatively low doses of these drugs. In those who do not, we add a directly acting dopamine agonist early, rather than pushing the dose of levodopa.

COMPLICATIONS OF THERAPY IN ADVANCED PARKINSON'S DISEASE

The treating clinician knows all too well about problems that develop in patients on long-term levodopa therapy, particularly fluctuations, dyskinesias and psychosis. Fortunately, an advance has been made in treating dopa-induced psychosis without worsening the state of parkinsonism or interfering with the effectiveness of levodopa. Clozapine is an atypical neuroleptic agent that does not cause drug-induced parkinsonism like the typical antipsychotics. Clozapine has been found to be effective in controlling dopa-induced psychosis (Friedman and Lannon, 1990; Pfeiffer *et al.*, 1990). Unfortunately, up to 2% of patients receiving clozapine develop agranulocytosis, which is life-threatening unless the drug is abruptly discontinued. Such a potential complication requires the treating physician to monitor the white blood count weekly.

The problems of dyskinesias and fluctuations are less easily brought under control and remain problems looking for solutions. The careful and scientific studies of Mouradian and Chase (Chapter 10), along with those of others such as Jay Nutt (1992) and Jose Obeso (1992), have provided insight into the pharmacokinetic and pharmacodynamic mechanisms involved in the emergence of these problems during long-term therapy. The practical problem, however, is what to do faced with patients with increasing wearing-off deterioration, on–off fluctuations and the range of off-period, diphasic and peak dose dyskinesias. Those not already taking deprenyl (selegiline), Sinemet CR or Madopar CR, or a directly acting dopamine agonist may be helped by the addition of such medications to begin with. One should resist the temptation to take levodopa in smaller doses at more frequent intervals. The critical pharmacodynamic changes during long-term therapy are:

1. The loss of a classical dose–response relationship of improvement in motor function to plasma levodopa level. This is replaced by the emergence of a critical threshold – patients are either on or off. Furthermore, increasing dosage is reflected not in extra degree of benefit, but in longer duration of response.
2. The threshold for dyskinesias drops so as to become closer and closer to that for motor improvement, and the impact of intermediate levels of dopaminergic stimulation causing diphasic dyskinesias becomes more and more apparent. In these circumstances, smaller individual doses of levodopa may be insufficient to switch patients on, and last for too short a period of time, and also may only reach the intermediate level, causing disabling diphasic dyskinesias.

Another practical problem is the failure of the delayed-release levodopa preparations of Sinemet CR and Madopar CR to produce adequate initial plasma levodopa levels to reach the critical theshold to turn patients on. Often a mixture of conventional levodopa (to give the kick-start) with the longer-acting preparations (to prolong the period of benefit) is required.

Despite all these manipulations, there is a cohort of patients, often young and intelligent, with disastrous motor and mental fluctuations, along with catastrophic dyskinesias. In Europe, the use of apomorphine (with domperidone to prevent peripheral side-effects if necessary) has proved of considerable value to such patients. Self- (or partner) administration of apomorphine by subcutaneous injection via preloaded Penjects can rapidly rescue patients from off periods within about 10 minutes, the benefit lasting for about an hour (Frankel *et al.*, 1990). Intranasal and sublingual preparations of apomorphine are being explored as alternatives to subcutaneous injections, as is levodopa methyl ester. In particularly difficult situations, continuous subcutaneous apomorphine infusions may give more stable relief.

References

Aziz TZ, Peggs D, Sambrook MA, and Crossman AR (1991). Lesion of the subthalamic nucleus for the alleviation of 1-methyl-4-phenyl-1,2,3,6-tetrahydropyridine (MPTP)-induced parkinsonism in the primate. *Movement Disorders*, **6**, 288–92

Bergmann H, Wichmann T, and DeLong MR (1990) Reversal of experimental parkinsonism by lesions of the subthalamic nucleus. *Science*, **249**, 1436–8

Calne DB (1992) The free radical hypothesis in idiopathic parkinsonism: evidence against it. *Ann Neurol*, **32**, 799–803

Duvoisin, RC (1993) The genetics of Parkinson's disease – a review. *Adv Neurol*, **60**, 306–15

Fahn S and Cohen G (1992) The oxidant stress hypothesis in Parkinson's disease: evidence supporting it. *Ann Neurol*, **32**, 804–12

Frankel JP, Lees AJ, Kempster PA, and Stern GM (1990) Subcutaneous apomorphine in the treatment of Parkinson's disease. *J Neurol Neurosurg Psychiatry*, **53**, 96–101

Freed CR, Breeze RE, Rosenberg NL, Schneck SA, Kriek E, Qi JX *et al.* (1992) Survival of implanted fetal dopamine cells and neurologic improvement 12 to 46 months after transplantation for Parkinson's disease. *N Engl J Med*, **327**, 1549–55

Friedman JH and Lannon MC (1990) Clozapine in idiopathic Parkinson's disease. *Neurology*, **40**, 1151–2

Jenner P, Schapira AHV, and Marsden CD (1992) New insights into the cause of Parkinson's disease. *Neurology*, **42**, 2241–50

Kurlan R (1988) International symposium on early dopamine agonist therapy of Parkinson's disease. *Arch Neurol*, **45**, 204–8

Laitinen LV, Bergenheim AT, and Hariz MI (1992) Leksell's posteroventral pallidotomy in the treatment of Parkinson's disease. *J Neurosurg*, **76**, 53–61

Myllyla VV, Sotaniemi KA, Vuorinen JA, and Heinonen EH (1992) Selegiline as initial treatment in *de novo* parkinsonian patients. *Neurology*, **42**, 339–43

Nutt J, Woodward WR, Carter JH, and Gancher ST (1992) Effect of long-term therapy on the pharmalodynamics of itrodopa – relation to the on–off phenomenon. *Arch Neurol*, **49**, 1123–30

Obeso JA, Luquin MR, Grandas I, Vamonde J, Laguna J, and Martinez-Lage JM (1992) Motor response to repeated dopaminergic stimulation in Parkinson's disease. *Clin Neuropharmacol*, **15**, 75–9

Parkinson Study Group (1989) Effect of deprenyl on the progression of disability in early Parkinson's disease. *N Engl J Med*, **321**, 1364–71

Parkinson Study Group (1993) Effects of tocopherol and deprenyl on the progression of disability in early Parkinson's disease. *N Engl J Med*, **328**, 176–83

Pfeiffer RF, Kang J, Graber B, Hofman R, and Wilson J (1990) Clozapine for psychosis in Parkinson's disease. *Movement Disorders*, **5**, 239–42

Rinne UK (1985) Combined bromociptine-levodopa therapy early in Parkinson's disease. *Neurology*, **35**, 1196–8

Rinne UK (1987) Early combination of bromocriptine and levodopa in the treatment of Parkinson's disease: a 5-year follow up. *Neurology*, **37**, 826–8

Schapira AHV, Mann VM, Cooper JM, Krige D, Jenner P, and Marsden CD (1992) Mitochondrial function in Parkinson's disease. *Ann Neurol*, **32**, S116–24

Sellal F, Hirsch E, Lisovoski F, Mutschler V, Collard M, and Marescaux C (1992) Contralateral disappearance of parkinsonian signs after subthalamic hematoma. *Neurology*, **42**, 255–6

Spencer DD, Robbins RJ, Naftolin F, Marek KL, Vollmer T, Leranth C *et al.* (1992) Unilateral transplantation of human fetal mesencephalic tissue into the caudate nucleus of patients with Parkinson's disease. *N Engl J Med*, **327**, 1541–8

Tetrud JW, and Langston JW (1989) The effect of deprenyl (selegiline) on the natural history of Parkinson's disease. *Science*, **245**, 519–22

Weiner WJ, Factor SA, Sanchez-Ramos JR, Singer C, Sheldon C, Cornelius L *et al.* (1993) Early combination therapy (bromocriptine and levodopa) does not prevent motor fluctuations in Parkinson's disease. *Neurology*, **43**, 21–7

Widner H, Tetrud J, Rehncrona S, Snow B, Brundin P, Gustavii B *et al.* (1992) Bilateral fetal mesencephalic grafting in two patients with parkinsonism induced by 1-methyl-4-phenyl-1,2,3,6-tetrahydropyridine (MPTP). *N Engl J Med*, **327**, 1556–63

7

Epidemiological clues to the cause of Parkinson's disease

Caroline M. Tanner

INTRODUCTION

In 1817, James Parkinson described 'the shaking palsy', characterized by resting tremor, stooped posture and propulsive gait, with sensation and cognition intact. Since then, many have sought without success a single cause for Parkinson's disease (PD), including stress (Charcot, 1878; Gowers, 1888), heredity (Mjones, 1949; Kondo *et al.*, 1973), infection (Poskanzer *et al.*, 1969; Elizan and Casals, 1987) and endocrine abnormality (Rinne, 1978). Recent observations suggest a different explanation for the cause of PD. Rather than being the result of any single factor, PD may result from the combination of metabolic susceptibility (which may be inherited) and toxicant exposure. Further modification of the risk of developing PD may be provided by exposure to protective agents. The percentage contribution of any individual factor may vary among PD cases, but all would result finally in a distinct clinical and pathological entity, PD. This review will briefly summarize recent laboratory work which contributes to this hypothesis, then review relevant epidemiological studies.

Although there is debate as to whether PD is a homogeneous or heterogeneous disorder (Calne, 1989), these issues will not be considered here. For the purpose of this discussion PD will be considered to be a distinct entity, characterized clinically by an insidious onset and slowly progressive course, with cardinal signs of resting tremor, bradykinesia, cogwheel rigidity and postural reflex impairment, and pathologically by degeneration of pigmented aminergic neurons and formation of Lewy bodies (Koller, 1987). Parkinsonism of known aetiology and parkinsonian syndromes with more extensive associated neuronal injury (including progressive supranuclear palsy, multiple system atrophy and olivopontocerebellar atrophy) are excluded. The clinical differentiation of PD from other parkinsonian syndromes is sometimes difficult, however, and error rates as high as 20% have been observed (Hughes *et al.*, 1992). The relatively low diagnostic accuracy of clinical examination in PD adds additional potential error to epidemiological studies, since none have universal autopsy confirmation.

RATIONALE FOR THE SEARCH FOR A TOXIC AETIOLOGY

MPTP-induced Parkinsonism

The hypothesis that Parkinson's disease might result from exposure to an environmentally present toxicant originally derived from an epidemiological observation. In 1983, Langston and colleagues described a cluster of parkinsonism in northern California. The cluster was identified as distinct from 'idiopathic' PD because the clinical syndrome differed in two major ways from the typical presentation of Parkinson's disease. Firstly, in each case, parkinsonism affected young subjects (26–42 years) in contrast to the usual onset of PD after the sixth decade of life. Secondly, the signs of parkinsonism developed abruptly, with severe disease manifesting within weeks, quite different from the insidious onset and slow progression over decades of PD. All of these parkinsonian patients were narcotics addicts, and an aetiology related to their addiction was sought. In each case parkinsonism developed after the intravenous use of an illicitly manufactured narcotic. Careful work identified the responsible toxin as the pyridine 1-methyl-4-phenyl-1,2,3,6-tetrahydropyridine (MPTP).

MPTP-induced parkinsonism is particularly remarkable because of the striking resemblance to PD (Langston *et al*., 1983). In contrast to other toxins producing parkinsonism, MPTP selectively reproduces the cardinal signs of PD, without signs suggesting injury of other nervous system structures. As in PD, persons with MPTP-induced parkinsonism improve with levodopa therapy, and later develop typical side-effects. A single human autopsy found prominent substantia nigra involvement, with one eosinophilic inclusion resembling a Lewy body (Davis *et al*., 1979).

However, the extent to which MPTP-induced neurotoxicity may serve as a model to suggest the pathogenesis or aetiology of PD remains unknown. MPTP-induced parkinsonism differs from PD in at least five major ways. Firstly, exposure to MPTP causes an acute toxic syndrome that does not include signs of parkinsonism, followed by the subacute evolution over several weeks of severe parkinsonism, in contrast to the insidious onset of PD (Langston *et al*., 1983). Secondly, although not all persons exposed to MPTP developed parkinsonism, a cluster of affected individuals did occur. Clusters of PD are not well-documented. Thirdly, MPTP has not yet been shown to cause progressive neurological disability, while a slowly progressive course is typical of PD. Fourthly, MPTP has been proved to cause parkinsonism in humans only after intravenous exposure, an unlikely route in most cases of PD. Finally, the pathological changes in the one human autopsy study of MPTP parkinsonism did not completely resemble those of PD (Davis *et al*., 1979), and this is also true of non-human primates, although these differences are less when older animals are studied (Forno *et al*., 1986; Ricaurte *et al*., 1987). Before the real utility of MPTP as a model for PD is understood, these differences must be explained.

None the less, the similarities between PD and MPTP parkinsonism suggest that similar pathophysiological abnormalities may underlie each disorder. Consequently, the mechanism of MPTP-induced neurotoxicity has been intensively sought. To summarize briefly current knowledge, MPTP becomes toxic after oxidation to the charged molecule, 1-methyl-4-phenylpyridinium (MPP+), by monoamine oxidase B (MAOB) (Chiba *et al*., 1984; Markey *et al*., 1984). Treating animals with MAOB inhibitors before MPTP exposure prevents toxicity (Heikkila *et al*., 1984). MPP+ appears to gain access to nigral dopaminergic neurons via the dopamine uptake system (Javitch *et al.*, 1985). MPP+ inhibits complex I of the mitochondrial respiratory chain (Nicklas *et al.*, 1985), and cell death may result from this action.

Selective vulnerability factors

Other characteristics of nigral neurons may explain their vulnerability in PD. For example, MPTP and MPP+ (D'Amato *et al.*, 1987) bind to melanin, and thus may be concentrated in melanin-containing neurons. Moreover, the formation of melanin may itself cause oxidative damage (Mann and Yates, 1983). Also, the relatively high metabolic activity of nigral neurons, as well as the relatively low concentration of reduced glutathione in the nigra, may increase vulnerability to oxidative stress (Perry *et al.*, 1982). Nigral iron is increased in postmortem PD brains (Dexter *et al.*, 1989; Sofic *et al.*, 1991) and ferritin is decreased (Dexter *et al.*, 1990), suggesting that iron may be present in a reactive form and provide a stimulus to oxidative reactions (Youdim *et al.*, 1989; Sengstock *et al.*, 1992; Youdim *et al.*, 1993). The occurrence of oxidative stress in PD is also suggested by increased activity of the protective enzyme superoxide dismutase in nigral mitochondria (Saggu *et al.*, 1989). Finally, the reduced capacity of the postmitotic central nervous system for DNA repair has been suggested to underlie neurodegenerative disorders such as Alzheimer's disease, amyotrophic lateral sclerosis and PD (Mazarello *et al.*, 1992). A similar hypothesis has been advanced for mitochondrial DNA (Linnane *et al.*, 1989). While little evidence for the latter hypotheses has been published, recent demonstration of an age-related decrease in dopamine transporter messenger RNA suggests that further exploration of the specific function of genes important to nigral neuron function may also provide clues to the pathogenesis of PD (Bannon *et al.*, 1992).

Evaluation of specific chemicals

The postulate that a compound structurally similar to MPTP may cause PD has been assessed by screening such compounds in mice. Although other neurotoxic pyridines have been described, none caused selective substantia nigra lesions (Perry *et al.*, 1988). Failure to succeed with this experimental approach, however, does not necessarily eliminate a role for such compounds in human PD, since factors such as dose, duration and route of exposure, animal species used, animal age and metabolic state may all influence the outcome of such investigations. Structurally similar herbicides such as paraquat or diquat may be environmentally present (Snyder and D'Amato, 1985), although no such agent has been shown to produce parkinsonism in humans or animals. Rather than seeking agents structurally similar to MPTP, agents with similar function might serve as PD-producing toxins. Of interest in this regard is rotenone, a compound that, like MPTP, is a specific inhibitor of mitochondrial complex I activity. Rotenone is a naturally occurring plant toxin used commercially as an insecticide (Windholz *et al.*, 1983).

Alternatively, parkinsonism-causing agents might be sought amongst those causing oxidative injury. Substances such as diquat and paraquat, certain quinones and certain phenols, for example, can cause the unregulated release of ferritin-bound iron (Reif, 1992). If iron-potentiated oxidative injury is important to the pathogenesis of PD, exposure to agents such as these could, theoretically, contribute to oxidative neuronal injuries. Finally, endogenous compounds, typically those resulting from metabolism of dopamine and serving as substrates of MAOB, may have similar mechanisms and may potentially contribute to nigral cell injury (Testa *et al.*, 1985; Jenner *et al.*, 1992).

Parkinsonism-causing toxicants need not be exclusive to one another. One interpretation of the available information is that the aetiology of PD is likely heterogeneous, with several possible routes to the final pathophysiological outcome. In this case, identification of a single causative agent would be difficult, but evaluation of categories of possible causative agents, all sharing similar mechanisms, might provide insights into the pathogenesis of PD.

Amyotrophic lateral scelerosis–Parkinsonism–dementia complex (ALS-PDC) in the Western Pacific

The classic evolution of a neurotoxic injury involves the development of clinical signs in immediate temporal relationship to a specific toxic exposure. In general, progressive injury is felt to be the result of continued exposure to the toxin. Since PD is a slowly progressive disorder, classical theory would suggest that, if PD is caused by toxic exposure, all patients must have continuous exposure to a putative toxin. An alternative mechanism is suggested by studies of the novel neurodegenerative disorder, ALS-PDC, prevalent in indigenous populations in several locations in the Western Pacific (Kurland, 1988). Extensive epidemiological studies over several decades suggest that ALS-PDC is the result of an exogenous exposure related to the traditional Guamanian lifestyle. Of interest is the observation that Guamanian men with ALS-PDC who join the US military as young adults and have minimal exposure to the Guamanian lifestyle throughout the remainder of their lives may none the less develop a progressive neurodegeneration identical to that experienced by lifelong residents of Guam (Garruto *et al.*, 1980). This observation suggests that exposure to a neurotoxin early in life may result in a progressive syndrome decades later. If this is correct, a similar exposure pattern may underlie PD.

EPIDEMIOLOGICAL INVESTIGATIONS

Epidemiological investigations of PD patients have also been used to address the issue of PD aetiology. Two general approaches have been used – firstly, the demographic characteristics of PD have been used to develop theories of disease aetiology; and secondly, case-control studies have been used to test hypotheses concerning specific risk factors. (Some epidemiological terms are defined in Table 7.1.) The following sections will first review the demographic characteristics of PD with respect to aetiological postulates. Next, studies testing specific hypotheses will be discussed.

Demographic characteristics

The demographic characteristics of PD are most accurately represented in community-based studies, rather than those drawn from clinic or hospital populations, where cultural practices, socioeconomic status, age, sex and degree of disability may all influence the composition of the group. Community-based studies

Table 7.1 Epidemiological terms

Cluster	Two or more people with a specific health event associated temporally and/or spatially
Community-based study	Study of an entire population defined by a geographical or political boundary
Clinic-based study	Study of a group of patients attending a medical care facility; not directly comparable to a community-based study
Case-control study	Persons with a particular disease compared to unaffected persons, with respect to specific factors thought to be related to the illness
Retrospective study	Information concerning exposures proposed to be related to the disease are collected *before* the development of illness
Prospective study	Information concerning exposures proposed to be related to the disease are collected *after* the development of illness
Incidence	New cases of a disease within a given time period
Prevalence	Total number of cases in a population at a given time
Relative risk (risk ratio, R)	Ratio of disease frequency in an exposed population to disease frequency in a theoretically identical unexposed population; if $R > 1$, disease is more likely in exposed subjects
Odds ratio	Ratio of the odds of disease in affected to the odds of disease in unaffected individuals; can be determined from case-control studies, and R can be estimated if disease is rare

are difficult, expensive and time-consuming, and only a few have been performed. This section will focus on studies performed using door-to-door surveys (Li *et al.*, 1985; Schoenberg *et al.*, 1985, 1988; Bharucha *et al.*, 1988; Rocca *et al.*, 1990), because the similarity of method facilitates comparisons among the studies (Table 7.2).

Age

PD is rare before age 40, and becomes increasingly common through subsequent decades. Although some studies have found lower PD prevalence in the very elderly, this is probably an artefact, caused by the small numbers of subjects in these categories (Rajput *et al.*, 1984; Schoenberg *et al.*, 1988). The association of increased risk for PD with increased age suggests either that age-specific factors, such as an expected senescent neuronal loss (Calne and Langston, 1983) and time-dependent factors such as duration of a toxic exposure or accumulation of DNA mutations (Linnane *et al.*, 1989; Mazzarello *et al.*, 1992) contribute to the development of PD.

Sex

With the exception of the door-to-door study conducted in China (Li *et al.*, 1985), most studies show PD to be only slightly more common in men (Table 7.2). Although

Table 7.2 Demographic characteristics of Parkinson's disease in door-to-door studies

	Prevalence (per 10⁵)		*Age-specific prevalence (per 10⁵)*			*Male:Female*
			Age groups			
			50–59	60–69	≥70	
Chinese cities (Li *et al.*, 1985)*	44		92	145	615	3.7:1
			Age groups			
			40–64	65–75	>75	
Copiah County, MS, USA (Schoenberg *et al.*, 1985)†	347	Blacks	236	430	640	1.01:1
		Whites	59	639	422	
Parsi Colony, Bombay, India (Bharucha *et al.*, 1988)‡	328.3	Progressive increase with age				1.59:1
Igbo-Ora, Nigeria (Schoenberg *et al.*, 1988)†	59	ND				ND
Sicily, Italy (Rocca *et al.*, 1990)‡	243	Progressive increase with age				No consistent sex difference

*Subjects' age >49 years.
†Subjects' age >39 years.
‡Subjects of all ages.
ND = Not determined.

the elderly Chinese population does not show the female sex predominance found in the USA (Population Census Office, People's Republic of China, 1982; Bogue, 1985), this difference is not sufficient to account for the 3.7 : 1 male:female prevalence ratio. One possible explanation for the dramatic male predominance of PD in China is that Chinese men have greater exposures to a PD-associated toxic factor, or Chinese women to a protective factor.

Race

US hospital-based surveys (Kessler, 1972; Paddison and Griffith, 1974) and death records (Kurtzke and Goldberg, 1988) have found PD to be much more common in whites than in blacks. When prevalence surveys from many countries are compared, PD prevalence is generally higher in areas where Caucasians constitute the majority of the population (Kurland, 1958; Marttila and Rinne, 1967; Rajput *et al.*, 1984; Sutcliffe *et al.*, 1985; Mutch *et al.*, 1986) and lower where other racial groups predominate (Harada *et al.*, 1983; Li *et al.*, 1985; Schoenberg *et al.*, 1988). Since both MPTP and MPP+ bind to melanin, these observations led to the postulate that non-neuronal melanin may bind a presumed toxin and thus protect against PD (Lerner and Goldman, 1987). One prominent exception to these observations is found in Copiah County, Mississippi, where PD prevalence was reported to be similar in blacks and whites (Schoenberg *et al.*, 1985). However, this determination is calculated based on both 'definite' and 'possible' PD cases. When only 'definite' cases are considered, age-adjusted prevalence in whites is higher than in blacks (280 versus 196 per 100 000), as has been observed in all other studies. Additional community-based studies in multiracial populations are needed to determine whether PD is more common in races with less cutaneous melanin.

Geography

Comparison of community-based prevalence studies generally shows PD to be more common in areas where industrialization is relatively long-standing (Kurland, 1958; Rosati *et al.*, 1980; Harada *et al.*, 1983; Sutcliffe *et al.*, 1985; Marttila and Rinne, 1967; Mutch *et al.*, 1986; Table 7.3). Others, using levodopa sales to approximate prevalence, found higher estimated prevalence in association with regions where wood pulp mills, vegetable farming or steel manufacture were important industries (Barbeau and Roy, 1985; Aquilonius and Hartvig, 1986). In Israel, a cluster of parkinsonism in three kibbutzim has been proposed (Goldsmith *et al.*, 1990). Death records from 1959 to 1961 showed more reported PD cases in northern than southern white US residents (Lux and Kurtzke, 1987). In contrast to these variations, an analysis of parkinsonism deaths among counties in the state of Georgia, USA, found no regional variation within the state (Meador *et al.*, 1987). In Michigan, however, PD deaths clustered in areas with high population density and farming density (Rybicki *et al.*, 1993). An association between PD mortality and the industrial use of heavy metals was suggested. Although the differences found in most of the death record studies may be produced by methodological artifacts, similar differences in door-to-door studies with comparable methods (Table 7.2) suggest that actual geographical variations in PD prevalence do occur. One explanation for these regional variations is that there is greater exposure to a PD-producing toxin in high-prevalence locations,

Table 7.3 Geographical distribution of Parkinson's disease in community-based studies

Location	*Study design*	*Prevalence/100 000*
Rochester, Mn, USA (Kurland, 1958)	Mayo Clinic records	187
Aberdeen, Scotland (Mutch *et al.*, 1986)	Public Health records MD exam verification	164.2
Turku, Finland (Marttila and Rinne, 1967)	Public Health records MD exam verification	120.1
Northampton, UK (Sutcliffe *et al.*, 1985)	Public Health records Some MD exams	108
Yonago, Japan (Harada *et al.*, 1983)	Public Health records MD exam verification	80.6
Sardinia, Italy (Rosati *et al.*, 1980)	Public Health records MD exam verification	65.6

or greater exposure to protective factors in low-prevalence areas. Alternatively, however, racial or genetic susceptibility may be greater in these high-prevalance areas.

Temporal changes

Evaluation of temporal changes in the distribution of disease may provide clues to the cause of disease. For example, if a single factor caused PD, changes in the distribution of that factor over time would be expected to correlate with changes in the distribution of PD. Examination of such possible changes is difficult in practice, however, since changes in disease diagnosis and reporting may also result in apparent changes in the occurrence of disease. Recently, two methods have been applied to examination of the question of temporal changes in the occurrence of PD. The first of these used death records to estimate PD incidence. In addition to misclassification errors in diagnosis and reporting, death records may underestimate disease, since PD may often not be listed as a cause of death (Chandra *et al.*, 1984). Two mortality studies suggested an increase in mortality from PD in elderly persons in the USA and in Italy during the last several decades (Lilienfeld *et al.*, 1990; Chio *et al.*, 1993), and were suggested to reflect an actual increase in disease occurrence as well as increased survival resulting from improved therapies. A second approach assessed the incidence of PD over a 50-year period in Olmsted County, Minnesota, USA, by classifying all cases using modern diagnostic criteria (Tanner *et al.*, 1992). A trend to higher PD incidence with increasing calendar year was observed for both sexes, which was statistically significant for men. While the latter study likely minimized misclassification and under-reporting of disease, the population surveyed is a homogeneous one (mostly descended from northern European immigrants) and may not be readily extrapolated to other populations.

Heredity and twin studies

In 1983 the first of a series of twin studies was published (Ward *et al.*, 1983). This study, as well as four subsequent reports, failed to demonstrate differences in concordance between monozygotic twins (expected to be 100% concordant for a genetic disorder) and dizygotic twins (expected to show the same frequency of disease as would other siblings, no more than 50% for an autosomal dominant disorder) (Marsden 1987; Marttila *et al.*, 1988; Zimmerman *et al.*, 1991; Vierregge *et al.*, 1992). Although there were methodological problems with each of these studies, some of which may have caused an underestimate of concordance, these results were interpreted to support a non-hereditary aetiology for PD.

Several recent observations have suggested that heredity may be important to the cause of PD. Firstly, three large kindreds with Parkinson's disease in multiple generations were described (Golbe *et al.*, 1990b, 1992; Waters, C. H., personal communication, 1992). Each had clinically atypical features – younger age at onset and more rapid progression – but autopsies in one or two members showed changes resembling typical PD. An autosomal dominant inheritance has been proposed in each case. Using a similar approach, Maraganore *et al.* (1991) identified 20 families with more than one case of Parkinson's disease and suggested an autosomal dominant pattern of inheritance. These reports caused a reanalysis of prior studies, with the conclusion that genetic influences cannot be excluded (Johnson *et al.*, 1990; Duvoisin and Johnson, 1992).

None the less, the presence of disease in families does not necessarily support a genetic aetiology. Although a number of studies have reported that relatives of persons with PD appear to have higher risk for the disorder than do members of the general population (Mjones, 1949; Kondo *et al.*, 1973; Martin *et al.*, 1973; Alonso *et al.*, 1986; Campanella *et al.*, 1990), few reported familial cases were evaluated by neurological examination. In some series, subjects were selected by positive family history, raising the question of their representativeness to the entire population (Barbeau and Pourcher, 1982; Maraganore *et al.*, 1991). Moreover, families also typically share common living and/or working environments, diets, hobbies and religious habits, any of which might alter exposure to an environmental cause of disease. Apparently Mendelian patterns of inheritance may be observed for outcomes such as attending medical school (Lilienfeld, 1959). The possible effect of a shared environment was emphasized in a recent report by Calne *et al.* (1987), who described six families in which both parents and children developed PD in close temporal association. The mean difference in disease onset across generations was 4.6 years, while the mean difference in age at disease onset was 25.2 years. This pattern could more easily be explained by a shared exposure to an environmental insult than by a purely genetic origin of disease, since the latter would be expected to occur at similar ages in each generation.

Gene–environment interaction

The failure to prove either a purely genetic or a purely environmental cause for PD suggests a third possibility – that both hypotheses are correct. PD could be the combined result of genetic predisposition (either acquired or inherited) and an environmental exposure to a toxicant. In such a scenario, disease occurs only if both the genetic predisposition and the environmental exposure occur. There are numerous precedents for such a mechanism for disease causation. In fact, in the case of some cancers, disease pathogenesis may be even more complex, involving both inherited and acquired injuries to several genes, as well as multiple toxicant exposures (Hollstein *et al.*, 1991). The analogy with cancer, however, points out the critical need for the identification of easily measured biomarkers for PD. Delineation of such a multistep process in carcinogenesis depended on the ability to analyse large quantities of tissue. In the case of PD, cell death, rather than cell proliferation, is the end-result of the disease process, limiting analysis of affected tissue. Moreover, the primary pathological lesions occur within the central nervous system, and hence tissue cannot be studied until after death.

These limitations highlight the critical need for relatively non-invasive, easily identified means of identifying persons at risk for PD, or those with presymptomatic disease. If biomarkers of susceptibility to PD can be identified, evaluation of exposures of interest in metabolically susceptible populations may be particularly important to the evaluation of gene–environment interaction in PD. Biomarkers for PD can be sought by explorations of proposed metabolic abnormalities underlying PD, such as impaired function of the mitochondrial respiratory chain, impaired function of the enzyme sulphotransferase and impaired function of the hepatic cytochrome P450 enzyme 2D6, or by identification of variant alleles of DNA encoding proteins important to nigral neuron function. The rationale and possible utility of some of these will be considered briefly.

The search for biomarkers

The activity of complex I of the mitochondrial respiratory chain was reported to be decreased in postmortem substantia nigra (Schapira *et al.*, 1989), and in platelets and muscle of living persons with PD, compared to control subjects (Bindoff *et al.*, 1989; Parker *et al.*, 1989; Shoffner *et al.*, 1991; Mann *et al.*, 1992). Attempts to determine the striatal content of complex I (Mizuno *et al.*, 1989), to characterize the polypeptide structure of complex I (Mizuno *et al.*, 1989; Schapira *et al.*, 1990a) or to identify a specific abnormality of mitochondrial DNA in PD (Ikebe *et al.*, 1990; Lestienne *et al.*, 1990; Schapira *et al.*, 1990b) have so far yielded contradictory results. Moreover, mitochondrial abnormalities are not specific for PD. Similar abnormalities of mitochondrial respiration have been identified in other neurological diseases (Rosing *et al.*, 1985; Wallace *et al.*, 1988), without associated parkinsonian signs. Rather than serving as a marker of susceptibility to disease, mitochondrial abnormalities may be the result of the pathophysiological process causing PD (Schoffner *et al.*, 1991). Since the presence of abnormal activity is not limited to PD, and was suggested to correlate with increasing PD severity, impaired activity of mitochondrial complex I may not provide a useful marker of susceptibility or of early disease.

Impaired activities of several detoxification enzymes have been associated with increased risk of PD, although most reports await confirmation. Cysteine dioxygenase activity, measured using S-carboxymethyl-L-cystine, and S-oxidation capacity was reduced in untreated PD patients as compared to controls (Steventon *et al.*, 1989). The ability to form the sulphate conjugation product of paracetamol was also found to be significantly reduced in PD patients versus controls in one study (Steventon *et al.*, 1989), suggesting a generalized problem in sulphation. Impaired phenytoin metabolism, mediated by hepatic cytochrome P450 enzymes, has been observed in some series (Ferrari *et al.*, 1986, 1990), but not others (Gudjonsson *et al.*, 1990). Although this phenotype may be inherited as an autosomal recessive, more than one closely related P450 gene may be involved (Guengerich, 1989). The utility of any of the preceding assays as biomarkers is likely limited, however. Firstly, the performance of such tests generally requires exposure to at least one pharmacological compound, and often long hours of specimen collection in a clinical setting, making them impractical as mass screening tools. Moreover, many enzyme systems may be induced, or their activities may be modified by numerous dietary, environmental and pharmacological factors, making categorization of metabolizer type imprecise and introducing significant intrasubject variability. In contrast, the identification of the gene coding for another detoxification enzyme, cytochrome P450 2D6 (CYP 2D6), has allowed the application of more rapid and precise molecular genetic techniques to a previously inconclusive association. Abnormal activity of this enzyme, as measured by hydroxylation of the drug debrisoquine, was associated with PD in some studies, but these results were controversial (Tanner, 1991). Recently, restriction fragment length polymorphism (RFLP) and polymerase chain reaction (PCR) analyses have identified allelic variants of CYP 2D6 associated with impaired enzyme activity (Daly *et al.*, 1991; Heim and Meyer, 1990). To date, two laboratories have used molecular genetic assays to observe that these allelic variants are associated with an increased risk for PD (Armstrong *et al.*, 1992; Smith *et al.*, 1992). More accurate techniques such as these may clarify the apparently contradictory results of other studies of enzyme activity, and help to determine if any of these abnormalities will prove useful as biomarkers of susceptibility for PD.

Two other strategies have been applied to the search for possible biomarkers of PD – the evaluation of oxidative enzymes, and of enzymes important to the neurons injured in PD. One recent study investigated the peripheral activity of oxidative enzymes in PD. Increased activity of the enzymes superoxide dismutase and glutathione peroxidase was observed in the serum of persons with PD, suggesting that a more generalized metabolic predisposition to free radical formation may be present in some persons with PD (Kalra *et al.*, 1992). Others have investigated allelic variants of genes coding for enzymes important to biogenic amine metabolism, such as monoamine oxidase A (Fink *et al.*, 1992) and MAOB (Kurth *et al.*, 1992) and tyrosine hydroxylase (Kurth and Kurth, 1992). While work with these proposed genetic markers of risk for PD is still preliminary, the ongoing evaluation of the relationship of these and other genetic polymorphisms to the risk of developing PD may provide important keys to understanding its aetiology.

Young-onset PD

Since PD is rare before age 40, study of young-onset patients may be particularly valuable, since they may have more prominent metabolic susceptibility factors, or greater exposure to a PD-associated toxin (Table 7.4). In Saskatchewan, Rajput *et al.* (1986) found that more than expected of the cases with young age at PD onset in a university hospital referral practice were born and raised in rural environments, and used well water for drinking, although attempts to identify specific toxins were not successful. Similarly, young-onset patients in a Chicago referral practice and early-onset respondents to a mail questionnaire also were more likely to have lived in a rural setting and to have used well water than PD patients with onset at an older age (Tanner *et al.*, 1987). In a case-control study comparing detailed lifelong occupational and residential exposures in 78 young-onset patients to age- and sex-matched controls without neurological disease, young-onset cases were

Table 7.4 Proposed risk factors for early Parkinson's disease (PD) onset

Location	*n*	*Onset age in cases*	*Control group*	*Proposed risk factor*
Saskatchewan (Rajput *et al.*, 1986)	22	<40	None	Rural residence, well water use
Chicago (Tanner *et al.*, 1987)	100	<48	PD onset >54	Rural residence, well water use
(Tanner *et al.*, 1987)	512	<48	PD onset >54	Rural residence, well water use
Chicago (Tanner *et al.*, 1990a)	78	<51	Non-PD; age-, sex-, race-matched	Farming
New Jersey, Philadelphia (Dulaney *et al.*, 1990)	73	<40	Non-PD; age-, sex-, race-matched	Head trauma

significantly more likely to have lived or worked on a farm, generally during the first two decades of life (Tanner *et al.*, 1990a). Although these studies vary in methods, they all suggest that some factor associated with rural living in North America may increase the risk for a young age at PD onset.

One exception is the study of Dulaney *et al.* (1990). When 73 young-onset (<40 years) PD patients were compared to 81 older onset (>60 years) patients, or to 73 matched controls, no significant differences were observed. The failure to observe an association with rural living in this population may reflect differences between the eastern seaboard and midwestern North America, where the previously cited studies were performed. A very common or very rare exposure might be missed in small studies such as these. Perhaps the apparent rural relationships noted above are artifacts of referral practices in the study areas, rather than factors actually associated with PD. Alternatively, a putative environmental toxicant might be distributed equally between rural and urban areas in the mid-Atlantic region of the USA, where Dulaney *et al.*'s subjects reside, but be concentrated primarily in rural areas in the Midwest.

Environmental risk factors

A number of researchers have used case-control studies to evaluate proposed risk factors for the development of PD (Table 7.5). All studies have varied somewhat in their choice of cases and controls, methods of verifying diagnosis and choice of proposed risks. In some, only very general questions were asked concerning residence, occupation or exposure, and these had largely negative results (Bharucha *et al.*, 1986; Rajput *et al.*, 1987). A comparison of specific occupational exposures to organic solvents, agricultural chemicals and mercury in Sweden found no difference between PD cases and controls (Ohlson and Hagstedt, 1981). Two studies were conducted in China, reasoning that the more recent industrialization here might facilitate the identification of any industry-related risks. One study of subjects from both north and south China found exposure to industrial chemicals (plants manufacturing chemicals, pesticides, herbicides or pharmaceuticals) to be associated with an increased risk for PD, but living in a village and participating in common farming practices to be associated with a decreased risk (Tanner *et al.*, 1989a). The second study, which included only subjects living in Hong Kong (Ho *et al.*, 1989), found exposure to herbicides or pesticides, and long duration (>20 years) of rural residence or farming to be associated with an increased risk of developing PD. Since villagers in the rural north likely had less exposure to farm chemicals than those in the south, Ho *et al.* (1989) proposed that differences between the two studies could reflect variations in farming practices or dietary habits between northern and southern China.

In a case-control comparison of PD cases and clinic-based controls, Kansas City researchers found that living in a rural environment and using well water as drinking water increased the risk of developing PD, particularly when exposures were in the first few decades (Koller *et al.*, 1990). However, farming or exposure to herbicides or pesticides was not associated with the development of PD. In New Jersey, a comparison of PD cases to spouse controls also found rural residence and use of herbicides or pesticides to be associated with PD (Golbe *et al.*, 1990a). In Campania, Italy, a comparison of 83 PD cases to 83 age- and sex-matched controls with other neurological diseases found drinking well water to be associated with an increased risk for PD, but other factors such as rural living or chemical exposure were not assessed (Campanella *et al.*, 1990). Hertzman *et al.* (1990) identified PD cases in

Table 7.5 Case-control studies testing the association between rural life, agricultural chemicals or well-water drinking and Parkinson's disease (PD)

Location	*Number cases/controls*	*Odds ratios for significant associations*			
		Rural home	*Farming*	*Well-water drinking*	*Herbicides/ pesticides*
China (Tanner *et al.*, 1989a)	100/200	0.57	0.17	NS	2.39
Hong Kong (Ho *et al.*, 1989)	35/105	2.1	5.2	NA	3.6
Kansas (Koller *et al.*, 1990)	150/150	1.9	NS	1.7	NS
New Jersey (Golbe *et al.*, 1990a)	106/106	2.0	NS	NS	7.0
Chicago (Tanner *et al.*, 1990a)	78/78*	NS	3.0	NS	NS
British Columbia (Hertzman *et al.*, 1990)	57/122	NA	NA	NS	6.62†
Campania, Italy (Campanella *et al.*, 1990)	83/83	NA	NA	2.6	NA
New Jersey (Dulaney *et al.*, 1990)	154/154	NS	NA	NS	NS
Calgary, Alberta (Semchuk *et al.*, 1992)	130/260	NS	NS	NS	3.06‡

NA = Not assessed; NS = not significantly different; *PD onset <51 years; †Chemical spraying; ‡Crude odds ratio for herbicide exposure.

rural British Columbia by physician report. In all 57 cases studied, diagnosis was confirmed by a single neurologist. Cases were compared to age-matched controls randomly selected from electoral rolls. Exposure to chemical spraying, work in an orchard and work in a planer mill were all associated with an increased risk of PD. Paraquat use was significantly more common in cases than in controls, but the number was small. Vierregge *et al.* (1992) found living in villages and harvesting mushrooms to be more common in persons with PD than in matched controls. Semchuk *et al.* (1992) studied 130 PD cases and 260 community controls in Calgary, Alberta, Canada. In a multivariate analysis controlling for confounding and possible interaction of exposures, they found a history of occupational herbicide use to be the only factor associated with an increased risk for PD (Semchuk *et al.*, 1992). Most had used primarily chlorphenoxy or thiocarbamate compounds, and only one had used paraquat.

Preliminary reports of three other case-control studies had similar findings. A study in Madrid identified an increased risk for PD associated with drinking well water for more than 40 years, and with exposure to pesticides (Jimenez-Jimenez *et al.*, 1988). In Quebec, occupational or residential exposures to heavy metal industries, pesticides, well water and cigarette smoke increased the risk of developing PD

(Campanella *et al.*, 1988). Finally, the previously cited Chicago-based study of young-onset subjects found early life exposure to farming to be associated with an increased risk for PD (Tanner *et al.*, 1990a).

Although all of these studies are limited by their small size, and differing methods prevent direct comparisons, the similar observations in most studies suggest that exposure to some factor associated with farming, rural residence or specific agricultural or industrial chemicals may be associated with an increased risk of developing PD.

Dietary protective factors

Dietary intake of factors which interfere with the pathogenetic mechanisms underlying PD might prevent disease development. For example, redox substances such as vitamins E, C or beta-carotene have been proposed to block free radical formation (Cross *et al.*, 1987). Alternatively, if the early stages of mitochondrial electron transport are impaired, the same compounds could theoretically serve as electron carriers, bypassing an early block and permitting adenosine triphosphate generation at subsequent stages. If diet can protect against PD, international differences in diet might contribute to variations in prevalence figures. Several case-control studies have evaluated the possible protective effects of one of these compounds, vitamin E (tocopherol). A case-control study of early life dietary habits in 81 PD patients and 81 same-sex siblings found an apparent protective effect of several foods with high vitamin E content (nuts, odds ratio=0.39; salad oil, odds ratio=0.30 and plums, odd ratio=0.24; Golbe *et al.*, 1988). In a follow-up study, the same investigators found that use of two categories of foods high in tocopherol in early life was associated with a decreased risk for PD in a case-control comparison of 106 PD patients and spouse controls (Golbe *et al.*, 1990a). Vierregge *et al.* (1992), however, asking questions similar to those used in the preceding studies, did not find a difference between PD cases and matched controls in Germany. Others compared supplemental vitamin use in 35 PD patients and 70 pair-matched controls (Tanner *et al.*, 1988). The use of supplemental multivitamins, vitamin E or cod liver oil was associated with a decreased risk for PD (odds ratio=0.25). A retrospective food-frequency interview in 100 PD cases and 200 controls in China, and in 35 cases and 70 controls in the USA, found no significant differences in dietary intake of vitamins E, C, beta-carotene, protein calories or total calories between cases and controls in either country (Tanner *et al.*, 1989b). However, the tocopherol content of many foods is not readily available, particularly those commonly eaten in China. Thus, this negative result may simply reflect limitations of study design.

Although the numbers studied to date are small, these studies suggest that tocopherol consumption or related behavioural or dietary factors may protect against the development of PD in some cases. One clinical trial found tocopherol supplementation to be ineffective in slowing the progression of PD (Parkinson's Study Group, 1993), but no study has systematically addressed the relationship of antioxidant nutrient intake and protection against developing PD. Few studies to date have explored the biological mechanisms which may underlie these observations, although tocopherol and beta-carotene may protect against MPTP toxicity and free radical-induced lipid peroxidation (Yong *et al.*, 1986). Susceptibility to oxidative stress may be greater in the substantia nigra of PD patients (Perry *et al.*, 1982; Olanow, 1990) and vulnerability to injury may be increased if dietary intake of antioxidants is inadequate. These observations allow the suggestion that areas with a low prevalence of PD may not be those with a lesser concentration of environmental toxins, but rather those in which there is higher dietary intake of protective substances.

Smoking

Smoking was first observed to have an inverse association with PD in a study of US military veterans in the late 1960s (Kahn, 1966). Nine subsequent case-control studies found cigarette smoking to be inversely associated with PD (Nefzinger *et al.*, 1968; Kessler and Diamond, 1971; Baumann *et al.*, 1980; Burch, 1981; Haack *et al.*, 1981; Godwin-Austin *et al.*, 1982; Bharucha *et al.*, 1986; Dulaney *et al.*, 1990; Tanner *et al.*, 1990b), while only three – one chart review performed in Olmsted County, Minnesota (Rajput *et al.*, 1987), and two performed in China (Tanner *et al.*, 1987; Ho *et al.*, 1989) – found no association between smoking and PD. In the Chinese patients studied, smoking was extremely rare in women with PD, although in China PD is much more common in men (Tanner *et al.*, 1987). If smoking exerted a truly protective effect in this population, a higher PD prevalence in women, rather than men, would be predicted.

Cigarette smoking could theoretically protect against an exogenous toxin by induction of enzyme systems such as hepatic or central nervous system cytochrome P450 mixed-function oxygenases. Alternatively, smoking could compete with an exogenous substrate at a specific enzyme system, such as cerebral MAOB. Rather than reflect an actual biological action, however, decreased smoking in PD could simply reflect the more conservative personality which may accompany PD (Golbe *et al.*, 1986). The failure to demonstrate an inverse association between smoking and PD in China may reflect culturally specific differences in the use of cigarettes, or genetic differences in nicotine metabolism between Chinese and non-Chinese. Also, if specific toxins are less prevalent in the environment, as may have been true in parts of China, a protective effect of smoking may be less apparent.

Infection

The association of parkinsonism with the pandemics of encephalitis lethargica early in this century led to the common belief that all parkinsonian syndromes resulted from occult infection with the causative agent (Poskanzer *et al.*, 1969). Two corollary predictons were: (1) that the mean age at PD onset would become increasingly older as the exposed cohort aged, until (2) PD ultimately disappeared in the 1980s, as survivors of that birth cohort died. The latter predictions have proven incorrect, and few cases of parkinsonism today are felt to be postencephalitic. In one study, however, Mattock *et al.* (1988) suggested that PD births coincided with influenza epidemics, proposing an *in utero* infection with consequent decrease in nigral neuron number. These observations await validation in other populations.

Until recently, efforts to link PD to any direct viral exposure using serum or cerebrospinal fluid antibody titres have failed (Marttila *et al.*, 1977; Elizan and Casals, 1987). In a preliminary report, Fazzini *et al.* (1992) described increased cerebrospinal fluid antibody titres to coronaviruses when 20 PD cases were compared to 18 controls and 29 subjects with other neurological illnesses. Although primarily a respiratory pathogen in humans, in animal studies coronavirus has an affinity for basal ganglia. Interesting, in view of the above-noted association between risk for PD and rural residence, is the fact that coronavirus commonly affects agricultural animals such as pigs. Recently, a second common rural pathogen, *Nocardia asteroides*, has been reported to cause a parkinsonism-like syndrome in mice, although investigations to date have not associated presence of antigens to *Nocardia* with PD (Hubble *et al.*, 1992). Rather than reflecting an exposure to a toxic environmental chemical, the association of PD with a rural environment may reflect environmental exposure to an infectious agent.

Trauma

Many retrospective case-control studies have reported an association between head trauma and an increased risk for PD (Bharucha *et al.*, 1986; Tanner *et al.*, 1987; Dulaney *et al.*, 1990). However, when prospectively collected information concerning the occurrence of trauma before PD onset was obtained from the medical records of all PD cases and age- and sex-matched controls in Rochester, Minnesota, trauma was not associated with an increased risk for PD (Rajput *et al.*, 1987). A similar failure to replicate retrospectively collected information when prospectively collected information is used has been reported for Alzheimer's disease (Chandra *et al.*, 1989). Subjects with an illness are typically more likely to remember injuries than controls, and consequently retrospective surveys will almost always identify increased injury in the cases. Unless other prospectively collected information is found to contradict the Rochester observations, trauma should not be considered to increase the risk for PD.

Emotional stress

Emotional stress, like trauma, was proposed to contribute to the development of PD over 100 years ago (Charcot, 1878; Gowers, 1888). In the laboratory, increased dopamine turnover is associated with increased oxidized glutathione (Spina and Cohen, 1989). In behaviourally normal animals with partial chemical lesions of the substantia nigra, various metabolic stresses transiently produced abnormal behaviour commonly seen after more extensive injuries of nigral dopaminergic neurons (Snyder *et al.*, 1985). Similarly, PD patients undergo transient worsening in association with stressful events such as auto accidents (Goetz, 1990).

Accurate evaluation of a possible role for stress in the development of PD, however, is subject to recall bias, as cited above in the discussion of trauma. Moreover, both the definition and quantitation of stress pose further difficulties. Information concerning stress can not be easily collected from a medical records review. None the less, two reports have linked the extreme emotional and physical hardship of concentration camp imprisonment with the subsequent development of PD (Gibberd and Simmons, 1980; Treves *et al.*, 1990). Whether these observations reflect an accelerated nigral injury as the result of stress-related increase in dopamine turnover with resultant increased oxidative injury, nutritional deficiencies of dietary protective agents or other factors cannot be determined. Evaluation of the relationship of less severe emotional or physical stress to the development of PD poses a methodoligical challenge.

Physical exercise

A case-control study conducted amongst men attending Harvard or the University of Pennsylvania between 1916 and 1950 found moderate but not heavy physical exercise to be associated with a mildly decreased risk of PD (Sasco *et al.*, 1992). Diagnosis of disease was by self-report on a mail questionnaire, and validated by a physician's report. Although exercise level was measured before disease onset, it is possible that the long preclinical period proposed for PD may have caused those ultimately developing PD to be less active earlier in life. Validation of this association in other populations has not yet been presented.

CONCLUSION

The hypothesis that PD is the combined result of metabolic predisposition and toxic exposure remains to be proven. A PD-producing toxin must replicate the criteria imposed by our knowledge of PD (Table 7.6). Although parkinsonism may be caused by many toxicants (Goetz, 1985; Tanner, 1992), none has been shown to produce a syndrome which exactly mimics PD. Possibly, failure to produce PD in experimental animals reflects an inability to reproduce a critical combination of metabolic abnormality, age and exposure to toxic and protective agents.

The growth of scientific interest in this area, and the development of new collaborative efforts between basic, clinical and epidemiological scientists is rapidly increasing scientific knowledge. Future work may permit the early identification of subjects at risk for PD, and the development of behavioural, dietary or pharmaceutical measures to delay or prevent PD.

Table 7.6 Requirements for a Parkinson's disease (PD)-producing toxin

Pathological specificity
Degeneration of pigmented neurons
Lewy bodies
Evidence of progressive degeneration
Injury limited to structures involved in PD
Clinical specificity
Susceptibility increases with age
Insidious onset of illness
Slow progression of illness
Variation in individual susceptibility?
Racial differences in susceptibility?
Geographic/temporal characteristics
Worldwide presence
Present since at least 1817
Varying geographical distribution?

References

Alonso ME, Otero E, D'Regules R, and Figueroa HH (1986) Parkinson's disease: a genetic study. *Can J Neurol Sci*, **13**, 248–51

Aquilonius SM and Hartvig P (1986) A Swedish county with unexpectedly high utilization of anti-parkinsonian drugs. *Acta Neurol Scand*, **74**, 379–82

Armstrong M, Daly AK, Cholerton S, Bateman DN, and Idle JR (1992) Mutant debrisoquine hydroxylation genes in Parkinson's disease. *Lancet*, **339**, 1017–18

Bannon MJ, Poosch MS, Xia Y, Goebel DJ, Cassin B, and Kapatos G (1992) Dopamine transporter mRNA content in human substantia nigra decreases precipitously with age. *Proc Natl Acad Sci*, **89**, 7095–9

Barbeau A and Pourcher E (1982) New data on the genetics of Parkinson's disease. *Can J Neurol Sci*, **9**, 53–60

Barbeau A and Roy M (1985) Uneven prevalence of Parkinson's disease in the province of Quebec. *Can J Neurol Sci*, **12**, 169

Baumann RJ, Jameson HD, McKean HE, Haack DG, and Weisburg LM (1980) Cigarette smoking and Parkinson's disease: I. A comparison of cases with matched neighbors. *Neurology*, **30**, 839–43

Bharucha NE, Stokes L, Schoenberg BS, Ward C, Ince S, Nutt JG, *et al.* (1986) A case-control study of twin pairs discordant for Parkinson's disease: a search for environmental risk factors. *Neurology*, **36**, 284–8

Bharucha NE, Bharucha EP, Bharucha AE, Bhise AV, and Schoenberg BS (1988) Prevalence of PD in the Parsi community of Bombay, India. *Arch Neurol*, **45**, 1321–3

Bindoff LA, Birch-Machin M, Cartlidge NEF, Parker WD, and Turnbull DM (1989) Mitochondrial function in Parkinson's disease. *Lancet*, **ii**, 49

Bogue DJ (1985) *The Population of the Unites States. Historical Trends and Future Projections*, New York, The Free Press

Burch PRJ (1981) Cigarette smoking and Parkinson's disease. *Neurology*, **31**, 500–3

Calne DB (1989) Is "Parkinson's disease" one disease? *J Neurol Neurosurg Psychiatry*, (suppl.), 18–21

Calne DB and Langston JW (1983) An etiology of Parkinson's disease. *Lancet*, **2**, 1457–9

Calne S, Schoenberg B, Martin W, Uitti RJ, Spencer P, and Calne DB (1987) Familial Parkinson's disease: possible role of environmental factors. *Can J Neurol Sci*, **4**, 303

Campanella G, Roy M, Masson H, Zayed J, Panisset JC, Ducic S *et al.* (1988) A case-control study of Parkinson's disease in southern Quebec: exposure to metals and pesticides. In *Proceedings of the Ninth International Symposium on Parkinson's Disease*, World Congress of Neurology, vol 57

Campanella G, Filla A, De Michele G, Zayed J, Roy M, and Barbeau A (1990) Etiology of Parkinson's disease: results of two case-control studies. *Movement Disorders*, **5** (suppl. 1), 31

Chandra V, Bharucha NE, and Schoenberg BS (1984) Mortality data for the U.S. for deaths due to and related to twenty neurologic diseases. *Neuropeidemiology*, **3**, 149–68

Chandra V, Kokmen E, Schoenberg B, and Beard MC (1989) Head trauma with loss of consciousness as a risk factor for Alzheimer's disease. *Neurology*, **39**, 1576–8

Charcot JM (1878) *Lectures on the Diseases of the Nervous System*, vol I. English translation by Sigerson G. London, New Sydenham Society

Chiba K, Trevor A, and Castagnoli N (1984) Metabolism of the neurotoxic tertiary amine, MPTP, by brain monoamine oxidase. *Biochem Biophys Res Commun*, **120**, 574–8

Chio A, Magnani C, Tolardo G, and Schiffer D (1993) Parkinson's disease mortality in Italy, 1951 through 1987. *Arch Neurol*, **50**, 148–53

Cross CE, Halliwell B, Borish ET, Pryor WA, Ames BN, Saul RL, *et al.* (1987) Oxygen radicals and human disease. *Ann Intern Med*, **107**, 526–45

Daly AK, Armstrong M, Monkman SC, Idle ME, and Idle JR (1991) Genetic and metabolic criteria for the assignment of debrisoquine 4-hydroxylation (cyctochrome P4502D6) phenotypes. *Pharmacogenetics*, **1**, 33–41

D'Amato RJ, Alexander GM, Schwartzmann RJ, Kitt CA, Price DL, and Snydey SH (1987) Evidence for neuromelanin involvement in MPTP neurotoxicity. *Nature*, **327**, 324–6

Davis GS, Williams AC, Markey SP, Ebert MH, Caine ED, Reichert CM *et al.* (1979) Chronic parkinsonism secondary to intravenous injection of meperidine analogues. *Psychiatry Res*, **1**, 249–59

Dexter DT, Wells FR, Agid Y, Lees AJ, Jenner P, and Marsden CD (1989) Increased nigral iron content and alterations in other metal ions occurring in brain in Parkinson's disease. *J Neurochem*, **52**, 1830–6

Dexter DT, Carayon A, Vidailhet M, Ruberg M, Agid F, Agid Y *et al.* (1990) Decreased ferritin levels in brain in Parkinson's disease. *J Neurochem*, **55**, 16–20

Dulaney E, Stern M, Hurtig H, Golbe L, Bergen M, Gruber S *et al.* (1990) The epidemiology of Parkinson's disease: a case-control study of young-onset versus old onset patients. *Movement Disorders*, **5**, (suppl 1), 12

Duvoisin RC and Johnson WG (1992) The genetics of Parkinson's disease. *Brain Pathol*, **2**, 309–20

Elizan TS and Casals J (1987) The viral hypothesis in Parkinson's disease and Alzheimer's disease: a critique. In Kurstak E, Lipowski SJ, and Morozov PV, eds, *Viruses, Immunity and Mental Disorders*, New York, Plenum Press, 47–59

Fazzini E, Fleming J, and Fahn S (1992) Cerebrospinal fluid antibodies to coronaviruses in patients with Parkinson's disease. *Movement Disorders*, **7**, 153–8

Ferrari MD, De Wolff FA, Vermey P, Veenema H, and Buruma OJS (1986) Hepatic cytochrome p450 function and Parkinson's disease. *Lancet*, **6**, 324

Ferrari MD, Peeters EAJ, Haan J, Roos RAC, Vermey P, de Wolff FA *et al.* (1990) Cytochrome P450 and Parkinson's disease. *J Neurol Sci*, **96**, 153–7

Fink JS, Hotamsigli GS, Girmen AS, Shalish C, Baezinger J, Sullivan *et al.* (1992) Allelic variants in the MAO-A gene mark activity state and may predict vulnerability to Parkinson's disease. *Neurology*, **42** (suppl 3), 173

Forno LS, Langston JW, DeLanney LE, Irwin I, and Ricaurte GA (1986) Locus coeruleus lesions and eosinophilic inclusions in MPTP-treated monkeys. *Ann Neurol*, **20**, 449–55

Garruto RM, Gajdusek DC, and Chen KM (1980) Amyotrophic leteral sclerosis among Chamorro migrants from Guam. *Ann Neurol*, **8**, 612–19

Gibberd FB and Simmons JP (1980) Neurological disease in ex-Far-East prisoners of war. *Lancet*, **ii**, 135–8

Godwin-Austin RB, Lee PN, Marmot MG, and Stern GM (1982) Smoking and Parkinson's disease. *J Neurol Neurosurg Psychiatry*, **45**, 577–81

Goetz CG (1985) *Neurotoxins in Clinical Practice*, New York, SP Medical and Scientific Books, xix

Goetz CG (1990) Motor vehicle accidents and Parkinson's disease disability. *Movement Disorders*, **5** (suppl 1), 16

Golbe LI, Cody RA, and Duvoisin RC (1986) Smoking and Parkinson's disease. Search for a dose–response relationship. *Arch Neurol*, **43**, 774–8

Golbe LI, Farrell TM, and Davis PH (1988) Case-control study of early life dietary factors in PD. *Arch Neurol*, **45**, 350–3

Golbe LI, Farrell TM, and Davis PH (1990a) Follow-up study of early life protective and risk factors in PD. *Movement Disorders*, **5**, 66–70

Golbe LI, Di Torio G, Bonavita V, Miller DC, and Duvoisin RC (1990b) A large kindred with autosomal dominant Parkinson's disease. *Ann Neurol*, **27**, 276–82

Golbe LI, De Irio G, Bonavita V, and Duovoisin RC (1992) A large kindred with Parkinson's disease, segregation ratios and anticipation. *Movement Disorders*, **7**, 24

Goldsmith JR, Herishanu Y, Abarbanel JM, and WeinBaum Z (1990) Clustering of Parkinson's disease points to environmental etiology. *Arch Environ Health*, **45**, 88–94

Gowers WR (1888) *Diseases of the Nervous System.* American edition, Philadelphia, P Blakiston

Gudjonsson O, Sanz E, Alván G, Aquilonius S-M, and Reviriego J (1990) Poor hydroxylator phenotypes of debrisoquine and S-mephenytoin are not over represented in a group of Parkinson's disease patients. *Br J Clin Pharmacol*, **30**, 301–2

Guengerich FP (1989) Polymorphism of cytochrome P450 in humans. *TIPS*, **10**, 107–9

Haack DG, Baumann RJ, McKean HE, Jameson HD, and Turbeck JA (1981) Nicotine exposure and Parkinson's disease. *Am J Epidemiol*, **114**, 119–200

Harada H, Nishikawa S, and Takahashi K (1983) Epidemiology of Parkinson's disease in a Japanese city. *Arch Neurol*, **40**, 151–4

Heikkila RE, Manzino L, Cabbat FS, and Duvoisin RC (1984) Protection against the dopaminergic neurotoxicity of 1-methyl-4-phenyl-1,2,3,6-tetrahydropyridine by monoamine oxidase inhibitors. *Nature*, **311**, 467–9

Heim M and Meyer UA (1990) Genotyping of poor metabolisers of debrisoquine by allele-specific PCR amplification. *Lancet*, **336**, 529–32

Hertzman C, Wiens M, Bowering D, Snow B, and Calne D (1990) Parkinson's disease: a case-control study of occupational and environmental risk factors. *Am J Indust Med*, **17**, 349–55

Ho SC, Woo J, and Lee CM (1989) Epidemiologic study of Parkinson's disease in Hong Kong. *Neurology*, **39**, 1314–18

Hollstein M, Sidransky D, Vogelstein B, and Harris CC (1991) Mutations in human cancers. *Science*, **253**, 49–53

Hubble J, Kjelstrom J, Beamann B, and Koller W (1992) Nocardia serology in Parkinson's disease. *Movement Disorders*, **7**, 292

Hughes AJ, Daniel SE, Kilford L, and Lees AJ (1992) The accuracy of the clinical diagnosis of Parkinson's disease: a clinico-pathological study of 100 cases. *J Neurol Neurosurg Psychiatry*, **55**, 181–4

Ikebe S, Tanaka M, and Ohno K (1990) Increase of deleted DNA in the striatum in Parkinson's disease and senescence. *Biochem Biophys Res Commun*, **170**, 1044–8

Javitch JA, D'Amato TJ, Strittmatter SM, and Snyder SH (1985) Parkinsonism-inducing neurotoxin MPTP: uptake of the metabolite MPP+ by dopaminergic neurons explains selective toxicity. *Proc Natl Acad Sci USA*, **82**, 2173–7

Jenner P, Schapira AHV, and Marsden CD (1992) New insights into the cause of Parkinson's disease. *Neurology*, **42**, 2241–50

Jimenez-Jimenez FJ, Gonzales DM, and Gimenez-Roldan S (1988) Exposure to well water drinking and pesticides in Parkinson's disease. A case-control study from the southeast area of Madrid. In *Proceedings of the Ninth International Symposium on Parkinson's Disease, World Congress of Neurology*, 118

Johnson WG, Hodge SE, and Duvoisin RC (1990) Twin studies and the genetics of Parkinson's disease – a reappraisal. *Movement Disorders*, **5**, 187–94

Kahn HA (1966) The Dorn Study of smoking among US veterans. In *National Cancer Institute, Epidemiologic Approaches to the Study of Cancer and other Diseases*. Washington, DC, US Government Printing Office, Monograph 19, 1–125

Kalra J, Rajput A, Massey KL, and Prasad K (1990) Increased production of oxygen free radicals in Parkinson's disease. *Neurology*, **40** (suppl 1), 169

Kessler II (1972) Epidemiologic studies of Parkinson's disease. II. A hospital-based survey. *Am J Epidemiol*, **95**, 308–18

Kessler II and Diamond EL (1971) Epidemiologic studies of Parkinson's disease. I. Smoking and Parkinson's disease: a survey and explanatory hypothesis. *Am J Epidemiol*, **94**, 16–25

Koller WC (1987) Classification of Parkinsonism. In Koller WC, ed, *Handbook of Parkinson's Disease*, New York, Marcel Dekker, 51–80

Koller W, Vetere-Overfield B, Gray C, Alexander C, Chin T, Dolezal J *et al.* (1990) Environmental risk factors in Parkinson's disease. *Neurology*, **40**, 1214–21

Kondo K, Kurland L, and Schull W (1973) Parkinson's disease: genetic analysis and evidence of a multifactorial etiology. *Mayo Clin Proc*, **48**, 465–75

Kurland LT (1958) Epidemiology: incidence, geographic distribution and genetic considerations. In Field W, ed, *Pathogenesis and Treatment of Parkinsonism*, Springfield, Charles C. Thomas, 5–43

Kurland LT (1988) Amyotrophic lateral sclerosis and Parkinson's disease on Guam linked to an environmental neurotoxin. *Trends Neurosci*, **11**, 51–5

Kurth JH and Kurth MC (1992) Allelic frequencies of tyrosine hydroxylase in Parkinson's disease patients. *Movement Disorders*, **7**, 290

Kurth JH, Podsulo SE, and Kurth MC (1992) Rapid identification of monoamine oxidase B alleles: possible predictors of increased risk for developing Parkinson's disease. *Neurology*, **42** (suppl 3), 379

Kurtzke JF and Goldberg ID (1988) Parkinsonism death rates by race, sex and geography. *Neurology*, **38**, 1558–61

Langston JW, Ballard PA, Tetrud JW, and Irwin I (1983) Chronic parkinsonism in humans due to a product of meperidine-analog synthesis. *Science*, **219**, 979–80

Lerner MR and Goldman RS (1987) Skin color, MPTP, and Parkinson's disease. *Lancet*, **ii**, 212

Lestienne P, Nelson J, Riederer P, Jellinger K, and Reichman H (1990) Normal mitochondrial genome in brain from patients with Parkinson's disease complex I defect. *J Neurochem*, **55**, 1810–12

Li SC, Schoenberg BS, Wang CC, Cheng X, Rui D, Bolis CL *et al.* (1985) A prevalence survey of Parkinson's disease and other movement disorders in the People's Republic of China. *Arch Neurol* **42**, 655–7

Lilienfeld AM (1959) A methodologic problem in testing a recessive genetic hypothesis in human disease. *Am J Public Health*, **49**, 199–204

Lilienfeld DE, Chan E, Ehland J, Godbold J, Landrigan PJ, Marsh G *et al.* (1990) Two decades of increasing mortality from Parkinson's disease among US elderly. *Arch Neurol*, **47**, 731–4

Linnane AW, Marzuki S, Ozawa T, and Tanaka M (1989) Mitochondrial DNA mutations as an important contributor to ageing and degenerative diseases. *Lancet*, **i**, 642–5

Lux WE and Kurtzke JF (1987) Is Parkinson's disease acquired? *Neurology*, **37**, 467–71

Mann DMA and Yates PO (1983) Possible role of neuromelanin in the pathogenesis of Parkinson's disease. *Mech Ageing Dev*, **21**, 193–203

Mann VM, Cooper JM, Krige D, Daniel SE, Schapira AHV, and Marsden CD (1992) Brain, skeletal muscle and platelet mitochondrial function in Parkinson's disease. *Brain*, **115**, 333–42

Maraganore DM, Harding AE, and Marsden CD (1991) A clinical and genetic study of familial Parkinson's disease. *Movement Disorders*, **6**, 205–11

Markey SP, Johannessen JN, Chiueh CC, Burns RS, and Herkenham MA (1984) Intraneuronal generation of a pyridinium metabolite may cause drug-induced parkinsonism. *Nature*, **311**, 464–7

Marsden CD (1987) Twins and Parkinson's disease. *J Neurol Neurosurg Psychiatry*, **50**, 105–6

Martin WE, Young WI, and Anderson VE (1973) Parkinson's disease: a genetic study. *Brain*, **96**, 495–506

Marttila RJ and Rinne UK (1967) Epidemiology of Parkinson's disease in Finland. *Acta Neurol Scand*, **43** (suppl 33), 9–61

Marttila RJ, Halonen P, and Rinne UK (1977) Influenza virus antibodies in parkinsonism. *Arch Neurol*, **34**, 99–100

Marttila RJ, Kaprio J, Koshewvuo M, and Rinne UK (1988) Parkinson's disease in a nationwide twin cohort. *Neurology*, **39**, 1217–19

Mattock C, Marmot M, and Stern G (1988) Could Parkinson's disease follow intrauterinal influenza?: a speculative hypothesis. *J Neurol Neurosurg Psychiatry*, **51**, 753–6

Mazzarello P, Poloni M, Spadari S, and Focher F (1992) DNA repair mechanisms in neurological diseases: facts and hypotheses. *J Neurol Sci*, **112**, 4–14

Meador KJ, Meador MP, Loring DW, Feldman DS, and Sethi KD (1987) Neuroepidemiology of Parkinson's disease. *Neurology*, **37** (suppl 1), 120

Mizuno Y, Ohta S, Tanaka M, Takamiya S, Suzuki K, Sato T *et al.* (1989) Deficiencies in complex I subunits of the respiratory chain in Parkinson's disease. *Biochem Biophys Res Commun*, **163**, 1450–5

Mjones H (1949) Paralysis agitans: a clinical and genetic study. *Acta Psychiatry Neurol*, **54** (suppl), 1–194

Mutch WJ, Dingwall-Fordyce I, Downie AW, Paterson JG, and Roy SK (1986) Parkinson's disease in a Scottish city. *Br Med J*, **292**, 534–6

Nefzinger MD, Quadfasel FA, and Karl VC (1968) A retrospective study of smoking and Parkinson's disease. *Am J Epidemiol*, **88**, 149–58

Nicklas WJ, Vyas I, and Heikkila RE (1985) Inhibition of NADH-linked oxidation in brain mitochondria by 1-methyl-4-phenyl-pyridine, a metabolite of the neurotoxin, 1-methyl-4-phenyl-1,2,3,6-tetrahydropyridine. *Life Sci*, **36**, 2503–8

Ohlson CG and Hagstedt C (1981) Parkinson's disease occupational exposure to organic solvents, agricultural chemicals and mercury: a case-referrent study. *Scand J Work Environ Health*, **7**, 252–6

Olanow CW (1990) Oxidation reactions in Parkinson's disease. *Neurology*, (**40** suppl 3), 32–7

Paddison RM and Griffith RP (1974) Occurrence of Parkinson's disease in black patients at Charity Hospital in New Orleans. *Neurology*, **24**, 688–90

Parker WD, Boyson SJ, and Parks JK (1989) Abnormalities of the electron transport chain in idiopathic Parkinson's disease. *Ann Neurol*, **26**, 719–23

Parkinson J (1817) *An Essay on the Shaking Palsy*, London, Sherwood, Neely and Jones

Parkinson's Study Group (1993) Effects of tocopherol and deprenyl on the progression of disability in early Parkinson's disease. *N Engl J Med*, **328**, 176–83

Perry TL, Godin DV, and Hansen S (1982) Parkinson's disease: a disorder due to nigral glutathione deficiency. *Neurosci Lett*, **33**, 305–10

Perry TL, Jones K, Hansen S, and Wall RA (1988) 2-Phenylpyridine and 3-phenylpyridine, constituents of tea, are unlikely to cause idiopathic Parkinson's disease. *J Neurol Sci*, **85**, 309–17

Population Census Office, People's Republic of China (1982) The 1982 Population Census of China (Major Figures). English edn, Hong Kong, Economic Information and Agency

Poskanzer DC, Schwab RS, and Fraser DW (1969) Further observations on the cohort phenomenon in Parkinson's syndrome. In Barbeau A and Brunnette JR, eds, *Progress in Neurogenetics*, Amsterdam, Excerpta Medica, 497–505

Rajput AH, Offord KP, Beard MC, and Kurland LT (1984) Epidemiology of Parkinson's disease. Incidence, classification and mortality. *Ann Neurol*, **16**, 278–87

Rajput AH, Uitti RJ, Stern W, and Laverty W (1986) Early onset of Parkinson's disease in Saskatchewan – environmental considerations for etiology. *Can J Neurol Sci*, **13**, 312–16

Rajput AH, Offord KP, Beard CM, and Kurland LT (1987) A case-control study of smoking habits, dementia, and other illnesses in idiopathic Parkinson's disease. *Neurology*, **37**, 226–32

Reif DW (1992) Ferritin as a source of iron for oxidative damage. *Free Radical Biol Med*, **12**, 417–27

Ricaurte GA, DeLanney LE, Irwin I, and Langston JW (1987) Older dopaminergic neurons do not recover from the effects of MPTP. *Neuropharmacology*, **26**, 97–9

Rinne UK (1978) Recent advances in research on parkinsonism. *Acta Neurol Scand*, **57** (suppl 67), 77–113

Rocca WA, Morgante M, Grigoletto F, Meneghini F, Reggio A, Savettieri G, *et al.* (1990) Prevalence of Parkinson's disease and other parkinsonisms: a door-to-door study in two Sicilian communities. *Neurology*, **40** (suppl 1), 422

Rosati G, Granieri E, Pinna L, Aiello I, Tola R, De Bastiani P *et al.* (1980) The risk of Parkinson's disease in Mediterranean people. *Neurology*, **30**, 250–5

Rosing HS, Hopkins LC, Wallace DC, Epstein CM, and Weidenheim K (1985) Maternally inherited mitochondrial myopathy and myoclonic epilepsy. *Ann Neurol*, **17**, 228–37

Rybicki BA, Johnson CC, Uman J, and Gorell JM (1993) Parkinson's disease mortality and the industrial use of heavy metals in Michigan. *Movement Disorders*, **8**, 87–92

Saggu H, Cooksey J, Dexter D, Wells FR, Lees AJ, Jenner P *et al.* (1989) A selective increase in particulate superoxide dismutase activity in Parkinsonian substantia nigra. *J Neurochem*, **53**, 692–7

Sasco AJ and Patternburger RS (1992) The role of physical exercise in the occurrence of Parkinson's disease, *Ann Neurol*, **49**, 360–3

Schapira AHV, Cooper JM, Dexter D, Clark JB, Jenner P, and Marsden CD (1989) Mitochondrial complex I deficiency in Parkinson's disease. *Ann Neurol*, **26**, 17–18

Schapira AHV, Cooper JM, Dexter D, Jenner P, Clark JB, and Marsden CD (1990a) Mitochondrial complex I deficiency in Parkinson's disease. *Lancet*, **1**, 1269

Schapira AHV, Holt IJ, Sweeney M, Harding AE, Jenner P, and Marsden CD (1990b) Mitochondrial DNA analysis in Parkinson's disease. *Movement Disorders*, **5**, 294–7

Schlesselman JJ (1982) *Case-Control Studies: Design, Conduct, Analysis*, New York, Oxford University Press

Schoenberg BS, Anderson DW, and Haerer AF (1985) Prevalence of Parkinson's disease in the biracial population of Copiah County, Mississippi, *Neurology*, **35**, 841–5

Schoenberg BS, Osuntokun BO, Adeuja AOG, Bademosi O, Nottidge V, Anderson DW *et al.* (1988) Comparison of the prevalence of Parkinson's disease in black populations in the rural US and in rural Nigeria: door-to-door community studies. *Neurology*, **38**, 645–6

Semchuk KM, Love EJ, and Lee RG (1992) Parkinson's disease and exposure to agricultural work and pesticide chemicals. *Neurology*, **42**, 1328–35

Sengstock GJ, Olanow CW, Dunn AJ, and Anderson GW (1992) Iron induces degeneration of nigrostriatal neurons. *Brain Res Bull*, **28**, 645–9

Shoffner JM, Watts RL, Juncos JL, Toroni A, and Wallace DC (1991) Mitochondrial oxidative phosphorylation defects in Parkinson's disease. *Ann Neurol*, **30**, 332–9

Smith CAS, Gough AC, Leigh PN, Summers BA, Harding AE, Maraganore DM *et al.* (1992) Debrisoquine hydroxylase gene polymorphism and susceptibility to Parkinson's disease. *Lancet*, **339**, 1375–7

Snyder SH and D'Amato RJ (1985) Predicting Parkinson's disease. *Nature*, **317**, 198

Snyder AM, Stricker EM, and Zigmond MJ (1985) Stress-induced neurological impairments in an animal model of parkinsonism. *Ann Neurol*, **18**, 544–51

Sofic E, Paulus W, Jellinger K, Riederer P, and Youdim MBH (1991) Selective increase of iron in substantia nigra zona compacta of parkinsonian brains. *J Neurochem*, **56**, 978–82

Spina MB and Cohen G (1989) Dopamine turnover and glutathione oxidation: implications for Parkinson's disease. *Proc Natl Acad Sci*, **86**, 1398–1400

Steventon GB, Heafield MTB, Waring RH and Williams RC (1989) Xenobiotic metabolism in Parkinson's disease. *Neurology*, **39**, 883–7

Sutcliffe RLG, Prior R, Mawby B, and McQuillan WJ (1985) Parkinson's disease in the district of the Northampton Health Authority, United Kingdom. *Acta Neurol Scand*, **72**, 363–79

Tanner CM (1992) Occupational and environmental causes of parkinsonism. In Shusterman D and Blanc P, eds, *Occupational Medicine: State of the Art Reviews. Unusual Occupational Diseases*, Philadelphia, Hanley & Belfus, 503–13

Tanner CM, Chen B, Wang W, Peng M, Liu Z, Liang X *et al.* (1987) Environmental factors in the etiology of Parkinson's disease. *Can J Neurol Sci*, **14**, 419–23

Tanner CM, Cohen JC, Summerville BC, and Goetz CG (1988) Vitamin use and Parkinson's disease. *Ann Neurol*, **233**, 182

Tanner CM, Chen B, Wang W, Peng M, Liu Z, Liang X *et al.* (1989a) Environmental factors and PD: a case-control study in China. *Neurology*, **39**, 660–4

Tanner CM, Chen B, Cohen JA, Wang W, Peng M, Summerville BC *et al.* (1989b) Dietary antioxidant vitamins and the risk of developing Parkinson's disease. *Neurology*, **39** (suppl), 181

Tanner CM, Grabler P, and Goetz CG (1990a) Occupation and the risk of Parkinson's disease: a case-control study in young onset patients. *Neurology*, **40** (suppl 1), 422

Tanner CM, Koller WC, Gilley DC, Goetz CG, Wang W, Peng M *et al.* (1990b) Cigarette smoking, alcohol drinking and Parkinson's disease: cross-cultural risk assessment. *Movement Disorders*, **5** (suppl 1), 11

Tanner CM, Thelen JA, Offord K, Rademacher D, Goetz CG, and Kurland LT (1992) Parkinson's disease incidence in Olmsted County, MN: 1935–1988. *Neurology*, **42** (suppl 1), 194

Testa B, Naylor R, Costall B, Jenner P, and Marsden CD (1985) Does an endogenous methylpyridinium analogue cause Parkinson's disease? *J Pharm Pharmacol*, **37**, 679–81

Treves TA, Rabey JM, and Korczyn AD (1990) Case-control study, with use of temporal approach, for evaluation of risk factors for Parkinson's disease. *Movement Disorders*, **5** (suppl 1), 11

Vierregge P, Maravic CV, and Friedrich HJ (1992) Lifestyle and dietary factors early and late in Parkinson's disease. *Can J Neurol Sci*, **19**, 170–3

Wallace DC, Sungh G, Lott MT, Hodge JA, Schurr TG, Lezza AMS *et al.* (1988) Mitochondrial DNA mutation associated with Leber's optic atrophy. *Science*, **242**, 1427–30

Ward CD, Duvoisin RC, Ince SE, Nutt JD, Eldridge R, and Calne DB (1983) Parkinson's disease in 65 pairs of twins and in a set of quadruplets. *Neurology*, **33**, 815–24

Windholz M, Budavari S, Blumetti RF, and Otterbein ES (1983) *The Merck Index. An Encyclopedia of Drugs and Biologicals*, 10th edn, Rahway, NY, Merck, 1191–2

Yong VW, Perry TL, and Krisman AA (1986) Depletion of glutathione in brainstem of mice caused by N-methyl-4-phenyl-1,2,3,6-tetrahydropyridine is prevented by antioxidant pretreatment. *Neuro Lett*, **63**, 56–60

Youdim MBH, Ben-Sachar D, and Riederer P (1989) Is Parkinson's disease a progressive siderosis of substantia nigra resulting in iron and melanin induced neurodegeneration? *Acta Neurol Scand*, **126**, 47–54

Youdim MBH, Ben-Sachar D, and Riederer P (1993) The possible role of iron in the etiopathology of Parkinson's disease. *Movement Disorders*, **8**, 1–12

Zimmerman TR, Bhatt M, Calne DB, and Duvoisin RC (1991) Parkinson's disease in monozgotic twins: a followup. *Neurology*, **41**, 255

8
Pathological clues to the cause of Parkinson's disease

W. R. G. Gibb and A. J. Lees

INTRODUCTION

James Parkinson (1817) speculated that the lesion in the shaking palsy might reside in the lower brain stem or upper cervical cord, and published his monograph in the hope that the anatomists of the day might be encouraged to determine the pathological substrate. In 1912 Lewy described neuronal inclusion bodies in the dorsal motor nucleus of the vagus and nucleus basalis of Meynert. Brissaud (1895) had already suggested that neuronal loss in the substantia nigra might be the cause of Parkinson's disease and 7 years after Lewy's observation, Tretiàkoff (1919) confirmed that the substantia nigra was severely damaged and that 'corps de Lewy' occurred in surviving nerve cells. This finding was not generally accepted, however, until the publication of Hassler's seminal paper in 1937 which described the neuroanatomy of the substantia nigra in great detail and drew attention to the predilection of the pathological process of Parkinson's disease for the ventrolateral pars compacta cell groups (Hassler, 1938).

One explanation for the reluctance to accept the loss of neuromelanin-containing nigral cells as an invariable and crucial pathological lesion in Parkinson's disease stems from the fact that the nigral cell loss may in milder cases be restricted predominantly to these ventrolateral nigral cell groups, and that even in patients dying after a long history of Parkinson's disease, up to a quarter of nigral neurons are preserved (Gibb and Lees, 1987). Similarly, the reluctance to exclude a diagnosis of Parkinson's disease if Lewy bodies could not be found was due in part to poor clinicopathological correlations and the inclusion of patients with postencephalitic Parkinson's syndrome in some pathological series. Most neuropathologists would now insist on pars compacta nigral cell loss of at least 60%, with Lewy bodies in surviving nerve cells, and a histologically normal striatum, as a prerequisite for the diagnosis of Parkinson's disease. Surprisingly the most influential neuropathological studies in Parkinson's disease (Tretiàkoff, 1919; Hassler, 1937; Greenfield and Bosanquet, 1953; Forno and Alvord, 1971) provide little, if any, clinical data.

Already by the time of Hassler's study it had become clear that the clinical features described by James Parkinson could be caused by a number of different pathologies, including cerebrovascular disease and postencephalitic Parkinson's syndrome. Until the 1960s there was a tendency for physicians to categorize (unjustifiably) all young-onset patients with Parkinson's syndrome as postencephalitic and those cases occurring in old age as being due to arteriosclerosis. Despite the decline in the number of cases of postencephalitic Parkinson's syndrome, differential diagnosis has become even more difficult. A number of distinct clinicopathological entities which may masquerade as Parkinson's disease have been described, including striatonigral degeneration (Adams *et al.*, 1964), Steele–Richardson–Olszewski disease (Richardson *et al.*, 1963) and corticobasal degeneration (Rebeiz *et al.*, 1968). Furthermore, up to 30% of patients presenting with Parkinson's syndromes in old age have received neuroleptic drugs in the year prior to presentation (Stephen and Williamson, 1984).

In the absence of any definitive biological markers for these conditions clinicopathological correlations are badly needed to improve diagnostic accuracy. Data from the Parkinson's Disease Society Brain Bank suggests that as many as 15% of patients diagnosed by consultant neurologists as having Parkinson's disease turn out at postmortem to have pathological findings incompatible with this diagnosis (Hughes *et al.*, 1992). Furthermore, some patients diagnosed as having other parkinsonian syndromes turn out to have Lewy body disease at autopsy (Sage *et al.*, 1990). In one of the few clinicopathological studies in the literature, Stadlan and colleagues (1965) suggested that, in the presence of bradykinesia, a resting tremor is a useful pointer to the diagnosis of Parkinson's disease and to this can probably be added a sustained response to L-dopa therapy of more than 5 years with the development of dyskinesias and on–off oscillations. Patients who present with a rapidly progressive, symmetrical, bradykinetic–rigid syndrome without any resting tremor or a benign tremulous disorder with duration of disease of longer than 30 years are unlikely to have Parkinson's disease.

This chapter examines some currently fashionable aetiological theories in the light of our current understanding of the neuropathology of Lewy body disease.

WHAT IS LEWY BODY DISEASE?

The Lewy body is a neuronal inclusion which is always present in areas of neuronal degeneration in Parkinson's disease. In its classical form in the substantia nigra it consists of a central core staining deeply with haematoxylin and eosin, surrounded by a body which stains less intensely, and then a peripheral halo which stains lightly or not at all. This appearance is relatively uncommon and more usually Lewy bodies have no core. Considerable variation in shape occurs, including elongated and serpiginous forms, and their appearance depends to some degree on their location within the nervous system. However, for the purpose of definition a Lewy body must be intracytoplasmic and eosinophilic and possess a halo. The predominant structural component of the Lewy body is filamentous material arranged in circular and linear profiles, often radiating from an electron-dense core. Immunohistochemistry has identified epitopes common to neurofilament polypeptides as well as to tubulin and ubiquitin within the Lewy body (Galloway *et al.*, 1988). Although its content is unique, the arrangement of a core, body and halo is not, being seen in other inclusions such as corpora amylacea, Marinesco bodies and neuroaxonal spheroids. A second inclusion body is frequently, but not invariably, found in neurons in the substantia nigra in Parkinson's disease; we have called this the pale body. This is a weakly staining neuronal inclusion with a finely granular and vacuolated texture which consists of very sparse accumulations of neurofilament interspersed with vacuoles and granular bodies. The cause for the excessive accumulation of filamentous material within surviving neurons in patients with Parkinson's disease is unknown; one possibility might be that it results from failure of normal neurofilament transport due to chemical modification of the cytoskeletal protein or impaired energy supply.

Although Lewy bodies always occur in Parkinson's disease, they are not absolutely specific as they may be found in a few other rare hereditary diseases, such as Hallervorden–Spatz disease and ataxia telangiectasia (Gibb and Lees, 1988a). However, they serve as a reliable marker of neuronal degeneration and may be found before there is clear histological evidence of nerve cell loss.

The loss of nerve cells in Parkinson's disease is quite specific, although widespread, and includes damage to the locus coeruleus, the ventral tegmentum, the thalamus, the nucleus basalis of Meynert, the raphé nucleus, limbic regions and throughout the autonomic nervous system including the hypothalamus, Edinger–Westphal nucleus, dorsal vagal nucleus, intermediolateral cell columns and sympathetic and parasympathetic ganglia such as the myenteric plexus in the walls of the oesophagus and colon. Most neuromelanin-containing neurons are affected in Parkinson's disease, but not all, as there appears to be sparing of the arcuate nuclei in the anterior hypothalamus. Although monoaminergic and cholinergic neurons are particularly affected, some nerve cell groups which contain these chemical messengers are preserved. Lewy bodies are not only associated with other disorders, but in some cases of sporadic and familial motor neuron disease, they are restricted to motor cranial nerve nuclei and anterior horn nerve cells (Takahashi *et al.*, 1972). Thus the Lewy body itself is not specific to Parkinson's disease, nor to the neurons which degenerate in Parkinson's disease.

Although the clinical spectrum is enlarging, the concept of Lewy body disease remains valid. In addition to the classical presentation with bradykinesia, rigidity and resting tremor, two other presentations are now recognized. A significant number of patients present with an Alzheimer-type dementia or symptoms and signs suggestive of an organic psychosis, including visual and auditory hallucinations, delusions and fluctuating confusion (Gibb *et al.*, 1987). These patients have at postmortem large numbers of Lewy bodies in the neocortex, in addition to brain stem pathology similar in distribution to that seen in those patients who present with a parkinsonian picture. These cases have been referred to as diffuse Lewy body disease or Lewy body dementia. Although correlations have been carried out showing that the severity of the dementia is related to the number of cortical Lewy bodies (Lennox *et al.*, 1987), most cases have additional Alzheimer-type changes in the cerebral cortex. A proportion of these patients develop parkinsonian features during the course of their illness. A second much rarer presentation of Lewy body disease is with autonomic failure and neuronal loss and Lewy body formation in the intermediolateral columns of the spinal cord. However, virtually all of these patients have additional parkinsonian features with neuronal loss in the substantia nigra (Rajput and Rozdilsky, 1976). It seems reasonable to look on these as different clinical presentations of the same underlying pathological process in the same way that multiple system atrophy can present with cerebellar, parkinsonian or autonomic features.

There are no wholly convincing reports which show a clear pathological association between Lewy body disease and Alzheimer's disease, although there are numerous published instances where the two diseases have occurred together in patients over the age of 60 years. The problem lies with the high prevalence of these pathological lesions in the population and the difficulty in providing age-related pathological data for the diagnosis of Alzheimer's disease. We have found nigral Lewy bodies in 7.8% of controls and 14% of Alzheimer's disease cases over the age of 60 years. However, cortical Alzheimer pathology was much reduced in the cases of 'Alzheimer's disease' with Lewy bodies compared to those without, although cortical choline acetyltransferase activities were similar (Gibb *et al.*, 1989). It is possible therefore that Lewy body neuronal degeneration in the nucleus basalis might contribute to the lowering of cholinergic activity and to the dementia, but not to the cortical Alzheimer pathology. However, there are a few reports of Lewy body and Alzheimer's disease pathologies coexisting in patients dying before the age of 60 years, suggesting an association at least in these individuals (Kosaka *et al.*, 1973).

THE RELEVANCE OF LEWY BODIES IN THE BRAINS OF PATIENTS DYING WITHOUT SIGNS OF PARKINSON'S DISEASE

Lewy bodies were first noted in patients dying without symptoms of Parkinson's disease or other central nervous system degenerative disorder in the locus coeruleus (Beheim-Schwarzbach, 1952) and were then later isolated in the substantia nigra and other locations of typical Lewy body disease. Forno (1969) suggested that the incidental finding of Lewy bodies might represent a preclinical stage of Parkinson's disease. She observed active nerve cell loss in the substantia nigra but less cell depletion than was associated with Parkinson's disease. The size of this putative preclinical population was initially overestimated due to the inclusion of patients with dementia, psychosis and early Parkinson's disease in some studies. Reported prevalence rates have varied from 6.8 to 12.2% over the age of 60 years (Lipkin, 1959; Woodard, 1962; Forno, 1969; Forno and Alvord, 1971; Tomonaga, 1983). In two smaller studies even higher rates of 21 and 16% respectively were reported (Hamada and Ishii, 1963; Hirai, 1968). When the age-specific data from five of these studies is combined, the prevalence of Lewy bodies increases from approximately 1.8% in the sixth decade to 18.2% in the ninth decade (Gibb and Lees, 1988a). We have examined 308 control subjects, strictly excluding patients with clinical evidence of mild parkinsonism or Alzheimer-type dementia (Gibb 1987; Gibb and Lees, 1988a). Only 1 of the 15 cases with Lewy bodies had neocortical tangles and plaques and the numbers in this case were insufficient for a diagnosis of Alzheimer's disease. The prevalence of Lewy bodies in the substantia nigra in our study increased to 11.5% in the 80–89-year age group and fell slightly to 11.1% in the 90–99-year age group (Gibb, 1987). It is of course impossible to be absolutely sure that many of these patients did not have mild signs of parkinsonism in life.

If these incidental Lewy body cases do indeed represent the earliest stages of the pathological process of Parkinson's disease then one might predict a comparable regional distribution of cell loss to that seen in the fully fledged disease and that the degree of nigral loss would fall between that seen in age-matched controls without Lewy bodies and that seen in Parkinson's disease. In a recent study carried out at the Parkinson's Disease Society Brain Bank, 7 incidental Lewy body cases have been compared with age-matched controls and parkinsonian brains. The midbrain was examined in a plane from the exit of the third nerve ventrally to the lower margin of the superior colliculus dorsally. Particular attention was paid to ensure that all the sections were taken at the same level using well-demarcated anatomical landmarks. Half midbrains were used and only 30% of all the control brains screened were suitable for the study. A 7 μ section of the substantia nigra stained with haematoxylin and eosin was divided into subregions (Fig. 8.1). The morphometrist counted pigmented neurons blind twice under $\times 400$ magnification using alternatively the cell body and nucleolus as the counting units. In the incidental Lewy body cases there

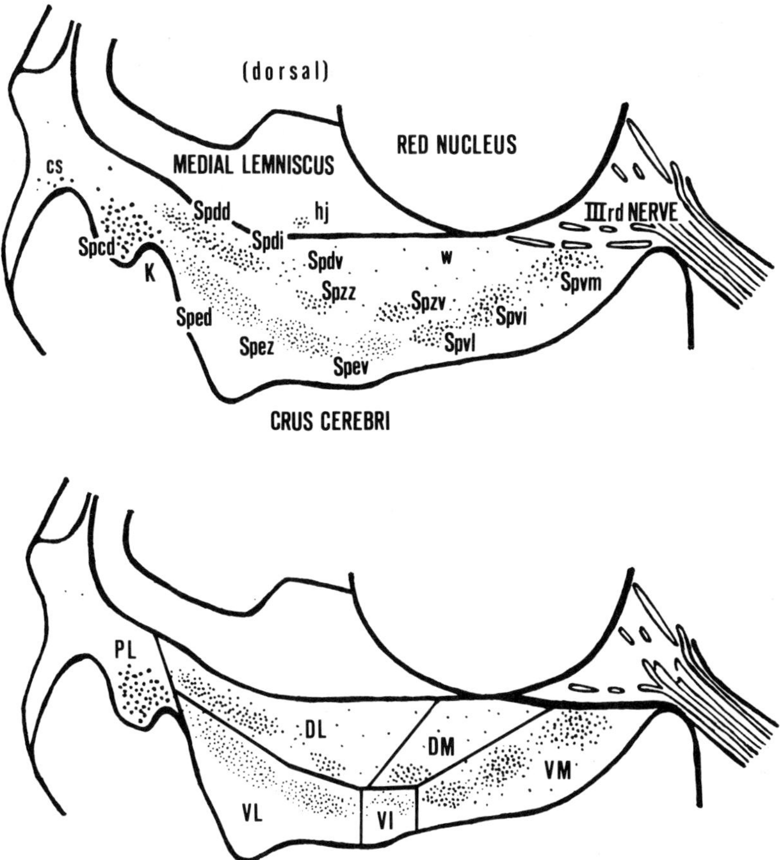

Figure 8.1 The subregional divisions of the pars compacta used at the Parkinson's Disease Brain Bank (bottom), compared with the divisions originally proposed by Hassler (top). DL = Lateral dorsal; DM = medial dorsal; PL = pars lateralis; VI = intermediate ventral; VL = lateral ventral; VM = medial ventral.

was a selective reduction of pigmented neurons in the ventrointermediate and ventrolateral nigral regions of 52%. Furthermore, signs of active cell loss were also seen with the presence of extraneuronal melanin, gliosis and neuronal fragmentation (Fearnley and Lees, 1991). This would support the notion that the pathological process in Parkinson's disease begins and remains more severe in the ventrointermediate and ventrolateral nigral cell groups.

These observations seem to support the concept of Lewy body disease (Forno and Alvord, 1971) and determinations of the prevalence of incidental Lewy body disease might provide more reliable information about the epidemiology of Parkinson's disease that can be obtained at the present time by clinical surveys. Errors inherent in the clinical diagnosis of Parkinson's disease mean that at the present time only 85% of patients given this diagnosis in life fulfil pathological criteria. Prevalence rates of incidental Lewy body disease in Japan, Europe and North America are remarkably similar, suggesting that geographical differences are unlikely to be great.

Among eight clinical studies quoting age-specific prevalence of Parkinson's disease for the population aged over 75 years (Marttila and Rinne, 1986; Mutch *et al.*, 1986), five show a decline in prevalence in the ninth decade (Marttila and Rinne, 1986; Schoenberg, 1987). However, it is possible that the case detection rate could fall in old age, because fewer elderly persons seek treatment and because early parkinsonian features may be attributed to ageing. The real prevalence of clinical disease might also fall because of decreasing survival duration with increasing age and because of early death, such as from accidents and chest infections, in patients without definite Parkinson's disease. The prevalence of incidental Lewy bodies in postmortem brains increases steadily with age, implying that even if the frequency of Parkinson's disease actually falls, the population at risk continues to increase.

THE MICROARCHITECTURE OF THE SUBSTANTIA NIGRA

The most detailed anatomical description of neuronal populations within the substantia nigra was provided by Hassler (1937). He divided the pars compacta into 21 different neuronal groups based on examination of 29 brains in a coronal plane perpendicular to the axis of Forel, which differs slightly from the more commonly used transverse plane by approximately 30–40°. Hassler found a natural division of the substantia nigra into an anterior (oral) and a posterior (caudal) part and his nuclear groupings fall broadly into three tiers in the ventrodorsal plane. The complex nomenclature employing anatomical acronyms and the presence of duplication have led to a reluctance of subsequent neuroanatomists to use Hassler's system, despite its accuracy. More simplified schemes have attempted to divide the pars compacta into three (Olszewski and Baxter, 1954) or seven divisions (Braak and Braak, 1986). Hassler's second major observation of the substantia nigra concerned the selective pattern of nerve cell loss in the pars compacta in 9 cases of Parkinson's disease (Hassler, 1938). Neuronal subpopulations, which he termed Spez, Sped and Spedd, corresponding to the ventrolateral region of the pars compacta, were destroyed in Parkinson's disease, whereas other subpopulations were only partially lost, suggesting different degrees of neuronal injury. This selective loss of the ventrolateral cell groups has subsequently been confirmed by others (Greenfield and Bosanquet, 1953) and verified by computer analysis (German *et al.*, 1989). The ventral tier dominates in the mid-substantia nigra region and cells are more compact and less diffusely spread than the dorsal tier. Available neuroanatomical evidence from animal studies would suggest that the nigrostriatal projection is organized in three ways. Firstly, the ventral tier projects mainly to striatal striosomes which then project back to the cell bodies and proximal dendrites of the ventral tier (Gerfen *et al.*, 1987a,b). The dorsal tier may project to the matrix, which projects back to the pars reticulata. It appears that the striatal patches and matrix are histochemically distinct areas with separate dendritic fields and, together with the ventral and dorsal nigral tiers identified in animals, seem to form two functionally separate units. In the cat the striosomal projection neurons have a high concentration of sigma receptors (Graybiel *et al.*, 1989), whereas the dorsal tier of the rat is marked by the presence of calcium-binding protein (Gerfen *et al.*, 1985; Fig. 8.2).

A second division of the substantia nigra projections is into alternating clusters of neurons projecting either to the putamen or the caudate (Parent *et al.*, 1983; Gerfen *et al.*, 1985). The lateral ventral tier in the monkey appears to project predominantly

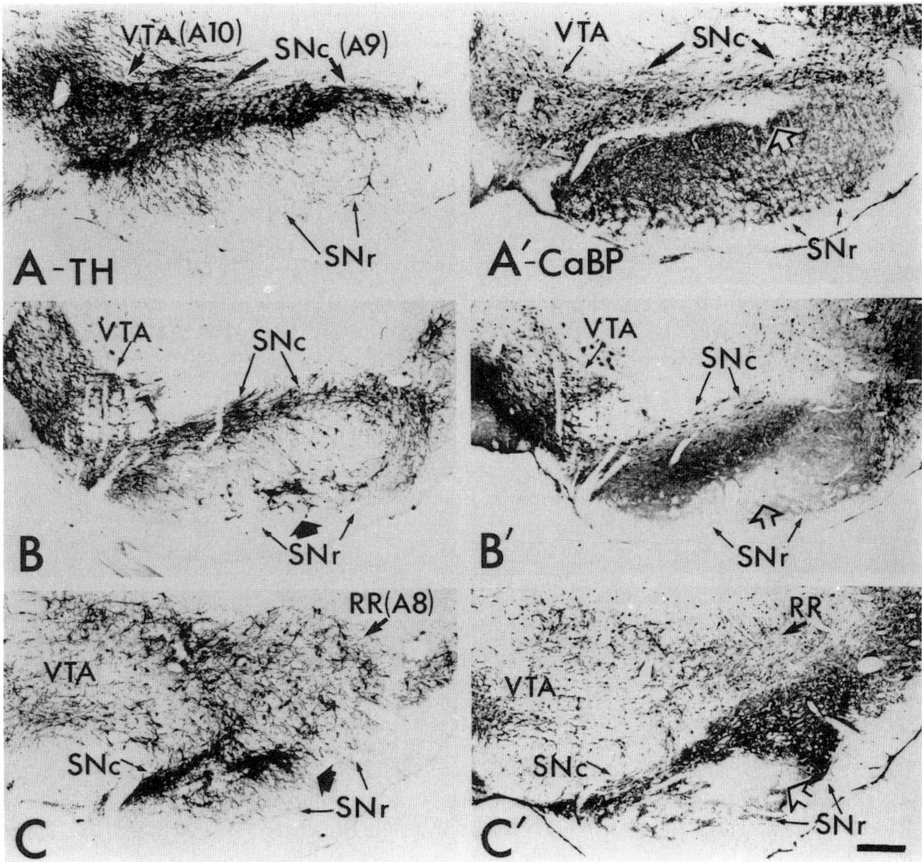

Figure 8.2 Adjacent sections through rostral (A, A′), mid (B, B′) and caudal (C, C′), levels of the ventral midbrain showing tyrosine hydroxylase (TH) immunostaining of dopaminergic neurons, particularly in substantia nigra pars compacta (SNc) (A–C). Calbindin (CaBP) immunoreactivity (A′–C′) is expressed in many ventral tegmental areas (VTA) and dorsal tier nerve cells and at the rostral level in terminals in the substantia nigra pars reticulata (SNr). RR = Retrorubral area. Scale bar = 500 μm. From Gerfen *et al.* (1987b) with permission.

to the dorsal putamen whereas the medial ventral tier projects to the dorsal caudate (Jimenez-Castellanos and Graybiel, 1987). Finally there is a weak topographical correlation with a mediolateral, orocaudal and inverted dorsoventral relationship between the nigra and striatum with the ventrolateral nigra projecting to the dorsolateral putamen (Szabo, 1980). If the human projection pathways are similar, one might predict that the dorsal tier and pars lateralis of the substantia nigra would project predominantly to the striatal matrix and that the ventrointermediate and ventrolateral groups of the ventral tier would go predominantly to the striosomes of the dorsal putamen. Parkinson's disease predominantly affects the ventrolateral nigra and neurochemical dopamine analyses have shown that putamen dopamine falls to 2% of normal, whereas caudate dopamine is 16% of normal at the time of death (Bernheimer *et al.*, 1973). The dorsal regions of the putamen and caudate nucleus are more severely depleted of dopamine than the ventral parts with a slight emphasis on the caudal putamen and the rostral caudate (Kish *et al.*, 1988).

The striosome and matrix divisions of the corpus striatum differ in their development, extrastriatal connections and neurochemistry (Penney and Young, 1986; Langer and Graybiel, 1989). Animals studies have shown a lower rate of dopamine release from nigral neurons projecting to striosomes, which corresponds to the less efficient presynaptic dopamine uptake in striosomal regions compared with matrix (Graybiel *et al.*, 1987; Graybiel and Moratalla, 1989). Using a microdialysis model, acetylcholine releases dopamine from striosomes, but not from matrix (Leigh, 1989). This suggests that the relative selectivity of the nigral lesion in early Parkinson's disease might be related to neurochemical differences in the ventral and dorsal tier neurons and differences in dopamine turnover, and that specific somatotopic effects can be expected in the striatum.

THE NIGRAL LESION IN PARKINSONIAN SYNDROMES

At least 60% of pigmented nigral neurons in the pars compacta of the substantia nigra are lost in Parkinson's disease and it is this lesion which is probably responsible for the cardinal motor abnormalities of bradykinesia, rigidity and tremor. Even in patients with a duration of disease of 20 years or more, 20% of nigral cells survive, which is in striking contrast to postencephalitic disease where there is a virtual wipe-out of all pigmented nigral neurons. The surviving nerve cells are, however, mainly in the dorsal tier and the ventral tegmental area and studies with incidental Lewy body disease and patients with different disease durations at the time of death suggest that there is a spread of nerve cell loss from the ventrolateral and ventrointermediate nuclear nigral groups to other nigral regions as the disease progresses. The cell loss, however, is never as great in the dorsal tier as in the ventral tier (Gibb and Lees, 1990; Fearnley and Lees, 1991).

This predilection for the ventrolateral nuclear pars compacta cell groups is not specific for Parkinson's disease. Cases of striatonigral degeneration also show more involvement of the ventrolateral nigra but have a greater involvement of the dorsal tier and a lesser involvement of the ventromedial nigral cell groups when compared with Parkinson's disease (Fearnley and Lees, 1990). In contrast, the nigral lesion in Steele–Richardson–Olszewski disease shows no ventrolateral selectivity, with marked involvement of the dorsal tiers and a tendency to involve the more medial parts of the nigra. The preferential ventral tier depletion in multiple system atrophy is not the cause or consequence of the striatal nerve cell loss because cell counts in the ventral tier do not correlate closely with those in the putamen (Fearnley and Lees, 1990). However the dorsal putamen and dorsal caudate are the most severely lesioned areas.

The most striking reported example of differential vulnerability in the pars compacta is a case of juvenile parkinsonism with dystonia reported by Yokochi and colleagues in 1984. This patient developed dystonia of the foot at the age of 6 and increasing rigidity in her second decade. During life she had two thalamotomies and with the addition of L-dopa her motor function was regarded as normal. She died from peritonitis at the age of 39 years. The ventral tier of the pars compacta was devoid of nerve cells and replaced by gliosis, while dorsal tier nerve cells were not depleted, although some contained Lewy bodies (Gibb *et al.*, 1989).

IS AGEING RESPONSIBLE FOR THE NIGRAL LESION IN PARKINSON'S DISEASE?

It has been suggested that the preclinical phase of Parkinson's disease is due to an acute exogenous or endogenous insult to the substantia nigra followed by slow age-related nigral cell attrition leading to the onset and progression of symptoms with increasing frequency after the sixth decade (Calne and Langston, 1983). In control subjects over the age of 40 without disease of the basal ganglia the substantia nigra shows occasional fragmenting cells and extraneuronal melanin deposits, whereas in patients younger than 40 years there is little or no evidence of neuronal destruction (McGeer *et al.*, 1988). In a study carried out by Hirai in 1968 in which he looked at age-related cell loss in the brains of patients without Lewy bodies, cell counts from one mid nigral section fell by 13.9% between the third and seventh decades and by a further 25% in the eighth decade and 4.4% in the ninth decade. In two smaller studies total nigral cell loss due to ageing was reported to be 48% (McGeer *et al.*, 1977) and 36% (Mann *et al.*, 1984) respectively.

Neurochemical analyses of dopamine levels in the corpus striatum have generally corroborated an age-related attrition of nigrostriatal projection neurons (Riederer and Wuketich, 1976; Carlsson *et al.*, 1984). In one published study it has been estimated that the mean neuronal loss at postmortem in patients with Parkinson's disease compared with age-matched controls (mean age 68) is 65% (Pakkenberg and Brody, 1965). Combining these findings, total neuronal loss from the age of 20 in a parkinsonian patient dying at 70 would be: ageing 29% and Parkinson's disease 46%. Recent histological studies from the Parkinson's Disease Society Brain Bank in London in control brains without Lewy bodies also indicate an approximate 30% loss of pigmented nigral neurons between the ages of 20 and 90 years (Gibb and Lees, 1990; Fearnley and Lees, 1991). Regional nigral cell counts in 36 control brains aged between 20 and 90 reveal a cell loss of 48% in the dorsal tier and pars lateralis, a 38% loss in the ventromedial region and a relative sparing of the ventrolateral region (15%; Fearnley and Lees, 1991). This pattern of regional neuronal loss is the opposite of that seen in Parkinson's disease and suggests that nigral cell loss in this disorder occurs by a mechanism other than ageing. This casts doubt on the notion that age-related nigral attrition contributes significantly to the pathological process.

THE RELEVANCE OF NEUROMELANIN ACCUMULATION TO THE PATHOGENESIS OF PARKINSON'S DISEASE

Neuromelanin is visible in the pars compacta cells of the substantia nigra by the age of 5 years and each nerve cell continues to accumulate pigment throughout life. The accumulation of neuromelanin is accompanied by a reduction of nucleolar volume and a selective loss of the more heavily pigmented nigral cells has been suggested to occur with age (Mann and Yates, 1974, 1979). The formation of neuromelanin occurs by the auto-oxidation of dopamine which leads to the production of toxic free radicals (Graham, 1979). Neuromelanin also traps a variety of toxic compounds, including 1-methyl-4-phenylpyridinium (MPP+) (Salazar *et al.*, 1978; Snyder and D'Amato, 1986). Its sheer physical bulk has also been claimed to disrupt normal cytoskeletal metabolism and lead to cell death. In contrast to most nigral cells, those of the locus coeruleus are larger and less pigmented. A study in 24 control subjects using multiple sections throughout the length of the locus coeruleus showed that loss of pigmented neurons in this structure only began after the age of 60, raising the possibility that this later age of onset of cell loss might relate to the lower melanin content in the locus coeruleus (Vijayashankar and Brody, 1979).

It has been suggested that neuromelanin might play a specific role in the pathogenesis of the nigral lesion in Parkinson's disease. The neuromelanin of 100 cells in the pars compacta of age-matched controls and 8 cases of Parkinson's disease was compared by staining with Schmorl's technique and light absorption was measured by spectrophotometry. The nigral cells surviving in Parkinson's disease were found to have 15% less pigment than in age-matched controls, suggesting that the most heavily pigmented cells were lost preferentially (Mann and Yates, 1982, 1983a). However there was a wide spread of results, including overlap with normal values. In a more recent study, tyrosine hydroxylase staining midbrain nerve cells were separated into five populations: the pars compacta, pars lateralis, central grey substance and A8 and A10 cell groups (Hirsch *et al.*, 1988).

The tyrosine hydroxylase-positive nerve cell populations with the highest proportion of melanized cells present in controls showed the greatest drop in tyrosine hydroxylase immunoreactive neurons in Parkinson's disease. Within these populations tyrosine hydroxylase cells without melanin were better preserved than those with melanin, although this non-melanized subgroup made up only 16% of the total pars compacta nerve cells in controls. The authors of this study suggested that neuromelanin conferred selective vulnerability on these midbrain nerve cells. However, no similar correlation occurred in the locus coeruleus and presumably melanized tyrosine hydroxylase cells possess functional differences compared with those which contain no pigment. This study also did not carry out any subregional cell counts (Hirsch *et al.*, 1988).

The ventrolateral region of the substantia nigra contains smaller quantities of melanin than the dorsal tier (Gibb *et al.*, 1990; Gibb and Lees, 1990; Fig. 8.3). The

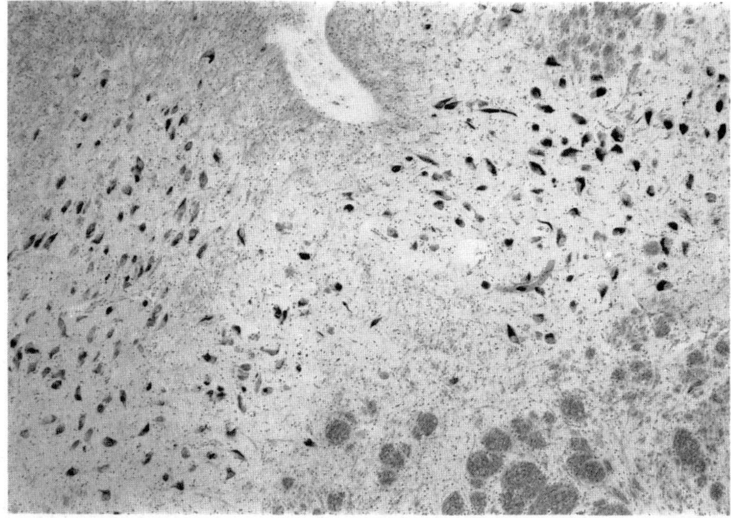

Figure 8.3 Poorly pigmented ventral tier cells in the substantia nigra (left) lie adjacent to heavily pigmented dorsal tier cells of the pars lateralis (right). Luxol fast blue-cresyl violet (×50). From Gibb *et al.* (1990) with permission.

difference in melanization between these two subpopulations is due to differences in the amount of melanin in each nerve cell, and not the proportion of nerve cells that contain melanin. It is the ventral tier of poorly melanized cells which is most vulnerable in Parkinson's disease, suggesting that neuromelanin accumulation is not a critical pathogenetic factor. However, neuromelanin may be important in the pathogenesis of age-related neuronal attrition as ageing seems to be more likely to affect the most heavily pigmented regions of the dorsal tier (Fearnley and Lees, 1991). This might also explain the findings of Mann and Yates (1982), who probably counted predominantly the surviving dorsal tier of heavily pigmented cells in the patients with Parkinson's disease.

A more general hypothesis linking the pathological lesions of Parkinson's disease to melanin can also be rejected. Areas such as the nucleus basalis of Meynert are not pigmented, yet they show substantial pathological lesions with nerve cell loss varying from 20 to 80% (Ezrin-Waters and Resch, 1986). In contrast, the arcuate and periventricular nuclei of the hypothalamus are pigmented but are not damaged in Parkinson's disease (Marsden, 1983; Matzuk and Saper, 1985). Furthermore, the locus coeruleus accumulates less pigment than the substantia nigra, but observed cell loss is approximately 75–80% in Parkinson's disease, which is the same magnitude as in the substantia nigra (Mann and Yates, 1983b).

THE RELEVANCE OF THE MPTP PARADIGM TO THE PATHOGENESIS OF PARKINSON'S DISEASE

1-Methyl-4-phenyl-1,2,3,6-tetrahydropyridine (MPTP) is converted within the central nervous system by monoamine oxidase type B to MPP+, the toxic pyridinium ion which destroys nigral cells in non-human primates. Higher doses or administration to older animals can also produce lesions in the ventral tegmental area, the locus coeruleus, the hypothalamus and the periamygdaloid region of the hippocampus (Burns *et al.*, 1984; Langston *et al.*, 1984; Mitchell *et al.*, 1985; Forno *et al.*, 1986; Gibb *et al.*, 1989; Langston, 1989). MPP+ has a high affinity for melanin (Snyder and D'Amato, 1986), which in part correlates with the pattern of lesions in monkeys, and in primates destruction of the pars compacta is greater in the lateral and dorsal parts which contain the most melanin (Deutch *et al.*, 1986; Gibb *et al.*, 1986). Chloroquine also has a high affinity for melanin and can protect against MPTP damage by preventing the binding of MPP+ (D'Amato *et al.*, 1986, 1987). Melanin might therefore provide a reservoir for MPTP which could then lead to slow cell death, but the potential for toxicity probably depends on other factors, including the distribution of dopamine reuptake sites by which MPP+ gains access to dopamine nerve terminals and is retrogradely transported to the nerve cell body. The precise cause of cell death due to MPTP is thought to be inhibition of mitochondrial complex I (Nicklas *et al.*, 1985; Denton and Howard, 1987). A selective depletion of complex I in the substantia nigra of patients dying with Parkinson's disease has been reported (Schapira *et al.*, 1989), raising the possibility that toxic mechanisms underlying the MPTP-induced lesion may be similar to those seen in Parkinson's disease. However there are a number of differences between the MPTP-induced lesion and Parkinson's disease. The cholinergic nuclear cell groups which are frequently damaged in Parkinson's disease, including the nucleus basalis of Meynert and the pedunculopontine nucleus, appear to be undamaged by MPTP, and although most

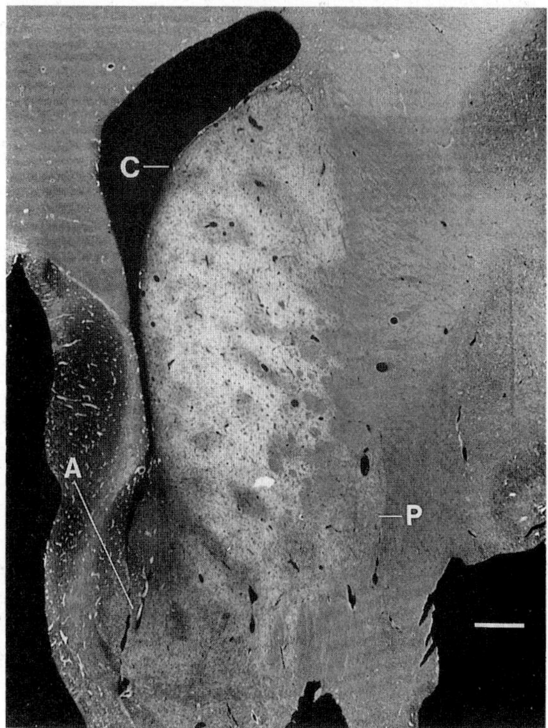

Figure 8.4 Dark-field photomicrograph stained for terminal degeneration 8 days after a single injection of 1-methyl-4-phenyl-1,2,3,6-tetrahydropyridine in the dog. Terminal and preterminal degeneration appears white. A = Nucleus accumbens; C = caudate nucleus; P = putamen. Bar = 1 mm. From Wilson *et al.* (1987) with permission.

neuromelanin-containing neurons are involved in Parkinson's disease, no reports have occurred of damage to the pigmented nuclei in the raphé or the dorsal nucleus of the vagus. In the dog, MPTP produces greater degeneration of dopamine terminals in the matrix than in the striosome compartment (Fig. 8.4), particularly in the anterior caudate nucleus (Turner *et al.*, 1988), which may be due to a greater concentration of presynaptic dopamine receptors in matrix compared with striosomes (Graybiel and Moratalla, 1989) (Fig. 8.5). Although it is not absolutely clear at this point whether the dorsal tier neurons, which in humans contain more neuromelanin than the ventral tier, are more affected by MPTP, it would appear that the ventral tier is not unduly susceptible to the toxin, which one might expect if the pathological process were the same as occurs in Parkinson's disease. In rhesus monkeys given MPTP mesolimbic dopamine was spared (Jacobowitz *et al.*, 1984) and dopamine levels in the caudate nucleus and putamen were severely and equally reduced (Pifl *et al.*, 1988), differing therefore from what occurs in Parkinson's disease. Present evidence therefore would suggest that although the acute MPTP lesion provides a superb animal model for the assessment of new treatments for Parkinson's disease, certain differences exist between the pathological lesion and that seen in Parkinson's disease. This in turn raises the possibility that the mechanism of cell death may also be different.

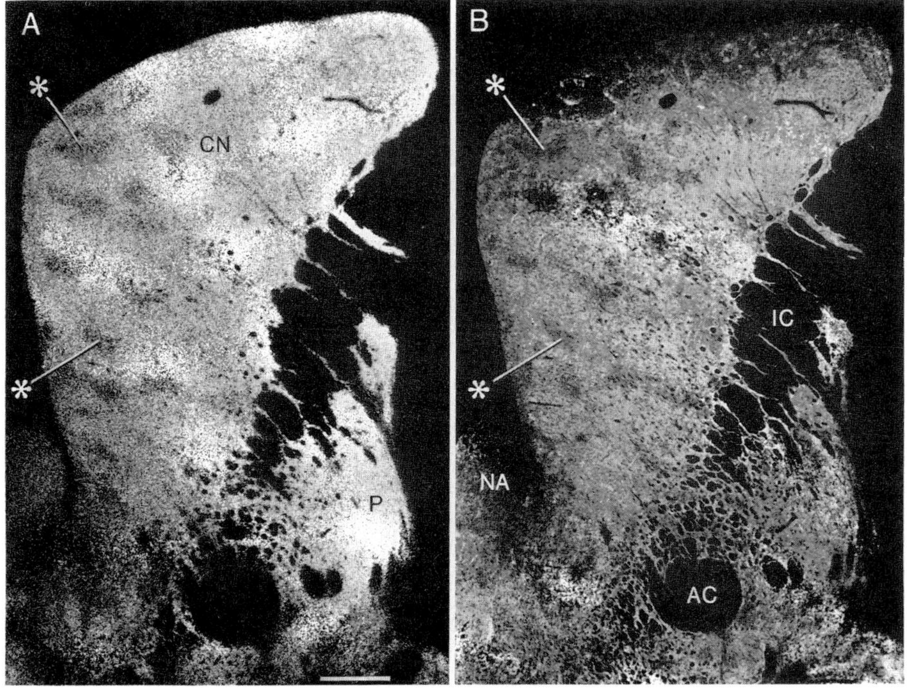

Figure 8.5 Tritiated mazindol binding (A) and acetylcholinesterase activity (B) as a measurement of dopamine uptake sites and acetylcholinesterase binding in the striatum of the cat. Patches of reduced mazindol binding seen in the central part of the caudate (asterisks) correspond to the acetylcholinesterase-poor zones (striosomes; B). AC = Anterior commissure; CN = caudate nucleus; IC = internal capsule; NA = nucleus accumbens; P = putamen. Bar = 1 mm. From Graybiel and Moratalla (1989) with permission.

THE RATE OF PROGRESSION OF PARKINSON'S DISEASE

The pathological changes seen in the substantia nigra of patients with Parkinson's disease and in incidental Lewy body cases are more active than occurs with normal ageing. There is increased neuronal fragmentation, extraneuronal melanin and gliosis which is independent of age. A comparison of the number of reactive microglia in the substantia nigra expressing HLA-DR in controls and in Parkinson's disease showed six times as many neurons being actively phagocytosed in the Parkinson's disease cases (McGeer *et al.*, 1988).

The speed of progression of clinical symptoms seems probably to be independent of age. Comparison of 359 patients with onset under 50 years, between 50 and 59 years, and over 60 years, showed that the youngest group had the lowest observed to expected mortality ratio, but that this was not statistically significant (Diamond *et al.*, 1989). A slightly greater mortality ratio in older patients could be explained by the disability of Parkinson's disease being compounded by the problems of old age. However, it has been claimed that younger-onset patients with Parkinson's disease are more likely to develop frequent motor fluctuations with L-dopa therapy

(Lima *et al.*, 1987; Quinn *et al.*, 1987), although not all studies have confirmed this (Gibb and Lees, 1988b; Diamond *et al.*, 1989). Dementia is commoner in old-onset patients, but this difference may be due to increasing Alzheimer pathology with age rather than Lewy body pathology (Gibb, 1989). A comparison of the nigral lesion in 12 patients with a median age at onset of 34 years and 22 with a median onset at 76 years, surviving for 15 years and 3 years respectively, has shown 24% fewer nerve cells in the young onset cases (Gibb and Lees, 1988b).

The density of [^{3}H]dihydrotetrabenazine binding sites in the caudate nucleus, which reflects dopaminergic innervation, increased with age at death in Parkinson's disease (Scherman *et al.*, 1989). However, the relative preservation of nigrostriatal dopaminergic innervation and shorter disease duration in older patients is compatible with them dying earlier in the course of the disease rather than a reflection of different rates of nigral degeneration. The study of Scherman and colleagues in fact identified similar rates of nigrostriatal neuron loss in patients older and younger than 60 years of age. These data provide some evidence to suggest that the speed of the pathological process in young-onset and old-onset patients with Parkinson's disease is probably the same and faster than that seen in normal ageing (Fig. 8.6).

Considerable controversy exists over the likely speed of nigral cell death before the appearance of clinical symptoms. Based on serial fluorodopa scans carried out in established Parkinson's disease and postmortem nigral cell counts in patients dying with different durations of disease, it would appear that nigral cell loss is relatively slow in established disease. For example, it is known that about 50–60% of pigmented

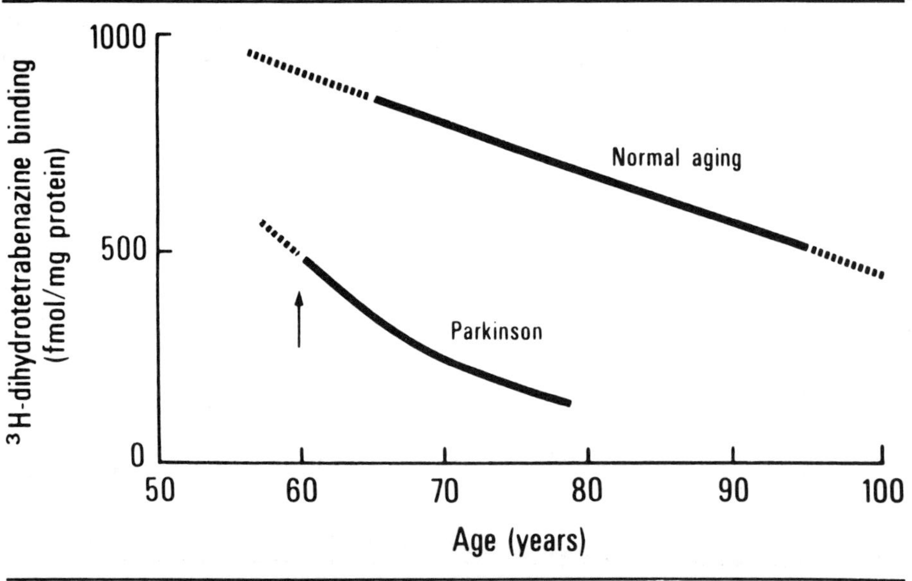

Figure 8.6 Schematic representation of age-related decrease in tritiated alpha-dihydrotetrabenazine binding in the caudate nucleus in control subjects and in a patient developing Parkinson's disease at the age of 60 years (the regression curve is based on data from 54 patients). The arrow indicates the threshold value of binding corresponding to the onset of Parkinson's disease and the dotted lines represent extrapolated values. From Scherman *et al.* (1989) with permission.

nigral cells are lost before the first signs of Parkinson's disease appear and even after 25 years of disease as many as 20% of nigral cells may be preserved (Fearnley and Lees, 1991). Corroborative evidence supporting a slow rate of cell loss in the substantia nigra in Parkinson's disease comes from comparisons of the age-specific prevalence of incidental Lewy body disease and Parkinson's disease. The frequency of incidental cases increases from about 2% in the sixth decade to over 10% in the ninth decade, whereas the frequency of Parkinson's disease increases from a very low level in middle age to almost 2% in the ninth decade. The three-decade difference in the 2% prevalence figures suggests that histological changes might begin some three decades before neurological symptoms (Gibb and Lees, 1988a; Fig. 8.7). For patients presenting at age 60, onset may have occurred between 25 and 35 years of age, thus pointing to an insult occurring or commencing much earlier in life. Furthermore, retrospective neurobehavioural studies in young-onset Parkinson's disease and twin studies have suggested that there may be a distinctive behavioural profile including mental inflexibility, introspection and non-smoking which antecedes the onset of motor symptoms by two or three decades (Ward *et al.*, 1984; Eatough *et al.*, 1990). Riederer and Wuketich (1976) speculated that if nigrostriatal degeneration of dopaminergic neurons was linear, on the basis of caudate dopamine levels Parkinson's disease might begin 20–30 years before the appearance of bradykinesia, rigidity and tremor.

However, the nigral damage seen in some patients with Parkinson's disease suggests a more active destructive lesion and the data published by McGeer and colleagues (1988) comparing the number of reactive microglia in the substantia nigra of patients with Parkinson's disease also suggests that a silent period of cell death of 20–30 years may be an over-estimate. In a recent study carried out in the Parkinson's Disease Society Brain Bank, 16 pathologically confirmed cases of Lewy body Parkinson's disease with different disease durations (1.5–39 years) and a mean age of 60 ± 11

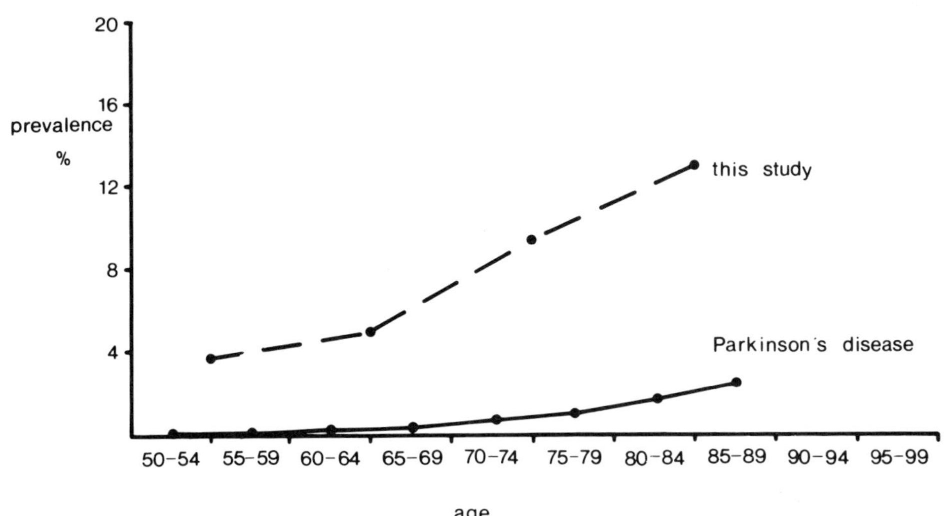

Figure 8.7 Graph combining pathological data on the age-specific prevalence of incidental Lewy body disease (interrupted line) and clinical data on the prevalence of Parkinson's disease. From Gibb and Lees (1990) with permission.

years were studied. In each case a count of the number of pigmented neurons was performed on a 7 μm section of the caudal nigra. Regional counts were carried out and the counts adjusted for age-related nerve cell loss. Thirty-six control cases without Lewy bodies aged between 21 and 91 were also counted and a linear regression equation calculated. The Parkinson's disease adjusted counts were calculated as a percentage of the value derived from the control regression equation and a good correlation existed between the adjusted count and the duration of symptoms. Based on these data, and using the regression equation, the preclinical phase seemed more likely to be of the order of 5–10 years (Fearnley and Lees, 1991).

CONCLUDING REMARKS

The nigral lesion in Parkinson's disease begins in the ventrolateral cell groups and spreads as the disease progresses to the dorsal tier. Incidental Lewy body brains have nigral cell loss restricted to the ventrolateral cell groups, suggesting that they represent a presymptomatic phase of Parkinson's disease. Age-related attrition has a predilection for the more heavily pigmented dorsal tier of the substantia nigra and the speed of cell loss is slower than that responsible for Parkinson's disease. Although tyrosine hydroxylase-positive non-pigment-containing midbrain neurons appear to be relatively resistant to the pathological process of Parkinson's disease, the fact that the ventral tier of the substantia nigra pars compacta appears to contain less melanin than the dorsal tier would argue against neuromelanin being an important aetiological factor. Increased understanding of the mechanism of MPP+ toxicity will undoubtedly throw further light on potential mechanisms of nigral cell death, but neuropathological observations suggest that there may be crucial differences between the MPTP-induced lesion and that occurring in Parkinson's disease. The incubation period and the rate of progression of the nigral lesion following the appearance of clinical symptoms are unclear at the present time and clearly are of crucial importance. Greater understanding of the microarchitecture of the substantia nigra and its highly specific projections to striatal areas may help to explain many of the baffling clinical phenomena which occur in this disorder. However, the cause of death in Parkinson's disease may be unrelated to progressive nigral cell death as patients with even relatively mild clinical symptoms from postencephalitic Parkinson's syndrome may die with an almost complete loss of pigmented nigral cells. Although the corpus striatum is histologically normal in the large majority of cases with Parkinson's disease, immunohistochemical techniques may illustrate important selective abnormalities. In the absence of any biological markers for Parkinson's disease the clinicopathological concept of Lewy body disease seems to us reasonable. Further clinicopathological correlations are urgently required in order to delineate the broadening clinical phenomenology of Lewy body disease. Until this becomes available, clinicians should probably venture no further than a diagnosis of probable Parkinson's disease or probable multiple system atrophy.

Acknowledgement

We acknowledge Dr Julian Fearnley's contribution to the work described in this review.

References

Adams RD, Bogaert van L, and Eecken HV (1964) Striato-nigral degeneration. *J Neuropathol Exp Neurol*, **24**, 584–608

Beheim-Schwarzbach D (1952) Uber Zelleib-veranderungen im nucleus coeruleus bei Parkinsonian-symptomem. *J Nerv Ment Dis*, **116**, 619–32

Bernheimer H, Birkmayer W, Hornykiewicz O, Jellinger K, and Seitelberger F (1973) Brain dopamine and the syndromes of Parkinson and Huntington. *J Neurol Sci*, **20**, 415–55

Braak H and Braak E (1986) Nuclear configuration and neuronal types of the nucleus niger in the brain of the human adult. *Hum Neurobiol*, **5**, 71–82

Brissaud E (1895) Leçons sur les Maladies Nerveuses (Salpètriére 1893–4) Paris

Burns RS, Chiueh CC, Markey SP, Ebert MH, Jacobowitz DM, and Koplin IJ (1984) A primate model in parkinsonism: selective destruction of dopaminergic neurons in the pars compacta of the substantia nigra by n-methyl-4-phenyl-1,2,3,6-tetrahydropyridine in the monkey and man. *Can J Neurol Sci*, **11**, 166–8

Calne DB and Langston JW (1983) Aetiology of Parkinson's disease. *Lancet*, **ii**, 1457–9

Carlsson A, Nyberg P, and Winblad B (1984) The influence of age and other factors on concentrations of monoamines in the human brain. In Nyberg P, ed, *Brain Monoamines in Normal Ageing and Dementia*. Sweden, Umea Medical Dissertations, 53–84

D'Amato RJ, Lipman ZP, and Snyder SH (1986) Selectivity of the parkinsonian neurotoxin MPTP: toxic metabolite MPP+ binds to neuromelanin. *Science*, **231**, 987–9

D'Amato RJ, Alexander GM, Schwartzman RJ, Kitt CA, Price DL, and Snyder SH (1987) Evidence for neuromelanin involvement in MPTP-induced neurotoxicity. *Nature*, **327**, 324–6

Denton T and Howard BD (1987) A dopaminergic cell line variant resistant to the neurotoxin MPTP. *J Neurochem*, **49**, 622–30

Deutch AY, Elsworth JD, Goldstein M, Fuxe K, Redmond DE, Sladek JR *et al.* (1986) Preferential vulnerability of A8 dopamine neurons in the primate to the neurotoxin 1-methyl-4-phenyl-1,2,3,6-tetrahydropyridine. *Neurosci Lett*, **68**, 51–6

Diamond SG, Markham CG, Hoehn MM, McDowell FH, and Muenter MD (1989) Effect of age at onset on progression and mortality of Parkinson's disease. *Neurology*, **39**, 1187–90

Eatough V, Kempster PA, Lees AJ, and Stern GM (1990) The pre-morbid personality of patients with Parkinson's disease. In Streifler M, ed, *Advances in Neurology*, New York, Raven Press

Ezrin-Waters C and Resch L (1986) The nucleus basalis of Meynert. *Can J Neurol Sci*, **13**, 8–14

Fearnley JM and Lees AJ (1990) Striatonigral degeneration: a clinicopathological study. *Brain*, **113**, 1823–42

Fearnley JM and Lees A (1991) Ageing is not involved in the pathophysiology of Parkinson's disease. *Brain*, **114**, 2283–301

Forno LS (1969) Concentric hyalin intraneuronal inclusions of Lewy type in the brains of elderly persons (50 incidental cases): relationship to parkinsonism. *J Am Geriatr Soc*, **17**, 557–75

Forno LS and Alvord EC (1971) The pathology of parkinsonism. In McDowell FH, Markham CH, eds, *Recent Advances in Parkinson's Disease*, Oxford, Blackwell, 120–61

Forno LS, Langston JW, DeLanney LE, Irwin I, and Ricaurte GA (1986) Locus coeruleus lesions and eosinophilic inclusions in MPTP-treated monkeys. *Ann Neurol*, **20**, 449–55

Galloway PG, Grundke-Iqbal I, Iqbal K, and Perry G (1988) Lewy bodies contain epitopes both shared and distinct from Alzheimer's neurofibrillary tangles. *J Neuropathol Exp Neurol*, **47**, 654–63

Gerfen CR, Baimbridge KG, and Miller JJ (1985) The neostriatal mosaic: compartmental distribution of calcium-binding protein and parvalbumin in the basal ganglia of the rat and monkey. *Proc Natl Acad Sci USA*, **82**, 8780–4

Gerfen CR, Herkenham M, and Thibault J (1987a) The neostriatal matrix: II. Patch- and matrix-directed mesostriatal dopaminergic and non-dopamineric systems. *J Neurosci*, **7**, 3915–34

Gerfen CR, Baimbridge KG, and Thibault J (1987b) The neostriatal mosiac: III. Biochemical and developmental dissociation of patch-matrix nigrostriatal systems. *J Neurosci*, **7**, 3935–44

German DC, Manaye K, Smith WK, Woodward DJ, and Saper CB (1989) Midbrain dopaminergic cell loss in Parkinson's disease: computer visualisation. *Ann Neurol*, **26**, 507–14

Gibb WRG (1987) The epidemiology of Lewy bodies. In Fahn S, Marsden CD, Calne DB, Goldstein M, eds, *Recent Developments in Parkinson's Disease*. vol 2, New Jersey, Macmillan, 1–13

Gibb WRG (1989) Dementia and Parkinson's disease. *Br J Psych*, **154**, 596–614

Gibb WRG and Lees AJ (1987) The progression of idiopathic Parkinson's disease is not explained by age-related changes. Clinical and pathological comparisons with post-encephalitic parkinsonian syndrome. *Acta Neuropathol*, **73**, 195–201

Gibb WRG and Lees AJ (1988a) The relevance of the Lewy body to the pathogenesis of idiopathic Parkinson's disease. *J Neurol Neurosurg Psychiatry*, **51**, 745–52

Gibb WRG and Lees AJ (1988b) A comparison of clinical pathological features of young- and old-onset Parkinson's disease. *Neurology*, **38**, 1402–6

Gibb WRG and Lees AJ (1991) Anatomy, pigmentation, ventral and dorsal subpopulations of the substantia nigra and differential cell death in Parkinson's disease. *J Neurol Neurosurg Psychiatry*, **54**, 388–96

Gibb WRG, Terruli M, Lees AJ, Jenner P, and Marsden CD (1989) The evolution and distribution of morphological changes in the nervous system of the common marmoset following the acute administration of 1-methyl-4-phenyl-1,2,3,6-tetrahydropyridine. *Movement Disorders*, **4**, 53–74

Gibb WRG, Lees AJ, Jenner P, and Marsden CD (1986) Effects of MPTP in the midbrain of the marmoset. In Markey SP, Castagnoli N, Trevor AJ, Kopin IJ, eds, *MPTP: A Neurotoxin Producing a Parkinsonian Syndrome*. London, Academic Press, 607–14

Gibb WRG, Esiri MM, and Lees AJ (1985) Clinical and pathological features of diffuse cortical Lewy body disease (Lewy body dementia). *Brain*, **110**, 1131–53

Gibb WRG, Narabayashi H, Yokochi M, and Izuka R (1989a) Additional pathological observations in juvenile onset parkinsonism with dystonia. *Neurology*, **39** (suppl 1), 139

Gibb WRG, Fearnley JM, and Lees AJ (1990) The anatomy and pigmentation of the human substantia nigra in relation to selective neuronal vulnerability. *Adv Neurol*, **53**, 31–4

Graham DG (1979) On the origin and significance of neuromelanin. *Arch Pathol Lab Med*, **103**, 359–62

Graybiel AM and Moratalla R (1989) Dopamine uptake sites in the striatum are distributed differentially in striosome and matrix compartments. *Proc Natl Acad Sci USA*, **86**, 9020–4

Graybiel M, Hirsch E, and Agid YA (1987) Differences in tyrosine hydroxylase-like immunoreactivity characterize the mesostriatal innervation of striosomes and extrastriosomal matrix at maturity. *Proc Natl Acad Sci USA*, **84**, 303–7

Graybiel AM, Besson M, and Weber E (1989) Neuroleptic-sensitive binding sites in the nigrostriatal system: evidence for differential distribution of sigma sites in the substantia nigra pars compacta of the cat. *J Neurosci*, **9**, 326–38

Greenfield JG and Bosanquet FD (1953) The brain-stem lesions in parkinsonism. *J Neurol Neurosurg Psychiatry*, **16**, 213–16

Hamada S and Ishii T (1963) The Lewy body in the brain of the aged. *Adv Neurol Sci*, **7**, 184–6

Hassler R (1937) Zur Normalanatomie de Substantia nigra. *J Psychol Neurol*, **48**, 1–55

Hassler R (1938) Zur Pathologie de Paralysis agitans und des postenzephalitischen Parkinsonismus. *J Psychol Neurol*, **48**, 387–455

Hirai S (1968) Ageing of the substantia nigra. *Adv Neurol Sci*, **12**, 845–9

Hirsch E, Graybiel AM, and Agid YA (1988) Melanized dopaminergic neurons are differentially susceptible to degeneration in Parkinson's disease. *Nature*, **334**, 345–8

Hughes AJ, Daniel SE, Kilford L, and Lees AJ (1992) The accuracy of clinical diagnosis of idiopathic. Parkinson's disease. *J Neurol Neurosurg Psychiatry*, **55**, 181–4

Jacobowitz DM, Burns RS, Chiueh CC, and Kopin IJ (1984) N-methyl-4-phenyl-1,2,3,6-tetrahydropyridine (MPTP) causes destruction of the nigrostriatal but not the mesolimbic dopamine system in the monkey. *Psychopharmacol Bull*, **20**, 416–22

Jimenez-Castellanos J and Graybiel AM (1987) Subdivisions of the dopamine-containing A8–A9–A10 complex identified by their differential mesostriatal innervation of striosomes and extrastriosomal matrix. *Neuroscience*, **23**, 223–42

Kish SJ, Shannak K, and Hornykiewicz O (1988) Uneven pattern of dopamine loss in the striatum of patients with idiopathic Parkinson's disease. *N Engl J Med*, **318**, 876–80

Kosaka K, Shibayama H, Kobayashi H, Hoshino RT, and Iwase S (1973) An autopsy case of unclassifiable presenile dementia. *Psychiatr Neurol Jap*, **75**, 18–34

Langer LF and Graybiel AM (1989) Distinct nigrostriatal systems innervate striosomes and matrix in the primate striatum. *Brain Res*, **498**, 344–50

Langston JW (1989) Mechanisms underlying neuronal degeneration in Parkinson's disease: an experimental and theoretical treatise. *Movement Disorders*, **4** (suppl 1), 15–25

Langston LW, Forno LS, Rebert CS, and Irwin I (1984) Selective nigral toxicity after systemic administration of 1-methyl-4-phenyl-1,2,3,6-tetrahydropyridine (MPTP) in the squirrel monkey. *Brain Res*, **292**, 390–4

Leigh PN (1989) Functional organization of the basal ganglia. In Quinn NP, Jenner PG, eds, *Disorders of Movement. Clinical, Pharmacological and Physiological Aspects*, London, Academic Press, 11–32

Lennox G, Love J, Morrell K, Landon M, and Mayor RJ (1987) Anti-ubiquitin immunocytochemistry is more sensitive than conventional techniques in the detection of diffuse Lewy body disease. *J Neurol Neurosurg Psychiatry*, **52**, 67–71

Lewy FH (1912) Paralysis agitans. I. Pathologisches Anatomie. In *Handbuch der Neurologie III*, Berlin, Springer, 920–33

Lima B, Neves G, and Nora M (1987) Juvenile parkinsonism: clinical and metabolic characteristics. *J Neurol Neurosurg Psychiatry*, **50**, 345–8

Lipkin LE (1959) Cytoplasmic inclusions in ganglion cells associated with parkinsonian states. *Am J Pathol*, **35**, 1117–33

McGeer PL, McGeer EG, and Suzuki JS (1977) Aging and extrapyramidal function. *Arch Neurol*, **34**, 33–5

McGeer PL, Itgaki S, Akiyama H, and McGeer EG (1988) Rate of cell death in parkinsonism indicates active neuropathological process. *Ann Neurol*, **24**, 574–6

Mann DMA and Yates PO (1974) Lipoprotein pigments – their relationship to ageing in the human nervous system. II. The melanin content of pigmented nerve cells. *Brain*, **97**, 489–98

Mann DMA and Yates PO (1979) Ageing, nucleic acids and pigments. In Smith WT, Cavanagh JB, eds, *Recent Advances in Neuropathology*, vol 1, London, Churchill Livingstone, 109–38

Mann DMA and Yates PO (1982) Pathogenesis of Parkinson's disease. *Arch Neurol*, **39**, 545–9

Mann DMA and Yates PO (1983a) Possible role of neuromelanin in the pathogenesis of Parkinson's disease. *Mech Ageing Dev*, **21**, 193–203

Mann DMA and Yates PO (1983b) Pathological basis for neurotransmitter changes in Parkinson's disease. *Neuropathol Appl Neurobiol*, **9**, 3–19

Mann DMA, Yates PO, and Marcynuik B (1984) Monoamiergic neurotransmitter systems in presenile Alzheimer's disease and in senile dementia of Alzheimer type. *Clin Neuropathol*, **3**, 199–205

Marsden CD (1983) Neuromelanin and Parkinson's disease. *J Neutral Transm* (suppl 19), 121–41

Marttila RJ and Rinne IK (1986) Epidemiology of Parkinson's disease. In Poeck K, Freind H-J, Ganshirt H, eds, *Proceedings of the XIIth World Congress of Neurology*. Heidelberg, Springer Verlag, 274–81

Matzuk MM and Saper CB (1985) Preservation of hypothalamic dopaminergic neurons in Parkinson's disease. *Ann Neurol*, **18**, 552–5

Mitchell IJ, Cross AJ, Sambrook MA, and Crossman AR (1985) Sites of the neurotoxic action of 1-methyl-4-phenyl-1,2,3,6-tetrahydropyridine in the macaque monkey include the central tegmental area and the locus coeruleus. *Neurosci Lett*, **61**, 195–200

Mutch WJ, Dingwall-Fordyce I, Downie AW, Paterson JG, and Roy SK (1986) Parkinson's disease in a Scottish city. *Br Med J*, **292**, 534–6

Nicklas WJ, Vyas I, and Heikkila RE (1985) Inhibition of NADH-linked oxidation in brain mitochondria by 1-methyl-4-phenyl-pyridine: a metabolite of the neurotoxin 1-methyl-4-phenyl-1,2,3,6-tetrahydropyridine. *Life Sci*, **36**, 2503–8

Olszewski J and Baxter D (1954) *Cytoarchitecture of the Human Brain Stem*, Basel, S. Karger

Pakkenberg H and Brody H (1985) The number of nerve cells in the substantia nigra in paralysis agitans. *Acta Neuropathol*, **5**, 320–6

Parent A, Mackey A, and De Bellefeville L (1983) The subcortical afferents to caudate nucleus and putamen in primate: a fluorescence retrograde double labelling study. *Neuroscience*, **10**, 1137–50

Parkinson J (1817) An Essay on the Shaking Palsy. Sherwood, Neely, Jones; London

Penney JB and Young AB (1986) Striatal inhomogeneities and basal ganglia function. *Movement Disorders*, **1**, 3–15

Pifl CH, Schingnitz G, and Hornykiewicz O (1988) The neurotoxin MPTP does not reproduce in the rhesus monkey the interregional pattern of striatal dopamine loss typical of human idiopathic Parkinson's disease. *Neurosci Lett*, **92**, 228–33

Quinn N, Critchley, P, and Marsden CD (1987) Young onset Parkinson's disease. *Movement Disorders*, **2**, 73–91

Rajput AH and Rozdilsky B (1976) Dysautonomia in parkinsonism: a clinico-pathological study. *J Neurol Neurosurg Psychiatry*, **39**, 1092–100

Rebeiz JJ, Kolodny EH, and Richardson EP (1968) Corticodentatonigral degeneration with neuronal achromisia. *Arch Neurol*, **18**, 20–33

Richardson JC, Steele J, and Olszewski J (1963) Supranuclear ophthalmoplegia, pseudobulbar palsy, nuchal dystonia and dementia: a clinical report on eight cases of heterogeneous system degeneration. *Trans Am Neurol Assoc*, **88**, 25–9

Riederer P and Wuketich ST (1976) Time course of nigrostriatal degeneration in Parkinson's disease. *J Neural Trans*, **38**, 277–301

Sage JI, Miller DC, Golbe LI, Walters A, and Duvoisin RC (1990) Clinically atypical expression of pathologically typical Lewy-body parkinsonism. *Clin Neuropharmacol*, **13**, 36–47

Salazar M, Sokoloski TD, and Patil PN (1978) Binding of dopaminergic drugs by the neuromelanin of the substantia nigra, synthetic melanins and melanin granules. *Fed Proc*, **37**, 2403–7

Schapira AHV, Cooper JM, Dexter D, Jenner P, Clark JB, and Marsden CD (1989) Mitochondrial complex I deficiency in Parkinson's disease. *Lancet*, **i**, 1269

Scherman D, Desnos C, Darchen F, Pollak P, Javoy-Agid, and Agid Y (1989) Striatal dopamine deficiency in Parkinson's disease: role of ageing. *Ann Neurol*, **226**, 551–7

Schoenberg BS (1987) Environmental risk factors for Parkinson's disease: the epidemiological evidence. *Can J Neurol Sci*, **14**, 407–13

Snyder SH and D'Amato RJ (1986) MPTP: a neurotoxin relevant to the pathophysiology of Parkinson's disease. *Neurology*, **36**, 250–8

Stadlan EM, Duvoisin RC, and Yahr MD (1965) The pathology of Parkinsonism. In *Proceedings of the 5th International Congress of Neuropathology*, vol 100, Excerpta Medica, 569–71

Stephen PJ and Williamson J (1984) Drug-induced parkinsonism in the elderly. *Lancet*, **ii**, 1082–3

Szabo J (1980) Organization of the ascending striatal afferents in monkeys. *J Comp Neurol*, **189**, 307–21

Takihashi K, Nakamura H, and Okada E (1972) Hereditary amyotrophic lateral sclerosis. Histochemical and electron microscopic study of hyaline inclusions in motor neurons. *Arch Neurol*, **27**, 292–9

Tomonaga M (1983) Neuropathology of the locus coeruleus: a semiquantitative study. *J Neurol*, **230**, 231–40

Tretiàkoff C (1919) Contribution a l'etude de l'anatomie pathologique du locus niger der Soemmering avec quelques deductions relatives a la pathogenie des troubles du tonus musculaire et de la maladie de Parkinson. Thesis, University of Paris

Turner BH, Wilson JS, McKenzie JC, and Richtand N (1988) MPTP produces a pattern of nigrostriatal degeneration which coincides with the mosaic organization of the caudate nucleus. *Brain Res*, **473**, 60–4

Vijayashankar N and Brody H (1979) A quantitative study of the pigmented neurons in the nuclei locus coeruleus and subcoeruleus in man as related to ageing. *J Neurol Exp Neuropathol*, **38**, 490–7

Ward CD, Duvoisin RC, and Ince SE (1984) Parkinson's disease in twins. In Hassler RG, Christ JF, eds, *Advances in Neurology*, vol. 40, Raven Press, New York, 341–6

Wilson JS, Turner BH, Morrow GD, and Hartmann PJ (1987) MPTP produces a mosaic-like pattern of terminal degeneration in the caudate nucleus of the dog. *Brain Res*, **423**, 329–32

Woodard JS (1962) Concentric hyhalin inclusion body formation in mental disease. Analysis of twenty-seven cases. *J Neuropathol Exp Neurol*, **21**, 442–9

Yokochi M, Narabayashi H, Iizuka R, and Nagatsu T (1984) Juvenile parkinsonism – some clinical, pharmacological and neuropathological aspects. *Adv Neurol*, **40**, 407–13

9
Protective therapy for Parkinson's disease

Ira Shoulson

In the context of Parkinson's disease (PD), *symptomatic* therapy refers to an intervention that ameliorates the clinical features of illness, but benefits are only temporary as the neurodegenerative process progresses. In contrast, *protective* therapy represents an intervention that substantively protects the population of vulnerable neurons and thereby slows the underlying progression of neurodegeneration. Both types of therapy may be associated with short-term improvement in clinical signs and symptoms, but the benefits of protective therapy are more enduring and generally reflect a substantial slowing of functional decline. Short of examining the substantia nigra prior to and following an intervention, the designations symptomatic and protective are inferred on the basis of the nature and time course of improvement (Shoulson, 1989).

Levodopa is an example of symptomatic therapy for PD. Symptoms are lessened temporarily by levodopa and exacerbated upon its withdrawal (e.g. wearing-off effects). There is no evidence that levodopa slows the underlying progression of PD, and theoretically levodopa may hasten nigral dysfunction and loss. While deprenyl (selegiline) has been suggested to slow nigral degeneration, protective therapy has not yet been established for PD. Decoppering interventions for Wilson's disease remain the hallmark of genuine protective (and even preventive) therapies for a neurodegenerative disorder.

PATHOGENESIS

The rational development of symptomatic and protective therapies for PD depends respectively on an understanding of underlying pathology (the consequences of neuronal loss) and pathogenesis (the process of neuronal dysfunction and degeneration). To develop successful symptomatic therapies, the consequences (e.g. dopamine loss) of neuronal (e.g. nigral) degeneration must be identified. Replenishing nigrostriatal dopaminergic activity therefore forms the basis of dopaminergic symptomatic therapy for PD. Meaningful protective therapies for PD depend on understanding the pathogenesis by which the vulnerable neuronal population degenerates. The development of protective strategies for PD is not necessarily dependent on determining aetiology. However, prevention of neuronal degeneration will ultimately depend upon identifying what appear to be the multifactorial causes of PD (see Chapter 7).

In the past decade, the pathogenesis of nigral degeneration in PD has been linked increasingly to oxidative-mediated mechanisms of intrinsic neural and extrinsic environmental origins (Parkinson Study Group, 1989a). As nigral neurons and dopamine content decline normally with age and pathologically in PD, remaining neurons compensate by increasing the production and release of dopamine. In turn, deamination of dopamine by monoamine oxidase (MAO) may result in increased formation of hydrogen peroxide and other potentially toxic byproducts such as hydroxyl radicals, superoxide, 6-hydroxydopamine and quinones. Increased lipid peroxidation and oxidized iron have also been observed in the postmortem PD brain, suggesting that heightened oxidative activity accompanies the neurodegenerative process. More recently, abnormalities of complex I (NADH: ubiquinone oxidoreductase) of the mitochondrial respiratory chain have been identified in circulating platelets and in the postmortem brain of PD patients (Parker *et al.*, 1989). Depletion of free radical scavenger enzymes may contribute further to the intrinsic vulnerability underlying oxidative-mediated nigral degeneration.

A variety of environmental factors may predispose nigral neurons to failure and death (Tanner, 1989). Protoxins, such as 1-methyl-4-phenyl-1,2,5,6-tetrahydropyridine (MPTP), may be transformed by MAO to toxic derivatives which disrupt the functions of nigral neurons and result in clinical and pathological features of PD. When oxidative biotransformation of MPTP in non-human primates and other experimental animals is blocked by MAO B-type inhibitors, nigral toxicity and parkinsonism are prevented (Heikkila *et al.*, 1984; Langston *et al.*, 1984). These collective observations form the basis for antioxidative protective strategies in PD aimed at slowing nigral degeneration and clinical decline through inhibition of MAO and/or detoxification of free radicals.

Deprenyl (selegiline) is a MAO B-type inhibitor, which in humans is relatively devoid of pressor effects when administered at a dosage of 10 mg/day (Knoll, 1983; Chrisp *et al.*, 1991). Alpha-tocopherol is a biologically active component of vitamin E which attenuates the effects of lipid peroxidation by quenching hydroxyl radicals (Halliwell and Gutteridge, 1985). To the extent that MAO B-mediated activity and free radical formation contribute to the pathogenesis of nigral degeneration, deprenyl and tocopherol, through different but complementary antioxidative mechanisms, may be expected to slow the clinical decline of PD (Parkinson Study Group, 1989a).

Many adverse effects of levodopa therapy, especially on–off motor fluctuations, have been attributed to loss of transmitter buffering capacity in presynaptic nigrostriatal neurons, resulting in uneven and unpredictable stimulation of dopamine receptors (Marsden, 1990). It has been postulated that long-acting and relatively selective dopamine agonists may buttress the capacity of nigrostriatal neurons and slow nigral degeneration by stimulating presynaptic dopamine autoreceptors, thus reducing the demands of presynaptic nigrostriatal neurons and sparing the amount of levodopa required to attain symptomatic relief (Mouradian *et al.*, 1988; see Chapter 10). Thus, dopamine agonists acting directly to stimulate postsynaptic D_2 receptor sites and presynaptic autoreceptors, alone or in combination with low-dose levodopa therapy, may also be expected to slow the progression of early PD.

PHARMACOLOGY

Deprenyl (selegiline)

Deprenyl (selegiline, Eldepryl) is a levorotatory acetylenic derivative of phenethylamine which irreversibly inhibits MAO by acing as a 'suicide substrate' for the enzyme. At a daily dosage of 10 mg in humans, deprenyl is a relatively selective inhibitor of type B MAO. Types A and B MAO differ in their substrate specificity and tissue distribution. Intestinal MAO is predominately type A and provides protection from exogenous amines (e.g. tyramine) that have the capacity to cause hypertensive crisis ('cheese effect') if absorbed intact. Brain MAO, especially in association with glial cells, is predominately type B. Deprenyl may also enhance nigrostriatal dopamine by interfering with presynaptic reuptake as well as inhibition of catabolism (Chrisp *et al.*, 1991). Deprenyl has been shown in mice to suppress the oxidant stress associated with increased dopamine turnover as measured by the accumulation of glutathione disulphide (Cohen and Spina, 1989).

L-Deprenyl is rapidly and well-absorbed with maximum plasma concentrations occurring 0.5–2 hours following administration. The parent compound is rapidly metabolized to L-desmethyldeprenyl (the major metabolite with mean half-life of 2 hours), L-amphetamine (mean half-life of 17.7 hours) and L-methamphetamine (mean half-life of 20.5 hours). Approximately 45% of an administered dose of deprenyl appears in the urine over 48 hours in the form of these three metabolites. Unchanged deprenyl is not detected. Although considered to be less biologically active than their D-isomers, L-amphetamine and L-methamphetamine may interfere with neuronal uptake and enhance release of endogenous catecholamines.

Platelet MAO activity, which is exclusively type B, is nearly 90% inhibited after a single dose of deprenyl 10 mg and remains inhibited for several days. In the setting of 100% inhibition of platelet MAOB activity, approximately 85–95% of dopamine-sensitive MAO activity is depleted in the postmortem brain of deprenyl-treated PD patients (Riederer and Youdim, 1986). The rate of MAOB regeneration following discontinuation of deprenyl is dependent upon *de novo* synthesis of MAO. In rodents, nearly full MAOB activity is restored within 1–2 weeks of deprenyl discontinuation (Elsworth *et al.*, 1978), but the rate of MAOB regeneration may be longer in non-human primates (Arnett *et al.*, 1987).

Tocopherol (alpha-tocopherol)

Alpha-tocopherol is one of the eight naturally occurring tocopherols with vitamin E activity; it comprises the largest percentage of tocopherols in animal tissue and the greatest degree of biological activity. Antioxidant effects, including free radical scavenger properties and inhibition of oxidation of unsaturated fatty acids, appear to be the most important biological property of tocopherols. Tocopherol has a better profile for both electron and hydrogen transfer reactions than do ascorbate, beta-carotene or glutathione (Willson, 1983).

Vitamin E is absorbed from the gut by a bile-dependent mechanism similar to that for other fat-soluble vitamins. Only 20–40% of orally ingested tocopherol is absorbed, and solubilization by bile salts is essential for absorption. In humans, blood levels of tocopherol peak 8 hours after administration and then remain the same or decline slightly by 24 hours (Baker *et al.*, 1980). Concentrations are higher when the free tocopherol (alcohol) is administered rather than the acetate. It is necessary to treat humans with high levels of vitamin E for at least 1–3 weeks in order to attain maximal plasma levels. Within 3 weeks of discontinuing vitamin E supplementation, plasma levels fall significantly and are virtually undetectable at 4 weeks. In rats placed on supplemental vitamin E 1000 mg/kg for 18 weeks, vitamin E levels doubled in the plasma and increased by 40% in the striatum (Brin and Traver, 1985).

Dopamine agonists

Directly acting dopamine agonists have several theoretical advantages over levodopa. Agonists are largely independent of the integrity of presynaptic nigral neurons, generally exert a long duration of action, and may selectively stimulate subtypes of dopamine receptors (Goetz, 1990). Bromocriptine is an ergot alkaloid which is absorbed rapidly in the gut, largely undergoes first-pass hepatic metabolism, and has a plasma half-life varying between 4 and 8 hours. Pergolide is an ergoline derivative which is absorbed rapidly and has a duration of action of 8–12 hours. Bromocriptine exerts agonist effects predominantly at the D_2 receptor site, while pergolide also stimulates D_1 receptors. Both agonists appear to stimulate D_2 presynaptic autoreceptors, resulting in reduced presynaptic dopamine release, as well as postsynaptic dopamine receptors. The adverse effects of bromocriptine and pergolide are similar to levodopa, although dyskinesias are rarely induced in PD patients by agonists alone. Lisuride is an ergot derivative, marketed in Europe, which can be administered intravenously and has a pharmacological profile similar to bromocriptine.

CLINICAL TRIALS

In most levodopa-treated PD patients, deprenyl attenuates dose-related wearing-off effects. The symptomatic benefits of deprenyl in levodopa-treated patients seem to be mild and often short-lived. However, retrospective analyses by Birkmayer and colleagues (1985) have suggested that, over the long term, deprenyl may slow the clinical decline and extend the life span of levodopa-treated patients.

Based on retrospective survey data, Goetz *et al.* (1987) reported that approximately 75% of non-levodopa-treated PD patients, some treated with amantadine and anticholinergics, required levodopa therapy within 2 years of follow-up. Fahn (1989) followed 12 early PD patients who were treated chronically with vitamin E (3200 IU/day) and vitamin C (3000 mg/day) and found durations of benefit, extending from 2.5 to 7.5 years, before dopaminergic therapy was required to treat disability. Other investigators have found that the intake of food or supplements containing high levels of vitamin E was inversely associated with the occurrence of PD (Parkinson Study Group, 1989a). These pilot studies suffer from retrospective analyses and lack of controls; however, they have prompted more rigorous examination of the therapeutic effects of deprenyl and vitamin E in early PD.

DATATOP

To the extent that MAO activity and the formation of oxygen radicals contribute to the pathogenesis of nigral degeneration, deprenyl, tocopherol, or both may be expected to slow the clinical progression of PD. Deprenyl and Tocopherol Antioxidative Therapy of Parkinsonism (DATATOP) is a placebo-controlled, double-blind, multicentre clinical trial which has been designed and conducted by the Parkinson Study Group. The aim of the trial is to determine whether long-term therapy with deprenyl or tocopherol extends the interval before sufficiently severe disability requires the initiation of levodopa therapy.

Eight hundred subjects with early, otherwise untreated PD were enrolled in DATATOP between September 1987 and November 1988. Subjects were assigned randomly by a 2×2 factorial design to one of four treatment groups: deprenyl (10 mg/day) and tocopherol placebo; deprenyl placebo and tocopherol (2000 IU/day); deprenyl 10 mg/day and tocopherol (2000 IU/day); or deprenyl placebo and tocopherol placebo. A stratified randomization helped ensure that each of the 34 participing investigators was assigned an approximate numerical balance of subjects in each of the four treatment groups. Thirteen investigators each enrolled between 21 and 44 subjects, and 21 investigators each enrolled 19 or 20 subjects (Parkinson Study Group, 1989a).

Following baseline evaluation and randomization, subjects were re-evaluated at 1 and 3 months and then at approximately 3-month intervals with respect to a variety of standardized clinical measures relevant to PD. The primary end-point of the trial occurred when, in the judgement of the enrolling investigator, a subject reached a level of functional disability sufficient to warrant the initiation of levodopa therapy. In arriving at this judgement, the investigator considered: (1) compromise to the subject's employability; (2) threat to the subject's ability to manage domestic or financial affairs; (3) an appreciable decline in activities of daily living; and (4) worsening of gait or balance (Parkinson Study Group, 1989a).

The DATATOP trial was designed for completion in December 1990, approximately 25 months after the 800th subject was enrolled. An independent safety monitoring committee reviewed the end-point data periodically, using predetermined guidelines for recommendation of an early termination of the trial if the results showed significant adverse effects ($P<0.05$), or evidence of efficacy ($P<0.001$ for the primary hypotheses and $P<0.0005$ for the interaction effects). In February 1989, the Safety Monitoring Committee informed the principal investigator that guidelines for efficacy had been reached for subjects assigned to deprenyl compared to subjects not assigned to deprenyl.

The preliminary data analysis, carried out after 12 ± 5 months of follow-up, disclosed that the 401 subjects who did not receive deprenyl (treatment group A) and the 399 subjects who received deprenyl (treatment group B) were highly comparable with respect to clinical and demographic measures attained at baseline. No differences were observed between these treatment groups with respect to the 95–99% compliance with assigned treatments (Parkinson Study Group, 1989b).

At the time of analysis, 176 subjects in treatment group A (not receiving deprenyl) had reached the end-point of disability while only 97 subjects in treatment group B (receiving deprenyl) had reached the end-point ($P<10^{-8}$). In survival terms, the hazard ratio comparing subjects in group B to group A with respect to the risk of reaching the end-point per unit of time was 0.43, representing a 57% reduction in the risk of reaching the end-point ($P<10^{-10}$; Fig. 9.1). When the 292 subjects who

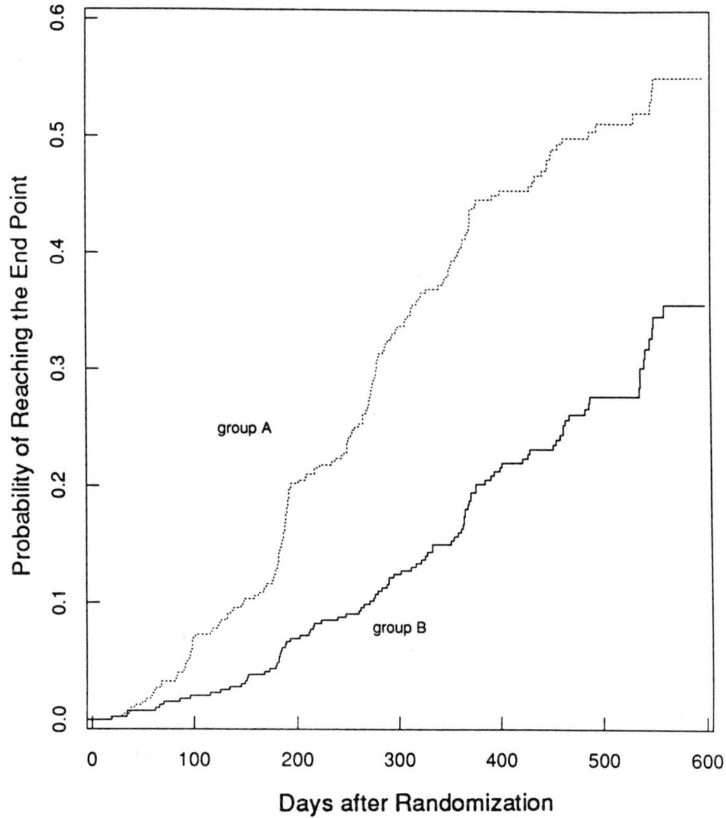

Figure 9.1 Cumulative probability of reaching end-point (Kaplan–Meier estimate), according to treatment group. The hazard ratio for the comparison of group B to group A with respect to the risk of reaching end-point per unit of time is 0.43 ($P<10^{-10}$; 95% confidence limits, 0.33 and 0.55). From Parkinson Study Group (1989b) with permission.

were fully employed upon entry into the study were analysed with respect to cessation of full-time employment, a hazard reduction of 0.5 ($P=0.01$) was found favouring subjects assigned to deprenyl (Fig. 9.2).

For the 682 subjects who completed at least 6 months of evaluation, those not assigned to deprenyl declined significantly – about 10% faster – than those assigned to deprenyl with respect to standardized clinical measures of PD. Subjects who reached end-point showed a similar extent of clinical decline, regardless of treatment group.

At 1 and 3 months after baseline evaluation, deprenyl-treated subjects showed significant improvement in measures of the Unified Parkinson's Disease Rating Scale (UPDRS); however, the magnitude of the total change was slight (improvement by 1.75 units at 1 month and 1.48 units at 3 months) and probably not clinically meaningful in the context of a scale which ranges from 0 (normal) to 125 (very abnormal). Changes in secondary response variables between the end-point and final

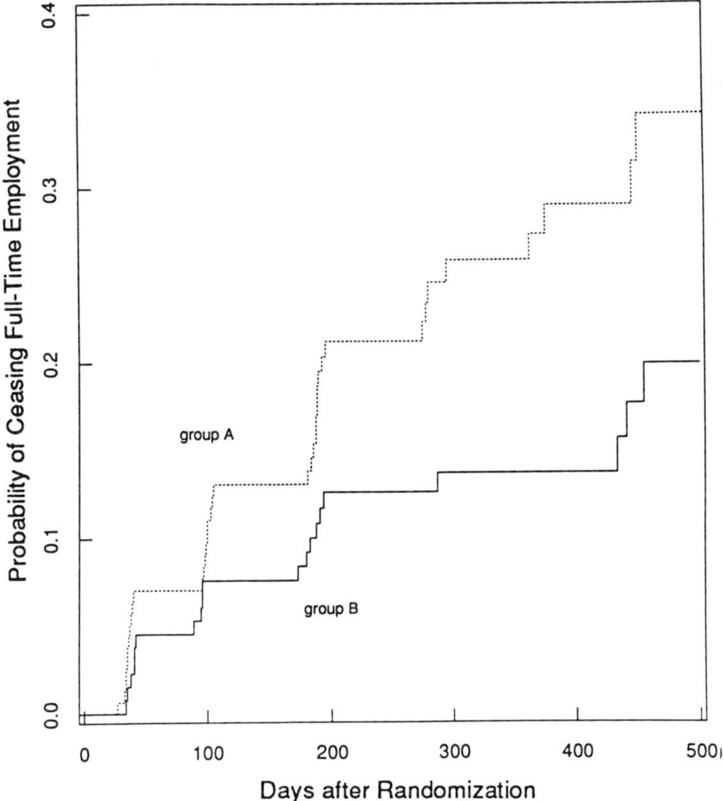

Figure 9.2 Cumulative probability of ceasing full-time employment (Kaplan–Meier estimate), according to treatment group. This analysis was restricted to the 292 subjects who were fully employed at baseline. The outcome event was the first report of cessation of full-time employment made at any follow-up visit, including the final evaluation. The difference between the treatment groups was statistically significant ($P=0.01$; hazard ratio, 0.50; 95% confidence limits, 0.29 and 0.86). From Parkinson Study Group (1989b) with permission.

evaluations (washout effects) were slight and revealed no significant differences between treatment groups (Parkinson Study Group, 1989b).

Tetrud and Langston trial of deprenyl

Tetrud and Langston (1989) reported on 51 PD subjects, different from those in DATATOP, who were enrolled in a placebo-controlled trial of deprenyl and followed to the same end-point as employed in DATATOP. This double-blind trial was initiated approximately 9 months prior to DATATOP and was intended as a pilot study to help assess feasibility and safety. In contrast to the DATATOP study, which followed patients to a maximum of 18 months, the Tetrud and Langston study followed subjects to maximum of 3 years. The results of Tetrud and Langston were strikingly similar to the preliminary DATATOP findings, showing a clear and statistically significant delay in the time until end-point ($P < 0.002$). The average time to end-point was 312 days in the 25 placebo-treated subjects and 549 days in the 26 deprenyl-treated subjects. No significant wash-in or wash-out effects were found.

Other clinical trials of deprenyl

Table 9.1 summarizes trials of deprenyl as monotherapy (10 mg/day) in early PD patients. While the trials varied considerably in design, duration and sample size, a few general conclusions can be drawn. Assessment of parkinsonian features in these relatively small samples has detected modest or negligible amelioration of PD features due to deprenyl, on the order of 10% change (Eisler *et al.*, 1981; Csandra and Tarczy, 1987; Elizan *et al.*, 1989; Myllyla *et al.*, 1989; Teravainen, 1990). While deprenyl obviously does not prevent the progression of clinical features, functional benefits are striking – on the order of 50% improvement (Parkinson Study Group, 1989b; Tetrud and Langston, 1989).

Interpretation of the deprenyl trials

The effect of deprenyl in delaying the onset of a predetermined level of disability was strong and unequivocal. However, the benefits of deprenyl may well derive from symptomatic effects. Deprenyl could have exerted an anti-PD effect by increasing the availability of nigrostriatal dopamine through inhibition of MAO catabolism of dopamine and inhibition of presynaptic reuptake of dopamine.

While short-term anti-PD effects can be reasonably ascribed to deprenyl, such effects do not adequately explain the long-term reduction in the rate of reaching end-point. For example, when the DATATOP subjects in each treatment group were subdivided into those who showed initial improvement in the total UPDRS score between baseline and 1-month evaluations (402 subjects; 189 in group A and 213 in group B) and those who showed a decline or no change within 1 month (379 subjects; 202 in group A and 177 in group B), the difference in the rate of reaching end-point favouring those taking deprenyl remains strong and statistically significant within subgroupings. Even when 'improved' subjects not taking deprenyl are compared with 'unimproved' subjects taking deprenyl, a significant ($P = 0.001$) benefit attributable to deprenyl remained in reducing the risk of reaching end-point (Parkinson Study Group, 1989b).

Other mechanisms may account for symptomatic anti-PD benefits of deprenyl. The L-amphetamine and L-methamphetamine metabolites of L-deprenyl may produce anti-PD effects. Parkes *et al.* (1975) reported that L-amphetamine produced an approximate 20% improvement in PD patients who were also treated with levodopa and anticholinergics ($n = 19$); in otherwise untreated patients ($n = 3$), L-amphetamine produced no change in parkinsonian features. Stern *et al.* (1983) have demonstrated that the effects of L-deprenyl in patients treated with levodopa did not depend on the pharmacological properties of its L-amphetamine metabolites. It remains unclear whether L-amphetamine induces clinically relevant anti-PD effects in otherwise untreated patients such as those enrolled in the DATATOP and the Tetrud and Langston trials.

Table 9.1 Trials of deprenyl (10 mg/day) as monotherapy in (early) Parkinson's disease

Trial	*Design*	*Duration*	*n*	*Primary end-point or outcome measure(s)*	*Effect*
Csandra and Tarczy (1987)	Open-label	At least 6 months	30	Webster score	Progressive overall decline 10/30 improved transiently
Elsler *et al.* (1981)	Parallel, placebo-controlled	4 weeks	2	Parkinsonism score	Negligible
Elizan *et al.* (1989)	Open-label	7–84 months	22	Clinical progression (new signs or worsening)	Fails to *halt* progression
Tetrud and Langston (1989)	Parallel, placebo-controlled, double-blind; survival analysis	To end-point (up to 3 years)	51	Need for levodopa (end-point)	1. Significant ($P<0.002$) delay to end-point 2. No significant wash-in or wash-out effects at 1 month
Parkinson Study Group DATATOP (1989b)	2 × 2 factorial, placebo-controlled, double-blind, multicentre; survival analysis	12 ± 5 months (in progress)	800	Need for levodopa (end-point)	1. Significant ($P<10^{-10}$) delay to end-point and to loss of full-time employment 2. Statistically significant, ? clinically meaningful wash-in effects at 1 and 3 months 3. No wash-out effects (among subjects who reached end-point after 1 month)
Myllyla *et al.* (1989)	Parallel, placebo-controlled double-blind; interim analysis	Up to 12 months	52	'Disability' rating scales (Webster, Columbia, Northwestern)	Significant ($P<0.05$–0.01) lessening of disability
Teravainen (1990)	Placebo-controlled, double-blind crossover	8 weeks on deprenyl 10–30 mg/day 4 weeks on placebo	20	Motor component of UPDRS and 'Columbia score'	Insignificant 10% reduction in Columbia score

UPDRS = Unified Parkinson's Disease Rating Scale.

Deprenyl may also exert symptomatic anti-PD effects through its potential antidepressant properties; however, patients with mild depression were excluded from DATATOP, and only trivial degrees of antidepressant change on the Hamilton scale among deprenyl-treated subjects (0.25 units out of a range of 53 units) were detected comparing baseline to 1-month and 3-month evaluations (Parkinson Study Group, 1989b). Deprenyl 10 mg/day has not been shown to produce antidepressant effects in patients with depression who do not have PD (Mann *et al.*, 1989). However, deprenyl may have produced a general improvement in sense of well-being, similar to that observed in patients with Alzheimer's disease who have been treated with this MAO inhibitor (Tariot *et al.*, 1987).

Trials of dopamine agonists

Dopaming agonists have been evaluated in several trials involving previously untreated PD patients (Giovanni *et al.*, 1981; Lees and Stern, 1981; Grimes and Delgado, 1985; Rinne, 1985; Staal-Schreinemachers *et al.*, 1986; Hely *et al.*, 1989; Rinne, 1989; Goetz, 1990; Langtry and Clissold, 1990). Outcome measures varied considerably, and average (symptomatic) improvement in PD clinical scores ranged from 15 to 50%. Since these trials did not measure a time-related end-point of disability, it is difficult to assess whether the improvement was symptomatic, protective or both.

THERAPEUTIC CONSIDERATIONS

The deprenyl studies of patients in the early stages of PD support a recommendation for considering treatment of these patients with deprenyl 10 mg/day. A lower dosage may be as effective or more effective because of the irreversible inhibition of MAOB by deprenyl. In view of the limited clinical experience with deprenyl, treated patients should be re-evaluated at 3–6-month intervals to assess efficacy and adverse effects and to consider the need for levodopa therapy (Parkinson Study Group, 1989b). Because of the uncertainty regarding the mechanism of deprenyl's therapeutic effect, additional placebo-controlled trials are warranted in patients with early PD.

Although early therapy with levodopa has not been shown to accelerate adverse effects and clinical progression, it seems prudent to delay levodopa until significant functional impairment develops. Initiation of dopamine agonists should be considered if and when such disability emerges. Deprenyl and dopamine agonists should also be considered in low dosage as symptomatic adjuvant therapies in levodopa-treated patients who have developed wearing-off effects, on–off responses or declining responsivity. No recommendations can as yet be made regarding tocopherol therapy.

FUTURE RESEARCH

The possibility remains that deprenyl may exert a genuine protective effect in slowing the underlying progression of PD through inhibition of MAO B and suppression of the putative toxic effects mediated by this enzyme. This possibility was supported largely by the failure to detect meaningful symptomatic anti-PD effects in the subjects enrolled in the DATATOP and Tetrud and Langston trials.

However, the continued DATATOP trial provided extra clues regarding the mechanism of deprenyl's effect in early PD. After the initial analysis carried out following 12 ± 5 months of follow-up (Parkinson Study Group, 1989b), the protocol was modified such that all active research subjects were withdrawn from originally assigned treatments for up to two months and then changed to active deprenyl. The blindness of original treatment assignments was maintained. Treatment with deprenyl (10 mg per day) was restarted during the two months after treatment was withdrawn if the investigator determined that features of PD has worsened sufficiently as a consequence of the withdrawal of experimental treatment. Subjects were followed for a mean of 14 ± 6 months after randomization, before withdrawal of experimental treatments. The results (Parkinson Study Group, 1993) showed that the beneficial effects of deprenyl which occurred largely during the first 12 months of treatment remained strong and significantly delayed the onset of disability requiring levodopa therapy (Hazard ratio, 0.50; $p<0.001$). The difference in the estimated median time to the end point was about 9 months. There was no beneficial effect of alpha-tocopherol or any interaction between tocopherol and deprenyl).

The new analysis (Parkinson Study Group, 1993) revealed that ratings for Parkinson's disease improved during the first 3 months of deprenyl treatment, and the motor performance of deprenyl-treated patients worsened after treatments were withdrawn. This suggests that the observed beneficial effect of deprenyl in delaying disability is at least partly related to a symptomatic amelioration of PD. There was no evidence that deprenyl has appreciable antidepressant effects during this extended period of observation. There was some evidence to indicate that, in addition, deprenyl might have exerted a true protective influence on PD. Thus, there was superior survival with respect to the primary end point even amongst deprenyl-treated subjects who initially had no improvement in rating scores. In addition, the overall persisting benefit (as compared with base-line status) among deprenyl-treated subjects who did not reach the end point and who did not require deprenyl during the two months after withdrawal suggested a protective influence. Nevertheless, the small but definite symptomatic effect of deprenyl hampered a clear-cut detection of potentially protective action of this agent in early PD.

It is unlikely that the ongoing DATATOP trial will provide conclusive data regarding the mechanism of deprenyl's benefit in PD. Further insight may come from studies using reversible, short-acting MAOB inhibitors that are not metabolized to potentially active anti-PD derivatives. Use of *in vivo* techniques such as positron emission tomography may also aid in clarifying the mechanism of deprenyl's action.

It appears that dopamine agonists administered alone exert discernible symptomatic benefits in early PD. However, the impact of agonists on functional milestones of disability seems less robust, at least when compared with levodopa monotherapy. Controlled clinical trials should be considered directly to compare agonists to deprenyl in previously untreated patients. The recent report by Felten *et al.* (1991), indicating that pergolide slows the age-related loss of nigral neurons in rats, supports the contention that dopamine agonists may exert protective as well as symptomatic benefits.

Acknowledgements

Preparation of this manuscript was supported by USPHS grant NS 24778 from the National Institutes of Health (NINDS).

References

Arnett CD, Fowler JS, MacGregor RR *et al.* (1987) Turnover of brain monoamine oxidase measured *in vivo* by positron emission tomography using L-[^{11}C] deprenyl. *J Neurochem*, **49**, 522–7

Baker HO, Frank O, DeAngelis B *et al.* (1980) Plasma tocopherol in man at various time after ingesting free or acetylated tocopherol. *Nutr Rep Int* **21**, 531–6

Birkmayer W, Knott J, Riederer P *et al.* (1985) Increased life expectancy resulting from addition of L-deprenyl to Madopar® treatment in Parkinson's disease: a longterm study. *J Neural Trans*, **64**, 113–27

Brin MF and Traver MG (1985) Vitamin E deficiency and human neurological disease. *Lab Management*, **23**, 57–67

Chrisp P, Mammen GJ and Sorkin EM (1991) Selegiline: a review of its pharmacological properties, and symptomatic and protective potential in Parkinson's disease. *Drugs Aging*, **1**, 228–48

Cohen G and Spina MB (1989) Deprenyl suppresses the oxidant stress associated with increased dopamine turnover. *Ann Neurol*, **26**, 689–90

Csandra E and Tarczy M (1987) Selegiline in the early and later phases of Parkinson's disease. *J Neural Trans* (suppl 25), 105–13

Eisler T, Teravainen H, Nelson R *et al.* (1981) Deprenyl in Parkinson disease. *Neurology*, **31**, 19–23

Elizan TS, Yahr MD, Moros DA *et al.* (1989) Selegiline use to prevent progression of Parkinson's disease. *Arch Neurol*, **46**, 1275–9

Elsworth JD, Glover V, Reynolds GP *et al.* (1978) Deprenyl administration in man: a selective monoamine oxidase B inhibitor without the 'cheese effect'. *Psychopharmacology*, **57**, 33–8

Fahn S (1989) The endogenous toxin hypothesis of the etiology of Parkinson's disease and a pilot trial of high-dosage antioxidants in an attempt to slow the progression of illness. *Ann NY Acad Sci*, **570**, 186–96

Felten DL, Felten SY, Fuller RW *et al.* (1992) Chronic dietary pergolide preserves nigrostriatal neuronal integrity in aged Fischer 344 rats. *Neurobiol Aging*, **13**, 339–51

Giovanni P, Scigliano G, Piccolo I *et al.* (1981) Lisuride in Parkinson's disease: 4-year follow-up. *Clin Neuropharmacol*, **11**, 201–11

Goetz CG (1990) Dopaminergic agonists in the treatment of Parkinson's disease. *Neurology*, **40** (suppl 3), 50–4

Goetz CG, Tanner CM, and Shannon KM (1987) Progression of Parkinson's disease without levodopa. *Neurology*, **37**, 695–8

Grimes JD and Delgado MR (1985) Bromocriptine: problems with low-dose *de novo* therapy in Parkinson's disease. *Clin Neuropharmacol*, **8**, 73–7

Halliwell B and Gutteridge JMC (1985) Oxygen radicals and the nervous system. *Trends Neurosci*, **8**, 22–6

Heikkila RE, Manzino L, Cabbat FS *et al.* (1984) Protection against the dopaminergic neurotoxicity of 1-methyl-4-phenyl-1,2,5,6-tetra-hydropyridine by monoamine oxidase inhibitors. *Nature*, **311**, 467–9

Hely MA, Morris JGL, Rail D *et al.* (1989) The Sydney Multicentre Study of Parkinson's disease: a report on the first 3 years. *J Neurol, Neurosurg Psychiatry*, **52**, 324–8

Knoll J (1983) Deprenyl (selegiline): the history of its development and pharmacological action. *Acta Neurol Scand* (suppl 95), 57–80

Langston JW, Irwin I, and Langston EB (1984) Pargyline prevents MPTP-induced parkinsonism in primates. *Science*, **225**, 1480–2

Langtry HD and Clissold SP (1990) Pergolide: a review of its pharmacological properties and therapeutic potential in Parkinson's disease. *Drugs*, **39**, 491–506

Lees A and Stern GM (1981) Sustained bromocriptine therapy in previously untreated patients with Parkinson's disease. *J Neurol, Neursurg Psychiatry*, **44**, 1020–3

Mann JJ, Aarons SF, Wilner PJ *et al.* (1989) A controlled study of the antidepressant efficacy and side effects of (–) deprenyl. *Arch Gen Psychiatry*, **46**, 45–50

Marsden CD (1990) Parkinson's disease. *Lancet*, **i**, 948–52

Myllyla VV, Sotaniemi KA, Touminen J *et al.* (1989) Selegiline as primary therapy in early phase Parkinson's disease – an interim report. *Acta Neurol Scand*, **126**, 177–82

Mouradian MM, Juncos JL, Fabbrini G *et al.* (1988) Motor fluctuations in Parkinson's disease: central pathophysiological mechanisms, Part II. *Ann Neurol*, **24**, 372–8

Parker WD, Boyson SJ, and Parks JK (1989) Abnormalities of the electron transport chain in idiopathic Parkinson's disease. *Ann Neurol*, **26**, 719–23

Parkes JD, Tarsy D, Marsden CD *et al.* (1975) Amphetamines in the treatment of Parkinson's disease. *J Neurol Neurosurg Psychiatry*, **38**, 232–7

Parkinson Study Group (1989a) DATATOP: a multi-center controlled clinical trial in early Parkinson's disease. *Arch Neurol*, **46**, 1052–60

Parkinson Study Group (1989b) Effect of deprenyl on the progression of disability in early Parkinson's disease. *N Engl J Med*, **321**, 1364–71

Parkinson Study Group (1993) Effect of tocopherol and deprenyl on the progression of disability in early Parkinson's disease. *N Engl J Med*, **328**, 176–83

Riederer P and Youdim MBH (1986) Monoamine oxidase activity and monoamine metabolism in brains of parkinsonian patients treated with L-deprenyl. *J Neurochem*, **46**, 1359–65

Rinne UK (1985) Combined bromociptine-levodopa therapy in early Parkinson's disease. *Neurology*, **35**, 1196–8

Rinne UK (1989) Lisuride, a dopamine agonist in the treatment of early Parkinson's disease. *Neurology*, **39**, 336–9

Shoulson I (1989) Experimental therapeutics directed at the pathogenesis of Parkinson's disease. In Calne DB, eds, *Handbook of Experimental Pharmacology: Drugs for the Treatment of Parkinson's Disease*, Berlin, Springer-Verlag, 289–305

Staal-Schreinemachers AL, Wesseling H, Kamphuis DL *et al.* (1986) Low-dose bromocriptine therapy in Parkinson's disease: double-blind, placebo-controlled study. *Neurology*, **36**, 291–3

Stern GM, Lees AJ, Hardie R *et al.* (1983) Clinical and pharmacological aspects of (–)deprenyl treatment in Parkinson's disease. *Mod Probl Pharmacopsychiatry*, **19**, 215–19

Tanner CM (1989) The role of environmental factors in the etiology of Parkinson's disease. *Trends Neurosci*, **12**, 49–54

Tariot PN, Cohen RM, Sunderland T *et al.* (1987) L-deprenyl in Alzheimer's disease: preliminary evidence for behavioral change with monoamine oxidase B inhibition. *Arch Gen Psychiatry*, **44**, 427–33

Teravainen H (1990) Selegiline in Parkinson's disease. *Acta Neurol Scand*, **81**, 333–6

Tetrud JW and Langston JW (1989) The effect of deprenyl (selegiline) on the natural history of Parkinson's disease. *Science*, **245**, 519–22

Willson RL (1983) Free radical protection: why vitamin E, not vitamin C, beta-carotene or glutathione? in Porter R and Whelan J, eds, *Biology of Vitamin E: Ciba Foundation Symposium 101*, London, Pitman Books, 19–44

10

Improved dopaminergic therapy of Parkinson's disease

M. Maral Mouradian and Thomas N. Chase

Considerable progress has been made over the past three decades in the pharmacotherapy of Parkinson's disease. The initial discoveries that reserpine depletes striatal dopamine causing a parkinson-like syndrome in experimental animals which could be reversed by the dopamine precursor levodopa (Carlsson *et al.* 1957), the finding of marked dopaminergic depletion in the striatum of patients dying of Parkinson's disease (Hornykiewicz, 1963), and the subsequent dramatic improvement of patients with the disease with levodopa made Parkinson's disease the first neurodegenerative disorder to be treated effectively with transmitter replacement (Cotzias *et al.*, 1967). To date, levodopa continues to be the most effective antiparkinsonian agent known, more often than not producing dramatic results. In fact, lack of a clinically appreciable motor response to this amine precursor should raise doubt about the diagnosis of Parkinson's disease. The drug initially provides a stable motor response to all parkinsonian patients, even when taken only three or four times daily. Unfortunately, these salutary effects of levodopa do not last (Barbeau, 1974; Fahn, 1974; Marsden and Parkes, 1976). After about 5 years of therapy, half of the patients begin to manifest motor response fluctuations, initially characterized by an end-of-dose type of deterioration, often referred to as wearing-off phenomenon. These fluctuations necessitate taking levodopa more frequently to bridge the gaps between each dose. Later, another type of fluctuation appears, known as on–off phenomenon, which is unrelated to the timing of levodopa intake, and results in abrupt, dramatic shifts between states of mobility (on) and severe immobility (off). To make matters even worse, a variety of abnormal involuntary movements often complicate the clinical picture, with their appearance generally heralding the onset of motor fluctuations. These movements are most commonly choreiform in nature and occur at peak levodopa levels, but they can also be athetoid and dystonic, and emerge when levodopa levels are at trough (Muenter *et al.*, 1977; Luquin *et al.*, 1992). One or any combination of these manifestations of motor instability ultimately develops in a majority of parkinsonian patients chronically treated with levodopa, and substantially contribute to disability to a degree that may rival the basic disease itself.

Efforts to develop improved dopaminomimetic therapy of Parkinson's disease have, thus, focused on the treatment and prophylaxis of the motor fluctuations. Attempts to understand the nature and pathophysiolgy of these motor complications have been instrumental in accomplishing considerable progress towards this goal. These studies centre largely around the pharmacology of levodopa and its interaction with the central nervous system (Hornykiewicz, 1979; Nutt, 1987; Wooten, 1987; Mouradian and Chase, 1988).

PERIPHERAL PHARMACOLOGICAL ASPECTS OF LEVODOPA

The absorption of levodopa occurs primarily in the proximal small intestine (Wade, Mearrick and Morris, 1973). Although the stomach does not absorb levodopa, its mucosa can rapidly decarboxylase the prodrug and control its delivery to its absorption site by changes in gastric motility (Rivera-Calimlim *et al.*, 1970). Factors that slow gastric emptying, including meals, excessive acidity and anticholinergic drugs thus can facilitate local metabolism and result in smaller, delayed and sometimes multiple peaks in plasma levodopa levels (Rivera-Calimlim *et al.*, 1971; Wade *et al.*, 1974; Anderson *et al.*, 1975; Evans *et al.*, 1980). Attempts to bypass the gastric barrier, by delivering the drug directly into the duodenum, have ameliorated erratic plasma levodopa levels and consequently improved motor performance in some patients (Kurlan *et al.*, 1988; Sage *et al.*, 1988; Cedarbaum *et al.*, 1990).

Levodopa has a short plasma half-life due to its rapid metabolism (Nutt and Fellman, 1984; Hardie *et al.*, 1986). Its clearance from circulation follows a biphasic model with an early distribution phase with a half-life of 5–10 minutes, and a subsequent elimination phase with a half-life of around 90 minutes (Nutt *et al.*, 1985; Fabbrini *et al.*, 1987a). The co-administration of peripheral decarboxylase inhibitors, like carbidopa, improves the bioavailability of levodopa primarily by inhibiting its decarboxylation in the gut, and tends to prolong the elimination half-life but not to a clinically appreciable degree (Nutt *et al.*, 1985). Several observations have raised suspicion that perhaps alterations in levodopa peripheral pharmacokinetics may underlie the motor fluctuation in advanced disease: (1) patients with motor response instability tend to have more oscillations in their plasma levodopa levels compared to those with a stable response to the drug (Tolosa *et al.*, 1975; Papavasiliou *et al.*, 1979); (2) the presence of temporal relation between clinical fluctuations, oral dosing, and plasma levodopa levels in patients with pure wearing-off phenomenon (Fahn, 1974; Sweet and McDowell, 1974; Shoulson *et al.*, 1975; Tolosa *et al.*, 1975; Rossor *et al.*, 1980; Eriksson *et al.*, 1984; Nutt and Woodward, 1986); and (3) the improvement of wearing-off fluctuations to stabilization of plasma levodopa levels (Shoulson *et al.*, 1975; Hardie *et al.*, 1984; Nutt *et al.*, 1984; Quinn *et al.*, 1984; Juncos *et al.*, 1987; Mouradian *et al.*, 1987a, 1990). Yet, several studies have confirmed that all pharmacokinetic parameters for levodopa – including its plasma half-life, clearance and volume of distribution – are essentially identical in all stages of the disease, regardless of the presence or absence of motor fluctuations (Fabbrini *et al.*, 1987a; Gancher *et al.*, 1987; Fig. 10.1). In fact, the short half-life of levodopa seems to be inconsequential in the early stages of the disease, when its efficacy is actually much longer than expected from its circulating half-life. But the short half-life becomes an issue in advanced stages (Fabbrini *et al.*, 1988; Mouradian *et al.*, 1989c). When motor fluctuations are mild and mainly of the wearing-off type, shortening the interdose interval to every 2 hours or even less can provide substantial clinical benefit initially, only to fail when the fluctuations become more complex.

Levodopa is an amino acid which is transported across the blood–brain barrier by means of the large neutral amino acid transport carrier which is saturable (Wade

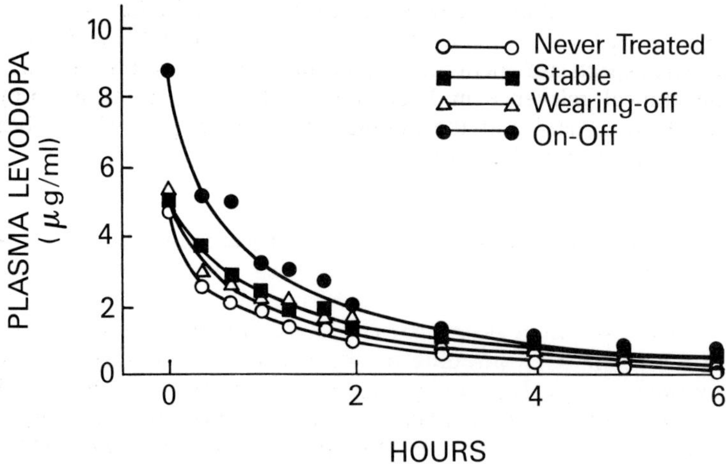

Figure 10.1 Decline in plasma levodopa levels following discontinuation of a steady-state, optimal-dose intravenous infusion. No differences were found between levodopa-naive patients, those treated with levodopa without motor fluctuations, those with simple wearing-off phenomenon and those with complex on–off fluctuations. From Fabbrini *et al.* (1987a).

and Katzman, 1975). Thus, other dietary amino acids that utilize the same transport system can readily compete with levodopa and diminish its access to target sites Cotzias *et al.*, 1967; Mena and Cotzias, 1975; Nutt *et al.*, 1984; Leenders *et al.*, 1986b). Consequently, limiting protein intake increases the availability of levodopa to the brain, improves its efficacy and decreases its requirements (Nutt *et al.*, 1984; Pincus and Barry, 1987). Dietary regimes severely restricting protein intake during the day and allowing proteins liberally at supper has been advocated (Pincus and Barry, 1987). By following such a schedule, patients can have more 'on' hours during the day but turn 'off' after dinner when they are generally immobile in bed. Implementation of such extreme measures should be carried out with appropriate caution to avoid undue catabolism.

Other aspects of the peripheral pharmacology of levodopa do not seem to play a role in the pathophysiology of motor response variability. A major metabolite of levodopa, 3-*O*-methyldopa, which is transported via the same transport system across biological membranes as the parent compound, tends to accumulate with chronic dosing due to its long half-life of around 15 hours (Fahn, 1974; Bartholini *et al.*, 1970; Muenter *et al.*, 1972). Nevertheless, levels achieved in parkinsonian patients are not high enough for this competition to impede the motor effects of levodopa (Fabbrini *et al.*, 1987b; Nutt *et al.*, 1987). In addition, levodopa is extensively stored in muscle tissue, and patients frequently report increased levodopa requirements with physical exercise. This is likely to be due to altered gastric emptying and decreased mesenteric blood flow (Nutt and Fellman, 1984), since strenuous physical exercise does not seem to affect either the pharmacokinetics or the efficacy of levodopa (Mouradian *et al.*, 1987b).

The peripheral pharmacokinetic characteristics of levodopa cannot, however, account for all forms of response complications. Some patients continue to experience resistant shifts between 'on' and 'off' states even while having stable and adequate circulating levels of levodopa taken parenterally and no interference by dietary proteins (Quinn *et al.*, 1984; Mouradian *et al.*, 1987a, 1990). Furthermore, these pharmacokinetic aspects are operational at all stages of Parkinson's disease, yet they only assume clinical relevance in later stages. The role of disease progression, chronicity of its treatment and the interaction of levodopa with the brain have consequently received critical attention.

CENTRAL PHARMACOKINETIC AND PHARMACODYNAMIC ASPECTS OF LEVODOPA

Levodopa, being a prodrug, is decarboxylated in nigrostriatal nerve terminals to dopamine which enters two main compartments: a short half-life synthetic pool and a slower-turnover storage one (Javoy and Glowinski, 1971). Under physiological conditions, dopaminergic neurons comprising this system fire tonically, thus stimulating postsynaptic dopamine receptors steadily (Bunney *et al.*, 1973). In early stages of Parkinson's disease, the surviving nigral neurons that are in a state of increased metabolic turnover appear to transform levodopa to dopamine and store it satisfactorily. Thus, levodopa taken orally at an interval much longer than its plasma half-life results in continuous availability of dopamine to postsynaptic receptors. Clinically, this is manifested as a stable motor response. With progressive neuronal degeneration in advanced disease, levodopa is still decarboxylated, albeit less efficiently (Spencer and Wooten, 1984), as evidenced by its continued antiparkinsonian efficacy. Under the circumstances, dopamine is presumably synthesized by other aromatic amino acid decarboxylase-containing cells that cannot store the transmitter or release it under appropirate neural control, and consequently cannot buffer the swings in circulating levodopa levels (Melamed *et al.*, 1980). Striatal dopamine receptors, therefore, become exposed to oscillations in plasma levodopa levels that attend intermittent oral therapy (Ogasahara *et al.*, 1984; Fabbrini *et al.*, 1987a, 1988). The clinical correlate of this phenomenon is wearing-off type of motor fluctuations, whereby the swings between the 'on' and 'off' states are a direct reflection of the availability of levodopa in plasma and brain (Fabbrini *et al.*, 1988; Mouradian *et al.*, 1989c; Fig. 10.2). Positron emission tomography using fluorinated levodopa has suggested severe limitations in the capacity of the striatum to retain the tracer in parkinsonian patients, particularly those with motor fluctuations (Leenders *et al.*, 1986a). Measures of levodopa efficacy duration correlate best with the degree of disease severity, further strengthening the hypothesis that wearing-off reflects severe loss of nigral neurons due to natural disease progression (Fabbrini *et al.*, 1988). Therefore, this form of motor response instability should and does promptly ameliorate upon stabilization of plasma dopaminomimetic levels (see below).

With continued denervation of the striatum and chronic levodopa therapy, additional changes in central dopamine pharmacodynamics occur (Mouradian and Chase, 1988). The recent observation that the efficacy duration of the direct-acting dopamine agonist, apomorphine, also shortens with the development of fluctuations suggests that secondary postsynaptic changes contribute importantly to the wearing-off phenomenon (Roberts *et al.*, 1992). In addition, the dose–response relationship for acutely administered levodopa becomes gradually more steep, and eventually nearly vertical so that even minute changes in levodopa availability result in dramatic shifts in motor performance (Mouradian *et al.*, 1988; Fig. 10.3). This phenomenon underlies the abrupt on–off switches that appear to have no temporal

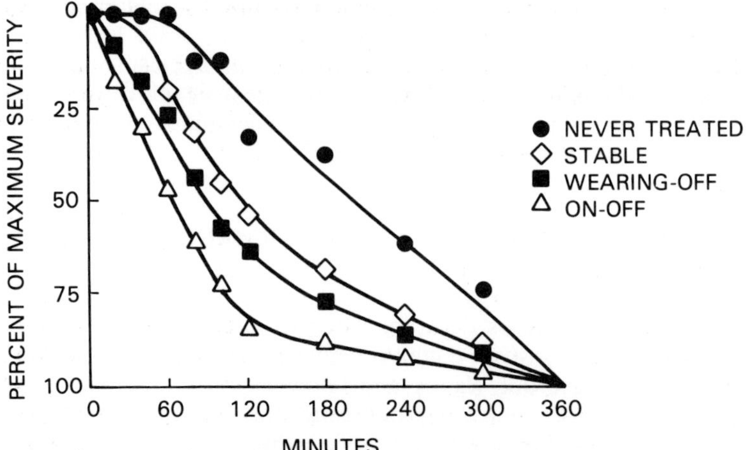

Figure 10.2 Decline of parkinsonian motor scores by percentage of maximum severity following discontinuation of steady-state, optimal-dose intravenous infusion of levodopa. Repeated measures ANOVA: $P < 0.0001$. From Mouradian *et al.* (1989c).

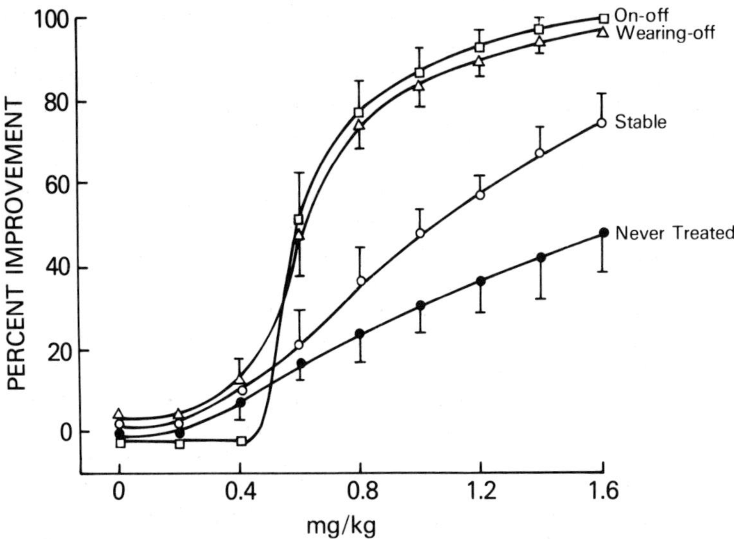

Figure 10.3 Levodopa dose–response relationship by groups defined in the legend to Figure 10.1. Levodopa is administered as intravenous boluses. Response is defined as the percentage improvement at peak action of each dose compared to complete obliteration of parkinsonian signs. From Mouradian *et al.* (1988).

relationship to levodopa intake. Since newly synthesized dopamine is released preferentially (Besson *et al.*, 1969), acute intravenous dose–response studies presumably assess the functional state of postsynaptic dopamine receptor-bearing cells and their downstream neuronal connections (Agid *et al.*, 1989). Heightened sensitivity of the dopamine receptors is a long-recognized sequel of denervation and is likely the case in *de novo* parkinsonian patients (Rinne *et al.*, 1990).

The effects of chronic dopaminomimetic therapy in experimental animals have yielded variable and confusing results with great difficulties in extrapolating findings to Parkinson's disease. These discrepancies are largely due to differences in dosage schedule and duration of drug administration (Jenner *et al.*, 1986). In addition, no good correlations exist between receptor binding studies and behavioural outcome measures, in part due to changes in second messenger systems, and downstream neuronal systems that contribute to the pathophysiology of Parkinson's disease. Recent, well-controlled preclinical studies, however, point to behavioural supersensitivity of the dopaminergic system as a consequence of chronic intermittent, but not continuous, levodopa therapy (Costall *et al.*, 1983; Engber *et al.*, 1989; Juncos *et al.*, 1989; Weick *et al.*, 1990). Currently available evidence suggests that a similar phenomenon occurs in parkinsonian patients chronically treated with standard oral levodopa. Frequent oscillations in plasma drug levels with this form of therapy result in stimulating the postsynaptic receptors only intermittently since the presynaptic cells have largely disappeared and can no longer store sufficient dopamine to buffer swings in levodopa availability. The slope of the levodopa dose–response curve is best correlated with years of its intake, suggesting that levodopa itself plays an important role in alterations in central dopamine pharmacodynamics (Mouradian *et al.*, 1988; Horstink *et al.*, 1990). These changes evolve over a long time, and not acutely within hours (Davis *et al.*, 1991). Long-term studies using bromocriptine alone or in combination with levodopa report a lower incidence of motor fluctuations compared with levodopa alone, perhaps due to the longer half-life of bromocriptine and thus the more steady stimulation of the dopamine receptors, or possibly due to the lower dose requirements of levodopa (Lees and Stern, 1981; Rinne, 1987, 1989) and consequently less accumulation of radicals from oxidative deamination of dopamine (Spina and Cohen, 1989).

In addition to fluctuations in parkinsonian symptoms, abnormal involuntary movements frequently complicate the therapeutic response to levodopa in patients with advanced disease (Nutt, 1990). Marked degeneration of nigral cells seems to be a prerequisite for the development of levodopa-induced dyskinesias, since these movements are essentially limited to parkinsonian patients (Barbeau, 1989; Chase *et al.*, 1973). Moreover, dyskinesias develop only after a prolonged period of levodopa administration in 1-methyl-4-phenyl-1,2,5,6-tetrahydropyridine (MPTP)-treated monkeys. Since these primates have a fixed, non-progressive nigral lesion (Boyce *et al.*, 1990a), both denervation and long-term levodopa therapy appear to be required for the genesis of these movements. Choreiform dyskinesias have generally been considered to represent a continuum of the antiparkinsonian action of levodopa based on a unified underlying pharmacological system. However, dyskinesias can occur simultaneously with parkinsonian symptoms and not all dyskinesias appear at peak drug levels. Such clinical observations have raised suspicion that these two motor effects of levodopa may be mediated through pharmacologically different systems. In fact, with the development of motor response complications, the minimum levodopa dose that can induce dyskinesias decreases markedly, while that for improving parkinsonism does not change significantly, thus narrowing the therapeutic window of levodopa (Mouradian *et al.*, 1988, 1989b; Fig. 10.4). Furthermore, the decline in the dyskinetic response following withdrawal of a steady-state levodopa infusion proceeds more rapidly than that for the antiparkinsonian action (Mouradian *et al.*, 1989b, Fig. 10.5). Additional biochemical and pathological data from other

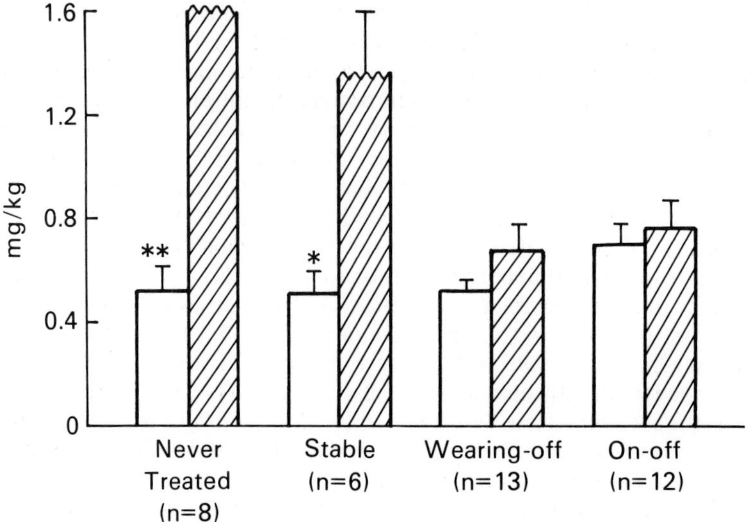

Figure 10.4 Threshold doses for the antiparkinsonian effect (open blocks) and the dyskinetic action (hatched blocks) of levodopa given as intravenous boluses. $*P<0.006$; $**P<0.0001$ for difference from dyskinesia threshold. From Mouradian *et al.* (1989b).

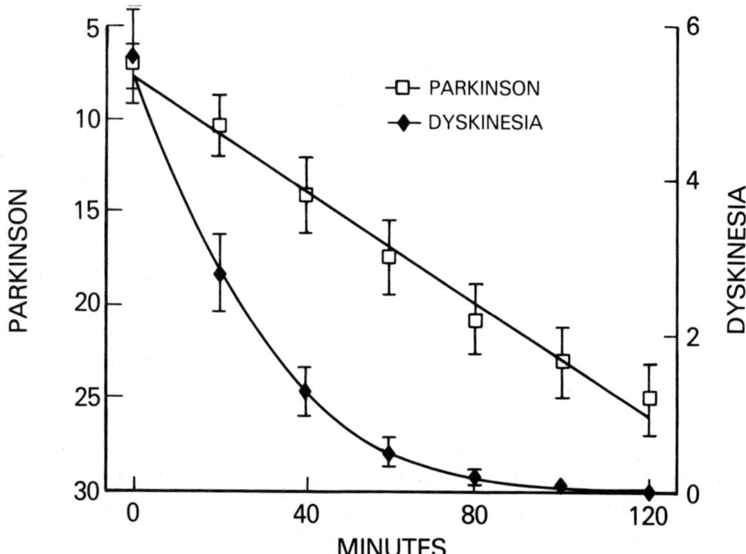

Figure 10.5 Decay of the antiparkinsonian and dyskinetic effects of levodopa after discontinuation of a steady-state, optimal-dose levodopa infusion. From Mouradian *et al.* (1989b).

choreiform movement disorders support the view that levodopa-induced dyskinesias may represent the preferential inhibition of a subpopulation of putaminal neurons that are mostly enkephalinergic and project to the lateral globus pallidus (Crossman, 1990). The recent observation of decreased proencephalin product but not dynorphin in spinal fluid of parkinsonian patients may relate to the genesis of these movements (Baronti *et al.*, 1991). With respect to the important role of other peptide transmitters, cholecystokinin appears to ameliorate levodopa-induced dyskinesias in parkinsonian monkeys (Boyce *et al.*, 1990b). Furthermore, D_1 and D_2 dopamine receptor-bearing neurons appear to project preferentially to different anatomical target sites (Trugman and Wooten, 1987). The differential stimulation of the D_1 versus D_2 subclasses of dopamine receptors may be involved in the generation of these movements; perhaps excessive D_1 tone predisposes to them (Rinne *et al.*, 1985; Groppetti *et al.*, 1986; Boyce *et al.*, 1990c). The lower incidence of dyskinesias in patients chronically treated with relatively selective D_2 agonists, bromociptine, pergolide and lisuride, supports this hypothesis (Lees and Stern, 1981; Rinne, 1987, 1989). Once again, intermittently, but not continuously, administered levodopa is associated with stereotypical behaviours in experimental animals (Costall *et al.*, 1983), and the threshold dose for dyskinesias in parkinsonian patients is best correlated with the duration of standard levodopa intake (Mouradian *et al.*, 1988).

The apparent alterations in the responsiveness of striatal cells to dopaminomimetics that underlie certain motor complications in patients with advanced Parkinson's disease are partially reversible. After several days of continuous round-the-clock infusions of levodopa intravenously, and especially after 3 months of lisuride subcutaneously, an improvement of the therapeutic index of levodopa occurs with heightened antiparkinsonian efficacy without increased dyskinesias (Mouradian *et al.*, 1990; Baronti *et al.*, 1992b). In addition, a state of relative tolerance to levodopa develops, with a slight increase in its requirements, and a shift of its dose–response curve to the right (Cedarbaum *et al.*, 1990; Mouradian *et al.*, 1990; Baronti *et al.*, 1992b; Fig. 10.6). Tolerance to continuous drug delivery compared with intermittent administration is known to occur with other agents as well, including apomorphine and amphetamine in rats (Nelson and Ellison, 1978; Post, 1980; Castro *et al.*, 1985). Some concerns have been raised about the issue of tolerance (Nutt, 1988); however, the efficacy of levodopa does not deteriorate with continuous therapy (Mouradian *et al.*, 1990; Baronti *et al.*, 1992b).

The aforementioned pharmacokinetic and pharmacodynamic data taken together form the rationale for continuous levodopa administration in the treatment as well as in the prophylaxis of motor response complications (Chase *et al.*, 1989). The next critical question is which pharmacological agent is best suited for this form of therapy. This issue is largely related to the efficacy of the drug, the therapeutic window and the physicochemical properties that determine practical aspects of the delivery route. Of all the agents available either for general use or experimentally, levodopa is still the most efficacious (Parkes *et al.*, 1976; LeWitt *et al.*, 1983; De Yebenes *et al.*, 1987; Lang, 1987; Stibe *et al.*, 1988; Mouradian *et al.*, 1991). The most plausible explanation for this observation is that levodopa is converted to dopamine, the normal endogenous transmitter that stimulates its receptors at a physiological ratio, while direct-acting dopamine agonists have a predilection to stimulate one subtype of receptors more than others. D_2 dopamine receptor stimulation appears necessary for the antiparkinsonian efficacy of dopaminomimetics; most clinically effective agents are predominantly D_2 agonists, including bromocriptine, pergolide, lisuride and PHNO

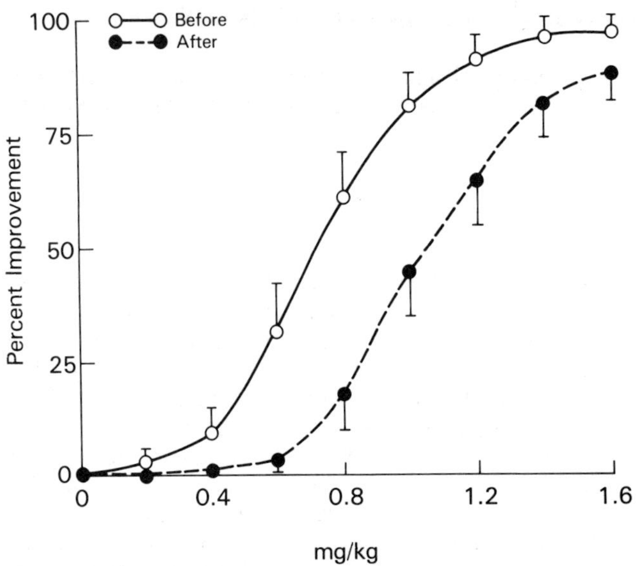

Figure 10.6 Levodopa dose–response profile before and after a mean of 10 days of continuous, round-the-clock levodopa infusions at optimal dose levels. $n = 12$. From Mouradian *et al.* (1990).

(Stoessl *et al.*, 1985). Studies with selective D_1 agonists have yielded mixed results. SKF 38393 is ineffective in parkinsonian patients (Braun *et al.*, 1987), perhaps because it is only a partial D_1 agonist, while CY 208-243 has both antiparkinsonian and dyskinetic effects (Temlett *et al.*, 1989). The question of therapeutic window relates to the potential of a particular drug to induce abnormal involuntary movements. For example, long-term bromocriptine, pergolide and lisuride therapy results in less dyskinesias than levodopa, while (−)-N-n-propyl-norapomorphine, a relatively selective D_2 agonist with partial D_1 agonism, can generate the same degree of dyskinesias as levodopa but has an inferior antiparkinsonian efficacy (Mouradian *et al.*, 1991). Thus, the issue of stimulating D_1 and/or D_2 subclasses of dopamine receptors is complex. On one hand, stimulating both receptor types seems necessary for full antiparkinsonian efficacy, and on the other hand, excessive D_1 stimulation may potentiate abnormal involuntary movements. Additional work using pharmacological agents with selective profiles based on molecularly defined receptor subtypes (Bunzow *et al.*, 1988; Minowa *et al.*, 1992a,b) and their use in combination should ultimately facilitate understanding the role of each in the different clinical manifestations of advanced Parkinson's disease.

The foregoing data also provide insight into the long-debated issue about whether to initiate levodopa therapy early or late, for fear of the drug causing some harm (De Jong *et al.*, 1987; Diamond *et al.*, 1987; Duvoisin, 1987). Both natural disease progression and chronic pulsatile levodopa therapy provided by standard oral levodopa play important and synergistic roles in the development of motor response complications. Efforts are currently underway to test potential neuroprotective agents (The Parkinson Study Group, 1989), and considerably more progress has been made towards long-term continuous dopaminomimetic therapy.

CONTINUOUS DOPAMINOMIMETIC THERAPY

A number of pharmacological agents and various routes of administration (Stahl, 1988) have been tried for the treatment of motor response complications.

Levodopa

In addition to standard oral levodopa/dopa decarboxylase inhibitor formulations that have been in wide clinical use for the past two decades, levodopa has been successfully used in different formulations and routes in an attempt to achieve stable plasma levels. The most effective and direct means to this goal is continuous intravenous infusion, the gold standard against which other formulations are tested for their adequacy in stabilizing circulating drug levels.

Levodopa infused intravenously results in an immediate and total amelioration of wearing-off phenomenon (Shoulson *et al.*, 1975; Hardie *et al.*, 1984; Nutt *et al.*, 1984; Quinn *et al.*, 1984; Juncos *et al.*, 1987, 1990; Mouradian *et al.*, 1987a, 1990), while complex on–off fluctuations require several days of continuous infusions before beginning their gradual decline (Mouradian *et al.*, 1987a, 1990). Furthermore, even after discontinuation of levodopa infusions and resumption of standard oral therapy, motor fluctuations continue at an improved level for several days before returning to preinfusion severity (Mouradian *et al.*, 1990; Fig. 10.7). Despite the attractive pharmacological features of levodopa, its intravenous administration is not practical for long-term use, mainly due to its poor solubility and the low pH of solutions

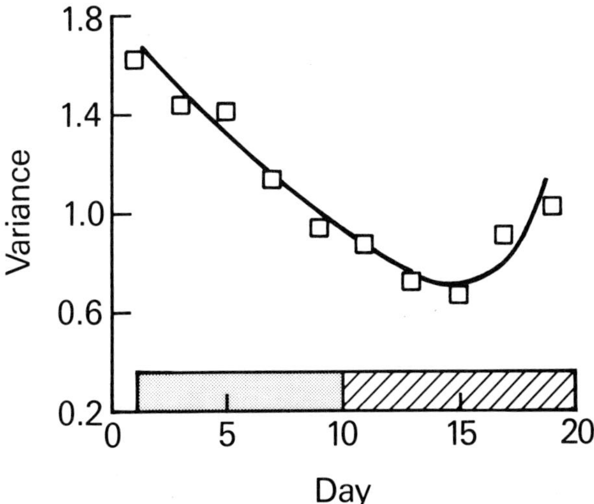

Figure 10.7 Gradual improvement of motor fluctuations during continuous, round-the-clock levodopa infusions at optimal dose levels. The solid bar refers to intravenous infusion; the hatched bar refers to standard oral levodopa therapy. From Mouradian *et al.* (1990).

resulting in frequent superficial phlebitis at the infusion site; the average volume of infusate of levodopa per 24 hours is 1 litre. A more soluble alternative tested in Parkinson's disease is levodopa methylester with an infusate volume of only about 50 ml per 24 hours. The intravenous administration of this analogue, which has a lower bioavailability than the parent drug, is also plagued by superficial phebitis (Juncos *et al.*, 1987). Another route of continuous levodopa delivery tried with some success in parkinsonian patients is the duodenal route (Kurlan *et al.*, 1988; Sage *et al.*, 1988; Cedarbaum *et al.*, 1990). A more practical approach is the oral controlled-release levodopa/carbidopa formulations, such as Sinemet-CR and Madopar HBS. These preparations stabilize plasma levodopa levels only modestly, much less than intravenous infusion, and are generally more effective in patients with simple wearing-off fluctuations (Nutt *et al.*, 1986; Poewe *et al.*, 1987; Goetz *et al.*, 1988; Cedarbaum, 1989; Lewitt *et al.*, 1989). Early-morning dystonias tend to respond favourably to these formulations. Due to the prolonged release, each dose requires a longer time to be effective, is more susceptible to changes in gastric emptying, and periods of under- or over-medication tend to last longer than with standard levodopa. Although Sinemet-CR is far inferior to intravenous infusion, the convenience of taking a tablet every 3 or 4 hours is clear.

More recent promising efforts that are still at the preclinical stage are long-term delivery of dopaminomimetics via implantable polymer matrices that have been used to deliver dopamine directly into brains of experimental animals with long-lasting behavioural effects (McRae-Degueurce *et al.*, 1988; During *et al.*, 1989; Winn *et al.*, 1989). This technology can be utilized in more practical and less invasive means by implanting different agents in polymer matrices for systemic delivery, such as the skin.

Lisuride

This relatively selective D_2 dopamine agonist is highly water-soluble, and thus practical for delivery via portable infusion pumps. It has been administered orally, intravenously and subcutaneously to parkinsonian patients with encouraging results. Its antiparkinsonian efficacy is equivalent to that of bromocriptine and pergolide (LeWitt *et al.*, 1982), and its chronic oral use is reportedly associated with a lower incidence of motor complications than levodopa (Rinne, 1989). When infused continuously, lisuride diminishes motor fluctuations occurring with oral levodopa (Obeso *et al.*, 1986, 1988; Critchley *et al.*, 1988; Ruggieri *et al.*, 1988; ; Baronti *et al.*, 1992b). However, not all patients respond favorably to lisuride, and most require the co-administration of some levodopa for an adequate antiparkinsonian response, once again pointing to the superior antiparkinsonian efficacy of levodopa (Ruggieri *et al.*, 1988). In addition to the usual dopaminomimetic side-effects that are generally well-controlled with domperidone, the main adverse effects of lisuride have been psychiatric, which reportedly occur in as many as one-third of patients and are more common in those with a previous history of psychosis (Critchley *et al.*, 1988; Obeso *et al.*, 1988). Interruption or decreased infusion rate during the sleeping hours may diminish the incidence of this untoward effect. The development of subcutaneous nodules at the infusion site is another common problem; frequent changes of the needle and skin site is recommended. Other infrequent side-effects include cardiopressor effects with diminished postural reflexes upon standing and atrial arrhythmias (Capria *et al.*, 1989).

Apomorphine

Apomorphine is a relatively non-selective dopamine agonist acting at both the D_1 and D_2 subfamilies receptors that was used for the treatment of parkinsonian patients of decades ago (Schwab *et al.*, 1951; Cotzias *et al.*, 1970), but quickly abandoned mainly due to the azotaemia associated with its oral administration. More recently, it has been more successfully used when given parenterally in combination with the peripheral dopamine antagonist domperidone, which blocks its peripheral side-effects and allows the administration of centrally effective doses. Currently, apomorphine is used primarily because of its ability to be administered parenterally, especially by means of continuous infusion pumps. Following subcutaneous injection, its antiparkinsonian effects occur within 5–15 minutes and last around 40–90 minutes (Stibe *et al.*, 1988). It has a plasma elimination half-life of 33 minutes (Gancher *et al.*, 1989). It can used for repeated subcutaneous injections using a Penject system, or sublingually, to rapidly alleviate 'off' periods and associated dystonia (Stibe *et al.*, 1988; Poewe *et al.*, 1988; Lees *et al.*, 1989b; Frankel *et al.*, 1990), and by continuous infusions to minimize motor fluctuations (Obeso *et al.*, 1987; Stibe *et al.*, 1988; Frankel *et al.*, 1990). Apomorphine appears to be more effective than lisuride, perhaps due to its non-selective agonism at both classes of dopamine receptors. Nevertheless, levodopa may still be required in some patients for full antiparkinsonian response (Obeso *et al.*, 1987; Poewe *et al.*, 1988; Stibe *et al.*, 1988; Frankel *et al.*, 1990). As with levodopa and lisuride, patients with simple wearing-off fluctuations tend to respond more readily to apomorphine infusion than those with complex on–off fluctuations (Obeso *et al.*, 1987). Unlike lisuride, hallucinations are generally not as much a problem with apomorphine, but subcutaneous nodules are also encountered at the infusion site (Stibe *et al.*, 1988; Poewe *et al.*, 1989; Frankel *et al.*, 1990). Gastrointestinal side-effects are effectively suppressed by co-administration of domperidone; tolerance to these adverse effects eventually develops in most patients and domperidone can be discontinued (Frankel *et al.*, 1990). With continuous apomorphine therapy, no tolerance to the antiparkinsonian efficacy appears to develop, contrary to earlier reports with its oral use (Cotzias *et al.*, 1976; Frankel *et al.*, 1990). More recently, there has been increasing interest to use subcutaneous injections of apomorphine for aiding the diagnosis of Parkinson's disease, and differentiating it from Parkinson-plus syndromes that do not show an appreciable response to apomorphine (Barker *et al.*, 1989; Oertel *et al.*, 1989). Despite the attractive features of apomorphine compared to levodopa and lisuride, long-term use of infusion pumps is still a cumbersome task, especially for a patient population with impaired motor skills. In addition, although frequent subcutaneous injections of apomorphine using Penject can be quite effective in reversing 'off' periods rapidly, the pulsatile nature of this therapy is disconcerting for its potential long-term changes in dopamine receptor sensitivity. Thus, efforts are ongoing to deliver dopaminomimetics continuously in more convenient ways.

Lipid-soluble dopaminergic agents

The transcutaneous route using a skin patch is a convenient means of administering therapeutic agents continuously. From this perspective, there has been increasing interest in the development of highly lipid-soluble agents. Two such drugs have been tested thus far in parkinsonian patients: PHNO and N-0437 (Hazelhoff *et al.*, 1986;

Van der Weide *et al.*, 1988). PHNO is a potent, highly selective D_2 dopamine receptor agonist which showed promising antiparkinsonian efficacy in patients when given orally, intravenously or transdermally (Stoessl *et al.*, 1985; Grandas Perez *et al.*, 1986; Lieberman *et al.*, 1988; Coleman *et al.*, 1990a). Despite the promising pharmacological features of PHNO, its clinical use was discontinued due to toxicity in experimental animals. N-0437 is less selective at the D_2 site compared to PHNO, and is a racemic mixture, with the negative enantiomer, N-0923, having postsynaptic agonist activity, and the positive enantiomer having mild antagonist properties. Because of this, plus the fact that it has very poor oral bioavailability due to first-pass effects, its antiparkinsonian efficacy has been modest in parkinsonian patients (Mouradian *et al.*, 1989a). Efforts are currently underway to administer the active isomer, N-0923, parenterally.

Long half-life dopamine agonists

The use of direct-acting dopamine agonists with very long plasma half-lives allowing the administration of tablets once or twice per day and assuring steady and effective plasma levels is another convenient route of providing continuous dopaminomimetics. Cabergoline is a dopamine agonist with a half-life of about 96 hours (Ferrari *et al.*, 1986; Jori *et al.*, 1990). It is currently being studied in clinical trials.

AGENTS AFFECTING DOPAMINE METABOLISM

Blocking the catabolism of dopamine to enhance its availability at postsynaptic receptor sites was proposed as an adjunct to levodopa soon after the limitations of the dopamine precursor was realized (Birkmayer *et al.*, 1975). Selegiline (deprenyl) is a selective monoamine oxidase B inhibitor, and thus free of the tyramine-induced hypertensive effect. Several studies have confirmed the mild antiparkinsonian efficacy of selegiline (deprenyl) both as monotherapy in previously untreated parkinsonian patients and as an adjunct to levodopa (Lees *et al.*, 1977, 1989a; Schachter *et al.*, 1980; Golbe, 1988; Myllyla *et al.*, 1989; Yahr *et al.*, 1989). It has a modest beneficial effect on motor fluctuations of the wearing-off type and lowers levodopa requirements by about 20%. In addition to monoamine oxidase B inhibition, deprenyl has other potential mechanisms of action; one of its metabolites is amphetamine which is known to modulate dopamine transmission (Heinonen *et al.*, 1989), as well as other central biochemical effects (Knoll, 1989). The potential neuroprotective effects of deprenyl are currently under investigation (The Parkinson Study Group, 1989).

Catechol-*O*-methyltransferase (COMT) is another enzyme that catabolizes dopamine both centrally and peripherally to 3-*O*-methyldopa. Clinical studies with COMT inhibitors, which may potentially prolong the half-life of levodopa, have been largely disappointing in the past (Ericsson, 1971; Reches and Fahn, 1984), likely due to lack of selectivity (Mannisto and Kaakkola, 1989). Recent preliminary studies using nitecapone report improved bioavailability of levodopa, decreased plasma 3-*O*-methyldopa and improved clinical performance (Teravainen *et al.*, 1990). Clinical studies with Ro 40-7592, the potent inhibitor acting both peripherally and centrally (Maj *et al.*, 1990; Mannisto *et al.*, 1992) revealed effective prolongation of the antiparkinsonian action of levodopa without raising peak plasma drug levels or worsening dyskinesias (Roberts *et al.*, 1993).

PARTIAL DOPAMINE AGONISTS

The altered dopamine receptor sensitivity in advanced Parkinson's disease as well as the accumulating evidence that abnormal involuntary movements may be mediated through a different pharmacological mechanism than the antiparkinsonian efficacy of dopaminomimetics provide some hope that stimulating certain dopamine receptors preferentially might ameliorate the dyskinesias without compromising the antiparkinsonian effects. Partial dopamine agonists are a class of compounds that act as antagonists at normosensitive receptors and as agonists at denervated, or supersensitive, ones (Clark *et al.*, 1985; Koller and Herbster, 1987). Furthermore, different biochemical and behavioural responses can be elicited with these agents at different dosage levels, and in the presence or absence of a strong agonist. Preliminary studies with one such partial agonist, ciladopa, suggested improved antiparkinsonian efficacy without more dyskinesias (Lieberman *et al.*, 1987); the human use of this agent has been terminated since because of carcinogenicity in experimental animals. Another partial dopamine agonist is the semisynthetic derivative of lisuride, 9,10-dihydrolisuride (terguride; Wachtel and Dorow, 1983). Studies using relatively small doses of terguride, either alone or in combination of levodopa, have reported net agonist effects, with improved parkinsonism and increased dyskinesias (Corsini *et al.*, 1985; Brucke *et al.*, 1986; Critchley and Parkes, 1987). However, a dose-ranging study in combination with levodopa has shown a mild antagonist effect at higher doses, manifested as decreased severity of abnormal involuntary movements without complete obliteration of the antiparkinsonian effects of levodopa (Baronti *et al.*, 1992a). Thus, this class of agents holds some promise in minimizing dyskinetic movements that contribute substantially to patient disability.

CONCLUSIONS

The motor response complications of chronic levodopa therapy are presumably a consequence of the progressive loss of nigrostriatal dopamine neurons plus the effects of long-term, non-physiological, intermittent levodopa therapy. These motor fluctuations can be treated by means of providing steady dopaminomimetic concentrations to the brain, and current evidence suggests that their incidence and/or severity might even be minimized by introducing such forms of treatment from the outset of pharmacotherapy. Nevertheless, the failure of appropriate dopaminomimetic therapies to provide total relief of parkinsonian signs without adverse effects suggests an important role for other neurotransmitter systems, especially striatal peptidergic systems receiving nigrostriatal inputs. Certain of these systems appear affected by the degenerative process as well as by long-term dopaminergic therapy. The role of these systems in the generation of motor response complications will receive increasingly critical attention in the coming years in terms of exploiting them for therapeutic purposes.

References

Agid Y, Cervera P, Hirsch E, Javoy-Agid F, Lehericy S, Raisman R *et al.* (1989) Biochemistry of Parkinson's disease 28 years later: a critical review. *Movement Disorders*, **4** (suppl 1), 126–44

Anderson I, Granerus AK, Jagenburg R, and Svanborg A (1975) Intestinal decarboxylation of orally administered L-dopa. *Acta Med Scand*, **198**, 415–20

Barbeau A (1969) L-dopa therapy in Parkinson's disease: a critical review of nine years' experience. *Can Med Assoc J*, **101**, 791–800

Barbeau A (1974) The clinical physiology of side effects in long-term L-dopa therapy. In McDowell FH and Barbeau A, eds, *Second Canadian–American Conference on Parkinson's Disease. Advances in Neurology*, vol 5, New York, Raven, 347–65

Barker R, Duncan J, and Lees A (1989) Subcutaneous apomorphine as a diagnostic test for dopaminergic responsiveness in parkinsonian syndromes. *Lancet*, **1**, 675

Baronti F, Conant KE, Giuffra M, Davis TL, Brughitta G, Iadarola MI *et al.* (1991) Opioid peptides in Parkinson's disease: effects of dopamine repletion. *Brain Research*, **560**, 92–6

Baronti F, Mouradian MM, Davis TL, Giuffra M, Brughitta G, Conant KE, and Chase TN (1992b) Continuous lisuride effects on central dopaminergic mechanisms in Parkinson's disease. *Ann Neurol* **32**, 776–81

Baronti F, Mouradian MM, Conant KE, Giuffra M, Brughitt G, and Chase TN (1992a) Partial dopamine agonist therapy of levodopa-induced dyskinesias. *Neurology*, **42**, 1241–3

Bartholini G, Kuruma I, and Pletscher A (1970) Distribution and metabolism of L-3-O-methyldopa in rats. *Br J Pharmacol*, **40**, 461–7

Besson MJ, Cheramy A, Feltz P, and Glowinski J (1969) Release of newly synthesized dopamine from dopamine-containing terminals in the striatum of the rat. *Proc Natl Acad Sci*, **62**, 741–8

Birkmayer W, Riederer P, Youdim MBH, and Linauer W (1975) Potentiation of anti-akinetic effect after L-dopa treatment by an inhibitor of MAO-B, L-deprenyl. *J Neural Transm*, **36**, 303–23

Boyce S, Clarke CE, Luquin R, Peggs D, Roberston RG, Mitchell IJ *et al.* (1990a) Inductihon of chorea and dystonia in parkinsonian primates. *Movement Disorders*, **5**, 3–7

Boyce S, Rupniak NMJ, Steventon MJ, and Iversen SD (1990b) CCK-8S inhibits L-dopa-induced dyskinesias in parkinsonian squirrel monkeys. *Neurology*, **40**, 717–18

Boyce S, Rupniak NMJ, Steventon MJ, and Iversen SD (1990c) Differential effects of D_1 and D_2 agonists in MPTP-induced primates: functional implications for Parkinson's disease. *Neurology*, **40**, 927–33

Braun A, Fabbrini G, Mouradian MM, Serrati C, Barone P, and Chase TN (1987) Selective D-1 dopamine receptor agonist treatment of Parkinson's disease. *J Neural Transm*, **68**, 41–50

Brucke T, Danielczyk W, Simanyi M, Sofic E, and Riederer P (1986) Terguride: partial dopamine agonist in the treatment of Parkinson's disease. In Yahr MD and Bergmann KJ, eds, *Parkinson's Disease. Advances in Neurology*, **45**, New York, Raven, 573–6

Bunney BS, Walters JR, Roth RH, and Aghajanian K (1973) Dopaminergic neurons: effect of antipsychotic drugs and amphetamine on single cell activity. *J Pharmacol Exp Ther*, **185**, 560–71

Bunzow JR, Van Tol HHM, Grandy DK, Alber P, Salon J, Christie M *et al.* (1988) Cloning and expression of a rat D2 dopamine receptor cDNA. *Nature*, **336**, 783–7

Capria A, Attanasio A, Quatrana M, Cannata D, Fioravanti M, Stocchi F *et al.* (1989) Cardiovascular effects of lisuride continuous intravenous infustion in fluctuating Parkinson's disease. *Clin Neuropharmacol*, **12**, 331–8

Carlsson A, Lindqvist M, and Magnusson T (1957) 3,4-Dihydroxy-phenylaline and 5-hydroxytryptophan as reserpine antagonists. *Nature*, **180**, 1200

Castro R, Abreu P, Calzadilla CH, and Roderiguez M (1985) Increased or decreased locomotor response in rats following repeated administration of apomorphine depends on dosage interval. *Psychopharmacology*, **85**, 333–9

Cedarbaum JM (1989) The promise and limitations of controlled-release oral levodopa administration. *Clin Neuropharmacol*, **12**, 147–66

Cedarbaum JM, Silversti M, and Kutt H (1990) Sustained enteral administration of levodopa increases and interrupted infusion decreases levodopa dose requirements. *Neurology*, **40**, 995–7

Chase TN, Holden EM, and Brody JA (1973) Levodopa-induced dyskinesias. Comparison in parkinsonism-dementia and amyotrophic lateral sclerosis. *Arch Neurol*, **29**, 328–30

Chase TN, Baronti F, Fabbrini G, Hueser IJE, Juncos JL, and Mouradian MM (1989) Rationale for continuous dopaminomimetic therapy of Parkinson's disease. *Neurology*, **39** (suppl 2), 7–10

Clark D, Hjorth S, and Carlsson A (1985) Dopamine-receptor agonists: mechanisms underlying autoreceptor selectivity. I. Review of the evidence. *J Neural Transm*, **62**, 1–52

Coleman RJ, Lange KW, Quinn NP, Loper AE, Bondi JV, Hichens M *et al.* (1990a) The antiparkinsonian actions and pharmacokinetics of transdermanal (+)-4-propyl-9-hydroxynaphthoxazine (PHNO): preliminary results. *Movement Disorders*, **4**, 129–38

Coleman RJ, Quinn NP, Traub M, and Marsden CD (1990b) Nasogastric and intravenous infusions of (+)-4-propyl-9-hydroxynaphthoxazine (PHNO) in Parkinson's disease. *J Neurol Neurosurg Psychiatry*, **53**, 102–5

Corsini GU, Bonuccelli U, Rainer E, and Del Zompo M (1985) Therapeutic efficacy of a partial dopamine agonist in drug-free parkinsonian patients. *J Neural Transm*, **64**, 105–11

Costall B, Domeney AM, and Naylor RJ (1983) A comparison of the behavioral consequences of chronic stimulation of dopamine receptors in the nucleus accumbens of rat brain effected by a continuous infusion or by single daily injections. *Naunyn-Schmiedeberg's Arch Pharmacol*, **324**, 27–33

Cotzias GC, Van Woert HH, and Schiffer LM (1967) Aromatic amino acids and modification of parkinsonism. *N Engl J Med*, **276**, 374–9

Cotzias GC, Papavasiliou PS, Fehling C, Kaufman B, and Mena I (1970) Similarities between neurologic effects of L-dopa and of aporphines. *N Engl J Med*, **282**, 31–3

Cotzias GC, Papavasiliou PS, Tolosa ES, Mendez JS, and Bell-Midura M (1976) Treatment of Parkinson's disease with apomorphines: possible role of growth hormone. *N Engl J Med*, **294**, 567–72

Critchley P and Parkes D (1987) Transdihydrolisuride in parkinsonism. *Clin Neuropharmacol*, **10**, 57–64

Critchley PHS, Grandas Perez F, Quinn NP, Parkes JD, and Marsden CD (1988) Continuous subcutaneous lisuride infusions in Parkinson's disease. *J Neural Transm*, **27** (suppl), 55–60

Crossman AR (1990) A hypothesis on the pathophysiological mechanisms that underlie levodopa- or dopamine agonist-induced dyskinesia in Parkinson's disease: implications for future strategies in treatment. *Movement Disorders*, **5**, 100–8

Davis TL, Brughitta G, Baronti F, and Mouradian MM (1991) Acute effects of pulsatile levodopa administration on central dopamine pharmacodynamics, *Neurology*, **41**, 630–3

De Jong GJ, Meerwaldt JD, and Schmitz PIM (1987) Factors that influence the occurrence of response variations in Parkinson's disease. *Ann Neurol*, **22**, 47

de Yebenes JG, Fahn S, Lovelle S, Jackson-Lewis V, Jorge P, Mena MA *et al.* (1987) Continuous intracerebroventricular infusion of dopamine agonists through a totally implanted drug delivery system in animal models of Parkinson's disease. *Movement Disorders*, **2**, 143–58

Diamond SG, Markham CH, Hoehn MM, McDowell FH, and Muenter MD (1987) Multi-center study of Parkinson mortality with early versus later dopa treatment. *Ann Neurol*, **22**, 8–12

During MJ, Freese A, Sabel BA, Saltzman WM, Deutch A, Roth RH *et al.* (1989) Controlled release of dopamine from a polymeric brain implant: *in vivo* characterization. *Ann Neurol*, **25**, 351–6

Duvoisin RC (1987) To treat early or to treat late. *Ann Neurol*, **22**, 2–3

Engber TM, Susel Z, Jorge JL, and Chase TN (1989) Continuous and intermittent levodopa differentially affect rotation induced by D-1 and D-2 dopamine agonists. *Eur J Pharmacol*, **168**, 291–8

Ericsson AD (1971) Potentiation of the L-dopa effect in man by the use of catechol-*O*-methyltransferase inhibitors. *J Neurol Sci*, **14**, 193–7

Eriksson T, Magnusson T, Carlsson A, Linde A, and Granerus AK (1984) 'On-off' phenomenon in Parkinson's disease: correlation to the concentration of L-dopa in plasma. *J Neural Transm*, **59**, 229–40

Evans MA, Triggs EJ, Broe GA, and Saines N (1980) Systemic availability of orally administered L-dopa in the elderly parkinsonian patient. *Eur J Clin Pharmacol*, **17**, 215–21

Fabbrini G, Juncos J, Mouradian MM, Serrati C, and Chase TN (1987a) Levodopa pharmacokinetic mechanisms and motor fluctuations in Parkinson's disease. *Ann Neurol*, **21**, 370–6

Fabbrini G, Juncos JL, Mouradian MM, Serrati C, and Chase TN (1987b) 3-O-Methyldopa and motor fluctuations in Parkinson's disease. *Neurology*, **37**, 856–9

Fabbrini G, Mouradian MM, Juncos JL, Schlegel J, Mohr E, and Chase TN (1988) Motor fluctuations in Parkinson's disease: central pathophysiological mechanisms, Part I. *Ann Neurol*, **24**, 366–71

Fahn S (1974) 'On-off' phenomenon with levodopa therapy in parkinsonism. Clinical and pharmacological correlations and the effect of intramuscular pyridoxine. *Neurology*, **24**, 431–41

Ferrari C, Barbieri C, Caldara R, Mucci M, Codecasa F, Paracchi A. *et al.* (1986) Long-lasting prolactin-lowering effect of cabergoline, a new dopamine agonist, in hyperprolactinemia patients. *J Clin Endocrinol Metab*, **63**, 941–5

Frankel JP, Lees AJ, Kempster PA, and Stern GM (1990) Subcutaneous apomorphine in the treatment of Parkinson's disease. *J Neurol Neurosurg Psychiatry*, **53**, 96–101

Gancher ST, Nutt JG, and Woodward WR (1987) Peripheral pharmacokinetics of levodopa in untreated, stable and fluctuating parkinsonian patients. *Neurology*, **37**, 940–4

Gancher ST, Woodward WR, Boucher B, and Nutt JG (1989) Peripheral pharmacokinetics of apomorphine in humans. *Ann Neurol*, **26**, 232–8

Goetz CG, Tanner CM, Shannon KM, Carroll VS, Klawans HL, Carvey PM *et al.* (1988) Long-acting levodopa/carbidopa combination in Parkinson's disease patients with and without motor fluctuations. *Neurology*, **38**, 1143–5

Golbe LI (1988) Deprenyl as symptomatic therapy in Parkinson's disease. *Clin Neuropharmacol*, **11**, 387–400

Grandas Perez FJ, Jenner PG, Nomoto M, Stahl S, Quinn NP, Parkes JD *et al.* (1986) (+)-4-propyl-9-hydroxynaphthoxazine in Parkinson's disease. *Lancet*, **1**, 906

Groppetti A, Flauto C, Parati E, Vescovi A, Rusconi L, and Parenti M (1986) Dopamine receptor changes in response to treatment with L-dopa. *J Neural Transm*, **22** (suppl), 33–45

Hardie RJ, Lees AJ, and Stern, GM (1984) On-off fluctuations in Parkinson's disease: a clinical and neuropharmacological study. *Brain*, **107**, 487–506

Hardie RJ, Malcolm SL, Lees AJ, Stern GM, and Allen JG (1986) The pharmacokinetics of intravenous and oral levodopa in patients with Parkinson's disease who exhibit on-off fluctuations. *Br J Clin Pharmacol*, **22**, 429–36

Hazelhoff B, De Vries JB, Dijkstra D, Mulder TBA, Timmermans PBMWM, Wynberg H *et al.* (1986) Neuropharmacological profile of a new series of dopamine agonists: N-n-propyl-hexahydro-naphthoxazines. *Eur J Pharmacol*, **124**, 93–106

Heinonen EH, Myllyla V, Sotaniemi K, Lammintausta R, Salonen JS, Anttila M *et al.* (1989) Pharmacokinetics and metabolism of selegiline. *Acta Neurol Scand*, **126**, 93–9

Hornykiewicz O (1963) Die Topische Lokalisation und das Verhalten von Noradrenalin und Dopamin in der substantia nigra des normalen und Parkinsonkranken Menschen. *Wien Klin Wochenschr*, **75**, 309–12

Hornykiewicz O (1979) Compensatory biochemical changes at the striatal dopamine synapse in Parkinson's disease – limitations of L-dopa therapy. In Poirer LJ, Sourkes TL, and Bedard PJ, eds, *The Extrapyramidal System and its Disorders. Advances in Neurology*, vol 24, New York, Raven, 275–81

Horstink MWIM, Zijlmans JCM, Pasman JW, Berger HJC, Korten JJ, and Van't Hof MA (1990) Which risk factors predict the levodopa response in fluctuating Parkinson's disease? *Ann Neurol*, **27**, 537–43

Javoy F and Glowinski J (1971) Dynamic characteristics of the 'functional compartment' of dopamine in dopaminergic terminals of the rat striatum. *J Neurochem*, **18**, 1305–11

Jenner P, Bojce S, and Marsden CD (1986) Effect of repeated L-dopa administration on striatal dopamine receptor function in the rat. In Fahn S, Marsden CD, Jenner P, and Teychenne P, eds, *Recent Developments in Parkinson's Disease*, New York, Raven Press, 189–203

Jori MC, Franceschi M, Giusti MC, Canal N, Piolti R, Frattola L *et al.* (1990) Clinical experience with cabergoline, a new ergoline derivative, in the treatment of Parkinson's disease. *Adv Neurol*, **53**, 539–43

Juncos JL, Mouradian MM, Fabbrini G, Serrati C, and Chase TN (1987) Levodopa methylester treatment of Parkinson's disease. *Neurology*, **37**, 1242–4

Juncos JL, Engber TM, Raisman R, Susel Z, Thibaut F, Ploska A *et al.* (1989) Continuous and intermittent levodopa differentially affect basal ganglia function. *Ann Neurol*, **25**, 473–8

Juncos JL, Mouradian MM, Fabbrini G, and Chase TN (1990) Levodopa infusion therapy. In Koller WC and Paulson G, eds, *Therapy of Parkinson's Disease*, New York, Marcel Dekker, 185–203

Knoll J (1989) The pharmacology of selegiline ((–)deprenyl). New aspects. *Acta Neurol Scand*, **126**, 83–91

Koller WC and Herbster G (1987) Terguride, a mixed dopamine agonist–antagonist, in animal models of Parkinson's disease. *Neurology*, **37**, 723–7

Kurlan R, Nutt JG, Woodward WR, Rothfield K, Lichter D, Miller C *et al.* (1988) Duodenal and gastric delivery of levodopa in parkinsonism. *Ann Neurol*, **23**, 589–95

Lang AE (1987) Update on dopamine agonists in Parkinson's disease: 'beyond bromocriptine'. *Can J Neruol Sci*, **14**, 474–82

Leenders KL, Palmer AJ, Quinn N, Clark JC, Firnau G, Garnett ES *et al.* (1986a) Brain dopamine metabolism in patients with Parkinson's disease measured with positron emission tomography. *J Neurol, Neursurg Psychiatry*, **49**, 853–60

Leenders KL, Poewe WH, Palmer AJ, Brenton DP, and Frackowiak RSJ (1986b) Inhibition of L-[^{18}F]fluorodopa uptake into human brain by amino acids demonstrated by positron emission tomography. *Ann Neurol*, **20**, 258–62

Lees AJ and Stern GM (1981) Sustained bromocriptine therapy in previously untreated patients with Parkinson's disease. *J Neurol Neurosurg Psychiatry*, **44**, 1020–3

Lees AJ, Shaw KM, Kohout LJ, Stern G, Elsworth JD, Sandler M *et al.* (1977) Deprenyl in Parkinson's disease. *Lancet*, **2**, 791–5

Lees AJ, Frankel J, Eatough, V, and Stern G (1989a) New approaches in the use of selegiline for the treatment of Parkinson's disease. *Acta Neurol Scand*, **126**, 139–45

Lees AJ, Montastruc JL, Turjanski N, Rascol O, Kleedorfer B, Peyro Saint-Paul H *et al.* (1989b) Sublingual apomorphine and Parkinson's disease. *J Neurol Neurosurg Psychiatry*, **52**, 1140

LeWitt PA, Gopinathan G, Ward CD, Sanes JN, Dambrosia JM, Durso R *et al.* (1982) Lisuride versus bromocriptine treatment in Parkinson's disease: a double-blind study. *Neurology*, **32**, 69–72

LeWitt PA, Ward CD, Larsen TA, Raphaelson MI, Newman RP, Foster N *et al.* (1983) Comparison of pergolide and bromocriptine therapy in parkinsonism. *Neurology*, **33**, 1009–14

LeWitt PA, Nelson MV, Berchou RC, Galloway MP, Kesaree N, Kareti D, and Schlick P (1989) Controlled-release carbidopa/levodopa (Sinemet 50/200 CR4): clinical and pharmcokinetic studies. *Neurology*, **39** (suppl 2), 45–53

Lieberman A, Gopinathan G, Neophytides A, Pasternack P, and Goldstein M (1987) Advanced Parkinson's disease: use of partial dopamine agonist, ciladopa. *Neurology*, **37**, 863–5

Lieberman A, Chin L, and Baumann G (1988) MK 458, a selective and potent D_2 receptor agonist in advanced Parkinson's disease. *Clin Neuropharmacol*, **11**, 191–200

Luquin MR, Scipioni O, Vaamonde J, Gershanik O, and Obeso JA (1992) Levodopa-induced dyskinesias in Parkinson's disease: clinical and pharmacological classification. *Movement Disorders*, **7**, 117–24

McRae-Degueurce A, Hjorth S, Dillon DL, Mason DW, and Tice, TR (1988) Implantable microencapsulated dopamine (DA): a new approach for slow DA delivery into brain tissue. *Neurosci Lett*, **92**, 303–9

Maj J, Rogoz Z, Skuza G, Sowinska H, and Superata J (1990) Behavioural and neurochemical effects of Ro 40-7592, a new COMT inhibitor with a potential therapeutic activity in Parkinson's disease. *J Neural Transm*, **2**, 101–12

Mannisto PT and Kaakkola S (1989) New selective COMT inhibitors: useful adjuncts of Parkinson's disease. *Trends Pharmacol Sci*, **10**, 54–6

Mannisto PT, Tuomainen P, and Tuominen K (1992) Different *in vivo* properties of three new inhibitors of catechol *O*-methyltransferase in the rat. *Br J Pharmacol*, **105**, 569–74

Marsden CD and Parkes JD (1976) 'On-off' effects in patients with Parkinson's disease on chronic levodopa therapy. *Lancet*, **1**, 292–6

Melamed E, Hefti F, and Wurtman RJ (1980) Nonaminergic striatal neurons convert exogenous L-dopa to dopamine in parkinsonism. *Ann Neurol*, **8**, 558–63

Mena I and Cotzias GC (1975) Protein intake and treatment of Parkinson's disease with levodopa. *N Engl J Med*, **292**, 181–4

Minowa MT, Minowa T, Monsma FJ Jr, Sibley DR and Mouradian MM (1992a) Characterization of the 5′ flanking region of the human D_{1A} dopamine receptor gene. *Proc Natl Acad Sciences USA*, **89**, 3045–9

Minowa T, Minowa MT, and Mouradian MM (1992b) Analysis of the promotor region of the rate D_2 dopamine receptor gene. *Biochemistry*, **31**, 8389–96

Mouradian MM and Chase TN (1988) Central mechanisms and levodopa response fluctuations in Parkinson's disease. *Clin Neuropharmacol*, **11**, 378–85

Mouradian MM, Juncos JL, Fabbrini G, and Chase TN (1987a) Motor fluctuations in Parkinson's disease: pathogenetic and therapeutic studies. *Ann Neurol*, **22**, 475–9

Mouradian MM, Juncos JL, Serrati C, Fabbrini G, Palmeri S, and Chase TN (1987b) Exercise and the antiparkinsonian response to levodopa. *Clin Neuropharmacol*, **10**, 351–5

Mouradian MM, Juncos JL, Fabbrini G, Schlegel J, Bartko JJ, and Chase TN (1988) Motor fluctuations in Parkinson's disease: central pathophysiological mechanisms, part II. *Ann Neurol*, **24**, 372–8

Mouradian MM, Heuser IJE, Baronti F, and Chase TN (1989a) Selective dopamine agonist therapy of Parkinson's disease. *Neurology*, **39** (suppl 1), 228

Mouradian MM, Heuser IJE, Baronti F, Fabbrini G, Juncos JL, and Chase TN (1989b) Pathogenesis of dyskinesias in Parkinson's disease. *Ann Neurol*, **25**, 523–6

Mouradian MM, Juncos JL, Fabbrini G, and Chase TN (1989c) Motor fluctuations in Parkinson's disease. *Ann Neurol*, **25**, 633–4

Mouradian MM, Heuser IJE, Baronti F, and Chase TN (1990) Modification of central dopaminergic mechanisms with continuous levodopa infusion therapy for advanced Parkinson's disease. *Ann Neurol*, **27**, 18–23

Mouradian MM, Heuser IJE, Baronti F, Giuffra M, Conant K, Davis TL, and Chase TN (1991) Comparison of the clinical pharmacology of (−)NPA and levodopa in Parkinson's disease. *J Neurol Neurosurg Psychiatry*, **54**, 401–5

Muenter MD, Sharpless NS, and Tyce GM (1972) Plasma 3-*O*-methyldopa in L-dopa therapy of Parkinson's disease. *Mayo Clin Proc*, **47**, 389–95

Muenter MD, Sharpless NS, Tyce GM, and Darley FL (1977) Patterns of dystonia ("I-D-I" and "D-I-D") in response to L-dopa therapy for Parkinson's disease. *Mayo Clin Proc*, **52**, 163–74

Myllyla VV, Sotaniemi KA, Tuominen J, and Heinonen EH (1989) Selegiline as primary treatment in early phase Parkinson's disease – an interim report. *Acta Neurol Scand*, **126**, 177–82

Nelson JR and Ellison G (1978) Enhanced stereotypies after repeated injections but not continuous amphetamines. *Neuropharmacology*, **17**, 1081–4

Nutt JG (1987) On-off phenomenon: relation to levodopa pharmacokinetics and pharmacodynamics. *Ann Neurol*, **22**, 535–40

Nutt JG (1988) The case for and concerns about continuous dopamine stimulation in Parkinson's disease. *J Neural Transm*, **27** (suppl), 11–15

Nutt JG (1990) Levodopa-induced dyskinesias: review, observations, and speculations. *Neurology*, **40**, 340–5

Nutt JG and Fellman JH (1984) Pharmacokinetics of levodopa. *Clin Neuropharmacol*, **7**, 35–49

Nutt JG and Woodward WR (1986) Levodopa pharmacokinetics and pharmacodynamics in fluctuating parkinsonian patients. *Neurology*, **36**, 739–44

Nutt JG, Woodward WR, Hammerstad JP, Carter JH, and Anderson JL (1984) The 'on-off' phenomenon in Parkinson's disease: relation to levodopa absorption and transport. *N Engl J Med*, **310**, 483–8

Nutt JG, Woodward WR, and Anderson JL (1985) The effect of carbidopa on the pharmacokinetics of intravenously administered levodopa: the mechanism of action in the treatment of parkinsonism. *Ann Neurol*, **18**, 537–43

Nutt JG, Woodward WR, and Carter HJ (1986) Clinical and biochemical studies with controlled-release Sinemet. *Neurology*, **36**, 1206–11

Nutt JG, Woodward WR, Gancher ST, and Merrick D (1987) 3-*O*-methyldopa and the response to levodopa in Parkinson's disease. *Ann Neurology*, **21**, 584–8

Obeso JA, Luquin MR, and Martinez-Lage JM (1986) Intravenous lisuride corrects motor oscillations in Parkinson's disease. *Ann Neurol*, **19**, 31–5

Obeso JA, Grandas F, Vaamonde J, Luquin MR, and Martinez-Lage JM (1987) Apomorphine infusion for motor fluctuations in Parkinson's disease. *Lancet*, **1**, 1376–7

Obeso JA, Luquin MR, Vaamonde J, and Martinez Lage JM (1988) Subcutaneous administration of lisuride in the treatment of complex motor fluctuations in Parkinson's disease. *J Neural Transm*, **27** (suppl), 17–25

Oertel WH, Gasser T, Ippisch R, Trenkwalder C, and Poewe W (1989) Apomorphine test for dopaminergic responsiveness. *Lancet*, **1**, 1262–3

Ogasahara S, Nishikawa Y, Takahashi M, Wada K, Nakamura Y, Yorifuji S *et al.* (1984) Dopamine metabolism in the central nervous system after discontinuation of L-dopa therapy in patients with Parkinson's disease. *J Neurol Sci*, **66**, 151–63

Papavasiliou PS, McDowell FH, Wang YY, Rosal V, and Miller ST (1979) Plasma DOPA and growth hormone in parkinsonism: oscillations in symptoms. *Neurology*, **29**, 194–200

Parkes JD, Debono AG, and Marsden CD (1976) Bromocriptine in parkinsonism: long-term treatment, dose response, and comparison with levodopa. *J Neurol Neurosurg Psychiatry*, **39**, 1101–8

Pincus JH and Barry K (1987) Protein redistribution diet restores motor function in patients with dopa-resistant 'off' periods. *Neurology*, **38**, 481–3

Poewe WH, Lees AJ, and Stern GM (1987) Clinical and pharmacokinetic observations with Madopar HBS in hospitalized patients with Parkinson's disease and motor fluctuations. *Eur Neurol*, **27** (suppl 1), 93–7

Poewe W, Kleedorfer B, Gerstenbrand F, and Oertel W (1988) Subcutaneous apomorphine in Parkinson's disease. *Lancet*, **1**, 943

Poewe W, Kleedorfer B, Wagner M, Benke T, Gasser T, and Oertel W (1989) Side effects of subcutaneous apomorphine in Parkinson's disease. *Lancet*, **1**, 1084–5

Post RM (1980) Intermittent versus continuous stimulation: effects of time interval on the development of sensitization or tolerance. *Life Sci*, **26**, 1275–82

Quinn N, Parkes JD, and Marsden CD (1984) Control of on/off phenomenon by continuous intravenous infusion of levodopa. *Neurology*, **34**, 1131–6

Reches A and Fahn S (1984) Catechol-*O*-methyltransferase and Parkinson's disease. In Hassler RG and Christ JF, eds, *Parkinson's-Specific Motor and Mental Disorders, Role of the Pallidum: Pathophysiological, Biochemical and Therapeutic Aspects. Advances in Neurology*, vol 40, New York, Raven, 171–9

Rinne JO, Rinne JK, Laakso K, Lonnberg P, and Rinne UK (1985) Dopamine D-1 receptors in the parkinsonian brain. *Brain Res*, **359**, 306–10

Rinne UK (1987) Early combination of bromocriptine and levodopa in the treatment of Parkinson's disease: a 5-year follow-up. *Neurology*, **37**, 826–8

Rinne UK (1989) Early dopamine agonist therapy in Parkinson's disease. *Movement Disorders*, **4** (suppl 1), 86–94

Rinne UK, Laihinen A, Rinne JO, Nagren K, Bergman J, and Ruotsalalnen U (1990) Positron emission tomography demonstrates dopamine D_2 receptor supersensitivity in the striatum of patients with early Parkinson's disease. *Movement Disorders*, **5**(1), 55–9

Rivera-Calimlim L, Morgan JP, Dujovne CA, Bianchine JR, and Lasagna L (1970) L-dopa absorption and metabolism by the human stomach. *Clin Invest*, **49**, 79a

Rivera-Calimlim L, Dujovne CA, Morgan JP, Lasagna L, and Bianchine JR (1971) Absorption and metabolism of levodopa by the human stomach. *Eur J Clin Invest*, **1**, 313–20

Roberts JW, Bravi D, Davis TL, Mouradian MM, and Chase TN (1992) Comparison of apomorphine pharmacodynamics in parkinsonian patients with and without fluctuations. *Neurology*, **42** (suppl 3), 441

Roberts JW, Cora-Locatelli G, Bravi D, Amantea MA, Mouradian MM, Chase TN (1993) catechol-O-methyltrasferase inhibitor, Ro 40-7592, prolongs levodopa/carbidopa action in parkinsonian patients. *Neurology*, in press

Rossor MN, Watkins J, Brown MJ, Reid JL, and Dollery CT (1980) Plasma levodopa, dopamine and therapeutic response following levodopa therapy of parkinsonian patients. *J Neurol Sci*, **46**, 385–92

Ruggieri S, Stocchi F, Carta A, Bravi D, Bragoni M, Giorgi L *et al.* (1988) Comparison between L-dopa and lisuride intravenous infusions: a clinical study. *Movement Disorders*, **3**, 313–19

Sage JI, Trooskin S, Sonsalla PK, Heikkila R, and Duvoisin RC (1988) Long-term duodenal infusion of levodopa for motor fluctuations in parkinsonism. *Ann Neurol*, **24**, 87–9

Schachter M, Marsden CD, Parkes JD, Jenner P, and Testa B (1980) Deprenyl in the management of response fluctuations in patients with Parkinson's disease on levodopa. *J Neurol Neurosurg Psychiatry*, **43**, 1016–21

Schwab RS, Amador LV, and Lettvin JY (1951) Apomorphine in Parkinson's disease. *Trans Am Neurol Assoc*, **76**, 251–3

Shoulson I, Glaubiger GA, and Chase TN (1975) On-off response: clinical and biochemical correlations during oral and intravenous levodopa administration in parkinsonian patients. *Neurology*, **25**, 1144–8

Spencer SE and Wooten GF (1984) Altered pharmacokinetics of L-dopa metabolism in rat striatum deprived of dopaminergic innervation. *Neurology*, **34**, 1105–8

Spina MB and Cohen G (1989) Dopamine turnover and glutathione oxidation: implications for Parkinson's disease. *Proc Natl Acad Sci*, **86**, 1398–400

Stahl SM (1988) Applications of new drug delivery techniques to Parkinson's disease and dopaminergic agents. *J Neural Transm*, **27** (suppl), 123–32

Stibe CMH, Lees AJ, Kempster PA, and Stern GM (1988) Subcutaneous apomorphine in parkinsonian on-off oscillations. *Lancet*, **1**, 403–6

Stoessl AJ, Mak E, and Calne DB (1985) (+)-4-propyl-9-hydroxynaphthoxazine (PHNO), a new dopaminomimetic, in treatment of parkinsonism. *Lancet*, **2**, 1330–1

Sweet RD and McDowell FH (1974) Plasma dopa concentrations and the 'on-off' effect after chronic treatment of Parkinson's disease. *Neurology*, **24**, 953–6

Temlett JA, Quinn NP, Jenner PG, Marsden CD, Poucher E, Bonnet A-M *et al.* (1989) Antiparkinsonian activity of CY 208-243, a partial D-1 dopamine receptor agonist, in MPTP-treated marmosets and patients with Parkinson's disease. *Movement Disorders*, **4**, 261–5

Teravainen H, Kaakola S, Jarvinen M, and Gordin A (1990) Selective COMT inhibitor, nitecapone, in Parkinson's disease. *Neurology*, **40** (suppl 1), 271

The Parkinson Study Group (1989) Effect of deprenyl on the progression of disability in early Parkinson's disease. *N Engl J Med*, **321**, 1364–71

Tolosa ES, Martin WE, Cohen NP, and Jacobson RL (1975) Patterns of clinical response and plasma dopa levels in Parkinson's disease. *Neurology*, **25**, 117–83

Trugman JM and Wooten GF (1987) Selective D1 and D2 dopamine agonists differentially alter basal ganglia glucose utilization in rats with unilateral 6-hydroxydopamine substantia nigra lesions. *J Neurosci* **7**, 2927–35

Van der Weide J, De Vries JB, Tepper PG, Krause DN, Dubocovich ML, and Horn AS (1988) N-0437: a selective D-2 dopamine receptor agonist in *in vitro* and *in vivo* models. *Eur J Pharmacol*, **147**, 249–58

Wachtel H and Dorow R (1983) Dual action on central dopamine function of transdihydrolisuride, a 9,10-dihydrogenated analogue of the ergot dopamine agonist lisuride. *Life Sci*, **32**, 421–32

Wade LA and Katzman R (1975) Synthetic amino acids and the nature of L-dopa transport at the blood–brain barrier. *J Neurochem*, **25**, 837–42

Wade DN, Mearrick PT and Morris JL (1973) Active transport of L-dopa in the intestine, *Nature*, **242**, 463–5

Wade DN, Mearrick PT, Birkett DJ, and Morris J (1974) Variability of L-dopa absorption in man. *Aust NZ J Med*, **4**, 138–43

Weick BG, Engber TM, Susel Z, Chase TN, and Walters JR (1990) Responses of substantia nigra pars reticulata neurons to GABA and SKF 38393 in 6-hydroxydopamine-lesioned rats are differentially affected by continuous and intermittent levodopa administration. *Brain Res*, **523**, 16–23

Winn SR, Wahlberg L, Tresco PA, and Aebischer P (1989) An encapsulated dopamine-releasing polymer alleviates experimental parkinsonism in rats. *Exp Neurol*, **105**, 244–50

Wooten GF (1987) Pharmacokinetics of levodopa. In Marsden CD, Fahn S, eds, *Movement Disorders 2*, London, Butterworths, 231–48

Yahr MD, Elizan TS, and Moros D (1989) Selegiline in the treatment of Parkinson's disease – long term experience. *Acta Neurol Scand*, **126**, 157–61

11
Neural transplantation in the dopamine system – basic and clinical research

Kathy Steece-Collier and John R. Sladek

In 1979, reports by Perlow and colleagues and Björklund and Stenevi (1979a) demonstrated that embryonic dopamine (DA) neurons transplanted into lesioned rats could replace DA in a behaviourally significant manner. Two years later, Freed and colleagues demonstrated that transplanted adrenal chromaffin cells could similarly ameliorate behavioural deficits associated with DA-depleting lesions (Freed *et al.*, 1981). Years of research in rodents and non-human primates have led to application of neural grafting in human Parkinson's patients. This chapter will attempt to summarize the work that forms the research basis for these clinical trials, outline clinical progress, and highlight the significant research questions that remain.

Initial research that served as an essential background to the current clinical experiments began as early as the 1890s when Thompson (1890) performed what is believed to be the first attempt to graft central nervous system (CNS) tissue from adult cats into adult dogs. Although success was reported, little evidence existed to support the claim that adult brain tissue survived this xenograft attempt. Elizabeth Dunn began a now classic experiment in 1903 that demonstrated survival of neurons grafted between immature rats (Dunn, 1917). The early developmental age of these neurons is credited with leading to the observed viability of grafted neurons. Modest progress (by today's standards) was made throughout the next 60 years and the field remained relatively quiescent until Scandinavian investigators began to test the characteristics of histochemically identified catecholaminergic neurons following implantation either into the anterior eye chamber or directly into CNS tissue (Sieger and Olson, 1977; Björklund and Stenevi, 1979b).

NEURAL TRANSPLANTATION IN RODENTS – FETAL DOPAMINE NEURONS

The anterior chamber of the eye proved a favourable environment that could support transplanted tissue and thus was used extensively in initial studies of tissue grafting in mammals. Intraocular grafting was advantageous because it allowed *in vivo* observation of the transplant as well as detailed qualitative and quantitative assessment of neurite outgrowth. Central monoamine neurons, including those from the developing substantia nigra, were first transplated into the anterior chamber of the eye in 1972 by Olson and Seiger. These neurons survived, developed an internal organization similar to their normal brain counterparts and partially reinnervated the sympathetically denervated host iris. The yield of fibres from younger embryonic donor tissue was more extensive than with older embryos or neonatal tissue. When embryonic nigral tissue was co-transplanted intraocularly with its normal target tissue, e.g. the immature striatum, both cell survival and fibre outgrowth, particularly into the target graft, were increased (Olson *et al.*, 1980). Using intraocular cerebellar homografts, Hoffer and colleagues (1974) were able to show that both electrophysiological and complex histological characteristics normally observed *in situ* were retained despite the lack of appropriate connections with the host brain. Importantly, the timetable for the development of these characteristics followed that observed normally in the brain.

Early grafting studies also examined the extent to which cerebral tissue could survive transplantation directly into the brain. Cerebral tissue from fetal or newborn mammals was observed early on to survive grafting into the brain of infant or young recipients (Dunn, 1917; LeGros Clark, 1940; Das, 1974). In one of the first systematic experiments, Stenevi and colleagues (1976) were able to obtain consistent survival of transplanted central monoaminergic tissue into an adult mammalian brain. Survival of neural tissue in adult brain appeared to be dependent on two factors. Firstly, in agreement with earlier reports, embryonic tissue survived transplantation better than neonatal tissue, and adult tissue did not survive. Secondly, neuronal transplants survived well only when grafted in contact with a vessel-rich tissue, for example, the pia in the choroidal fissure. Survival was less optimal with placement of solid pieces of tissue into the striatum or into a freshly made cavity overlying the striatum. In this pioneering study, under optimal conditions, neuronal survival at up to 6 months ranged from about 10 to 500 DA neurons, and over time, neurite outgrowth became extensive. The outgrowing fibres from the surviving peripheral and central monoaminergic neurons formed patterns in the nearby, previously denervated, dentate gyrus and hippocampus, which was suggestive of the formation of terminal contacts in the host brain (Stenevi *et al.*, 1976). In a separate study, Björklund *et al.* (1976) demonstrated that a variety of fetal monoaminergic neurons placed adjacent to the denervated hippocampus could form distinctly different and highly consistent patterns of reinnervation characteristic of the intact hippocampus. Concomitant with this reinnervation, elevated DA levels were observed in the hippocampus, an area normally lacking any significant DA innervation (Stenevi *et al.*, 1977). Curiously, there was also a development of DA-sensitive adenylate cyclase in the hippocampus following grafting, possibly indicative of DA receptor induction in this region (Stenevi *et al.*, 1977).

Thus, initial studies from several laboratories provided evidence that immature mammalian neural tissue could survive transplantation into an ectopic site. The grafted tissue could grow, differentiate, display some normal electrophysiological properties and even maintain organotypic organization inherent to the tissue as seen *in situ*. It appeared that grafted neurons could extend processes which could reinnervate the host in a manner similar to that seen under normal conditions. Up to this point, transplantation was primarily viewed as a tool for studying mechanisms of neural plasticity and regeneration. However, the stage was being set for examining the potential as well as the limitation of neural grafting as a therapeutic intervention in the treatment of neurodegenerative diseases.

Perlow and co-workers (1979) were the first directly to address the issue of transplantation as a tool to restore a functional deficit by investigating the efficacy of grafted DA neurons in reversing lesion-induced behavioural asymmetries in a rat model of Parkinson's disease. Parkinson's disease is a progressive neurodegenerative disorder characterized by a loss of DA neurons in the zona compacta of the substantia nigra, with a resulting decrease in concentrations of nigral and striatal DA (Bernheimer *et al.*, 1975). The syndrome is primarily characterized by abnormalities in movement and posture. An important animal model that mimics some of the neurochemical abnormalities of Parkinson's disease involves a toxin-induced unilateral lesion of the ascending nigrostriatal DA system in the rat. This lesion results in a compensatory unilateral increase in DA receptors in the lesioned striatum (Ungerstedt, 1974). As a result, these animals manifest severe behavioural asymmetry after systemic injection of a DA agonist. Perlow and colleagues (1979) reasoned that transplanted fetal nigral tissue, a replacement source of DA, adjacent to the DA-denervated caudate nucleus, might compensate for neurological deficits in a more physiological manner than conventional drug therapy which was associated with undesired side-effects. When embryonic nigral tissue was placed into the lateral ventricle of unilaterally lesioned adult rats, there was good survival of grafted tissue (average number of surviving neurons = 1974). Monoamine-containing fibres were abundant not only within the grafts but also extended into the adjacent striatum. Most importantly, for the first time, grafted neurons were shown to have a beneficial functional effect; there was a significant reduction (~50%) in apomorphine-induced rotational asymmetry 1 month after grafting. These investigators also were able to demonstrate that in conjunction with the decrease in motor asymmetry, there was a normalization of supersensitive DA receptors in the dorsomedial striatum (Freed *et al.*, 1983). In comparison, a control tissue was not observed to affect behaviour or receptor binding (Perlow *et al.*, 1979; Freed *et al.*, 1983).

That grafted tissue could improve a functional deficit accompanying a neurological lesion opened a new way of thinking about grafting. Research progressed rapidly over the next several years and many important issues were addressed. For example, if grafting was to be considered a viable alternative to drug treatment in human disease, it was necessary to determine the long-term effectiveness of transplanted neurons. Freed and co-workers (1980) followed their preliminary study with a long-term behavioural, biochemical and histochemical study. Although others had been able to demonstrate that grafted cells could survive over extended periods of time, these authors were able to correlate long-term survival with long-term functional and biochemical benefit. Attenuation of apomorphine-induced rotational behaviour was found to be stable for up to 6 months. There was also an increase in DA concentration in the striatum adjacent to the graft, which decreased as distance from the graft increased. An interesting observation in this long-term study was that despite increased accumulation of lipofuscin in the host brain, the grafted tissue looked 'younger'; there was very little lipofuscin accumulation, suggesting that the grafts aged independently of the host. In a parallel study, Björklund and Stenevi (1979) showed that embryonic substantia nigra transplanted into a richly vascularized precavitation site overlying the caudate nucleus also survived for up to 7 months and provided functional improvement in amphetamine-induced rotation for up to 16 weeks after grafting. These authors noted a correlation between cell survival (ranging from a few to approximately 4000 DA neurons), neurite outgrowth and attenuation of amphetamine-induced turning.

Another important issue which was addressed was the scope of functional benefit derived from grafting. In addition to drug-induced rotational behaviour, there are numerous spontaneous behavioural abnormalities which accompany unilateral and bilateral lesions of the nigrostriatal DA system in a rat (e.g. sensorimotor neglect, side bias in T-maze, akinesia, aphagia, adipsia). Thus, this experimental model was useful in examining the degree to which grafting of fetal DA neurons could affect the kind of multiple lesion-induced deficits that can be enountered in Parkinson's disease. Initial research indicated that grafting could induce recovery of some functional deficits, but not others (Dunnett *et al.*, 1981). It was hypothesized that the ability of transplanted neurons to affect only certain behaviours may be related to the topographic organization of the striatum and limited capacity of the transplant to reinnervate all of the appropriate areas. Unfortunately, there were limitations to exploring the importance of graft placement in affecting specific behaviours since evidence at that time indicated that solid grafts placed directly into the parenchyma of adult brain did not survive well.

In 1980, Björklund and colleagues reported a new method that resulted in enhanced neuron survival following grafting of fetal tissue directly into the brain parenchyma without the need for prior cavity formation. These investigators injected dissociated fetal nigral cell suspensions into the DA-denervated caudate. This approach put grafted cells in direct contact with host neuropil, circumventing the need for special vascular support. The results showed excellent cell survival and extensive neurite outgrowth. The ability of the suspension grafts fully to compensate for amphetamine-induced rotational behaviour was reported to be even more rapid than that seen previously with solid grafts (3–5 weeks versus 2–3 months; Björklund *et al.*, 1980). This methodological advance widened the possible investigations of functional reconstruction as it allowed varied and multiple placements of desired tissue.

Björklund and co-workers (1983) carried out a study comparing single versus multiple implants of nigral cell suspensions as well as the importance of placement site in improving various lesion-induced deficits. These investigators found that single grafts could alter particular behavioural abnormalities dependent on graft placement within the striatum. In particular, placement within the dorsal striatum was important for altering rotational behaviour whereas ventrolateral placement was important in sensorimotor function. As might be expected, multiple graft placement within the striatum provided a more complete restoration of lost innervation; up to two-thirds of the volume of the rostral striatum in the rat could be reinnervated with three placement sites (Björklund *et al.*, 1983). Accordingly, multiple placements were capable of reversing all behavioural asymmetries examined and abolished the increased rate of apomorphine-induced rotations seen in control animals (Dunnett *et al.*, 1983). Single placement of nigral tissue outside the striatal target into the lateral hypothalamus, along the trajectory of the ascending DA pathway, or substantia nigra showed good survival of grafted DA neurons but, interestingly, neurite outgrowth was restricted to the graft itself. There was no effect of these grafts on behavioural indices measured.

The results from behavioural studies in rats with unilateral nigral lesions were encouraging. However, examination of the bilaterally lesioned rat model suggested that grafting of cell suspensions into the lesioned striata may not be a panacea. Bilateral ablation of the nigrostriatal DA system results in severe adipsia, aphagia and akinesia with bilateral sensory neglect. Dunnett and co-workers (1983) used a paradigm of single versus multiple grafts, again with various placement strategies in these bilaterally lesioned rats. The results showed that, although grafts were capable of reversing sensorimotor and akinetic impairments, no single graft or combination grafts could induce a substantial recovery of aphagia, adipsia or body weight loss. These authors discussed possible reasons for their findings, which likely are important factors to consider for future studies. Briefly, some critical forebrain DA regions, other than the striatum, may not have been compensated by the grafting approach used in this study or simply the overall magnitude of DA recovery was insufficient to affect specific parameters. Further, the ectopic placement of grafted DA neurons, remote from their normal location, may result in deficency of afferent connections important in the neuronal modulation that yields normal consummatory behaviours.

The functional success of fetal transplantation appears to depend on continuous survival of appropriate neurons in appropriate target regions. No beneficial effect has been observed in animals with control grafts (non-dopaminergic tissue) or, as cited above, when DA neurons are placed into non-target regions in the adult brain such as the hypothalamus or substantia nigra (Perlow *et al.*, 1979; Dunnett *et al.*, 1983). That intentional rejection of a DA graft results in a return of pregraft behavioural abnormalities supports the idea that DA neuron graft effects are unique to this tissue and dependent on its survival (Dunnett *et al.*, 1988).

Biochemical measurements have been useful in quantifying graft-derived reinnervation. Implants of nigral cell suspensions into animals with approximately 99% striatal DA depletion can restore DA levels to between 13 and 18%, with the highest levels reaching about 50% of control in individuals with multiple graft placement (Schmidt *et al.*, 1983). These values are similar to those obtained with solid grafts placed into a cavitation site above the striatum (Schmidt *et al.*, 1982). Suspension grafts also appear to restore dopaminergic transmission toward normal, as demonstrated by an increase in levels of the DA metabolite 3,4-dihydroxyphenylacetic acid (DOPAC) and precursor dihydroxyphenylalanine (DOPA) from 5 to 20%, and 6 to 30% of control, respectively. Dopac/DA and dopa/DA ratios following grafting are in the range of those reported in the intrinsic DA system following partial lesion. Dopamine turnover rates, following either suspension or solid grafts, follow the same pattern of change seen with varying degrees of lesioning of the intrinsic nigrostriatal system (Schmidt *et al.*, 1983). This may suggest that mechanisms regulating transmitter function are similar in suspension and solid grafts and, to a degree, in the intrinsic nigral neurons.

Electrophysiological studies have demonstrated that mesencephalic tissue grafted into the lateral ventricle exhibit spontaneous firing rates reminiscent of those seen in the intact substantia nigra. In addition, these grafted cells exhibit reliable alterations in firing patterns after local application of DA agonists and antagonists which again mimic those seen in intact nigral neurons (Wuerthele *et al.*, 1981).

At the ultrastructural level, fetal DA neurons form synaptic contacts with host neurons (Freund *et al.*, 1985; Jaeger, 1985; Mahalik *et al.*, 1985). Host-to-graft connections also have been observed morphologically by Mahalik *et al.* (1985), but not by Freund *et al.* (1985). In support of host-to-graft communications, Arbuthnott and co-workers (1985) demonstrated electrophysiological evidence of host input from the frontal cortex, striatum and other brain regions to nigral grafts.

Another aspect of neural grafting which has gained much interest is the application of the expanding knowledge of neuronal survival and growth-promoting molecules to the augmentation of grafted neuron survival and function. Indeed, one of the areas of most intense activity in neurotrophic factor research is the search for substances active in the dopamine system. Several factors have been identified which promote survival of embryonic rat mesencephalic dopamine neurons in tissue culture. These include brain-derived neurotrophic factor (BDNF) (Hyman *et al.*, 1991; Knusel *et al.*, 1991), insulin-like growth factor 1 (IGF-1) (Knusel *et al.*, 1990), acidic and basic fibroblast growth factor (aFGF, bFGF) (Engele and Bohn, 1991; Knusel *et al.*, 1990, 1991), epidermal growth factor (EGF) (Casper *et al.*, 1991), and glial cell line-derived growth factor (GDNF) (Lin *et al.*, 1993). While the activity of these molecules in cultures of embryonic dopamine neurons suggests that they may be useful adjuncts to embryonic dopamine neuron grafts, work on combining grafts and growth factors is just beginning. bFGF has been reported to enhance survival and neurite extension of embryonic dopamine neurons grafted into lesioned rats (Steinbusch *et al.*, 1990). In this study, cell suspensions of embryonic ventral mesencephalon mixed with either bFGF or bFGF + heparin, resulted in better survival of grafted dopamine neurons and a doubling of the density of outgrowing dopaminergic fibers innervating the host striatum. Administration of bFGF alone had no effect on host dopamine fibers. Initial study of the effects of chronic intraventricular infusion, or daily intrastriatal injection of relatively high levels of BDNF in association with embryonic ventral mesencephalic grafts in lesioned rats indicated that while amelioration of rotational behavior to amphetamine was significantly enhanced in these animals, no effect on survival or neurite extension of grafted dopamine neurons could be detected (Sauer *et al.*, 1992).

At least two cellular sources of growth factors have been studied in co-graft paradigms with embryonic dopamine neurons in rats. Brundin and colleagues (1986) examined mixed cell suspension grafts of ventral mesencephalon and embryonic striatum. These nigral/striatal co-grafts yielded a transient acceleration of recovery of amphetamine-induced rotational behavior, increased area of the host striatum densely innervated by graft-derived fibers, but no increase in survival of grafted dopamine neurons. A similar co-grafting study by Yurek and colleagues (1990), found a sustained enhancement of recovery of amphetamine-induced rotational behavior in animals with nigral/striatal co-grafts, increased neurite extension and cell body size of grafted dopamine neurons, but no increase in grafted cell number. A second co-graft paradigm has combined embryonic dopamine neurons with peripheral nerve as a source of Schwann cell-derived growth factors. Collier and Springer (1991) found that intraventricular co-grafts of polymer-encapsulated adult rat peripheral nerve adjacent to intrastriatal dopamine neuron grafts yielded enhanced recovery of amphetamine-induced rotational behavior, a modest increase in grafted cell survival, and a marked increase in reinnervation of the host striatum. Van Horne and colleagues (1991) found that mixed intrastriatal implants of peripheral nerve fragments and embryonic dopamine neurons accelerated recovery of apomorphine-induced rotational behavior, but observed no morphological correlate of this effect. Thus, these early findings suggest that the combination of growth factors and neural grafts may be effective in improving survival and function of grafted neurons. Further evaluation of administration of individual molecules, as well as co-grafted cellular sources of growth factors is needed.

Finally, the efficacy of these survival and growth-promoting molecules in enhancing the viability and function of cultured and grafted embryonic dopamine neurons raises the possibility that these substances may be useful as potential stimuli for compensatory mechanisms in the host dopamine system. bFGF (Otto and Unsicker, 1989) and EGF (Hadjiconstantinou *et al.*, 1991) have been reported to ameliorate the neurochemical and anatomical deficits in the nigrostriatal dopamine system of mice treated with the neurotoxin MPTP. Similarly, GM1 ganglioside administration has been reported to ameliorate these deficits in MPTP-treated monkeys (Schneider *et al.*, 1992). All three of these molecules appear to exert a protective or cell rescue effect in these systems, as treatment immediately after the neurotoxic insult is required for best effect. In the case of bFGF, the authors demonstrated that delaying administration by 7 days eliminated the efficacy of the treatment in reversing the MPTP-induced deficits. Infusion of BDNF into the striatum, medial forebrain bundle, or substantia nigra of rats with knife-cut lesions of the nigrostriatal bundle failed to rescue nigral dopamine neurons from degeneration (Knusel *et al.*, 1992). Chronic infusion of Schwann cell conditioned medium into the lateral ventricle of rats has been reported to significantly increase the density of the dopamine terminal field in the adjacent lateral septal area, and intrastriatal grafts of Schwann cells attract dopamine fiber ingrowth in rats with partial nigrostriatal system lesions induced 4 weeks previously (Collier *et al.*, 1992). Clearly, further work needs to be done to establish whether certain molecules or combinations of molecules will be effective in cell rescue and are capable of inducing compensatory activity in a population of host dopamine neurons reduced in number by disease or experimental manipulation. This area holds promise for both establishing combined graft-growth factor therapies that may yield better outcomes than neural grafts alone, and in identification of survival and growth-promoting factors that may be active in the damaged host dopamine system.

Although experimental models of nerve cell grafting in parkinsonian animals shows great promise for providing a significant treatment option in Parkinson's disease, there are many factors which remain to be explored before optimal therapeutic benefit can be gained. Nearly all experimental protocols employed thus far have utilized young, adult animals. However, the average onset of symptoms in Parkinson's disease occurs during the sixth decade of life. Thus, investigation of graft integration and function in aged animals warrants examination. Initial studies in this regard have provided evidence that fetal DA neurons can survive intrastriatal implantation in the aged rat brain (Gage *et al.*, 1983a). Additionally, they can extend neuritic processes into the host striatum and produce a significant improvement in the motor coordination which normally deteriorates with age (Gage *et al.*, 1983a, b). However, it remains to be elucidated whether fetal DA grafts can reverse the many lesioned-induced changes which occur in experimental parkinsonism in aged rodents and importantly, nonhuman primates.

Another factor of Parkinson's disease that has yet to be investigated is the long-term relationship of the lesion relative to the time of implantation of fetal neurons. In the human disease, nigrostriatal degeneration may occur over a considerable number of years until a high percentage of cell is lost with a progressive worsening of symptoms. Studies to date in animal models of the disease have intervened with grafts several weeks to months after lesioning. It is possible that the damaged DA system may be more difficult to repair during advanced stages of the disorder due to changes in postsynaptic receptors as well as other factors. Thus, the ability of grafted DA neurons to alter long-term changes is an important issue which likewise needs investigation.

NEURAL TRANSPLANTATION IN PRIMATES – FETAL DOPAMINE NEURONS

The initiation of neural grafting experiments in primates occurred in reverse sequence of what many would have predicted: far more humans received autologous chromaffin cell grafts between 1985 and 1989 than monkeys. While this paradox has been the subject of numerous reviews and editorials (Sladek and Shoulson, 1988; Gash and Sladek, 1989; Lindvall, 1989), it is important to appreciate that considerable work with grafting of fetal neurons in non-human primates has been initiated in several laboratories with encouraging results, as highlighted below.

The discovery that 1-methyl-4-phenyl-1,2,5,6-tetrahydropyridine (MPTP), a protoxin derived as an unintended byproduct of the manufacture of illicit synthetic heroin, results in the selective destruction of DA neurons of the substantia nigra in primates prompted considerable research on the aetiology and treatment of Parkinson's disease. The symptoms of hypokinesia, tremor, rigidity and difficulty in initiation of movement produced in humans and monkeys by MPTP closely resembled those seen in human parkinsonism (Burns *et al.*, 1983; Langston *et al.*, 1983). This model provided unique opportunities for studying the potential therapeutic value of nerve cell grafts to alter a movement disorder produced by destruction of the nigrostriatal system.

An initial attempt at grafting fetal substantia nigra into primate brain did not support the feasibility of this procedure. Morisha and co-workers (1984, 1987) found no evidence of fetal nigral neuron survival 3 months after transplantation into the DA-denervated caudate nucleus of two rhesus monkeys. This lack of success was viewed not as a discouragement, but rather as a need for methodological refinement. Shortly thereafter, Bakey and colleagues (1985, 1987), using tissue suspension of earlier gestational age donor (35–37 days versus 59–71 days used by Morisha *et al.*) reported that nigral neurons could survive, reverse certain neurological deficits in MPTP-treated primates and enhance cerebrospinal fluid DA levels for up to 2 months post-transplantation.

Concurrently, short-term experiments, initiated in 1985 by Redmond and colleagues demonstrated that multiple bilateral placements of intrastriatal fetal mesencephalic DA neuron grafts could survive, grow and effect an improvement in the tremor and bradykinesia of experimental parkinsonism in African green monkeys for up to 10 weeks after transplantation (Redmond *et al.*, 1986; Sladek *et al.*, 1986). As seen in rodents, grafts were particularly robust when placed in proximity to the lateral ventricles. Control grafts of embryonic substantia nigra were positioned into the cerebral cortex, overlying the striatum in a single monkey and, although they showed excellent survival of DA neurons, they resulted in no improvement of the parkinsonian condition. This pilot project prompted similar tests in a greater number of monkeys and for longer post-transplantation survival times (up to 7.5 months; Sladek *et al.*, 1988). Also, an important control was added by grafting non-dopaminergic cerebellar tissue, derived from the same brains that yielded fetal substantia nigra grafts, into the striatum of MPTP-lesioned monkeys. This was done because of the possibility that the improvement observed after grafting in these monkeys may have resulted either from toxin or surgical-induced regeneration of the residual host DA system (Bohn *et al.*, 1987). After 5 months, a monkey that received grafts of fetal cerebellum showed no improvement and continued to require extensive care, including nasogastric feeding and physical therapy. Anatomical examination of their brains subsequently revealed the presence of well-defined grafts of cerebellar tissue within the striatum, but a lack of any evidence of DA fibre regeneration from host systems. An equally debilitated monkey showed behavioural improvement beginning within 5 weeks of grafting of ventral mesencephalic tissue into the same loci; this improvement gradually progressed to a level whereby this monkey appeared relatively normal by 5–7.5 months. These grafts contained impressive clusters of DA neurons that appeared to fulfil four criteria for fetal cell induced recovery. Specifically: (1) they contained numerous, chemically appropriate neurons; (2) their neurites extended from the grafts into host brain, providing a probable morphological link for graft–host interactions;

(3) they released DA as judged from elevated DA levels in microdissected regions of the caudate nuclei in proximity to grafts; and (4) they resulted in a marked improvement in DA-mediated function, as determined by significantly reduced parkinsonian scores on various behavioural observations (Redmond *et al.*, 1986; Sladek *et al.*, 1986, 1988). Recently Sladek and colleagues (1993) demonstrated that fetal DA cell survival is markedly improved at a specific and potentially critical donor gestional age in the same species of nonhuman primates by the demonstration of grafts that contained as many as 15,000 dopaminergic neurons collected from a single fetus. Other laboratories have also demonstrated that embryonic DA neurons, from different species of non-human primates, survive grafting into the parkinsonian brain, affect MPTP-induced behavioural deficits and enhance appropriate biochemical change in DA metabolism (Fine *et al.*, 1988; Annett *et al.*, 1990; Bankiewicz *et al.*, 1990).

In addition to the putative restorative effects of implanted embryonic cells, the work of Bankiewicz and colleagues (1990) raises some important questions about the ability of host dopaminergic neurons to respond to injury, perhaps in a compensatory way. Their grafting experiments in MPTP-treated rhesus monkeys involved precavitation, a technique first described by Stenevi and colleagues in 1976 for enhancing fetal nerve cell survival in rats. Again, this approach improves the host vascular bed at the intended site of nerve cell grafting. Bankiewicz and associates observed that the cavitation procedure itself can stimulate growth of tyrosine hydroxylase-positive fibres into the region of the eventual grafts. These fibres likely arise from collateral sprouts of mesolimbic DA axons that innervate the nucleus accumbens, situated immediately ventral to the implantation cavity. It is also possible that regenerative sprouting could occur from residual neurons of the nigrostriatal system. This is especially likely since MPTP does not destroy all neurons of the substantia nigra. In fact between 10 and 50% of nigral DA neurons can be spared in primates even after multiple doses that produce parkinsonian symptoms (German *et al.*, 1988). Thus, in spite of profound damage to the nigrostriatal system, there remain a sufficiently large number of neurons that may contribute to a regenerative response, at least in young animals that have been treated with MPTP for relatively short periods of time.

Could a similar regenerative response occur in parkinsonian humans after mesencephalic or adrenal intrastriatal grafts? Although there is no direct anatomical evidence to support this in the limited number of autopsy cases presented to date on graft recipients, some behavioural and historical information suggests a possible linkage. All of the reports of adrenal cell grafting in humans that used an open surgical approach instead of stereotaxic placement through a small (1.0–1.5 mm) cannula, described some degree of improvement in 'on–off' phenomena, and to some extent motor skills, in a large proportion of their patients. Based on autopsy information indicating poor survival of grafted chromaffin cells, and a similar lack of optimal survival of adrenal medullary cells grafted into monkeys (see following section), it follows that any functional improvement attributed to DA release in such patients could be the result of a host sprouting mechanism similar to that observed by Bankiewicz and colleagues (1990) and Fiandaca and colleagues (1988), who observed enhanced tyrosine hydroxylase fibre staining in the striatum following adrenal autografting in monkeys (see following section). It is well-known that parkinsonian symptoms can be manifested when part but not all of the nigral neurons have been destroyed; some accounts suggest, for example, that as high as an 80% cell loss must be achieved. Thus, the residual neurons represent a population that, in theory, could give rise to a regenerative response upon appropriate stimulation. In addition, the mesolimbic DA system is intact and could be the source of origin of putative regenerative fibres.

Historically, the early neurosurgical literature on attempts to ameliorate parkinsonian symptoms through surgical intervention reveals numerous accounts where extirpation of a number of sites in the basal ganglia resulted in some improvement in tremor and motor skills. Usually, such improvement lacked permanency, but this could be accounted for by continued progression of the disease that could counterbalance a 'last-gasp' attempt to reinnervate the striatum with DA terminals (Meyers, 1942). Another possible confound to this theory is the unknown capacity of DA neurons to sprout in humans of advancing age. In favour of this is the fact that catecholaminergic neurons exhibit profound plasticity in response to injury and were used as models to test the phenomenon in transmitter-identified neurons during the pioneering era of transmitter histochemistry (Björklund *et al.*, 1971; Moore *et al.*, 1974). These neurons have been shown to sprout following transection in aged rats and to resupply a distant target with catecholamine fluorescence-positive fibres (Phelps and Sladek, 1984). With respect to humans, it has been reported that dendrites of cortical pyramidal neurons continue to grow in human brain, even into the eighth decade of life (Buell and Coleman, 1979). That this growth was arrested in another neurodegenerative disorder, Alzheimer's disease, may be of relevance to the present discussion if, for example, the progression of symptomology seen in parkinsonism is in part due to failed growth of the (20%) residual DA cell pool of the substantia nigra.

Numerous significant questions should be addressed as we anticipate more widespread application of transplant technology to human disease. For example, Lindvall's review (1989) on the status of human experimentation points to the need to 'scale-up from rodents, through monkeys, to humans.' The fact that the human striatum is 200 times the volume of the rat striatum means that better cell survival must be achieved than the current 5–15% reported following grafting of human mesencephalic DA neurons into rats. This will most likely require the use of cells from several fetuses or, alternatively, the development of reproducible and constant cell lines. This is particularly important if maximal innervation of the caudate and putamen is to be achieved, which may be necessary to maintain graft-induced recovery in a progressive disease such as parkinsonism. Thus, a relatively modest number of neurons (e.g. 3000–6000) might be sufficient to cause an initial improvement in human parkinsonism by boosting the host DA capacity above the level of the 70–80% loss generally accepted as prerequisite to the manifestation of symptoms, but this number may be insufficient to maintain improved function in the event of continuing destruction of the residual nigrostriatal system.

When to intervene in the course of the human disease also may prove to be critical for successful application. Based on our current understanding in monkeys, the procedure appears effective in animals that have shown symptoms for 1–3 months, a relatively short period of time 'into the disease'. By comparison, the vast majority of patients who have received either adrenal or fetal grafts have been relatively late-stage. It is likely that striatal receptor changes occurring either with the disease or following several years of DA agonist therapy (Reisine *et al.*, 1977; Rinne *et al.*, 1983; Hagglund *et al.*, 1987) may render such individuals less favourable recipients for grafts. In these instances, even the introduction of new DA-producing cells may be ineffective if the receptors on striatal postsynaptic membranes are irreversibly altered. Moreover, many of these patients may be in their sixth or seventh decades of life. As such, the aged brain may be less capable of promoting graft–host integration or be less responsive to graft-induced sprouting (Date *et al.*, 1990a). The essential experiments have not yet been performed in rodents or monkeys to examine the potential of either the aged brain or the long-term debilitated host to accept and maintain grafted neurons.

ADRENAL MEDULLARY CELLS IN NEURAL TRANSPLANTATION – RODENT AND PRIMATE MODELS

Parallel experiments have been performed using alternative sources of DA-secreting cells, primarily adrenal chromaffin tissue, in attempts to circumvent legal, ethical and practical concerns associated with the use of fetal neural tissue. Chromaffin cells of the adrenal medulla offered several unique qualities which make them attractive as potential candidates for replacement therapy. Normally, chromaffin cells are round, endocrine cells that produce high concentrations of adrenaline and noradrenaline as well as DA. However, they become phenotypically more similar to neurons (elongated cell body, some neuritic processes) in the absence of the corticosteroids provided by the adrenal cortex, such as when isolated and grown in culture conditions or in grafts. The presence of nerve growth factor (NGF) further shifts chromaffin cells towards a more neuronal phenotype, such that they develop elaborate neuritic outgrowth (Perlow *et al.*, 1979). Additional qualities that make adrenal medullary tissue suitable for grafting are: (1) they share a common embryological origin with central catecholamine neurons; (2) again, they produce the desired neurotransmitter; and (3) a graft recipient can potentially act as an autologous donor, thereby reducing the possibility of tissue rejection.

As researchers began to investigate whether this peripheral tissue could serve as a DA replacement source in the treatment of Parkinson's disease, two pieces of early evidence seemed encouraging. Firstly, Olson and colleagues (Olson, 1980; Olson *et al.*, 1980) demonstrated that chromaffin cells could survive elaborate processes and innervate adjacent transplants of CNS tissue when transplanted to the anterior chamber of the eye. Next, Freed *et al.* (1981) found that intraventricular grafts of adrenal medulla in rats survived for 2 months (average number of surviving chromaffin cells/animal = 1535) and decreased behavioural asymmetry induced by the DA agonist apomorphine. The surviving cells were positive for catecholamine histofluorescence in a majority of the animals. As anticipated, there was a partial transformation of the chromaffin cells from an endocrine to a more neuronal phenotype; some cells had elongated processes but these were not seen to leave the graft. Freed and co-workers concluded that the beneficial behavioural effect of the grafted cells probably was due to a diffusion of catecholamine from the graft into the adjacent striatum rather than from morphological integration with the host.

If adrenal grafts have a beneficial effect due to diffusion, it was reasoned that the usefulness of these grafts may be improved by placing them directly into the DA-denervated striatum. In acute studies, intrastriatal chromaffin cells were shown to release large quantities of catecholamine which presumably diffused through adjacent regions of the neuropil to act on supersensitive DA receptors and caused acute rotational behaviour suggestive of DA release for up to 400 minutes (Herrera-Marschitz *et al.*, 1984; Stromberg *et al.*, 1984). However, long-term studies began to reveal that intraparenchymal placement did not provide as favourable an environment for chromaffin cells as did the lateral ventricle. The average number of surviving cells several months post-transplantation was in the range of 100–200 (Stromberg *et al.*, 1985; Freed *et al.*, 1986) versus the thousands seen with ventricular placement. Despite the lesser number of surviving chromaffin cells, one study (Stromberg *et al.*, 1985) found that there was still a significant behavioural effect on apomorphine-induced rotational asymmetry that lasted for up to 3 months; beyond the 3-month period, rotational behaviour returned to pregrafting levels. In addition, the decrease in rotational behaviour with intrastriatal grafts was of the order of a 25% reduction compared to approximately a 45% reduction with intraventrical placement (Freed *et al.*, 1981; Freed, 1983). This is consistent with the decrease in cell viability with intrastriatal placement.

In a parallel experiment, Stromberg *et al.* (1985) co-administered NGF to investigate what effect it would have on morphology and function of intrastriatal grafts. Long-term (14–28 days) infusion of NGF via an osmotic minipump increased both cell survival (average number of cells = ~450) and fibre outgrowth into the surrounding host striatum. These changes resulted in a large degree of functional benefit (44% decrease in rotational behaviour 3 months postgrafting) as well as increased duration (1 year versus 3 months). Several other investigators subsequently have verified the usefulness of NGF, either through direct infusion or from a variety of sources such as C6-glioma cells, peripheral nerve, and mouse submaxillary gland, as an important factor in enhancing survival and behavioural effect of grafted chromaffin cells (Freed, 1983; Bing *et al.*, 1988a, 1990; Pezzoli *et al.*, 1988; Kordower *et al.*, 1990).

The modest degree of chromaffin cell viability following transplantation into the striatum in initial rat studies also was confirmed in other species such as mice and non-human primates. In the first report of grafting into rhesus monkeys, graft survival ranged from less than 10 cells in 2 animals to 190 and 300 cells in another (Morihisa *et al.*, 1984). Likewise, in mice lesioned with the neurotoxin MPTP, although a few grafted cells survived intrastriatal placement, most of the cells appeared to be dying and the grafts were filled with macrophages 1 month post-transplantation (Bohn *et al.*, 1987). Despite poor survival of these grafts, an interesting phenomenon began to emerge from studies in these species. Bohn and colleagues were the first to report on a remarkable enhancement of tyrosine hydroxylase immunoreactive (TH-IR) fibres thoughout the dorsal striatum ipsilateral but not contralateral to the transplanted cells in MPTP-treated mice. This sprouting or regeneration of DA fibres was seen in mice that received adrenal grafts, but not in those receiving a sham graft. Similarly, Fiandaca *et al.* (1988) and Bankiewicz *et al.* (1988) observed enhanced ipsilateral expression of TH-IR fibres adjacent to adrenal implant sites in monkeys. In these studies, enhancement of immunoreactivity was not dependent on the presence of adrenal tissue. Bankiewicz and colleagues (1988) reported that adrenal medulla, adrenal cortex, adipose tissue or cavitation alone resulted in DA fibre enhancement. However, these authors observed a significant increase in volitional arm use and reduction in apomorphine-induced rotations 3 months after grafting only in the animals with adrenal medulla grafts. This beneficial effect was seen to diminish to the level of the other experimental animals, which were slightly improved over pregrafting levels when tested again 6 months postgrafting, a time when sprouting was still evident. In the study reported by Fiandaca *et al.* (1988) and Hansen *et al.* (1988), surviving chromaffin cells could be identified in only 2 to 7 monkeys with adrenal grafts, yet 8 of 9 total monkeys showed enhanced TH-IR fibres. These authors reported that the degree of host response was related to the degree of tissue damage; the more damage, the more intense the tyrosine hydroxylase immunoreactivity. No functional assessment of these monkeys was reported. Enhancement of fibre outgrowth has been observed in mice and non-human primates treated with MPTP (Bohn *et al.*, 1987; Bankiewicz *et al.*, 1988; Fiandaca *et al.*, 1988) and in one case in rats where grafting was done early (2-week interval versus a several-month interval most commonly employed) after lesioning with the neurotoxin 6-hydroxydopamine 6-OHDA (Bing *et al.*, 1988b). As mentioned previously, MPTP does not entirely destroy all nigral DA neurons but rather it is thought to spare some neurons and cause a temporary impairment of others, resulting in decreased tyrosine hydroxylase expression (Hallman *et al.*, 1985). It is possible then that nigral neurons in MPTP animals may be more responsive to trophic-induced sprouting. Likewise, in a 6-OHDA-lesioned animal grafted shortly after neurotoxin insult, neurons that are damaged (and would likely die with no intervention) may be responsive to trophic assistance from adrenal grafts.

Again, since the onset of Parkinson's disease generally occurs later in life, the usefulness of aged donor tissue and responsiveness of an aged host are important issues which have been examined in studies using adrenal medullary tissue. Freed (1983) showed in rats that chromaffin cells from young (5–7 weeks) and ageing (1 to 2 years) donors both showed intense catecholamine fluorescence, evidence of active catecholamine diffusion, and similar, 'healthy' morphology. However, only young donor grafts produced a significant effect on rational behaviour. Co-grafting mouse submaxillary glands, as a source of NGF, with ageing adrenal cells did not significantly enhance the behavioural efficacy of the grafts (Freed, 1983). The effect of mouse submaxillary glands on cell survival or its effect on young donor tissue was not examined in this study.

In contrast to these findings, Pezzoli *et al.* (1988) showed that adrenal autografts from 20-month-old rats had a small, statistically insignificant, transient effect on apomorphine-induced rotations. When combined with ventricular administration of NGF, behavioural efficacy of aged autografts was significantly improved, similar to that seen in young animals with young grafts plus NGF. Following cessation of NGF, behaviour remained significantly improved, but diminished to the level seen in young animals with adrenal grafts only. Adrenal cell survival with or without NGF was minimal in this study.

One factor that may account for the discrepancy between these two studies could be the quantity of NGF. Freed (1983) reported that, although a percentage of ageing chromaffin cells did develop processes, there was no significant effect of submaxillary gland on this parameter. This may suggest that ageing chromaffin cells are not as responsive to NGF, or simply that the concentration required for neuronal transformation was not present. Using a different model system, examining specifically host response, Date *et al.* (1990) found that the DA system in ageing mice has less regenerative capacity compared to young mice. In young mice (2–3 months), dense TH-IR fibres and a significant increase in striatal DA content were observed adjacent to chromaffin cell grafts 4 weeks following transplantation. This effect of chromaffin grafts was less robust in the 12-month-old mice; recovery was significantly greater than controls without grafts but significantly less than in young animals.

Finally, Kordower *et al.* (1990) observed good survival (8000–18 000 cells) of autologous adrenal medullary tissue implanted into the striatum of aged (>20 years) rhesus monkeys. Co-grafting adrenal tissue with sural nerve increased survival four- to eightfold. Although these authors do not report on the effects of these grafts on TH-IR fibres or behaviour, the excellent viability of these aged grafts 3 months post-transplantation into ageing donors is encouraging.

The understanding of how adrenal chromaffin grafts have a therapeutic effect remains unclear. Although chromaffin cells are surrounded by a halo of fluorescence, presumably due to diffusion of catecholamine from grafted cells (Freed, 1983; Stromberg *et al.*, 1984; Freed *et al.*, 1986) and grafted tissue as well as areas adjacent to the grafts contain elevated DA concentrations (Freed, 1983), *in vivo* microdialysis was unable to detect DA in the cerebrospinal fluid or adjacent striatum of animals with functionally effective grafts (Becker and Freed, 1988). An explanation for the lack of detection of DA in the cerebrospinal fluid may be due to a large degree of dilution. Therefore, although a paracrine function of grafted cells may be one attribute of grafted neurons, it does not seem likely that limited diffusion from a small number of cells could be accountable for the total benefit seen. This function of neurotransmitter release may become more important with concomitant NGF administration where cell number and neurite outgrowth can be increased. However, microdialysis does detect an increase in DA turnover and increased response to amphetamine-induced DA release, suggesting that the presence of grafted tissue could be acting in an indirect manner to promote host striatal DA activity (Becker and Freed, 1988).

There are several ways in which grafting of chromaffin tissue could influence the host striatum. Adrenal medullary cells are thought to release trophic factors known to enhance nigrostriatal function such as gangliosides and basic fibroblast growth factor (Date *et al.*, 1990b). Additionally, injury to the host brain associated with grafting results in gliosis and accumulation of macrophages in the vicinity of degenerating chromaffin cells. In addition to their role of scavengers of necrotic tissue, macrophages contain and release various trophic substances (Nathan *et al.*, 1980; Weber *et al.*, 1990). Microglia are also thought to be a source of trophic substance (Longo and Penhoet, 1974). In an attempt better to understand the contribution of the grafted tissue in adrenal cell transplants, Date *et al.* (1990c) placed syngeneic, allogeneic and xenogeneic adrenal medulla into the striatum of MPTP-treated mice and examined the number of cells that survived versus the recovery of the intrinsic host DA fibres. As usual, there was modest survival of chromaffin cells in the syngeneic group of animals (mean number of cells = 93). In both the allogeneic (12 and 14 grafted cells in 2 to 5 animals) and xenogeneic (no grafted cells) groups there were essentially no surviving chromaffin cells. Examination of TH-IR fibre recovery and striatal DA concentrations revealed that all three transplant groups showed a significant degree of recovery compared to sham grafted controls. However, the increase in both measures in the syngeneic group was significantly greater than those in either the allogeneic or xenogeneic animals (no difference between these two groups). The authors conclude that survivability of grafted chromaffin cells influences the degree of recovery of the host DA system over and above that produced by tissue implant-induced damage to the host. This is supported by several studies that have shown that increased survivability of cells co-grafted with a source of NGF increases the functional or biochemical efficacy of these transplants (Bing *et al.*, 1988, 1990; Pezzoli *et al.*, 1988).

Interestingly, Pezzoli *et al.* (1988) demonstrated that either chromaffin or non-chromaffin tissue (e.g. adipose tissue or sciatic nerve) grafted into the lateral ventricle, in the presence of NGF, produced a similar beneficial effect on behavioural asymmetry in unilaterally lesioned rats. In the absence of NGF only chromaffin tissue was effective and NGF alone had no functional benefit (Stromberg *et al.*, 1985; Pezzoli *et al.*, 1988). Pezzoli and colleagues (1988) suggested that a synergistic interaction may occur between the exogenous NGF and endogenous response to the transplanted tissue such that a persistent cellular reaction beyond that caused by cannula injury alone may be necessary. These authors saw no evidence of trophic-induced sprouting to account for their findings. This evidence further confuses the idea that a paracrine function is important in the therapeutic effectiveness of adrenal grafts.

There may be a variety of mechanisms by which implantation of adrenal medullary tissue can be therapeutic, and a lack of consensus on the importance of surviving grafted chromaffin cells remains. There are numerous examples, though, that suggest that increasing cell survival is an important variable for success of this procedure. Unfortunately, modest to poor survival of intrastriatal grafts has been common even in co-grafting situations. Using a novel technical approach, Dubach and German (1990) demonstrated survival of several thousand chromaffin cells placed into the 6-OHDA-lesioned striatum of young adult long-tail macaques 4–8 weeks following implantation. These authors contend that modification of technical aspects of the grafting procedure may be of critical importance in the survival of adrenal cells. In their study, the adrenal medulla was cut into long ribbons of tissue and implanted with minimal distortion or traumatization of either the adrenal tissue or the brain. Most monkeys in this study received concomitant intraventricular NGF; however, no difference in survival or morphology with or without NGF was observed, suggesting that NGF may not have been available to the grafted cells (Dubach and German, 1990). The report by Kordower *et al.* (1990), either with or without co-grafts of sural nerve, also provides encouragement that enhanced adrenal cell viability is feasible in intrastriatal grafts. Despite these encouraging findings of increased cell survival, a beneficial functional consequence is the goal of transplantation therapy for human patients. Both of these studies caution that conclusions regarding any behavioural benefit from these grafts are not yet definitive. Continued study in this respect as well as examination of long-term survival of the grafted cells and potential side-effects are needed in primates.

In summary, researchers have discovered that in animal models adrenal cells can: (1) survive grafting into a damaged host brain; (2) have a beneficial effect on a DA-related behavioural measure; and (3) affect local transmitter function. However, there are several unresolved aspects that need further examination prior to understanding the feasibility of adrenal cell grafting. For instance, although adrenal grafts can influence drug-induced rotational behaviour, they do not appear to have a significant effect on contralateral sensorimotor neglect in rats. The usefulness of these grafts on spontaneous behavioural parameters in parkinsonian monkeys also is unclear. Despite two recent reports of what could be considered to be excellent graft survival, most studies by a variety of investigators have shown modest survival of intrastriatal adrenal grafts. Furthermore, long-term effects and viability in rats appear to be dependent on NGF. A reliable, safe mode of NGF administration needs to be identified for primates. Finally, there is inconsistent evidence pertaining to the effectiveness of aged donor tissue and responsiveness of the aged host system. It will be important to elucidate more definitely these issues prior to application in human disease.

APPLICATIONS OF GRAFTING IN HUMAN PARKINSONISM

The first attempt of neural grafting in parkinsonian patients occurred in Sweden and the results were reported in 1985 (Backlund *et al.*, 1985). Adrenal medullary autografts were placed unilaterally into the caudate nucleus of two parkinsonian patients. This intervention resulted in transient minor improvement. A subsequent attempt by the Scandinavian researchers was made to implant medullary tissue into the putamen of two additional Parkinson's patients (Lindvall *et al.*, 1987). Again, only modest benefit from the procedure was observed in these patients. In spite of the careful approach taken in these early experiments, the field moved rapidly ahead following the publication of remarkable improvement in patients who received adrenal grafts through an open microsurgical approach in Mexico (Madrazo *et al.*, 1987). Apparent confirmation followed quickly from a study in Beijing, China (Jiao *et al.*, 1988) and stimulated considerable activity in the USA, as summarized by Goetz *et al.* (1989) who concluded from a multi-center effort involving six medical centers, that medullary transplants in 19 patients resulted in selective areas of improvement, primarily in the amount of 'on-time' versus 'off-time.' Although the results were viewed as encouraging, the degree of improvement was more modest than that reported earlier by Madrazo *et al.* (1987) and Jiao *et al.* (1988). There was no marked amelioration of the clinical signs of parkinsonism and the improvements occurred in patients while they were receiving stable doses of anti parkinsonian medication. Moreover, unlike the report from Mexico (Madrazo *et al.*, 1987), the patients in the subsequent multicenter study did not show benefits from reduced doses of medication. It is also noteworthy that significant medical complications frequently were experienced, e.g. a number of patients exhibited severe behavioral and psychological disabilities for extended periods after transplantation. In other studies, some mortalities occurred and post-mortem analysis of several of these patients reported the presence of only few surviving adrenal medullary cells at autopsy (Hurtig *et al.*, 1989; Kordower *et al.*, 1991; Hirsch *et al.*, 1990). Although Hurtig and coworkers (1989) identified adrenal cells with a relatively ubiquitous stain, chromagranin-A, they could not demonstrate these same cells with antibodies directed against TH in spite of the fact that the unoperated adrenal, as well as the residual substantia nigra, stained positively for TH in tissues taken at autopsy and prepared in a similar manner from this patient. Likewise, Hirsch *et al.*, (1990) found no evidence of TH positive cells in the necrotic graft 4 months post-transplantation. This may suggest a down-regulation of TH in surviving adrenal medullary cells following transplantation. In contrast, Kordower and colleagues (1991) did observe a few TH immunoreactive cells amidst large numbers of macrophages and tissue necrosis in their postmortem examination 30 months after implantation. Interestingly, Kordower *et al.*, (1991) and Hirsch *et al.*, (1990) observed enhanced host-derived TH-fiber staining in the striatum adjacent to the graft site, similar to that observed in mice and non-human primates (Bohn *et al.*, 1987; Fiandaca *et al.*, 1988; Bankiewicz *et al.*, 1988). Kordower and colleagues suggest that this potential 'graft-induced sprouting' may be a more likely mechanism for the transient 18 month period of behavioral improvement in their patient rather than catecholamine release from transplanted cells.

As clinical trials continued, the adrenal grafting experiments continued to provide equivocal results. At Vanderbilt University, investigators concluded that four of eighteen patients showed 'distinct improvement' in both signs and symptoms of parkinsonism one year after transplantation and that none showed a deterioration (Allen *et al.*, 1989). Six patients that were more severely debilitated were followed for only six months and did not show any improvement. Of these, four demonstrated deteriorated mental status that was interpreted to contraindicate the application of this approach to older patients with pre-existing cognitive deterioration.

Based on experimental findings in animal models of parkinsonism which demonstrated that NGF can enhance neurite outgrowth and viability of adrenal medullary cells, Olson and collagues (1991), infused this trophic factor into the site of a putamental adrenal autograft in a patient with Parkinson's disease. Similar to previous attempts there was a rapid albeit transient improvement in some symptoms. However, in contrast to other medullary graft recipients not receiving concomittent trophic support, there was a second, more gradual phase of improvement which lasted for one year. The definitive benefit of chronic infusion of NGF following adrenal transplantation, remains to be determined pending similar clinical trials. Despite some encouraging findings, the overall enthusiasm for adrenal medullary autografts for the treatment of Parkinson's disease has waned based on minimal and variable efficacy as well as transient benefit.

Several years after the advent of adrenal medullary grafting in patients, investigators began to explore whether embryonic mesencephalic DA neurons might be a more feasible treatment strategy for parkinsonism. These initial clinical trials were preceded by pilot studies testing the survival and function of human embryonic nerve cells following xenografting either into rats (Brundin *et al.*, 1986; Seiger *et al.*, 1988) or monkeys (Redmond *et al.*, 1988). In monkeys, the donor cells were first subjected to cryopreservation to test the feasibility of establishing a 'cell bank.' Although limited cell survival was seen, there was excellent quality of cell growth reflecting normal patterns of human neuronal development and capacity for grafted neurons to improve behavioral abnormalities (Brundin *et al.*, 1986; Redmond *et al.*, 1988).

The initial report of nigral cell grafting by Lindvall and colleagues (1989), described the unilateral stereotaxic implantation of human fetal substantia nigra of early gestational age (8–10 weeks gestation) into the caudate and putamen of two patients with advanced Parkinson's disease. In these as well as subsequent clinical trials, patients with moderate to severe Parkinson's disease were chosen largely because there was great need for therapeutic intervention in these patients in which drug therapy was no longer effective. In this initial study, immunosuppression was utilized, patients were maintained on antiparkinsonian medications and they were followed for six months pre- and post-operatively. In contrast to that observed following adrenal transplants, (1) there were no significant postoperative complications and (2) there was an initial worsening for both patients postoperatively followed by a small and gradual improvement in some clinical test parameters. There were indices suggestive of small grafts surviving twelve months after transplantation. These indices included enhanced premotor cortical electrical activity, primarily over the operated hemisphere and increased performance in neurophysiological measurements on the side contralateral to the transplant. The investigators theorized that the lack of significant improvement was most likely to be due to the survival of an insufficient number of nerve cells to provide an effective DA level in the grafted striatum. Many other reasons also could account for this, including a less than hospitable environment in the host striatum. Considering that a disease process may still be present, it is possible that grafted cells could be subjected to the same internal insult that destroyed the host nigrostriatal system. The advanced age of the recipient also could play a role. Lindvall and collagues (1989) also pointed out that the relatively large size of the implantation instrument could have caused too much tissue damage with resultant hemorrhage around the implanted tissue. Alternatively, tissue damage may be the one common denominator that links all of the reported 'successes' following adrenal, open surgical autografting. This may be consistent with early accounts in the neurosurgical literature of improvement in basal ganglia function following extirpation of large portions of the striatum or globus pallidus for example (Meyers

1942). It is possible that in response to tissue damage, neurotrophic factors or other elements that stimulate neuronal survival and regeneration may be released from the host system.

With cautious optimism, research employing embryonic nigral tissue continued and several groups reported some degree of symptomatic improvement (Hitchcock *et al.*, 1988; Madrazo *et al.*, 1988). More recently, the surgical procedure has been refined using smaller diameter cannulaes, reported to give better cell survival (see Freed *et al.*, 1933), and multiple drop sites. The first report providing evidence of significant graft-induced benefit in one patient that received unilateral nigral implants into the putamen was published in 1990 (Lindvall *et al.*). Again, success was attributed to the use of a greater amount of tissue (four embryonic midbrains at three putamenal sites) and reduced tissue damage as well as a reduction in the holding time for the embryonic cells.

These initial studies provided encouragement for more extensive trials with larger numbers of patients. Three recent reports (Freed *et al.*, 1993; Spencer *et al.*, 1993; Widner *et al.*, 1993), published simultaneously, have given cause for closer examination into the feasibility of human embryonic DA grafts for the treatment of Parkinson's disease. Freed and coworkers used up to 14 implant sites in 7 patients and reported improvements in activities of daily living from 3 to 12 months post-surgery as well as significant improvement on neurologic examination (e.g.: group mean Hoehn-Yahr value went from 3.71 to 2.50). In addition, drug doses were decreased and severity and duration of 'off' periods were reduced. Fluorodopa positron emission tomography (PET) in one patient gave evidence of graft survival 46 months after transplantation. Similarly, 3 of 4 patients receiving unilateral caudate grafts reported by Spencer *et al.*, (1993), also showed improved motor function and daily living activities; reduction in levodopa dosage and elimination of DA agonists; and importantly, improvements in drug free periods. There was one death related to complications unrelated to the surgery in this trial. Postmortem analyses revealed the presence of neuromelanin-containing neurons and evidence of synaptic connections, although no TH immunoreactivity was present. An important aspect of the clinical trials carried out by Spencer and coworkers was the inclusion of controls who would receive a graft after a one-year delay. Due to ethical concerns, controls in clinical trials have been problematic. The addition of 'one-year delay controls', managed identically to transplanted patients, provides valuable information on the course of the disease, daily fluctuations in diet, mood, medications, as well as expectation of the patient (Redmond *et al.*, 1993). Although these authors submit that the number of controls studied to date is too small to give a statistical evaluation, it does provide further evidence of graft-derived benefit over time.

Particularly interesting results were reported by Widner *et al.*, (1993) who transplanted embryonic mesecephalic DA neurons bilaterally into two patients with MPTP-induced parkinsonism. In effect these patients most closely approximated the condition reported by Redmond *et al.*, (1985) of reversal of MPTP-induced parkinsonism in non-human primates. In these patients, there was a substantial improvement in motor function which was sustained for 24 months after surgery. Both patients went from needing extensive assistance with daily activities such as eating, dressing, etc., to being able to perform most chores without assistance. Evidence of striatal DA uptake using PET imaging showed no change at 5–6 months post-transplant, however, at 12–13 and 22–24 months there was a marked elevation. These biochemical data correlated well with behavioral improvement seen in the patients and may have reflected the time course of maturation of the transplanted

DA neurons. The more dramatic recovery seen in these 2 MPTP-induced parkinsonian patients compared with that seen in the patients with idiopathic Parkinson's disease may have been related to several factors. The MPTP patients were logic candidates for graft replacement therapy for several reasons including: (1) their relative youth; (2) the relatively short duration of their lesion; (3) that the cause of degeneration was acute toxicity and not an ongiong disease process; (4) that the lesion is primarily localized in the nigrostriatal DA system; (5) the observation that previous work in MPTP treated non-human primates indicates feasibility of grafting to reverse lesion-induced deficits. Widner and coworkers point out that these patients may be a crucial bridge between work in non-human primates with MPTP-induced lesions and work in human patients with idiopathic Parkinson's disease.

The procedure is still experimental and a complete amelioration of parkinsonian symptoms has not been achieved. Despite the dramatic improvement in the MPTP lesioned patients, their Hoehn-Yahr scores, during practically defined off periods, only improved from 4–5 to 2.5–3. There are still numerous unresolved issues such as site of implantation, amount of tissue needed, optimal gestational age, method of tissue preparation, etc. There also has been great interest in defining growth factor(s) which may stimulate growth and viability of transplanted neurons as reviewed in the previous section. With the recent lifting of the government ban against the use of federal money to perform human fetal tissue research, there may be greater potential to resolve some of these remaining issues.

Finally, another possible barrier to the success of fetal cell grafts in humans is the need for continued precursor therapy which could potentially have a negative impact on the viability and function of grafted neurons. Specifically, we previously reported that twice daily injections of levodopa in rats with mesencephalic DA neuron grafts placed into their unilaterally lesioned striatum results in impaired morphological development (Steece-Collier *et al.*, 1990) and decrease effectiveness of grafted neurons to reverse DA agonist-induced rotational abnormalities associated with unilateral lesions (Yurek *et al.*, 1991). In contrast, Blunt and coworkers (1991) observed no detrimental effect of levodopa given in drinking water over 5 weeks to embryonic DA neurons. One factor which may be an important difference between these two studies is the route of administration. In our studies, we administered repeated boluses of drug whereas in the study by Blunt and colleagues, the animals were given the prescribed dosage over the entire day. Further investigation is needed to confirm the influence of route of administration and brain level of drug on viability of embryonic neurons.

While levodopa toxicity in a grafting paradigm remains unsettled, toxicity in cultured nigral DA neurons is well established (Steece-Collier *et al.*, 1990; Piano *et al.*, 1992; Kontur *et al.*, 1992). There is a dose-dependent decrease in neurite outgrowth and viability (Steece-Collier *et al.*, 1990) and reduction in DA levels and uptake sites (Kontur *et al.*, 1992) in monolayer cultures of mesencephalic DA neurons exposed to levodopa. There are several potential mechanisms by which these effects may occur. First, increased extracellular DA via levodopa treatment may impair neuronal function by decreasing synthesis and release of DA through feedback regulation. Second, elevated DA levels may result in increased generation of potentially neurotoxic oxidative metabolites of DA. Piano and coworkers (1992) have found that the antioxidant ascorbic acid can significantly reduce the negative effects of levodopa on cultured embryonic midbrain DA neurons. Thus, further examination of mechanism(s) by which levodopa can influence these neurons may be useful in developing treatment strategies which could circumvent problems of altered viability or function. Nevertheless, it would be premature at present to maintain that levodopa therapy is detrimental in human graft recipients. Clearly, continued examination of this phenomenon in both rodent and non-human primate models is needed.

Neural grafting has moved quickly within a short period of time since its rebirth in neurobiology laboratories about 25 years ago. It has provided critical information as a tool for studying the development and growth as well as the connectivity and maintenance of synapses of central neurons and has been aided by the development of transmitter and receptor-specific technologies to study the cellular mechanisms attendent to the growth process. Its clinical applications emerged quickly when improvements were seen following grafting into a number of neurologically deficient rodent models of endocrine disorders, motor abnormalities and cognitive defects (Sladek and Gash, 1988). A great need for intervention in debilitating neurodegenerative disorders prompted the application of grafting technology to the human condition, with reports of mixed success. Although this work was inevitable, the speed with which it moved was surprising. New frontiers involving the genetic engineering of immortalized cell lines offer great hope that ethical concerns about the use of human fetal tissue for transplantation can be circumvented at some point in the future (Gage *et al.*, 1987; Horellou *et al.*, 1990). Nevertheless, in spite of excellent progress by molecular engineering, the practical application of such cell lines may be several years away. In the interim, the addition of about 60 000 cases of parkinsonism in North America annually, coupled with the ever-increasing mean age of the population, signals the need seriously to consider the application of neural transplantation techniques in the clinics. A preventive strategy to delay the progression of neural degeneration report by the DATATOP study may obviate the need for neural grafting in early-onset patients (Shoulson *et al.*, 1989), but those individuals who either are unresponsive to protective therapies or whose nigrostriatal system has degenerated below threshold may, at some point, require surgical intervention to provide an essential boost to the host system. Additional and emerging strategies alternatively may signal the utility of implantation of cells that produce growth factors to stimulate or enhance the capacity of the residual DA system to provide a booster effect. These approaches alone or in combination may prove ultimately to be effective in the treatment of parkinsonism.

Acknowledgements

The authors thank Dr Timothy Collier for his constructive comments. This study was supported by The United Parkinson Foundation, and a grant from NINCDS (PO1-NS24032).

References

Allen GS, Burns S, Tulipan N, and Parker A (1989) Adrenal medullary transplantation to the caudate nucleus in Parkinson's disease. *Arch Neurol*, **46**, 487–91

Annett LE, Dunnett SB, Martel FL, Rogers DC, Ridley RM, Baker HF *et al.* (1990) A functional assessment of embryonic dopaminergic grafts in the marmoset. *Prog Brain Res*, **82**, 535–42

Arbuthnott G, Dunnett SB, and Macleod N (1985) Electrophysiological properties of single units in dopamine-rich mesencephalic transplants in rat brain. *Neurosci Lett*, **57**, 205–10

Backlund EO, Granberg PO, Hamberger B, Knutsson E, Martensson A, Sedvall G *et al.* (1985) Transplantation of adrenal medullary tissue to striatum in parkinsonism. First clinical trials. *J Neurosurg*, **62**, 169–73

Bakay RAE, Fiandaca MS, Barrow DL, Schiff A, and Collins DC (1985) Preliminary report on the use of fetal tissue transplantation to correct MPTP-induced Parkinson-like syndrome in primates. *Appl Neurophysiol*, **48**, 358–61

Bakey RAE, Barrow DL, Fiandaca MS, Iuvone PM, Schiff A, and Collins DC (1987) Biochemical and behavioral correction of MPTP Parkinson-like syndrome by fetal cell transplantation. *Ann NY Acad Sci*, **495**, 623–38

Bankiewicz KS, Plunkett RJ, Kopin IJ, Jacobowitz DM, London WT, and Oldfield EH (1988) Transient behavioral recovery in hemiparkinsonian primates after adrenal medullar allografts. *Prog Brain Res*, **78**, 543–9

Bankiewicz KS, Plunkett RJ, Jacobowitz DM, Porrino L, di Porzio U, London WT *et al.* (1990) The effect of fetal mesencephalon implants on primate MPTP-induced parkinsonism. *J Neurosurg*, **72**, 231–44

Becker JB and Freed SJ (1988) Adrenal medulla grafts enhance functional activity of the striatal dopamine system following substantia nigra lesions. *Brain Res*, **462**, 401–6

Bernheimer H, Birkmayer W, Hornykiewicz O, Jellinger K, and Seitelberger F (1975) Brain dopamine and syndromes of Parkinson and Huntington. *J Neurol Sci*, **30**, 415–55

Bing G, Jiao S, Notter MFD, Hansen JT, and Gash DM (1988a) Cografts of adrenal medulla with peripheral nerve in the dopamine-denervated rat striatum. *Soc Neurosci Abstracts* **14**, 735

Bing G, Notter MFD, Hansen JT, and Gash DM (1988b) Comparison of adrenal medullary, carotid body and PC12 cell grafts in 6-OHDA lesioned rats. *Brain Res Bull*, **20**, 399–406

Bing G, Notter MFD, Hansen JT, Kellogg C, Kordower JH, and Gash DM (1990) Co-grafts of adrenal medulla with C6 glioma cells in rats with 6-hydroxydopamine-induced lesions. *Neuroscience*, **34**, 687–97

Björklund A and Stenevi U (1979a) Reconstruction of the nigrostriatal dopamine pathway by intracerebral nigral transplants. *Brain Res*, **177**, 555–60

Björklund A and Stenevi U (1979b) Reconstruction of the nigrostriatal dopamine pathway by intracerebral nigral transplants. *Brain Res*, **177**, 555–60

Björklund A, Katzman R, Stenevi U, and West KA (1971) Development and growth of axonal sprouts from noradrenaline and 5-hydroxytryptamine neurons in the rat spinal cord. *Brain Res*, **31**, 21–33

Björklund A, Stenevi U, and Svendgaard NA (1976) Growth of transplanted monoaminergic neurons into the adult hippocampus along the perforant path. *Nature*, **262**, 787

Björklund A, Schmidt RH, and Stenevi U (1980) Functional reinnervation of the neostriatum in the adult rat by use of intraparenchymal grafting of dissociated cell suspensions from the substantia nigra. *Cell Tissue Res*, **212**, 39–45

Björklund A, Stenevi U, Schmidt RH, Dunnett S, and Gage FH (1983) Intracerebral grafting of neuronal cell suspensions. II. Survival and growth of nigral cell suspensions implanted in different brain sites. *Acta Physiol Scand*, **522** (suppl), 9–18

Blunt S, Jenner P, Marsden D (1991) The effect of chronic l-dopa treatment on the recovery of motor function in 6-hydroxydopamine-lesioned rats receiving ventral mesencephalic grafts. *Neurosci*, **40**, 453–64

Bohn MC, Cupit L, Marciano F, and Gash DM (1987) Adrenal medulla grafts enhance recovery of striatal dopaminergic fibers. *Science*, **237**, 913

Brundin P, Isacson O, Gage FH, and Björklund A (1986) Intrastriatal grafting of dopamine-containing neuronal cell suspensions: Effects of mixing with target or non-target cells. *Devel brain Res.*, **24**, 77–84

Brundin P, Nilsson OG, Strecker RE, Lindvall O, Astedt B, and Björklund A (1986) Behavioural effects of human fetal dopamine neurons grafted in a rat model of Parkinson's disease. *Exp Brain Res*, **65**, 235–40

Buell SJ and Coleman PD (1979) Dendritic growth in aged human brain and failure of growth in senile dementia. *Science*, **206**, 854–6

Burns RS, Chiueh CC, Markey SP, Ebert MH, Jacobowitz DM, and Kopin IJ (1983) A primate model of parkinsonism: selective destruction of dopaminergic neurons in the pars compacta of the substantia nigra by N-methyl-4-phenyl-1,2,3,6-tetrahydropyridine. *Proc Natl Acad Sci*, **80**, 4546–50

Casper D, Mytilineou C, and Blum M (1991) EGF enhances the survival of dopamine neurons in rat embryonic mesencephalon primary culture. *J Neurosci Res*, **30**, 372–81

Collier TJ and Springer JE (1991) Co-grafts of embryonic dopamine neurons and adult sciatic nerve into the denervated striatum enhance behavioral and morphological recovery in rats. *Exper Neurol*, **114**, 343–50

Collier TJ, Martin PN, Maguire BA, Springer JE (1992) Grafted Schwann cells and infusion of a Schwann cell-derived growth factor (DNTF) enhance morphological recovery in the damaged adult rat dopamine system. *Soc Neurosci*, **18**, 1292

Das GD (1974) Transplantation of embryonic neural tissue in the mammalian brain. I. Growth and differentiation of neuroblasts from various regions of the embryonic brain in the cerebellum of neonate rats. *Life Sci*, **4**, 93–124

Date I, Felten SY, Olschowka JA, and Felten DL (1990a) Limited recovery of striatal dopaminergic fibers by adrenal medullary grafts in MPTP-treated aging mice. *Exp Neurol*, **107**, 197–207

Date I, Felten SY, and Felten DY (1990b) Cografts of adrenal medulla with peripheral nerve enhance the survivability of transplanted adrenal chromaffin cells and recovery of the host nigrostriatal dopaminergic system in MPTP-treated young mice. *Brain Res* (in press)

Date I, Felten SY, and Felten DL (1990c) The nigrostriatal dopaminergic system in MPTP-treated mice shows more prominant recovery by syngeneic adrenal medullary graft than by allogeneic or xenogeneic graft. *J Neurosurg*,

Dubach M and German DC (1990) Extensive survival of chromaffin cells in adrenal medulla 'ribbon' grafts in the monkey neostriatum. *Exp Neurol*, **110**, 167–80

Dunn EH (1917) Primary and secondary findings in a series of attempts to transplant cerebral cortex in albino rat. *J Comp Neurol*, **27**, 565–82

Dunnett S, Björklund A, Stenevi U, and Iversen S (1981) Behavioural recovery following transplantation of substantia nigra in rats subjected to 6-OHDA lesions of the nigrostriatal pathway. I. Unilateral lesions. *Brain Res*, **215**, 147–61

Dunnett S, Björklund A, Schmidt RH, Stenevi U, and Iversen SD (1983) Intracerebral grafting of neuronal cell suspensions. IV. Behavioral recovery in rats with unilateral 60HDA lesions following implantation of nigral cell suspensions in different forebrain sites. *Acta Physiol Scand*, **522** (suppl), 29–38

Dunnett SB, Hernandez TD, Summerfield A, Jones, GH, and Arbuthnott G (1988) Graft-derived recovery from 6-OHDA lesions: specificity of ventral mesencephalic graft tissue. *Exp Brain Res*, **71**, 411–24

Engele J, Bohn MC (1991) The neurotrophic effects of fibroblast growth factors on dopaminergic neurons in vitro are mediated by mesencephalic glia. *J Neurosci*, **11**, 3070–78

Fiandaca MS, Kordower JH, Hansen JT, Jiao S-S, and Gash DM (1988) Adrenal medullary autografts into the basal ganglia of cebus monkeys: injury-induced regeneration. *Exp Neurol*, **102**, 76–91

Fine A, Hunt SP, Oertel WH, Nomoto M, Chong PN, Bond A *et al.* (1988) Transplantation of embryonic marmoset dopaminergic neurons to the corpus striatum of marmosets rendered parkinsonian by 1-methyl-4-phenyl-1,2,3,6-tetrahydropyridine. *Prog Brain Res*, **78**, 479–89

Freed CR, Breeze RE, Rosenberg NL, Schneck SA, Kriek E, Qi J-X, *et al.* (1993) Survival of implanted dopamine cells and neurologic improvement 12 to 46 months after transplantation for Parkinson's disease. *N Engl J Med*, **327**, 1549–55

Freed C, Breeze RE, Rodenberg NL, Schneck SA (1993) Embryonic dopamine cell implants as a treatment for the second phase of Parkinson's disease. *Adv Neurol*, **60**, 721–28

Freed WJ (1983) Functional brain tissue transplantation: reversal of lesion-induced rotation by intraventricular substantia nigra and adrenal medulla grafts, with a note on intracranial retinal grafts. *Biol Psychiatry*, **18**, 205–67

Freed WJ, Perlow MJ, Karoum F, Seiger A, Olson L, Hoffer B, and Wyatt RJ (1980) Restoration of dopaminergic function by grafting of fetal rat substantia nigra to the caudate nucleus: long-term behavioral, biochemical and histochemical studies. *Ann Neurol*, **8**, 510–19

Freed WJ, Morihisa JM, Spoor E, Hoffer B, Olson L, Seiger A *et al.* (1981) Transplanted adrenal chromaffin cells in rat brain reduce lesion-induced rotational behaviour. *Nature*, **292**, 351–2

Freed WJ, Ko GN, Niehoff D, Kuhar M, Hoffer BJ, Olson L *et al.* (1983) Normalization of spinoperidol binding in the denervated rat striatum by homologous grafts of substantia nigra. *Science*, **222**, 937–9

Freed WJ, Cannon-Spoor HE, and Krauthamer E (1986) Intrastriatal adrenal medulla grafts in rats. *J Neurosurg*, **65**, 664–70

Freund TF, Bolam JP, and Björklund A (1985) Efferent synaptic connections of grafted dopaminergic neurons reinnervating the host neostriatum: a tyrosine hydroxylase immunocytochemical study. *J Neurosci*, **5**, 603–16

Gage FH, Björklund A, Stenevi U, and Dunnett SB (1983a) Intracerebral grafting of neuronal cell suspensions VII. Survival and growth of implants of nigral and septal cell suspensions in intact brains of aged rats. *Acta Physiol Scand*, **522** (suppl), 67–75

Gage FH, Dunnett SB, Stenevi U, and Björklund A (1983b) Aged rats: recovery of motor impairments by intrastriatal nigral grafts. *Science*, **221**, 966–9

Gage FH, Wolff JA, Rosenberg MB, Xu L, Yee J-K, Shults C *et al.* (1987) Grafting genetically modified cells to the brain: possibilities for the future. *Neuroscience*, **23**, 795–807

Gash DM and Sladek JR Jr (1989) Neural transplantation: problems and prospects – where do we go from here? *Mayo Clin Proc*, **64**, 363–7

German DC, Dubach M, Askari S, Speciale SG, and Bowden DM (1988) 1-Methyl-4-phenyl-1,2,3,6-tetrahydropyridine-induced parkinsonian syndrome in *Macca fascicularis*: which midbrain dopaminergic neurons are lost? *Neuroscience*, **24**, 161–74

Goetz CG, Olanow CW, Koller WC, Penn RD, Cahill D, Morantz R *et al.* (1989) Multicenter study of autologous adrenal medullary transplantation of the corpus striatum in patients with advanced Parkinson's disease. *N Engl J Med*, **320**, 337–41

Hadjiconstantinou M, Fitkin JG, Dalia A, and Neff NH (1991) Epidermal growth factor enhances striatal dopaminergic parameters in the 1-methyl-4-phenyl-1,2,3,6-tetrahydropyridine-treated mouse. *J Neurochem*, **57**, 479–482

Hagglund J, Aquilonous SM, Eckernas SA, Hartvig P, Lundquist H, Gullberg P *et al.* (1987) Dopamine receptor properties in Parkinson's disease and Huntington's chorea evaluated by positron emission tomography using 11C-N-methyl-spiperone. *Acta Neurol Scand*, **75**, 87–94

Hallman H, Lange J, Olson L, Stromberg I, and Jonsson G (1985) Neurochemical and histochemical characterization of neurotoxic effects of 1-methyl-4-phenyl-1,2,3,6-tetrahydropyridine on brain catecholamine neurons in the mouse. *J Neurochem*, **44**, 117–27

Hansen JT, Kordower JH, Fiandaca MS, Jiao S-S, Notter MFD, and Gash DM (1988) Adrenal medullary autografts into the basal ganglia of cebus monkeys: graft viability and fine structure. *Exp Neurol*, **102**, 65–75

Herrera-Marschitz M, Stromberg I, Olsson D, Ungerstedt U, and Olson L (1984) Adrenal medullary implants in the dopamine-denervated rat striatum. II. Acute behavior as a function of graft amount and location and its modulation by neuroleptics. *Brain Res*, **297**, 53–61

Hirsch EC, Duyckaerts C, Javoy-Agid F, Hauw J-J, Agid Y (1990) Does adrenal graft enhance recovery of dopaminergic neurons in Parkinson's disease? *Ann Neurol*, **27**, 676–82

Hitchcock ER, Clough C, Hughes R, Kenny B (1988) Embryos and Parkinson's disease.*Lancet*, **1**, 1274

Hoffer B, Sieger Å, Ljungberg T, Olson L (1974) Electrophysiological and cytological studies of brain homografts in the anterior chamber of the eye: maturation of cerebellar cortex *in oculo*. *Brain Res*, **79**, 165–84

Horellou P, Brundin P, Kalen P, Mallet J, and Björklund A (1990) *In vivo* release of dopa and dopamine from genetically engineered cells grafted to the denervated rat striatum. *Neuron*, **5**, 393–402

Hurtig H, Joyce J, Sladek JR Jr and Trojanowski JQ (1989) Postmortem analysis of adrenal-medulla-to-caudate autograft in a patient with Parkinson's disease. *Ann Neurol*, **25**, 607–14

Hyman C, Hofer M, Barde Y-A, Juhasz M, Yancopoulos GD, Squinto SP, Lindsay RM (1991) BDNF is a neurotrophic factor for dopaminergic neurons of the substantia nigra. *Nature*, **350**, 230–32

Jaeger CD (1985) Cytoarchitectonics of substantia nigra grafts: a light and electron microscopic study of immunocytochemically identified dopaminergic neurons and fibrous astrocytes. *J Comp Neurol*, **231**, 121–35

Jiao S, Zhang W, Cao J, Zhang ZM, Wang H and Ding MC (1988) Study of adrenal medullary tissue transplantation to striatum in parkinsonism. *Prog Brain Res*, **78**, 575–80

Knusel B, Winslow JW, Rosenthal A, Burton LE, Seid DP, Nikolics K, Hefti F (1991) Promotion of central cholinergic and dopaminergic neuron differentiation by brain-derived neurotrophic factor but not neurotrophin 3. *PNAS* (USA), **82**, 6330–34

Knusel B, Beck KD, Winslow JW, Rosenthal A, Burton LE, Widmer HR, Nikolics K, and Hefti F (1992) Brain-derived neurotrophic factor administration protects basal forebrain cholinergic but not nigral dopaminergic neurons from degenerative changes after axotomy in the adult rat brain. *J Neurosci*, **12**, 4391–4402

Knusel B, Michel PP, Schwaber JS, and Hefti F (1990) Selective and nonselective stimulation of central cholinergic and dopaminergic development in vitro by nerve growth factor, basic fibroblast growth factor, epidermal growth factor, insulin and the insulin-like growth factors I and II. *J Neurosci*, **10**, 558–570

Kontur PJ, Marek KL, Redmond DE, Roth RH (1992) L-dopa toxicity in cultures of rat mesencephalic dopamine neurons. *Soc Neurosci*, **18**, 1576

Kordower JH, Cochran E, Penn RD, Goetz CG (1991) Putative chromaffin cell survival and enhanced host-derived TH-fiber innervation following a functional adrenal medulla autograft for Parkinson's disease. *Ann Neurol*, **29**, 405–12

Kordower JH, Fiandaca MS, Notter MFD, Hansen JT, and Gash DM (1990) NGF-like trophic support from peripheral nerve for grafted rhesus adrenal chromaffin cells. *J Neurosurg*, (in press)

Langston JW, Ballard P, Tetrud JW and Irwin I (1983) Chronic parkinsonism in humans due to a product of meperidineanalog synthesis. *Science*, **219**, 979–80

LeGros Clark WE (1940) Neuronal differentiation in implanted foetal cortical tissue. *J Neurol Psychiatry*, **3**, 263–72

Lin L-F H, Doherty DH, Lile JD, Bektesh S, Collins F (1993) GDNF: A glial cell line-derived neurotrophic factor for midbrain dopaminergic neurons. *Science*, **260**, 1130–32

Lindvall O (1989) Transplantation into the human brain: present status and future possibilities. *J Neurol Neurosurg Psychiatry* (suppl), 39–54

Lindvall O, Backlund EO, Farde L, Sedvall G, Freedman R, Hoffer B (1987) Transplantation in Parkinson's disease: two cases of adrenal medullary grafts to the putamen. *Ann Neurol*, **22**, 457–68

Lindvall O, Rehncrona S, Brundin P, Gustavii B, Astedt B, Widner H (1989) Human fetal dopamine neurons grafted into the striatum in two patients with severe Parkinson's disease. *Arch Neurol*, **46**, 615–31

Lindvall L, Brundin P, Widner H, Rehncrona S, Gustavii B, Frackowiak R *et al.* (1990) Intrastriatal grafts of fetal dopamine neurons survive and improve motor function in Parkinson's disease. *Science*, **247**, 574–7

Longo AM and Penhoet EE (1974) Nerve growth factor in rat glioma cells. *Proc Natl Acad Sci*, **71**, 2347–9

Madrazo I, Drucker-Colin R, Diaz V, Martinez-Mata J, Torress C and Becerril JJ (1987) Open microsurgical autograft of adrenal medulla to the right caudate nucleus in two patients with intractable Parkinson's disease. *N Engl J Med*, **316**, 831–4

Madrazo I, Leon V, Torres C, del Carmen Aguilera M, Varela G, Alvarez F *et al.* (1988) Transplantation of fetal substantia nigra and adrenal medulla to the caudate nucleus in tow patients with Parkinson's disease. *New Eng J Med*, **318**, 51

Mahalik TJ, Finger TE, Stromberg I, and Olson L (1985) Substantia nigra transplants into denervated striatum of the rat: ultrastructure of graft and host interconnections. *J Comp Neurol*, **240**, 60–70

Meyers R (1942) The modification of alternating tremors, rigidity and festination by surgery of the basal ganglia. *R Assoc Nerv Mental Dis*, **21**, 602–65

Moore RY, Björklund A, and Stenevi U (1974) Growth and plasticity of adrenergic neurons. In Schnitt FO and Worden FG, eds, *The Neurosciences: The Third Study Program*, Cambridge, MA, MIT Press, 961–77

Morihisa JM, Nakamura RK, Freed WJ, Mishkin M, and Wyatt RJ (1984) Adrenal medulla grafts survive and exhibit catecholamine specific fluorescence in the primate brain. *Exp Neurol*, **84**, 642–53

Morisha JM, Nakamura RK, Freed WJ, Mishkin M, and Wyatt RJ (1987) Transplantation techniques and the survival of adrenal medulla autografts in the primate brain. *Ann NY Acad Sci*, **495**, 599–605

Nathan CF, Murray HW, and Cohn ZA (1980) The macrophage as an effector cell. *N Engl J Med*, **303**, 622–6

Olson L (1970) Fluorescence histochemical evidence for axonal growth and secretion from transplanted adrenal medullary tissue. *Histochemie*, **22**, 1–7

Olson L, Backlund EO, Ebendal T, Freedman R, Hamberger B, Hansson P, Hoffer B, Lindblom U, Meyerson B, Stromberg I, Sydow O, Seiger A (1991) *Arch Neurol*, **48**, 373

Olson L and Sieger Å (1972) Brain tissue transplanted to the anterior chamber of the eye. 1. Fluorescence histochemistry of immature catecholamine and 5-hydroxytryptamine neurons reinnervating the rat iris. *Z Zellforsch*, **135**, 175–94

Olson L, Sieger Å, Freedman R, and Hoffer B (1980) Chromaffine cells can innervate brain tissue: evidence from intraocular double grafts. *Exp Neurol*, **70**, 411–26

Otto D, Unsicker K (1990) Basic FGF reverses chemical and morphological deficits in the nigrostriatal system of MPTP-treated mice. *J Neurosci*, **10**, 1912–1921

Paino CL, Pardo B, Mena MA (1992) L-dopa toxicity in embryonic mesencephalic neurons prevented by ascorbic acid. *Restorative Neurol and Neurosci*, **4**, 167

Perlow MJ, Freed WJ, Hoffer FM, Seiger A, Olson L and Wyatt RJ (1979) Brain grafts reduce motor abnormalities produced by destruction of nigrostriatal dopamine system. *Science*, **204**, 643–7

Pezzoli G, Fahn S, Dwork A, Truong DD, deYebenes JG, Jackson-Lewis V *et al.* (1988) Non-chromaffin tissue plus nerve growth factor reduces experimental parkinsonism in aged rats. *Brain Res*, **459**, 398–403

Phelps CJ and Sladek JR Jr (1984) Plasticity of catecholaminergic neurons in aged rat brain: reinnervation and functional recovery after axotomy. *Brain Res Bull*, **13**, 727–36

Redmond DE Jr, Sladek JR Jr, Roth RH, Collier TJ, Ellsworth JD, Deuthch AY and Haber S (1986) Fetal neuronal grafts in monkeys given methylphenyltetrahydropyridine. *Lancet*, **1**, 1125–7

Redmond DE, Naftolin F, Collier TJ, Leranth C, Robbins RJ, Sladek CD *et al.* (1988) Cryopreservation, culture, and transplantation of human fetal mesencephalic tissue into monkeys. *Science*, **242**, 768–71

Redmond DE, Robbins RJ, Naftolin F, Marck KL, Vollmer TL, Leranth C *et al.* (1993) Cellular replacement of dopamine deficit in Parkinson's disease using human fetal mesencephalic tissue:

preliminary results in four patients. In *Molecular and Cellular Approaches of Neurological Disease*, SG Waxman, ed, Raven Press, New York, 325–59

Reisine TD, Fields JZ, and Yamamura HI (1977) Neurotransmitter receptor alterations in Parkinson's disease. *Life Sci*, **21**, 335–44

Rinne UK, Rinne JO, Rinne JK, Laakso K, Laihinen A, and Lonnberg P (1983) Brain receptor bhanges in Parkinson's disease in relation to the disease process and treatment. *J Neural Transm*, **18**, (suppl), 279–86

Sauer H, Fischer W, Nikkhah G, Brundin P, Lindsay RM, and Björklund A (1992) Effects of BDNF-administration in rats grafted with fetal nigral tissue. *Restorative Neurol and Neurosci*, **4**, 197

Schneider JS, Pope A, Simpson K, Taggart J, Smith MG, DiStefano L (1992) Recovery from experimental parkinsonism in primates with GM1 ganslioside treatment. *Science*, **256**, 843–46

Schmidt RH, Ingvar M, Lindvall O, Stenevi U and Björklund A (1982) Functional activity of substantia nigra grafts reinnervating the striatum: neurotransmitter metabolism and [^{14}C]2-deoxy-D-glucose autoradiography. *J Neurochem*, **38**, 737–48

Schmidt RH, Björklund A, Stenevi U, Dunnett SB, and Gage FH (1983) Intracerebral grafting of neuronal cell suspensions III. Activity of intrastriatal nigral suspension implants assessed by measurements of dopamine synthesis and metabolism. *Acta Physiol Scand*, **522**, (suppl), 19–28

Seiger A, Bygdeman M, Goldstein M, Almqvist P, Hoffer B, Stromberg I *et al.* (1988) Human fetal catecholamine-containing tissues grafted intraocularly and intracranially to immuno-compromised rodent hosts. *Prog Brain Res*, **78**, 449–55

Shoulson I, Fahn S, Oakes D, Odoroff C, Lang A, Langstron JW *et al.* (the Parkinson Study Group) (1989) Effect of deprenyl on the progression of disability in early Parkinson's disease. *N Engl J Med*, **321**, 1364–71

Sieger Å and Olson L (1977) Quantitation of fiber growth in transplanted central monoamine neurons. *Cell Tissue Res*, **179**, 285–316

Sladek JR Jr and Gash DM (1988) Nerve-cell grafting in Parkinson's disease. *J Neurosurg*, **68**, 337–51

Sladek JR Jr and Shoulson I (1988) Neural transplantation: a call for patience rather than patients. *Science*, **240**, 1386–8

Sladek JR Jr, Collier TJ, Haber SN, Roth RH, and Redmond DE (1986) Survival and growth of fetal catecholamine neurons transplanted into primate brain. *Brain Res Bull*, **17**, 809–18

Sladek JR Jr, Redmond DE Jr, Collier TJ, Blount JP, Elsworth JD, Taylor JR and Roth RH (1988) Fetal dopamine neural grafts: extended reversal of methylphenyltetrahydropyridine-induced parkinsonism in monkeys. *Prog Brain Res*, **78**, 497–506

Sladek JR, Jr., Elsworth JD, Roth RH, Evans LE, Collier TJ, Cooper TJ, Taylor JR, Redmond DE, Jr. (1993) Fetal Dopamine Cell survival after transplantation is dramatically improved at a critical donor gestational age in non-human primates. *Exp Neurol*, **122**, 16–27

Spencer DD, Robbins RJ, Naftolin F, Marek KL, Vollmer T, Leranth C (1993) Unilateral transplantation of human fetal mesencephalic tissue into the caudate nucleus of patients with Parkinson's disease. *N Engl J Med*, **327**, 1541–48

Steece-Collier K, Collier TJ, Sladek CD, and Sladek JR Jr (1990) Chronic levodopa impairs morphological development of grafted embryonic dopamine neurons. *Exp Neurol*, **110**, 201–8

Steinbusch HWM, Vermeulen RJ, Tonnaer JADM (1990) Basic fibroblast growth factor enhances survival and sprouting of fetal dopaminergic cells implanted in the denervated rat caudate-putamen: Preliminary observations. In: Neural Transplantation From Molecular Basis to Clinical Applications, *Prog Brain Res*, **82**, 81–86, SB Dunnett and S-J Richards (Eds.), Elsevier, Amsterdam

Stenevi U, Björklund A, and Svendgaard NA (1976) Transplantation of central and peripheral monoamine neurons to the adult rat brain: techniques and conditions for survival. *Brain Res*, **114**, 1–20

Stenevi U, Emson P, and Björklund A (1977) Development of dopamine sensitive adenylate cyclase in hippocampus reinnervated by transplanted dopamine neurons: evidence for new functional contacts. *Acta Physiol Scand*, **452**, (suppl), 39–42

Stromberg I, Herrera-Marschitz M, Hultgren L, Ungerstedt U, and Olson L (1984) Adrenal medullary implants in the dopamine-denervated rat striatum. I. Acute catecholamine levels in grafts and host caudate as determined by HPLC-electrochemistry and fluorescence histochemical image analysis. *Brain Res*, **297**, 41–51

Stromberg I, Herrera-Marschitz M, Ungerstedt U, Ebendal T, and Olson L (1985) Chronic implants of chromaffin tissue into the dopamine-denervated striatum. Effects of NGF on graft survival, fiber growth and rotational behavior. *Exp Brain Res*, **60**, 335–49

Thompson WG (1890) Successful brain grafting. *NY Med J*, **51**, 701

Ungerstedt U (1974) Functional dynamics of central monoamine pathways. In Schmitt FO and Worden FG, eds, *The Neurosciences Third Study Program*, Cambridge, MA, MIT Press, 979–88

VanHorne CG, Stromberg I, Young D, Olson L, Hoffer B (1991) Functional enhancement of intrastriatal dopamine-containing grafts by the co-transplantation of sciatic nerve tissue in 6-hydroxydopamine-lesioned rats. *Exper Neurol*, **113**, 143–54

Weber RJ, Ewing SE, Zauner A, and Punkett RJ (1989) Recovery in hemiparkinsonian rats following intrastriatal implantation of activated leukocytes. *Soc Neurosci Abstracts*, **15**, 123

Widner H, Tetrud J, Rehncrona S, Snow B, Brundin P, Gustavii B *et al.* (1993) Bilateral fetal mesencephalic grafting in two patients with parkinsonism induced by 1-methyl-4-phenyl-1,2,3,6-tetrahydropyridine (MPTP). *N Engl J Med*, **327**, 1556–63

Wuerthele SM, Freed WJ, Olson L, Morisha J, Spoor L, Wyatt RJ and Hoffer BJ (1981) Effect of dopamine agonists and antagonists on the electrical activity of substantia neurons transplanted into the lateral ventricle of the rat. *Exp Brain Res*, **44**, 1–10

Yurek DM, Collier TJ, Sladek JR Jr (1990) Embryonic mesencephalic and striatal co-grafts: Development of grafted dopamine neurons and functional recovery. *Exper Neurol*, **109**, 191–99

Yuerk D, Steece-Collier K, Collier TJ, and Sladek JR Jr (1991) Chronic levodopa impairs the recovery of dopamine agonist-induced rotational behavior following neural grafting. *Exp Brain Res*, **86**, 97–107

12
Transplantation – the clinical position

Olle Lindvall

INTRODUCTION

The clinical application of neural transplantation in patients with Parkinson's disease (PD) and Huntington's disease (HD) was first suggested in 1979 (Björklund and Stenevi, 1979; Perlow *et al.*, 1979) and 1983–1984 (Deckel *et al.*, 1983; Isacson *et al.*, 1984), respectively, when intracerebral grafts of fetal central nervous system (CNS) tissue could be demonstrated to ameliorate motor and cognitive deficits in animal models of these disorders (for details, see Chapter 11). These major scientific achievements occurred early in the development of this research field and, in fact, the reversal of parkinsonian symptoms by implanted mesencephalic tissue was the first example of functional effects of neural grafts in an experimental model of a human disease state. The findings supported the possible clinical usefulness of the cell replacement paradigm, i.e. that specific cell populations that are lost in the host brain can be replaced by grafted neurons, which leads to partial or complete functional restoration. During the last decade much animal work has been devoted to basic problems related to the mechanisms of action of neural grafts, e.g. to clarify the level of integration of the grafts anatomically and functionally in the host neuronal circuitries, and whether they exert their effects via a synaptic release of transmitter or through a trophic action, stimulating sprouting of the recipient's own neuronal systems.

When looking back at the development of clinical neural transplantation, it may be argued that the application of this approach in patients should have waited until more animal experiments had been carried out (Landau, 1990). The introduction of cell transplantation as a possible treatment for PD and HD has, of course, been prompted by the lack of adequate medical therapy and the severity of symptoms in these disorders. It must be underscored, however, that the grafting in patients with PD performed so far cannot be viewed as clinical trials of procedures that have been optimized in animal experiments. It would be unfair, therefore, to compare the results with those obtained after established treatments. Instead, it must be remembered that the first clinical trials using grafting in PD have intended to test whether the basic principles of cell replacement established in animal experiments are also valid in the diseased human brain. The danger when viewing the clinical trials carried out so far as tests of a new therapy (and even considering starting randomized, placebo-controlled studies at this stage) is that such a classification could lead to the erroneous conclusion that the symptomatic relief induced by intracerebral grafts is only minor. It must therefore be clearly stated that the optimal clinical grafting procedure for PD has not yet been developed, and that no treatment for PD and HD based on cell transplantation is presently available. On the other hand, the animal experimental work performed during the last decade and the positive findings reported in PD patients with implants of fetal dopamine (DA)-rich mesencephalic tissue provide further support for the idea that neural grafting can be developed into a useful treatment in PD and possibly other neurological disorders.

The major objectives of the present chapter are fourfold: firstly, to summarize the results of clinical trials with grafting of fetal mesencephalic tissue and adrenal medulla autotransplantation, respectively, in patients with PD; secondly, to describe current basic and clinical research strategies in order to proceed further towards a transplantation therapy in PD; thirdly, to analyse the prospects for successful clinical application of neural grafting in patients with HD; and, fourthly, to discuss some more general issues of importance for the development of transplantation procedures in PD and HD.

GRAFTING OF FETAL DOPAMINE NEURONS IN PARKINSON'S DISEASE

Results from clinical trials

It is estimated that 140 patients with PD have so far received implants of human fetal mesencephalic tissue into the striatum. Tables 12.1 and 12.2 summarize the (often incomplete) data reported from clinical studies performed on 70 patients. Two major surgical approaches have been used (Fig. 12.1): either stereotaxic implantation of dissociated tissue directly into the striatum, or placement of pieces or fragments of nigral tissue into a cavity in the head of the caudate nucleus. The grafts have been placed unilaterally and, in 7 patients, bilaterally in the caudate nucleus and/or putamen. In most studies, tissue from only one fetus has been used in each patient, but Lindvall *et al.* (1989, 1990a,b, 1992) implanted tissue from four fetuses and the patients grafted bilaterally by Widner *et al.* (1992) received mesencephalic tissue from six to eight fetal cadavers. Fetal ages have varied from 6 to 19 weeks. The preoperative assessment period ranges from 1 to 12 months and in several cases has not been reported. In most studies (except in those of Lindvall *et al.*, 1989, 1990a,b, 1992 and Widner *et al.*, 1992), doses of antiparkinsonian medication have been changed at the time of transplantation and/or postoperatively. All patients have been subjected to immunosuppressive treatment, except those operated on by Hitchcock and co-workers (Henderson *et al.*, 1991), and 3 of the patients of Freed *et al.* (1990, 1992). Few attempts to show graft survival have been undertaken.

The reported results can be summarized as follows (Table 12.2):

1. Some general improvement of motor symptoms has been observed in almost all patients after implantation of fetal mesencephalic tissue. The degree of this functional change varies from minor to moderate but in no case there has been a full reversal of symptomatology.
2. The improvement has been observed as a prolonged duration of L-dopa response (Lindvall *et al.*, 1990a, 1992) and by several groups as increased percentage of

Table 12.1 Study design of clinical trials with grafting of human fetal mesencephalic tissue into the striatum of patients with Parkinson's disease

Authors	*Number of patients*	*Tissue preparation[a] surgical technique[b] uni- or bilateral*	*Location[c]/number[d] of implantations*	*Number[e]/age[f] of fetal cadavers*	*Duration of pre/postoperative assessment period[g]*	*Changes of antiparkinsonian medication during study period[h]*	*Immuno-suppression*	*Attempts to show graft survival*
Lindvall *et al.* (1989, 1990b)	2	Diss/ster/uni	Caud/1 + Put/2	4/8–10 weeks (m)	6/20 months	No	Yes	PET
Lindvall *et al.* (1990a, 1992, 1993)	2	Diss/ster/uni	Put/3	4/8–10 weeks (m)	6–11/36 months	No	Yes	PET
Madrazo *et al.* (1990c, 1991)	4	Fragm/open/uni	Caud/1	1/12–14 weeks (g)	NR/19–32 months	Yes	Yes	No
Molina *et al.* (1991)	30	Fragm/open/uni	Caud/1	1/6–12 weeks	30–45 days/ –24 months	Yes	Yes	CSF
Henderson *et al.* (1991)	12	Diss/ster/uni	Caud/1	1/11–19 weeks (g)	1–6 weeks/ 12 months	Yes	No	No
Freed *et al.* (1990, 1992)	7	Diss or strand/ster/ uni (2) or bi (5)	Caud + Put uni (2) or Put bi (5)/10–14	1 (6) or 2 (1)/ 7–8 weeks (g)	4–12/12–46 months	Yes	Yes (4), no (3)	PET
López-Loranzo *et al.* (1991b)	7	Fragm/open/uni	Caud/1	1/8–17 weeks (m)	NR/7 months	Yes	Yes	No
Widner *et al.* (1992)	2	Diss/ster/bi	Caud/1 + Put/3 bi (1) Caud/0–1 + Put/3 bi (1)	6–8/6–8 weeks (pc)	18/22–24 months	No	Yes	PET
Spencer *et al.* (1992)	4	Fragm (cryo)/ster/uni	Caud/2–4	1/7–11 weeks (g)	NR/18 months	Yes	Yes	PET

[a] Diss = cell suspension or dissociated tissue; fragm = tissue fragments; strand = strand of tissue; cryo = cryopreserved.
[b] Ster = stereotaxic implantation; open = open microsurgery with implantation into a cavity.
[c] Caud = caudate nucleus; put = putamen; uni = unilateral; bi = bilateral.
[d] Number of implantation sites.
[e] Number of fetal donors for tissue implanted in each patient.
[f] Age of fetal cadavers (weeks) as reported: m, menstrual; g, gestational; pc, post conception.
[g] Time period during which the patient is included in the transplantation program and subjected to regular clinical assessments: NR = not reported.
[h] Defined as from start of preoperative assessment to 6 months postoperatively.
Number of patients is given within parentheses.
CSF = Cerebrospinal fluid; PET = positron emission tomography.

Table 12.2 Results from clinical trials with grafting of human fetal mesencephalic tissue into the striatum of patients with Parkinson's disease[a]

Authors	*Number of patients*[b]	*Degree of reported improvement*[c]									*Latency to first signs/peak of improvement*	*Adverse effects*	*Evidence of graft survival*
		Overall motor performance	*% on time*[d]	*Duration of L-dopa response*[e]	*Tremor*	*Rigidity*	*Brady-/ hypokinesia*	*Gait*	*Dyskinesia*	*Balance*			
Lindvall *et al.* (1989, 1990b)	2	+	0	0	0	0	+	+	NO	0	1–3/5–6 months	No	(+)[h]
Lindvall *et al.* (1990a, 1992, 1993)	1 1	+ + + +(+)	+ + + + +	+ + + +	0 0	+ + + +(+)	+ + + +	0 0	NO NO	0 0	6 weeks/5 months 3/24 months	No Minor	+ + + + +
Madrazo *et al.* (1990c, 1991)	2 2	+ +(+) + +	+ +	NR	0	+ +	+ +	+ +	NR	+ +	1–2/8 months	Brain abscess (1)	No
Molina *et al.* (1991)	26 4	+ +(+) + +	+ +(+)	NR	+ +	+ +	+ +	+ +	+ +	+ +	12 hours/6 months	'Postsurgical syndrome'	No
Henderson *et al.* (1991)[g]	1 2 6	+ + +(+) 0	+	NR	NR	NR	+	NR	+	NR	Immediate/3 months	No[h]	No
Freed *et al.* (1990, 1992)	4 2 1	+ + + 0	+ +	NR	NR	NR	+ +	+(+)	+ +	+ +	6 weeks/6 months	No	(+) (1)
López-Lozano *et al.* (1991b)	7	+	NR	NR	NR	NR	NR	NR	NR	NR	3/7 months	No	No
Widner *et al.* (1992)	2	+ +(+)	+ +	+	+	+ +(+)	+ +(+)	+ +(+)	+ +	+ +	6/24 months	No	+ +
Spencer *et al.* (1992)	3 1	+ 0	NR	NR	+	+	+	+	NR	NR	NR/NR	Minor	No

[a]The results summarized in Table 12.2 refer to the clinical trials in Table 12.1.
[b]The patients are grouped according to the reported changes in overall motor performance.
[c]The symptomatic relief has been scored on the basis of the data presented as follows: 0 = no improvement; + = small improvement of no or minor therapeutic value; + + = moderate improvement of clear therapeutic value; + + + = excellent, of major therapeutic value, complete reversal of symptoms, no medication.
[d]Percentage of time awake spent in mobile phase. NR = not reported.
[e]In specific tests of motor response after a single dose of L-dopa.
[f]Changes of fluorodopa uptake in grafted striatum as assessed by positron emission tomography were scored on the basis of data presented as follows: 0 = no change; + = small increase; + + = moderate increase, but still with pathological uptake; + + + = major increase, uptake within the normal range.
[g]Clinical data reported in nine out of twelve operated patients.
[h]One patient died at 17 months of causes not related to grafting.
NO = Not observed.

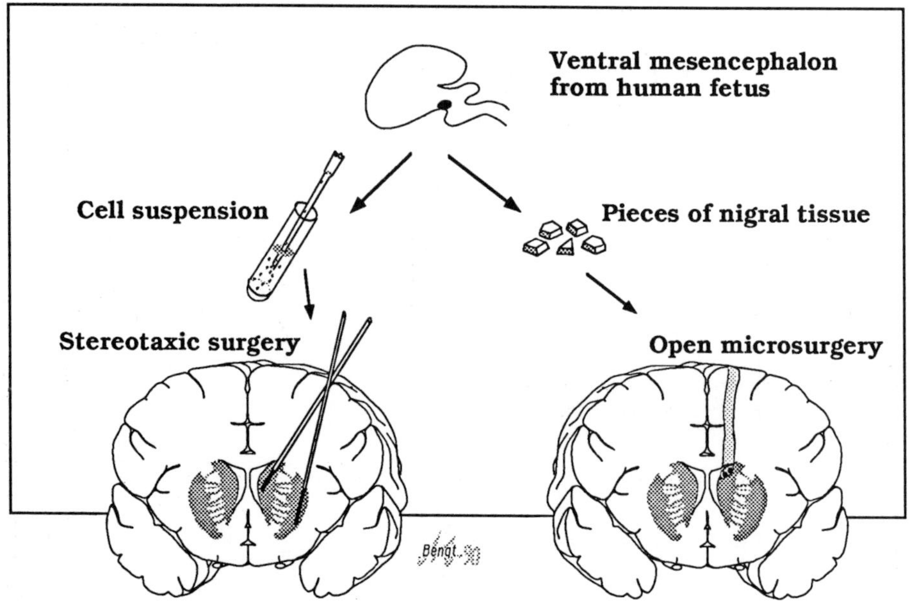

Figure 12.1 Schematic representation of the two alternative procedures used for grafting of human fetal dopamine neurons into the striatum of patients with Parkinson's disease. The ventral mesencephalon is either prepared as a cell suspension which is implanted stereotaxically into the caudate nucleus and/or putamen, or divided into pieces which are put into a premade cavity in the head of the caudate nucleus.

time spent in 'on' phase and reduction of the severity of symptoms, particularly during the 'off' time (Figs 12.2–12.5).

3. Regarding individual symptoms, tremor has shown little change except in the patients of Molina *et al.* (1991). The most consistent improvement has been observed for rigidity and hypo-/bradykinesia, but significant changes of gait and balance have also been reported by Madrazo *et al.* (1990c, 1991), Molina *et al.* (1991), Freed *et al.* (1992) and Widner *et al.* (1992).
4. Some studies have described therapeutically valuable reduction of the severity and duration of dyskinesias after transplantation.
5. The latency reported for the appearance of the first positive signs has varied considerably (from immediately after implantation up to 3–6 months) and improvement has continued up to 24 months postgrafting (Fig. 12.5 and Lindvall *et al.*, 1993).
6. No major adverse effects related to the implantation of fetal tissue have been reported. One patient developed a brain abscess (Madrazo *et al.*, 1991) and another partial motor seizures (Spencer *et al.*, 1992). One patient (Lindvall *et al.*, 1993) has shown increased blood pressure secondary to immunosuppressive treatment with cyclosporine. All patients operated on by Molina *et al.* (1991), using an open microsurgical technique, developed a transient 'postsurgical syndrome'. Some clinical features of this syndrome, which came regularly 1–3 times daily and lasted up to 3 months, were anxiety, hyperthermia, flushing, arterial hypertension, tachycardia and polyuria. Molina *et al.* (1991) have proposed that the postsurgical syndrome is directly related to the fetal DA-rich transplant, but this interpretation

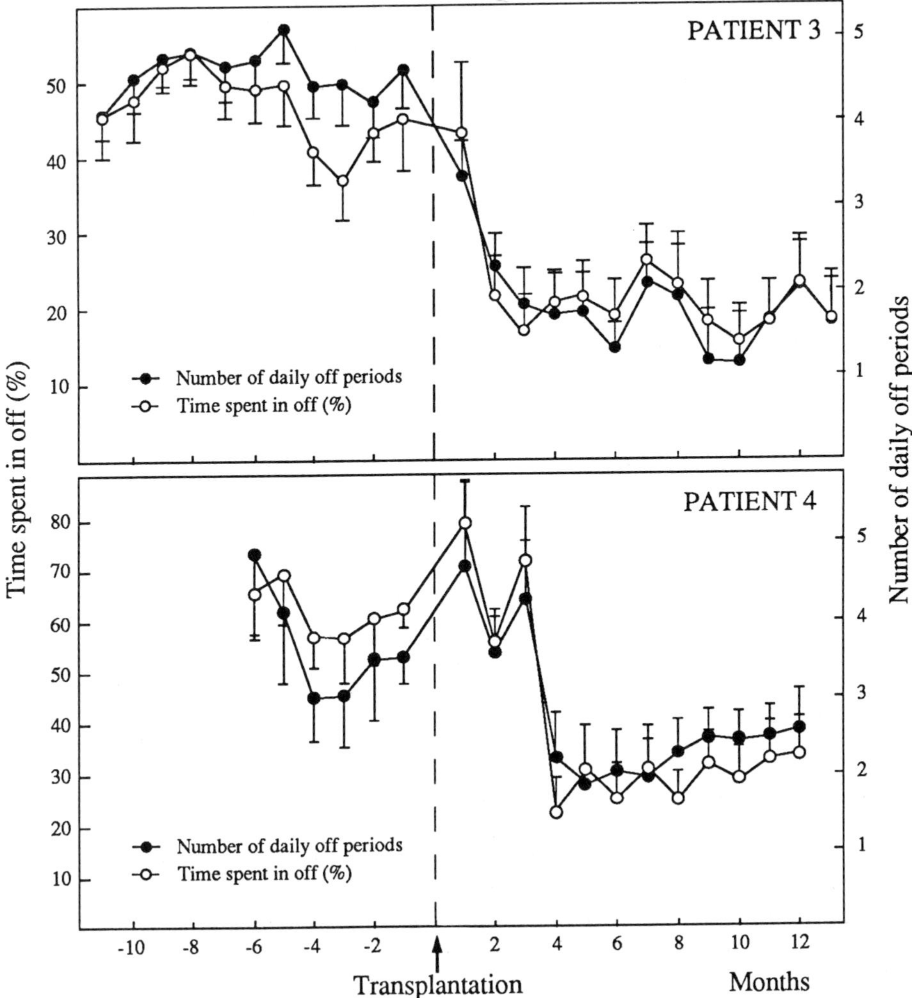

Figure 12.2 The mean monthly percentage of awake time spent in 'off' phase and the mean number of 'off' periods per day for each month (based on daily self-scoring by the patients) for 2 patients implanted with mesencephalic tissue from four 8–10-week-old fetuses into the putamen, either on the left (patient 3) or the right side (patient 4). Bars indicate 99% confidence limits. During the second and fourth postoperative month, respectively, there was a marked reduction of both the time spent in 'off' and the number of daily 'off' periods. Data from Lindvall *et al.* (1990a, 1992).

seems unlikely since these symptoms have not been observed in any other clinical grafting studies.

7. Evidence for survival of grafted DA neurons has been provided only for 5 patients (Lindvall *et al.*, 1990a, 1992; Freed *et al.*, 1992; Sawle *et al.*, 1992; Widner *et al.*, 1992). Autopsy studies on 2 patients who died of causes unrelated to grafting 1 and 4 months, respectively, after implantation of fetal mesencephalic tissue have been reported to show surviving CNS tissue, although no presumed DA neurons could be found (Redmond *et al.*, 1989; J. Dymecki, personal communication).

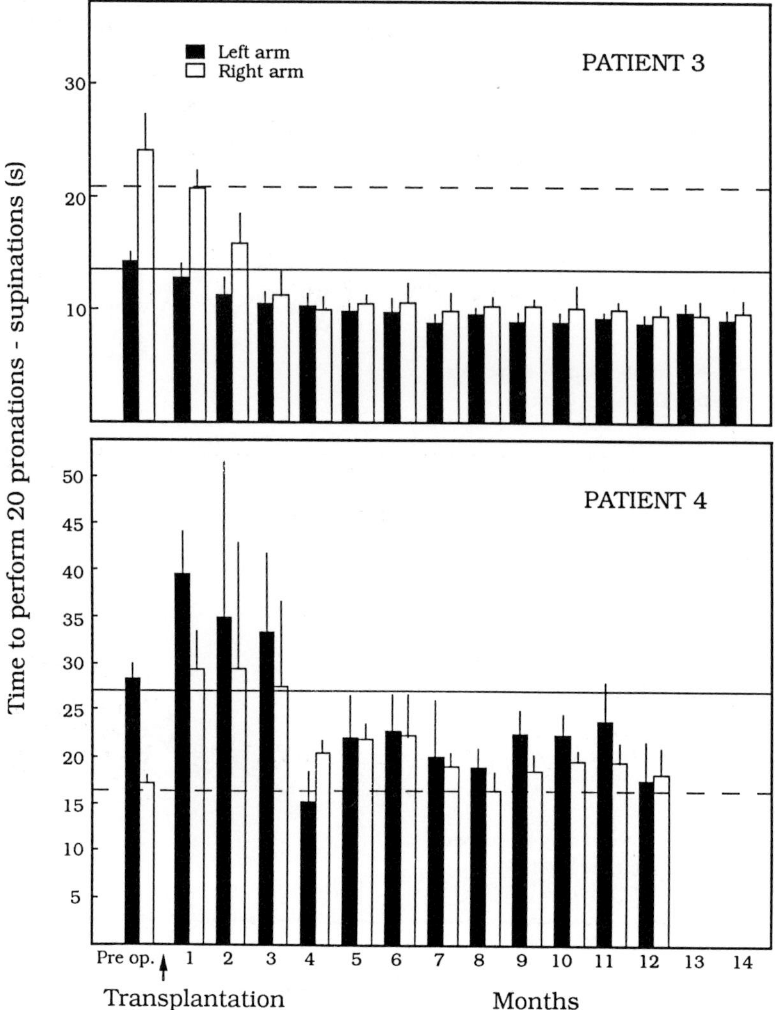

Figure 12.3 Time taken to perform 20 pronations-supinations with the left (solid blocks) and right (open blocks) arm in the 'off' state in patients 3 and 4 (see Fig. 12.2). Mean of measurements with 99% confidence limits. The horizontal lines show the preoperative means minus confidence limits for the left (continuous line) and right (dashed line) arm. From the second (patient 3) and fourth (patient 4) month after transplantation this task is performed more rapidly than preoperatively. The improvement is bilateral in patient 3, but most pronounced on the right side (contralateral to the graft); in patient 4, improvement is only observed on the left side (contralateral to the graft). Data from Lindvall *et al.* (1990a, 1992).

Positron emission tomography (PET) has demonstrated a significant increase of 6-L-(^{18}F) fluorodopa uptake confined to the grafted putamen in 2 patients with idiopathic PD who improved clinically (Fig. 12.6; Lindvall *et al.*, 1990a, 1992; Sawle *et al.*, 1992). Similarly, 2 patients with 1-methyl-4-phenyl-1,2,5,6-tetrahydropyridine (MPTP)-induced parkinsonism, who were grafted bilaterally

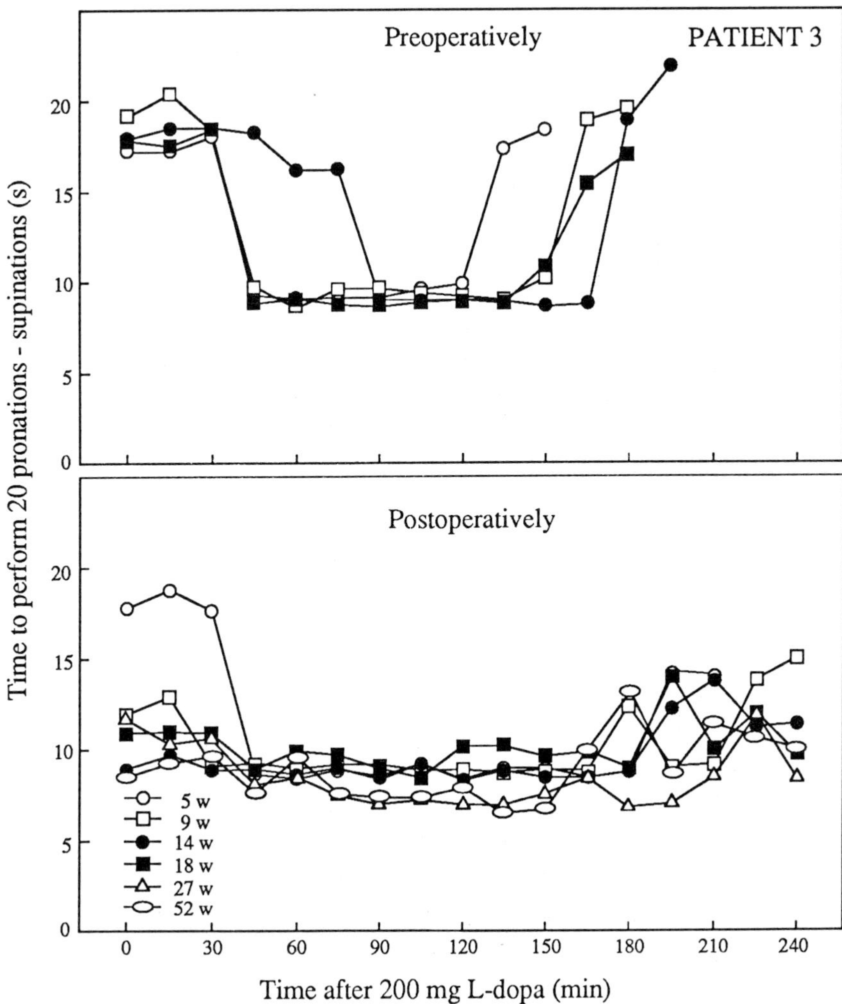

Figure 12.4 Effect on motor performance in patient 3 (see Fig. 12.2) of a single dose of L-dopa given after a 14-hour drug-free period. The time taken to perform 20 pronations-supinations with the right arm was recorded every 15 minutes up to 4 hours after administration of 200 mg L-dopa. Each line respresents an individual trial performed at 9.00 a.m. (the patient fasted overnight). Top: The performance in four trials conducted 2–4 months before grafting. Bottom: The performance in six trials performed at 5–52 weeks after transplantation. After the fifth postoperative week, the patient's motor performance before L-dopa intake improved, the duration of the drug-induced 'on' phase became longer, and there was no immediate major worsening of motor symptoms at the end of the 'on' period, as had always been seen preoperatively. Data from Lindvall *et al.* (1990a, 1992).

in the caudate nucleus and putamen, have exhibited a gradual and marked increase of striatal fluorodopa uptake on both sides (Widner *et al.*, 1992). Freed *et al.* (1992) have described significant increase of fluorodopa uptake in the grafted putamen at 33 months as compared to 9 months after surgery. Since there is no evidence for a breach in the blood–brain barrier (Lindvall *et al.*, 1990a, 1992;

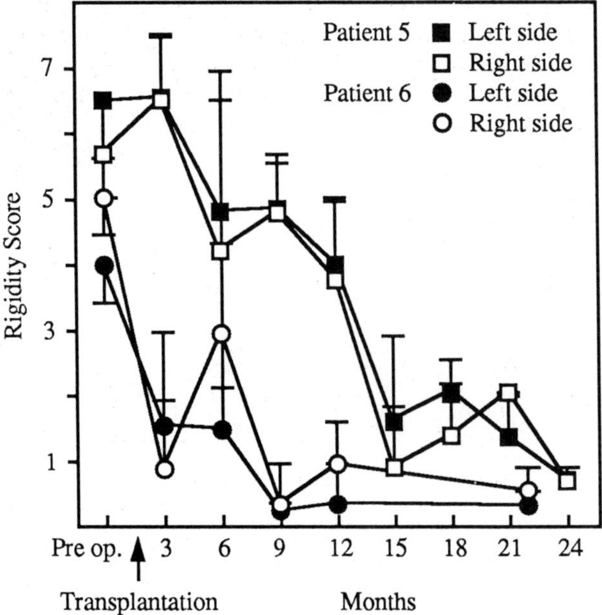

Figure 12.5 Rigidity scores in the 'off' state in 2 patients with 1-methyl-4-phenyl-1,2,5,6-tetrahydropyridine (MPTP)-induced parkinsonism (patients 5 and 6 in our own series) implanted bilaterally in the caudate and putamen with mesencephalic tissue from three to four fetuses on each side. The rigidity scale is a four-point scale of the degree of rigidity in the wrist, below and knee joints: 0 = no rigidity; 1 = slight rigidity; 2 = clear rigidity; 3 = severe rigidity. The total score is obtained by adding the scores for each joint. The maximal score is 9 per side. The lowest 25 percentiles are given for the preoperative values, and the highest 25 percentiles are given for the postoperative values. Beginning at about 6 months after grafting there was a gradual and marked bilateral decrease of muscle rigidity in both patients. Data from Widner *et al.* (1992).

Freed *et al.*, 1990; Sawle *et al.*, 1992), ths most likely explanation is that the grafts had restored DA synthesis and storage in the implanted region. This is probably due to survival and growth of grafted DA neurons, although a trophic effect of the fetal tissue leading to axonal sprouting of the host's own DA system cannot be excluded (see below).

In conclusion, the clinical trials reported so far indicate that fetal neural tissue can be implanted into the human brain without major risks. Improvements have been observed to a varying degree in almost all cases but the underlying mechanisms are often unclear. Even in the best cases, no complete reversal of multiple or single parkinsonian symptoms has been obtained. The differences in the design of available studies with regard to duration of preoperative assessment period, drug regimens and methods of evaluation and the lack of data on graft survival in most patients make the results from various groups difficult to compare. This variable design also

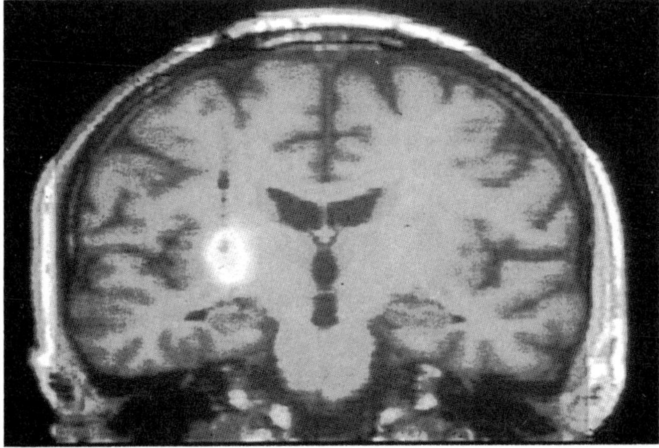

Figure 12.6 Combined magnetic resonance imaging (MRI)/positron emission tomography (PET) data from patient 3 (see Figure 12.2) acquired 3 years after operation. The MRI data (in grey scale) shows a coronal section through one of the operative needle tracks. The 6-L (^{18}F) fluorodopa PET data (in arbitrary colour scale) shows tracer uptake at the site of implantation in the left putamen, indicating the presence of a surviving dopaminergic graft. Data from Lindvall *et al.* (1993). Courtesy of Dr Guy Sawle.

means that it is impossible to draw any conclusions about the relative importance for graft survival and function of, for example, surgical and tissue preparation techniques, number of implantation sites, number and age of fetuses and use of immunosuppression.

Research strategies

Although there is now good evidence that grafts of human fetal DA neurons can survive and exert functional effects in the parkinsonian brain, this constitutes only a first step towards a transplantation therapy in PD. It remains to be clarified how frequently graft survival and function can be obtained in patients and whether nigral grafts survive permanently and have long-lasting functional effects. If the graft is destroyed, for example, due to the disease process itself, immunological mechanisms or the lack of trophic factors, new treatment strategies must be developed to prevent this degeneration. Further work is also necessary to optimize the transplantation procedures with respect to the yield of surviving DA neurons and the location and number of implantation sites necessary to achieve the largest possible symptomatic improvement. It seems highly warranted to agree on common principles for the design of clinical trials with fetal DA neuron transplantation, which would make the results obtained by different investigators directly comparable. It is of critical importance to establish with a non-invasive technique such as PET to what extent the graft has survived and restored DA transmission in the striatum. Verification of graft survival is necessary in order to be able to evaluate in detail different factors of possible importance for successful grafting in patients, such as fetal age, number of fetuses used, placement (caudate nucleus versus putamen versus both; unilateral versus bilateral grafts), time interval between abortion and implantation, whether antiparkinsonian drug treatment affects graft function and survival, and if immunosuppressive treatment is necessary. Some of the major scientific problems will be discussed in the following sections.

MONITORING GRAFT SURVIVAL AND FUNCTION

At present PET seems to be the only technique that can provide quantitative *in vivo* data regarding DA function within both the graft and the host brain. 6-L-(^{18}F)fluorodopa is the tracer most commonly used to demonstrate the functional integrity of the human DA system (see, for example, Leenders *et al.*, 1986b). After intravenous injection, this tracer accumulates in DA terminals and loss of nigral neurons in PD is accompanied by a reduction of striatal fluorodopa uptake on PET. For clinical studies with DA neuron grafting in PD the usefulness of the PET technique seems to be several-fold: firstly, PET allows characterization of the pattern of DA denervation in each patient before transplantation, which, in addition to providing a preoperative baseline, also could be of importance for the selection of implantation sites; secondly, PET provides the ability to monitor survival and possibly also growth of a graft; and, thirdly, with PET one can follow degeneration of intrinsic DA neurons in non-grafted regions. In fact, sequential fluorodopa scans in 2 PD patients have provided evidence not only for survival and growth of grafted DA neurons but also for disease progression, as suggested by reduced uptake of fluorodopa in parts of the striatum outside the graft (Sawle *et al.*, 1992).

A committee formed at the international symposium Intracerebral Transplantation in Movement Disorders – Experimental Basis and Clinical Experiences, Lund, Sweden, 1990, has proposed guidelines for how clinical trials with neural grafting should be standardized, mainly with respect to inclusion criteria and methods of assessment (Langston *et al.*, 1992). The main recommendations are the following: (1) the patient should have idiopathic PD and respond to L-dopa; (2) antiparkinsonian medication should be kept unchanged (if possible) for a minimum of 3 months preoperatively and 12 months postoperatively; (3) the patient should be observed for at least 6 months preoperatively and 12 months postoperatively. A minimum of three examinations before and three to four examinations after transplantation must be performed; (4) the clinical assessment protocol has to include self-scoring of time spent in 'on' and 'off' periods, scoring according to Hoehn and Yahr and Unified Parkinson's Disease Rating Scale (UPDRS), timed neurological tests such as repeated pronation-supination, and tests of the response to a single dose of L-dopa after drug withdrawal overnight; (5) if possible, a fluorodopa PET scan should be performed preoperatively and at 6 months after grafting; (6) the staging of the donor fetuses must be defined exactly.

YIELD OF SURVIVING DA NEURONS AND VOLUME OF REINNERVATION

It has been estimated that in rat-to-rat grafting experiments using the cell suspension technique a maximum of 10% of the fetal DA neurons survive in the adult striatum (Brundin and Björklund, 1987). When dissociated human fetal DA neurons are implanted into the DA-denervated striatum of immunosuppressed rats, the survival rate is about 5% (Brundin *et al.*, 1988b) – slightly lower than that observed when using fetal rat tissue. This figure forms the basis for estimations on the amount of fetal mesencephalic tissue needed to effect a significant symptomatic improvement in clinical trials (Lindvall *et al.*, 1987b), but the actual survival rate of fetal DA neurons in the human brain is unknown. It seems reasonable to assume that the functional effect in PD patients is correlated to the number of surviving DA neurons and the degree of reinnervation. The survival rate of DA neurons must therefore be increased in future transplantations to improve the clinical outcome and to allow for a significant DA reinnervation at multiple deposits, despite the limited availability of human fetal tissue. Presently, the low yield of surviving DA neurons after grafting is poorly understood. One important factor seems to be the degree of tissue damage at the implantation site (Brundin *et al.*, 1990), which suggests that the size of the implantation instrument may be of crucial importance for neuron survival.

Another possibility to increase graft survival has been raised by Finger and Dunnett (1989), who showed a significant increase of the volume of mesencephalic grafts if the rat hosts had been treated with the calcium channel antagonist, nimodipine. It was not clear, however, if there was also an increased number of DA neurons in the grafts.

In the future, the graft may be supplied with some trophic factor, not only to increase the number of DA neurons surviving transplantation, but also their volume of reinnervation in the striatum. It can be estimated that if human fetal DA neurons are implanted along three tracts in the putamen (as in the 4 patients of Lindvall *et al.*, 1992, and Widner *et al.*, 1992) still only about 25% of the total volume of this structure is reached by a graft-derived reinnervation with a density 25% or more of normal. In a nearly completely denervated human parkinsonian brain, a DA terminal density of 25% could represent a critical level for obtaining functional effects. Brain-derived neurotrophic factor (BDNF), basic fibroblast growth factor (bFGF) and platelet-derived growth factor (PDGF) have been shown to enhance DA uptake and the number of neurite-bearing cells in cultures of mesencephalic DA neurons (Ferrari *et al.*, 1989; Knüsel *et al.*, 1990, 1991; Hyman *et al.*, 1991; Nikkhah *et al.*, 1993). These trophic factors could be added to the graft tissue before and/or after implantation in order to enhance survival and axonal outgrowth of the DA neurons. However, the effects of BDNF, bFGF and PDGF after administration to DA grafts *in vivo* are yet unclear. Infusion of BDNF into the lateral ventricle or directly into the implant did not influence the survival of the grafted DA neurons or their axonal outgrowth in the striatum (Sauer *et al.*, 1993). Only minor effects of bFGF were found on sprouting from intrastriatal grafts of fetal DA neurons (Steinbusch *et al.*, 1990). Another approach to obtain a more complete reinnervation of the striatal complex is to distribute the graft material over larger areas and bilaterally, which may carry an additional surgical risk.

DRUG TREATMENT

The symptomatic drug treatment of patients with PD could be potentially harmful to the grafted tissue, particularly during its growth and development. It also seems possible that the chronic drug treatment could lead to postsynaptic changes, making the host brain less responsive to the action of the graft. In patients severely affected with PD, drug therapy must be maintained until beneficial effects appear, which may not occur until several months after the operation. It has been suggested that L-dopa treatment may accelerate the degeneration of remaining intrinsic nigrostriatal DA neurons in PD patients. One way this might occur is through an autoxidation of L-dopa, which has been reported to produce many cytotoxic substances such as free radicals and quinones (Graham *et al.*, 1978). In rat-to-rat grafting experiments, L-dopa treatment has either been described to have no detrimental affect (Blunt *et al.*, 1991; Chalmers and Fine, 1991) or to reduce maturation, growth and function of implanted

DA neurons (Steece-Collier *et al.*, 1991). If the latter is true for human fetal DA neurons, which should be tested in animal experiments, it will obviously have implications for the selection of patients for transplantation in the future. It may then be necessary to confine this procedure to patients who can manage without L-dopa, at least during the period of development and growth of the graft. However, the long-term data from clinical trials (Widner *et al.*, 1992; Lindvall *et al.*, 1993) indicate that grafted human DA neurons can survive, grow and function at least up to 3 years after implantation, despite ongoing antiparkinsonian drug therapy.

GRAFT PLACEMENT

In rat-to-rat grafting experiments, functional recovery has only been obtained if the mesencephalic DA-rich tissue has been placed near the target area, i.e. within or directly outside the striatum (Dunnett *et al.*, 1983). This is most probably due to the inability of the grafted DA neurons to extend their axons over a great distance, such as from the substantia nigra to the forebrain target region. However, in their ectopic striatal location, probably only part of the anatomical and functional connections characteristic for normal mesostriatal DA neurons are re-established by the grafts. This might then lead to a situation where nigral grafts would be effective for some but not all symptoms of PD. Experiments in rats support this idea by showing, for example, that the impairment in skilled movement with the contralateral limb after unilateral lesion of the mesostriatal DA system is not improved by fetal nigral grafts (Dunnett *et al.*, 1987). Furthermore, although such grafts reverse deficits in simple sensorimotor orientation observed in experimental PD, they do not ameliorate impairments in a more complex sensorimotor integrative task, in which the rat has to perform the orienting response while in the act of eating (Mandel *et al.*, 1990). Inability of a graft to reverse a DA-mediated behaviour might reflect an insufficient integration of the graft into the host brain. It seems highly warranted to clarify in more detail to what extent nigral grafts are effective and ineffective, respectively, on particular parkinsonian deficits in non-human primates and if a failure to compensate can be referred to a lack of integration or proper activation of the graft.

More complete integration would probably require implantation of the grafts in the ventral mesencephalon (where the neurons could receive their normal afferent inputs) which, in turn, would necessitate elongated growth of DA axons to reach the striatum. In a recent study (Wictorin *et al.*, 1992), human fetal DA neurons implanted into the substantia nigra of immunosuppressed rats were observed to grow along the mesostriatal pathway and give rise to a terminal plexus in the denervated striatum. Although the implications for human-to-human grafting trials are as yet unclear, the results indicate that the activity of presumed growth-inhibiting factors present along the pathway might be overcome under certain conditions.

It also seems possible, however, that the placement of the graft should be carefully selected to reverse a particular symptom in a PD patient and that insufficient relief could be explained by inappropriate choice of implantation site. Studies in the rat brain have clearly shown that DA neurons implanted into specific subregions of the denervated striatum compensate for specific features of the hemiparkinsonian syndrome (Dunnett *et al.*, 1981, 1983). Postural (rotational) asymmetry can be reversed by grafts reinnervating the dorsal caudate putamen, whereas grafts innervating the ventrolateral part of the striatum ameliorate deficits in sensorimotor attention but have no effects on rotational asymmetry. Given numerous other similarities between the primate and rodent basal ganglia, it is highly likely that such a topography also exists in the primate brain but it remains to be shown how it is organized. In a recent report (Dunnett and Annett, 1991), monkeys with caudate grafts (but not those with putamen grafts) showed good recovery of rotational asymmetry. In contrast, the data indicated that the monkeys with putamen grafts improved their skills in reaching into tubes and reduced the contralateral neglect. This also underscores the importance of graft placement in clinical transplantations for the pattern of functional recovery. It should be noted though, as stated by Dunnett and Annett (1991), that the 'degree of functional change in each animal still falls far short of optimal recovery'.

In most human trials the fetal nigral grafts have been placed unilaterally either in the caudate nucleus or the putamen, although some patients have received grafts in both structures. It seems unlikely that reinnervating one part of the striatal complex, on one side, would lead to optimal graft-induced recovery in PD. Therefore, one obvious change in order to increase symptomatic relief would be to implant nigral tissue on both sides. The current clinical findings indicate that grafts have bilateral effects, although the improvement has been most marked contralaterally. Implantation of DA-producing cells into the ventral striatum in some patients might be necessary, since it has been reported (Brundin *et al.*, 1987) that grafts in the rat nucleus accumbens are important for the amplitude of locomotion. In patients with marked disturbances of the locomotor component of movement, maximal recovery can therefore probably only be obtained with multiple graft placements also involving the nucleus accumbens.

GRAFTING OF ADRENAL MEDULLA IN PARKINSON'S DISEASE

Results from clinical trials

The first clinical trials with adrenal medulla autotransplantation were carried out using stereotaxic implantation (Fig. 12.7) in 4 PD patients between 1982 and 1985. Only very modest changes were observed (Backlund *et al.*, 1985; Lindvall *et al.*, 1987a). The major interest in this approach emerged from the study by Madrazo *et al.* (1987), in which they reported successful adrenal medulla autotransplantation in 2 young patients with PD. Instead of a stereotaxic approach, Madrazo and co-workers used open microsurgical techniques and implanted pieces of adrenal medullary tissue through the cerebral cortex into a premade cavity in the head of the caudate nucleus (Fig. 12.7). Madrazo *et al.* (1990a,b) have summarized their findings up to 1–3 years postoperatively in 42 consecutive cases with adrenal medullary autografts implanted unilaterally in the caudate nucleus. Four patients died and 4 others could not be followed up. As assessed by different rating scales, 60% of the 34 patients showed good response, 20% moderate improvement and only 20% responded poorly. The quality of life improved clearly in 53% of the patients. The improvement was always bilateral and affected primarily rigidity, bradykinesia, postural instability and gait disturbances. The mean L-dopa dose could be reduced by 60%. Morbidity and mortality were significantly reduced after the first 15 cases (among whom all the deaths occurred). Madrazo *et al.* (1989) have also summarized briefly the clinical outcome in 106 patients after adrenal medulla autotransplantation performed in Mexico, Chile, Cuba and Spain (so-called Hispanic Registry of Graft Procedures for Parkinson's Disease; see also López-Lazano *et al.*, 1991a). Nine patients died (8%), and the others were followed for 6 months or more. Of these, 32% showed a good

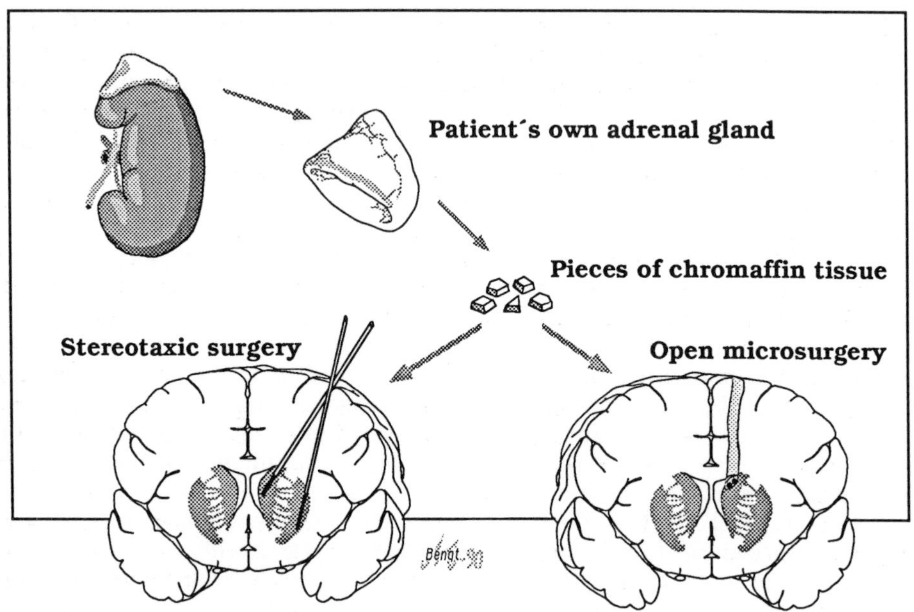

Figure 12.7 Schematic representation of the two alternative procedures used for grafting of adrenal medulla cells into the striatum of patients with PD. Pieces of chromaffin tissue have either been implanted into the caudate nucleus or putamen using stereotaxic surgical techniques or with open microsurgery into a premade cavity in the head of the caudate nucleus.

response (50–90% improvement), 27% a moderate response (30–50%), 15% had a poor response (5–30% improvement) and 9% showed no change. There were numerous complications.

Other groups have, however, not been able to replicate the dramatic results of Madrazo and co-workers using a similar surgical technique. In a series of 61 patients subjected to adrenal medulla autotransplantation at different centres in the USA and Canada (Goetz *et al.*, 1990a, 1991), 56 patients were followed up to 2 years postoperatively. They showed a significant though modest reduction of the severity and duration of 'off' periods. The mean percentage of 'off' time during the day decreased from 50% before transplantation to 39% at both 1 and 2 years after surgery. Even if the patients were more independent during 'off' periods and showed significant improvement of all measures of 'off' function, the changes were small and the patients remained prominently affected by their disease. For example, Hoehn and Yahr score during 'off' time only decreased from 4.18 to 3.74 and Schwab and England score increased from 35 to 44%. Motor fluctuations persisted in all patients. Moreover, the doses of antiparkinsonian medication could not be reduced after transplantation. Only 19% of patients were improved 2 years after surgery. There were numerous medical complications, including 6 deaths; 3 were judged as related or possibly related to the surgery. The morbidity involved several body systems, but was mostly focused on neurological, psychiatric and respiratory dysfunction. It was concluded that the current procedure for adrenal medulla implantation involves significant risk to seriously disabled PD patients (Goetz *et al.*, 1990a, 1991).

The detailed reports from different groups trying to replicate the findings of Madrazo *et al.* (1987) have also clearly shown the limited improvements achieved with this procedure. In 19 patients operated at three centres in the USA and followed for 18 months (Penn *et al.*, 1988; Goetz *et al.*, 1989, 1990b; Olanow *et al.*, 1990), percentage 'on' time increased from 48% preoperatively to a maximum of 75% at 6 months but then decreased to 55% at 18 months after transplantation. There was a modest reduction in the severity of symptoms during 'off' time, with maximal benefit for the patients occurring between the sixth and 12th months and deterioration thereafter. The dosages of medication could not be decreased. Postoperative morbidity was substantial. In the series of Allen *et al.* (1989), one group consisting of 12 patients was followed up to 1 year after adrenal medulla autotransplantation and another group of 6 older and more severely affected patients up to 6 months. None of the patients in the latter group improved, whereas 4 of the other 12 patients showed a significant reduction of parkinsonian symptoms (as assessed by the Columbia Rating Scale), although there were no significant changes of medication. Kelly *et al.* (1989) reported definite improvement of early-morning motor function in 1 out of 7 patients followed for 1 year after surgery. There was no significant change either in percentage 'off' time or Schwab and England and Hoehn and Yahr scores, and although 4 of the 7 patients were taking less L-dopa at 6 months postoperatively than preoperatively, the change in doses for the grafted group was not statistically significant. Kelly *et al.* (1989) concluded that they could not 'exclude a placebo effect contributing to any of this improvement'. Jankovic *et al.* (1989) reported 'modest improvement in motor function' in 3 patients with advanced PD. No major changes in medication could be made.

It has not yet been established whether survival of the adrenal medullary graft occurs and is essential for the reported improvements. In the few cases that have been subjected to autopsy, either no surviving graft (Dohan *et al.*, 1988; Forno and Langston, 1989; Jankovic *et al.*, 1989; Peterson *et al.*, 1989; Hirsch *et al.*, 1990) or a very limited number of presumed adrenal medulla cells (Hurtig *et al.*, 1989; Kordower *et al.*, 1991) have been demonstrated. It should be pointed out, though, that most of the cases analysed have shown very little clinical benefit from the operation (which agrees with a poor graft survival) and it can therefore not be excluded that in the more successful cases there is also a higher yield of surviving chromaffin cells. Analyses of cerebrospinal fluid from PD patients subjected to adrenal medulla autotransplantation have not demonstrated significant and consistent increases of catecholamines and their metabolites (Franco-Bourland *et al.*, 1988; Pezzoli *et al.*, 1988; Jankovic *et al.*, 1989; Tyce *et al.*, 1989), which would support the presence of a surviving graft acting through catecholamine release. Finally, attempts to use PET to show graft survival and/or increases of striatal DA innervation have not been successful. In the study of Guttman *et al.* (1989), 3 out of 5 patients showed accumulation of fluorodopa at the site of the implant, but this was probably due to leakage of the blood–brain barrier.

In conclusion, it has only been possible to document a modest improvement after adrenal medullary autotransplantation using the technique of Madrazo *et al.* (1987). The morbidity and mortality have been considerable. The mechanisms of improvement are largely unknown. Most investigators agree that this procedure should not be performed in more patients but that the further development of the approach using adrenal medulla grafting in PD should be pursued primarily in the laboratory.

Research strategies

While there seems to be a moderate improvement that can be reproduced in some patients subjected to adrenal medulla autotransplantation, the widespread clinical use of this procedure is definitely premature. Continued clinical trials would require a substantial reduction of the mortality and morbidity rate as well as a marked increase of both the degree and duration of the functional effects. The further development of the adrenal medulla transplantation procedure is, however, severely hampered by the fact that the mechanisms underlying the reported improvements are largely unknown. It seems unlikely (cf. above) that the reduction of PD symptoms is due to catecholamine release from the implanted cells, as originally intended. Also in animal experiments, it has not been possible to detect any spontaneous catecholamine release from intrastriatal implants of chromaffin cells (Decombe *et al.*, 1990). Much interest has recently been focused on the hypothesis that the adrenal medulla tissue contains some unknown trophic factor(s) or that the implantation induces the formation of such a factor, stimulating axonal sprouting from the remaining DA neurons in the host (Bohn *et al.*, 1987; Bankiewicz *et al.*, 1988, 1990). Morphological support for this phenomenon has been reported in autopsy studies on 2 PD patients subjected to adrenal medulla grafting (Hirsch *et al.*, 1990; Kordower *et al.*, 1991). However, the functional importance of the presumed sprouting-derived new striatal DA innervation is presently unknown and must be analysed in animal experiments. If the trophic factor(s) can be isolated and they are found to be responsible for the improvement after adrenal medulla autotransplantation in patients, then there will be possibilities for new treatment strategies in PD. However, in that case it seems unlikely that implantation of adrenal medulla tissue will be the most efficient way of delivering these factors. The possible involvement of bFGF has been suggested, since this factor is present in the adrenal gland and brain, increases in areas of injury and promotes survival and neurite extension of DA neurons in culture. In support of this idea, bFGF has been shown to stimulate recovery of nigral DA neurons in MPTP-treated mice (Otto and Unsicker, 1990).

Another possibility is to return to the original idea that adrenal medulla cells would supply the striatum with a new source of DA and other catecholamines. Given the data currently available, in order to develop an adrenal medulla-based treatment strategy for PD, the long-term survival and action of the grafts would require substantial improvement. Implantation of chromaffin tissue as long, narrow 'ribbons' into the monkey striatum has been reported to increase survival of grafted adrenal medullary cells (Dubach and German, 1990). Another approach to improve the long-term survival of these cells is to supply the graft tissue with nerve growth factor (NGF). Animal studies have shown that NGF supplied either by infusion (Strömberg *et al.*, 1985) or by co-grafts of NGF-secreting peripheral nerve (Kordower *et al.*, 1990) or genetically engineered cells (Cunningham *et al.*, 1991) induces a significant increase in the number of surviving chromaffin cells. On the basis of these data, clinical programmes with adrenal medulla autotransplantation and addition of NGF have been initiated. One patient has received NGF via intrastriatal infusion for 4 weeks after stereotaxic implantation of adrenal medulla cells and has been described as exhibiting improved motor function, although the therapeutic value was only modest (Olson *et al.*, 1991). Other series of patients are currently receiving adrenal medulla–peripheral nerve double grafts (see, for example, López-Lozano *et al.*, 1992) but no conclusive data are yet available.

There have been several attempts to reduce the morbidity and mortality after adrenal medulla autotransplantation: firstly, by using a retroperitoneal approach instead of frontal abdominal incision to take out the adrenal gland (Goetz *et al.*, 1990a), secondly, by operating on the patients in two steps using stereotaxic surgery (Pezzoli *et al.*, 1990). The adrenal medullary tissue has then been implanted in a cavity in the caudate nucleus prepared some weeks earlier. Pezzoli *et al.* (1990) have concluded from results in 2 patients that, in addition to increased safety, the precavitation technique also improves the functional outcome after adrenal medulla autotransplantation. Thirdly, the neurosurgical technique has been changed to an even less traumatic one, i.e. stereotaxic implantation using specially designed cannulas (Backlund *et al.*, 1985; Lindvall *et al.*, 1987a; Jiao *et al.*, 1988, 1989; Takeuchi *et al.*, 1990). No significant adverse effects have been reported in patients operated on with this technique. The improvements have been described as very modest and transient (4 patients, 2 of whom were implanted in the caudate nucleus and 2 in the putamen; Backlund *et al.*, 1985; Lindvall *et al.*, 1987a), moderate, lasting for 6 months (in 1 patient with putaminal implants; Takeuchi *et al.*, 1990), and, after implantation in the caudate nucleus, as permanent and slight (reduction by 20% on the Webster disability scale; 2 patients), moderate (reduction by 36%; 4 patients), or significant (reduction by 57%; 4 patients; Jiao *et al.*, 1988, 1989). It should be mentioned, though, that Tanner *et al.* (1989), after examining some of these latter patients, have reported that the improvements are, in fact, only moderate.

Following stereotaxic implantation of adrenal medullary tissue into or near the left caudate nucleus, Fazzini *et al.* (1991) observed modest improvement in 2 patients and 'dramatic' increase in percentage 'on' time and decrease in severity and duration of 'off' phases in 1 patient. This patient died of multifocal glioblastoma 1 year after grafting; autopsy showed no surviving adrenal medulla cells. No improvement was observed in a fourth patient with the graft misplaced in the medial thalamus. In the series of Apuzzo *et al.* (1990); (9 patients, 5 grafted unilaterally and 4 bilaterally in the caudate nucleus; 1 patient died of causes unrelated to transplantation), 50% of the cases showed modest improvement. No increased clincal response was detected after bilateral graft placement.

PROSPECTS FOR CLINICAL APPLICATION OF NEURAL GRAFTING IN HUNTINGTON'S DISEASE

Much of the experience gained in the clinical trials with neural grafting in PD will be of value also for the decision if and when this approach should be applied to patients with HD. Firstly, the procedures for obtaining non-contaminated fetal CNS tissue from routine elective abortions have been worked out. Secondly, there is good evidence that neural grafts can be implanted into the brains of immunosuppressed patients without major risks. Thirdly, at least in PD, fetal neural tissue seems to be able to survive in the human brain (however, see the section on impairment of graft function by disease process, below). The difference between PD and HD with regard to life expectancy and to availability of medical treatment are important issues when discussing the application of neural grafting to HD patients. In PD, L-dopa gives a marked symptomatic relief in a majority of patients, at least for some years. Furthermore, new therapeutic principles for protection of the remaining neurons in the PD patient's own DA system are being introduced (Tetrud and Langston, 1989; Shoulson and The Parkinson Study Group, 1989). Several reports have indicated that, as a consequence of L-dopa treatment, the mortality rate in PD has decreased to approximately the same as in control populations (Weiner and Lang, 1989). In contrast, therapeutics in HD are 'absymal' (Weiner and Lang, 1989). Although chorea can be ameliorated to some extent by drugs interfering with dopaminergic transmission, mainly neuroleptics, these agents do not improve the dementia. HD is a progressive fatal disorder with a duration from onset to death of approximately 13–15 years (Weiner and Lang, 1989).

The lack of serious adverse effects in the clinical trials performed so far on PD patients, with evidence of graft survival and function, together with the importance of even a minor symptomatic improvement in HD, clearly motivate the application of the transplantation approach to patients with HD. In the following paragraphs the animal experimental basis as well as some other important issues for such trials will be discussed, with the emphasis on what additional information is necessary before a clinical transplantation programme should be started in HD.

Evidence for graft-induced reduction of motor and cognitive deficits in animal models of Huntington's disease

There is no naturally occurring animal model of HD. However, injections of kainic acid, ibotenic acid or other excitotoxic acids directly into the striatum cause extensive neuronal cell loss in this structure, with many similarities to the neuropathology seen in HD (Coyle and Schwarcz, 1983). The lesions lead to selective destruction of striatal neurons while the cortical afferent and efferent fibres running in the internal capsule are spared. When made bilaterally in rats, such lesions produce a behavioural syndrome that has been considered to provide a good rodent model of HD: the lesioned animals are hyperkinetic (Mason and Fibiger, 1978; Dunnett and Iversen, 1981) and display cognitive impairments (Divac *et al.*, 1978; Dunnett and Iversen, 1981, 1982). In a recently developed model of HD for non-human primates (Hantraye *et al.*, 1990), a unilateral excitotoxic lesion is made in the caudate putamen, which leads to neurodegenerative changes in the striatum resembling those in HD. Administration of the DA agonist apomorphine to the lesioned animals produces a dyskinetic syndrome with features in common with HD: hyperkinesia, chorea, dystonia, postural asymmetries, and head and orofacial dyskinesias.

The experimental data obtained in rodents and non-human primates show that grafts of striatal tissue from rat fetuses can: (1) survive implantation into the excitotoxically lesioned striatum; (2) become integrated, at least to some extent into host neuronal circuitries; and (3) improve motor and cognitive behavioural deficits (Fig. 12.8). In rat recipients, the atrophy of the striatum, which is about 50–70% in the lesioned animals, is reduced to about 20–30% as a result of the growth of the implanted tissue. This reduced atrophy is accompanied by increases of a similar magnitude of major neurochemical markers in the grafted striata, such as the transmitter-synthesizing enzymes for gamma-aminobutyric acid (GABA) and acetylcholine (Isacson *et al.*, 1985).

The intrinsic organization of the striatal grafts resembles that of the intact neostriatum. The grafts contain characteristic GABAergic, cholinergic and peptidergic neurons (Clarke *et al.*, 1988; Graybiel *et al.*, 1989; Isacson *et al.*, 1987; Sirinathsinghji *et al.*, 1990). The two histochemical compartments, patch and matrix, which are normally present in the neostriatum, also develop in the striatal grafts (Isacson *et al.*, 1987; Graybiel *et al.*, 1989; Wictorin *et al.*, 1989a; Liu *et al.*, 1990).

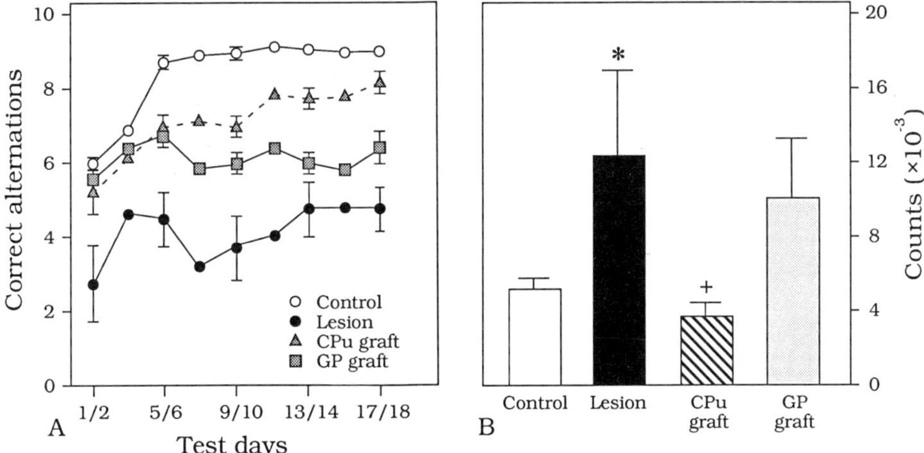

Figure 12.8 Examples of functional effects on cognitive and motor deficits induced by bilateral striatal or pallidal grafts in a rat model of Huntington's disease (bilateral ibotenic acid-induced lesions of the striatum). (A) Performance in a delayed alternation task (T-maze). Both grafts placed in the caudate putamen (CPu graft) and in the globus pallidus (GP graft) substantially ameliorated the learning deficits in animals with striatal lesions. (B) Locomotor activity recorded overnight. The lesions caused significant hyperactivity (*,$P<0.05$ compared to controls), which was reduced by the caudate putamen grafts (+, $P<0.05$ compared to lesion). Data from Isacson *et al.* (1986).

Neuroanatomical and electrophysiological studies have provided evidence that the intrastriatal striatal grafts can establish extensive reciprocal connections with the host brain (Pritzel *et al.*, 1986; Rutherford *et al.*, 1987; Wilson *et al.*, 1987; Clarke *et al.*, 1988; Wictorin *et al.*, 1988, 1989a,c, 1991; Wictorin and Björklund, 1989; Xu *et al.*, 1989, 1990, 1991). The striatal grafts have been shown to project to appropriate targets (such as the globus pallidus and, in some cases, probably also the substantia nigra) and to receive inputs from appropriate populations of host neurons in the frontal cortex, amygdala, thalamus, substantia nigra and the dorsal raphe. There is now good evidence that the rich dopaminergic input from the host substantia nigra plays an important role in the functional regulation of the grafted striata (Dunnett *et al.*, 1988; Norman *et al.*, 1989; Liu *et al.*, 1991; Mandel *et al.*, 1992).

The functional influence of the striatal grafts on the recipient has been observed in different ways: firstly, such grafts reduce the lesion-induced hypermetabolism (as assessed by local glucose utilization) in primary (e.g. globus pallidus) and secondary (e.g. subthalamic nucleus) striatal target areas, showing that they can normalize brain function in areas of the basal ganglia circuitry both close to and remote from the graft sites (Isacson *et al.*, 1984). Secondly, striatal grafts reinstate GABAergic neurotransmission within the globus pallidus, probably via the extensive axonal outgrowth from the grafted neurons into this structure. After implantation of striatal tissue, there is a significant recovery of both the activity of the GABA-synthesizing enzyme, GAD (Isacson *et al.*, 1985), and of GABA release (Sirinathsinghji *et al.*, 1988) in the globus pallidus of ibotenic acid-lesioned rats. Thirdly, striatal grafts reduce lesion-induced locomotor hyperactivity in rats and improve their performance in several behavioural tasks such as skilled paw-reaching and delayed alternation learning (Fig. 12.8; Deckel *et al.*, 1983, 1986; Isacson *et al.*, 1984, 1986; Dunnett *et al.*, 1988; Sanberg *et al.*, 1989).

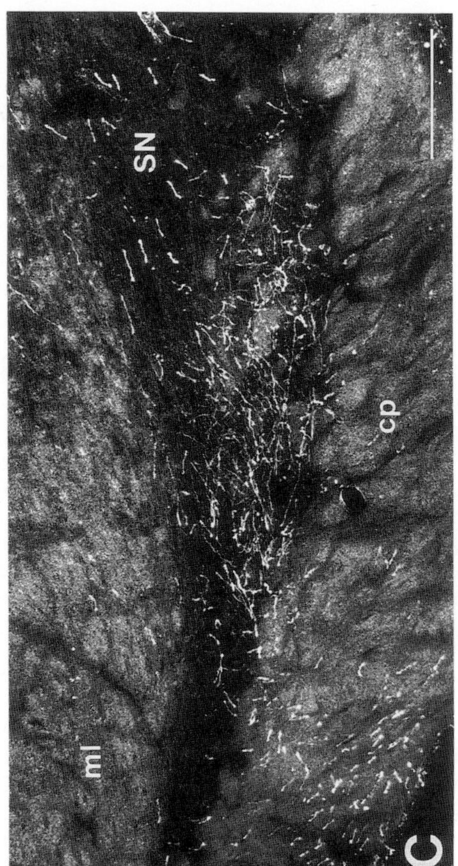
B
T
cc
H
lv
ic
gp
ac
th
ep
sn
cp

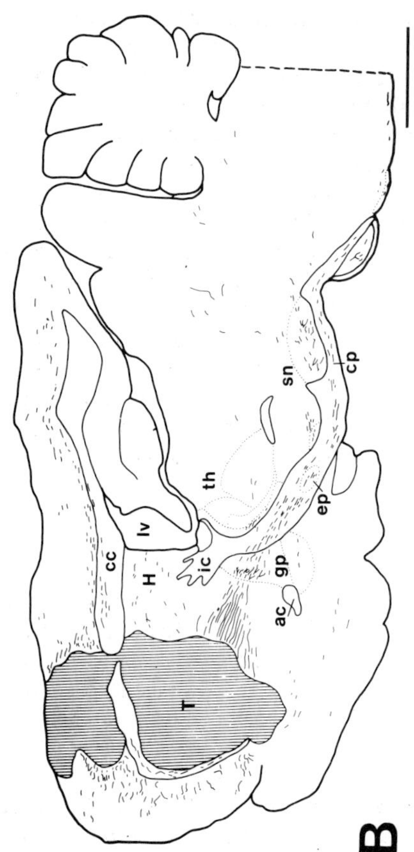
A
lv
cc
T
H

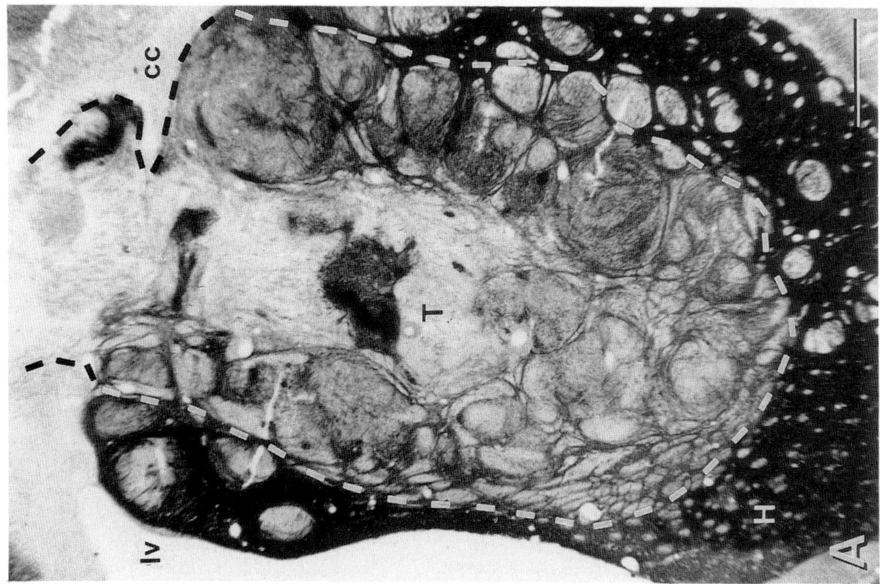
C
ml
SN
cp

Isacson *et al.* (1989, 1991) have reported symptomatic relief in 5 immunosuppressed baboons in which grafts of fetal rat striatal tissue were implanted into the ibotenic acid-lesioned striatum. All 5 baboons showed a gradual decline in apomorphine-induced dyskinesias, resulting in a 60–80% reduction of dyskinesia scores by 7–10 weeks after transplantation. In 2 monkeys where immunosuppression was discontinued the symptoms reappeared as the grafts were rejected.

From the results obtained in rats, it has been proposed that the striatal grafts reinstate a tonic inhibitory GABAergic control over the striatal output structures. For the clinical application it is of course important to know if human fetal striatal neurons have the same capacity. When implanted into the ibotenic acid-lesioned rat striatum, grafts from the striatal region of 8–10-week-old aborted human fetuses survive and grow extensively into the host brain (Fig. 12.9; Wictorin *et al.*, 1990). The axons reach the globus pallidus and substantia nigra, which are normally innervated by the striatum. Thus, human fetal striatal cells also reinnervate denervated target areas but whether this, similar to what has been observed in the rat and non-human primate, leads to functional improvement is not yet known.

Research strategies

The animal experimental data support the idea that intrastriatal implantation of human fetal striatal neurons should be tested in patients with HD. However, in order to obtain surviving grafts and induce functional improvement of therapeutic value to the patient, certain technical and scientific issues need to be clarified in more detail. Some of these issues will be discussed below.

DONOR AGE AND DISSECTION PROCEDURE

A detailed analysis of the optimal donor age for obtaining human fetal striatal tissue for transplantation purposes has to be carried out. In the successful human-to-rat grafting experiments reported so far (Fig. 12.9; Wictorin *et al.*, 1990), the age of the donors was 8–10 menstrual weeks. Two major factors limit the fetal ages suitable for clinical transplantations. Firstly, with brains from young fetuses (less than 8 weeks), a relatively selective dissection of the striatal anlage becomes exceedingly difficult and there is a high risk that the graft will contain significant portions of non-striatal, most likely neocortical, tissue (Fig. 12.9). On the other hand, tissue from fetuses older than 10–11 weeks is difficult to obtain in the amounts that seem

Figure 12.9 Examples of survival and growth of human striatal neurons (fetal age 8–10 weeks) implanted into the ibotenic acid-lesioned rat striatum. (A) Coronal section stained for acetylcholinesterase (AChE) showing a large graft containing some patches resembling normal striatal tissue (AChE-positive), but also areas with non-striatal features or looking more immature. (B) Semischematic drawing of 3–4 superimposed sagittal sections stained for human neurofilaments (HNF) taken from an adult rat brain with a 23-week-old intrastriatal implant (hatched area) of human fetal striatal tissue (fetal age 8–10 weeks). (C) Details of the HNF-immunoreactive projections extending into the host brain from striatal implants. Some HNF efferents extended into the substantia nigra (SN) and others continued in the medial part of the cerebral peduncle (cp) to reach even more caudal host brain regions. High-power bright field micrograph from a coronal section. Scale bars: A = 0.5 mm; B = 2 mm; C = 200 μm. ac = Anterior commissure; cc = corpus callosum; ep = entopeduncular nucleus; gp = globus pallidus; H = host striatum; ic = internal capsule; lv = lateral ventricle; SN = substantia nigra; T = striatal transplant; th = thalamus. Modified from Wictorin *et al.* (1990).

necessary for implantation into HD patients. With respect to the difficulty in obtaining a transplant consisting almost exclusively of striatal tissue, it should be mentioned that also under optimal conditions in rat-to-rat grafting experiments the grafts are composed of a mixture of striatal and non-striatal (in part neocortical) tissue (Wictorin *et al.*, 1989b).

TECHNIQUES AND TIMING OF TRANSPLANTATION

The target area and implantation site in patients with PD, i.e. the striatum, show no major morphological changes except a loss of dopaminergic afferents. In contrast, there are characteristically progressive morphological abnormalities in HD, leading to a marked atrophy of the striatum and a resultant dilatation of the lateral ventricle. In addition there is often mild to moderate atrophy of the cerebral cortex. It is obvious that several considerations will have to be taken into account when deciding the timing of the grafting in relation to the onset of symptoms of the disease. Firstly, to what extent can a graft survive and exert functional effects in the advanced stages of the disease? In almost all studies in rodents and non-human primates, the implantation of the fetal striatal tissue has been carried out acutely after the excitotoxic lesion was induced. Much less is known about the consequences of grafting in the chronically lesioned animal (being more comparable to patients with advanced pathological changes). It has been reported, though, from observations in 2 animals that human striatal grafts show similar axonal outgrowth into rats 1 year postlesion, as in animals with acute excitotoxic lesions (Wictorin *et al.*, 1990).

Another factor influencing whether transplantation should be performed early or late in HD relates to the possibility that fetal grafts implanted into the striatum may counteract secondary degenerative changes in other brain regions, e.g. in the cerebral cortex. If their intrinsic target neurons in the striatum are replaced by neural grafts when the first signs of striatal dysfunction appear, this might lead to preservation of afferent neuronal systems. Evidence for such a target-derived trophic support exerted by neural grafts have been provided by experimental studies in the excitotoxically lesioned rat neocortex. In this model, grafts of fetal neocortical tissue prevent the atrophy of cholinergic basal nucleus neurons induced by the lesion (Sofroniew *et al.*, 1986).

It also seems possible that fetal striatal grafts might counteract primary degenerative changes in the striatum induced by the progressive lesion in HD. Tulipan *et al.* (1986) have reported that striatal grafts can reduce the acute toxic damage caused by an excitotoxin. Furthermore, Schumacher *et al.* (1991) have found that NGF-secreting, genetically engineered fibroblasts implanted adjacent to the striatum can provide protection against the toxic effects of subsequent injection of quisqualic acid or quinolinic acid. It must be underscored, though, that the relevance of any of these lesion models for the progressive, genetically determined degenerative process in HD is presently unclear.

A major technical problem is to calculate how much fetal striatal tissue should be implanted in a HD patient. The size of the implant must be sufficient to induce a significant improvement but, on the other hand, must not exceed that of the normal striatum. The risk of overgrowth must be minimized; there is a substantial volume increase in striatal grafts (200–300%) when placed in the anterior chamber of the eye (Seiger, 1985). Another technical issue that needs further study concerns how the striatal tissue shall be implanted in the partly or completely atrophied human striatum, i.e. instrument design, number of implantation sites, and open or stereotaxic neurosurgery.

MONITORING OF GRAFT SURVIVAL AND FUNCTION

In the first clinical trials with neural grafting in HD it will be of utmost importance in order for the technique to progress to be able to detect any functional improvements, even subclinical, and to correlate those with the demonstration of a surviving graft. Careful clinical examination before and after grafting, including rating of choreatic movements, must be performed. It is important to develop protocols for neuropsychological tests that can be performed repeatedly and reveal graft-induced influences on cognitive deficits. Objective analyses of striatal function using electrophysiology, e.g. evoked potentials, should also be used. It seems possible that computed tomography and magnetic resonance imaging (MRI) scans may be of some value to monitor graft survival, although single photon emission computed tomography (SPECT) and, in particular, PET probably are more attractive for this purpose. For example, it may be possible to label the grafted striatal tissue with some DA receptor ligand, which can be monitored *in vivo* with PET (see, for example, Leenders *et al.*, 1986a). In addition, the PET technique combined with fluorodeoxyglucose as ligand might give additional information on graft-induced functional changes in different brain regions.

GENERAL ISSUES FOR CELL TRANSPLANTATION IN MOVEMENT DISORDERS

Use of immunosuppressive treatment

The brain is regarded as an immunologically privileged site (Barker and Billingham, 1977; Widner and Brundin, 1988; Nicholas and Arnason, 1989), but it has been clearly demonstrated that immunological rejection processes can occur also in the CNS (Mason *et al.*, 1986; Brundin *et al.*, 1989; Finsen *et al.*, 1991). Fetal neural tissue has been shown to be immunogenic (Mason *et al.*, 1986; Widner *et al.*, 1989a), although most cells in the immature as well as adult brain lack expression of major histocompatibility complex (MHC) class I and II antigens (the strong transplantation antigens). However, subgroups of glia cells can under certain circumstances be induced to express high levels of MHC I and II antigens. Microglia express both kinds of molecules and have, in addition, a function as antigen-presenting cells. Furthermore, endothelial cells constituently express class I antigens and can be induced to express class II MHC antigens. Any one of these cell types may thus be responsible for initiating a rejection response (Widner and Brundin, 1988; Nicholas and Arnason, 1989). Fetal neurons express several minor transplantation antigens, but the degree of host immunization against these molecules after grafting and their role in determining long-term survival of intracerebral grafts remain to be elucidated.

Several factors are of importance for the magnitude of the immune response in the recipient after intracerebral neural grafting (for discussion, see Widner *et al.*, 1990). Firstly, if the graft tissue is in a poor condition, e.g. large solid pieces with central necrotic areas, or if the implantation technique leads to major trauma and tissue necrosis, the inflammatory response will be extensive and cause massive accumulation of scavenger cells. These cells will induce enhanced MHC expression on different cells in the graft, which can lead to extensive host immunization. Secondly, fetal neural suspension grafts are vascularized by ingrowth of vessels from the host, whereas solid grafts develop intrinsic, donor-derived vessels that connect to the host vaculature. Due to the different origin of the vessels, intracerebral grafts of solid tissue can be expected to be more prone to immune responses than suspension grafts.

It is still not known whether immunosuppression is necessary in clinical trials with grafting of human fetal neural tissue. There is evidence of host immunization by fetal neural grafts of human origin in a xenograft situation (Brundin *et al.*, 1988b). Immune reactions as well as fulminant rejections have been observed in animal recipients of human fetal tissue (Brundin *et al.*, 1988b). On the other hand, implantation of allografts of fetal substantia nigra into the brains of MPTP-lesioned non-human primates has in most cases been performed without immunosuppression. The available reports have indicated good graft function up to at least 7 months postoperatively (Fine *et al.*, 1988; Sladek *et al.*, 1988). Only 1 case of regrafting has been described in monkeys, in which a prompt loss of graft function was observed on the previously implanted side (Freed *et al.*, 1988).

It is thus at present not possible to give any general recommendations regarding the use of immunosuppression in intracerebral transplantation. The reasons for using immunosuppression in our programme are as follows (Widner *et al.*, 1990):

1. Immunological rejection can occur in the CNS, and immunization of the host against donor tissue has been observed after intracerebral neural grafting.
2. By minimizing the risk for possible immune reactions, immunosuppression allows for optimal conditions for the evaluation of the functional effects of neural grafting. We have not, in rat experiments, detected any detrimental effects caused by administration of the immunosuppressive drugs, cyclosporin and azathioprine, on the development of transplanted fetal neural tissue.
3. Patients subjected to allografting of human CNS tissue should have the possibility of receiving a second graft at a later stage. The outcome of a second transplantation is much worse if the host is preimmunized (Medawar, 1948) but immunosuppression reduces the degree of host immunization. Experimental data obtained in rats support the idea that a second fetal CNS graft may fail to develop after implantation and also increase the risk of rejection of the first graft if the two grafts are genetically identical (Freed *et al.*, 1988; Widner *et al.*, 1989a).
4. The risk for unexpected adverse autoimmune reactions can be reduced by immunosuppression (Nicholas and Arnason, 1989).

In ongoing clinical trials with neural grafting in PD, cyclosporin, either alone or in combination with steroids and/or azathioprine, is given as immunosuppressive treatment (Table 12.1). We favour the triple-drug regime since the three components act on different mechanisms for the immune response. T cell-mediated responses, which probably are the most critical ones for graft rejection also in the brain, are preferentially controlled by cyclosporin. The inflammatory events are minimized by steroids. The critical proliferation of activated lymphocytes can be partly controlled by azathioprine. Furthermore, the toxicity observed after higher doses of the different drugs is considerably reduced by the combination, in which lower doses are used without loss of efficacy.

The duration of immunosuppressive treatment to ensure long-term graft survival can only be speculated upon since appropriate experimental and clinical data are lacking. With the uncertainty about the need for immunosuppression in intracerebral transplantation in humans, it is clear that if serious complications occur, the immunosuppressive treatment should be withdrawn. If patients have graft effects of significant therapeutical value, it seems at present recommendable to expect lifelong immunnosuppressive treatment. However, in 1 of our patients with idiopathic PD, cyclosporin was withdrawn at 31 months (Lindvall *et al.*, 1993) and 2 patients with

MPTP-induced parkinsonism were taken off cyclosporin at 12 months and azathioprine at 18 months (Widner *et al.*, 1992) without evidence of graft dysfunction over at least the subsequent year.

If immunosuppression is necessary, the present inability reliably and non-invasively to monitor rejection of grafted fetal tissue becomes a problem. A leaking blood–brain barrier could indicate an early phase of rejection and this might be detectable by MRI. If rejection were to precede any functional effects, it would probably pass unnoticed. If positive functional effects have developed, rejection would lead to a partial or complete disappearance of such graft-induced improvements. In either situation it would be desirable to detect the first signs of a rejection process in the brain in order to be able to prevent the complete destruction of the graft.

On the basis of estimations of the number of mesencephalic DA neurons normally innervating the human striatum (Lindvall *et al.*, 1987b) and with the present survival rate of grafted DA neurons, it seems likely that tissue from more than one fetus is necessary to ensure a graft-derived reinnervation inducing a significant therapeutic effect. This raises the question whether grafting of CNS tissue from several donors increases the risk for immunological rejection. At present, there are no conclusive experimental data supporting that this is the case. With four donors at each transplantation (as in our clinical programme) it seems more likely, considering MHC I and II antigen disparity (see Widner *et al.*, 1990 for discussion), that the risk for rejection is the same when tissue from each of the fetuses is implanted in the same host as if it had been grafted to different recipients. This idea is supported by the finding that mixed grafts of fetal mesencephalic tissue from two mouse donor strains showed no reduction of the number of DA cells after implantation into mice of a third strain (Widner *et al.*, 1989b). There is, however, an additive effect of minor transplantation antigens, which means that increasing the amount of tissue may lead to a stronger immune response.

Alternative sources of donor tissue

Fetal CNS tissue is presently the best or the only source of cells giving symptomatic relief after implantation in animal models of PD and HD. From the theoretical point of view it also seems most likely that the most efficient functional restoration after nerve cell degeneration is achieved by neuronal grafts. These can act through a synaptic release of transmitter which, at least to some extent, is physiologically regulated due to autoreceptors and the integration of the grafted cells in host neuronal circuitries. However, it is highly warranted to find alternative sources of donor tissue with the ultimate goal of becoming independent of a continuous supply of human fetal tissue. This will be even more important if, in the future, cell transplantation into the CNS will have a wider application, including other neurological disorders. The use of tissue from aborted human fetuses will always be a controversial ethical issue and in some countries this therapeutic approach will not be possible.

In HD there is no obvious alternative to fetal striatal tissue at present. However, in addition to fetal neurons and adrenal chromaffin cells, several catecholamine-producing tissues have been suggested to be potentially useful for grafting in PD patients and should be further explored in animal experiments. Superior cervical ganglion cells survive implantation into the striatum, show axonal outgrowth and ameliorate parkinsonian symptoms in MPTP-treated monkeys (Nakai *et al.*, 1990). Immortalized cell lines like PC 12 represent another potential source of graft tissue

(Bing *et al.*, 1988) which can provide a continuous supply of DA, but are unsuitable for clinical application since they either form tumours or are rejected after implantation. If the PC 12 cells are enclosed in polymer capsules, both uncontrolled growth and rejection by the host may, however, be prevented and long-term survival is then possible (Aebischer *et al.*, 1991).

Implantation of cells that have been genetically engineered to produce either DA or GABA might in the future be developed into clinically valuable therapeutic strategies in PD and HD, respectively. Fibroblasts and cell lines in which the tyrosine hydroxylase gene has been introduced either by infection or transfection can release L-dopa or DA and ameliorate apomorphine-induced rotational asymmetry after grafting into the denervated rat striatum (Wolff *et al.*, 1989; Horellou *et al.*, 1990; Fisher *et al.*, 1991). It should be underscored, though, that this research is still at a very early stage and that transplantation of genetically engineered cells is far from application in patients. Before any clinical trials can be carried out in PD, it must be shown in rodents and non-human primates that long-term survival and function of genetically engineered cells after transplantation are possible without major risks, and that these grafts can also reverse motor deficits resembling the symptoms in the PD patient.

Impairment of graft function by disease process

It may be hypothesized that in PD and HD patients subjected to neural transplantation, the ongoing disease process itself could interfere with the long-term survival and outgrowth of the grafted neurons. This problem can only be resolved in human trials since PD and HD are not observed in animals. In the animal models of these disorders the exposure to the neurotoxin occurs during a short period of time and has ceased at the time of cell implantation. In contrast, there is evidence for a progressive degeneration over several years of nigral and striatal neurons in idiopathic PD and HD, respectively. If the cell death is not due to an intrinsic defect in the patient's own nigral or striatal neurons, but instead caused by some other mechanism, this could elicit a degeneration also of grafted neurons. Both in PD and HD graft degeneration would probably occur if the patients lose nigral DA neurons and striatal neurons, respectively, because of a lack of trophic factors or due to a continuous exposure to some environmental (Langston *et al.*, 1984; Barbeau *et al.*, 1986) or endogenously produced neurotoxin (Olney, 1989).

Even if the disease also leads to degeneration of grafted nigral or striatal neurons but is a slow process, one would expect that patients with PD or HD could still benefit from neural transplantation, at least for a limited time period. One possibility to protect grafted DA neurons in idiopathic PD would be to use the monoamine oxidase inhibitor deprenyl which, according to recent clinical studies (Shoulson and The Parkinson Study Group, 1989; Tetrud and Langston, 1989), retards the disease process in PD patients. The possibility currently exists to clarify the influence of the disease process on the long-term survival and action of DA grafts by comparing the outcome after transplantation in patients with PD of unknown cause (i.e. idiopathic) with those having a known (MPTP-induced) aetiology.

Interestingly, recent data indicate that survival and function of grafted DA neurons are possible in patients with idiopathic PD at least up to 3 years postimplantation (Lindvall *et al.*, 1993). Two patients showed high fluorodopa uptake in the grafted putamen on repeated PET scans (Fig. 12.6) whereas there was a progressive fall of tracer uptake in non-grafted striatal regions. Clinical assessment demonstrated that improvement of motor function in the limbs contralateral to the graft persisted at 3 years whereas there was a worsening of parkinsonian symptoms on the ipsilateral side. It seems possible to conclude that the grafted DA neurons had survived despite ongoing degeneration of the patients' own DA system.

Storage of fetal tissue

With the current survival rate of grafted DA neurons, mesencephalic tissue from more than one human fetus is probably needed to achieve maximum symptomatic relief in each PD patient, especially with multiple implantation sites. Similarly, in future clinical trials in HD patients, striatal tissue from a single fetus is probably insufficient. With a technique for storage of fetal CNS tissue which does not significantly compromise graft viability, it may be possible to pool donor tissue obtained from routine abortions over several days and also to perform bacteriological examination of the tissue prior to implantation. Pretransplantation storage could also allow for preoperative manipulation of the graft tissue, such as addition of trophic factors (to increase graft survival and growth) or cell sorting. The latter technique would intend to make a more or less 'pure' population of DA or striatal neurons for implantation but could also allow for a removal of cells that have negative influences on graft survival, e.g. glial and endothelial cells expressing MHC antigens and thereby initiating immune responses in the host.

Whereas very little information exists on fetal striatal tissue, three major technical approaches are being explored for the storage of mesencephalic DA neurons – freezing (Collier *et al.*, 1987, 1988; Redmond *et al.*, 1988; Robbins *et al.*, 1990; Sauer *et al.*, 1992), refrigeration above freezing temperature (Sauer and Brundin, 1991) and cell culture (Brundin *et al.*, 1988a; Strecker *et al.*, 1989). Although surviving DA grafts can be obtained by all these methods, tissue preservation usually results in decreased DA neuron survival. Depending on the technique used, this could be due to different factors (for references see Sauer and Brundin, 1991), such as rate of freezing and thawing, storage temperature and medium, increased vulnerability of the preserved cells to mechanical stress, donor age and maturation of the fetal tissue in culture. The only storage technique used so far for human fetal mesencephalic tissue in clinical trials is cryopreservation at the temperature of liquid nitrogen (Redmond *et al.*, 1989; Spencer *et al.*, 1992). This technique reduces the number of surviving DA neurons (Collier *et al.*, 1988) but yields viable intrastriatal grafts after implantation of mesencephalic cell suspensions from rat, monkey and human fetal donors into the monkey brain (Collier *et al.*, 1988; Redmond *et al.*, 1988). In rat-to-rat transplantation experiments the number of DA neurons in the graft at 6 weeks after surgery was about 60% lower with cryopreserved as compared to fresh donor tissue (Sauer *et al.*, 1992). To what extent the cryopreserved human DA neurons survive in the brain of PD patients is presently unknown (Redmond *et al.*, 1989).

An alternative approach that seems to be potentially useful in clinical trials has been described by Sauer and Brundin (1991). Rat ventral mesencephalic tissue could be stored at 4°C in a 'hibernation medium' and then grafted within a few days, without significant morphological and functional impairment compared to fresh tissue. Similarly, volume assessment of fresh and hibernated grafts prepared from human fetal tissue and implanted into rats revealed no adverse effects of hibernation. This technique promises to be a convenient and simple tool for storage of mesencephalic tissue and possibly also for striatal tissue in clinical trials. In comparison with cryopreservation it has however the disadvantage that it does not allow for prolonged storage of the tissue (more than 5 days).

Fetal rat DA neurons can also be successfully grafted into the rat brain after short periods in culture, but after longer times (7 days) very poor graft survival has been observed (Brundin *et al.*, 1988a). It has been proposed that the maturation of the DA neurons in the cell culture, particularly the formation of axonal processes, and the dissociation before implantation compromise their ability to survive cell suspension grafting. Interestingly, Strecker *et al.* (1989) have obtained good survival and function of grafts of rat fetal DA neurons cultured for 9 days in rotating flasks. These aggregate cultures could be implanted without dissociation, which might explain the good survival of the grafts despite the maturation that had taken place *in vitro*.

CONCLUDING REMARKS

Although animal experimental data are very promising and clinical trials have given encouraging results, it must be underscored that there exists at present no treatment for PD or HD based on intracerebral transplantation. It is important that patients and relatives are informed that this research is still at an experimental stage and that widespread clinical trials with transplantation in PD are not warranted at this time. A number of scientific problems have to be clarified in more detail and this can only be achieved through the application of systematic scientific approaches. For the clinical studies, this means that intracerebral grafting should only be performed in few, well-characterized PD patients who are closely monitored before and after transplantation both functionally and with respect to graft survival. One step forward towards a transplantation therapy in PD seems to have been taken by the demonstration that grafts can survive and can have functional effects in the human parkinsonian brain. Available animal experimental data as well as ethical and medical considerations motivate further efforts also to apply neural grafting in patients with HD. However, for the further development of transplantation therapies in PD and HD, more animal research is needed in parallel to well-designed clinical trials.

Acknowledgements

Our research reviewed in this article was supported by the Swedish MRC (14X-8666), Riksbankens Jubileumsfond, and Thorsten and Elsa Segerfalks Stiftelse.

References

Aebischer P, Tresco PA, Winn SR, Greene LA, and Jaeger CB (1991) Long-term cross-species brain transplantation of a polymer-encapsulated dopamine-secreting cell line. *Exp Neurol*, **111**, 269–75

Allen GS, Burns RS, Tulipan NB, and Parker RA (1989) Adrenal medullary transplantation to the caudate nucleus in Parkinson's disease. Initial clinical results in 18 patients. *Arch Neurol*, **46**, 487–91

Apuzzo MLJ, Neal JH, Waters CH, Appley AJ, Boyd SD, Couldwell WT *et al.* (1990) Utilization of unilateral and bilateral stereotactically placed adrenomedullary-striatal autografts in parkinsonian humans: rationale, techniques and observations. *Neurosurgery*, **26**, 746–57

Backlund E-O, Granberg P-O, Hamberger B, Knutsson E, Mårtensson A, Sedvall G *et al.* (1985)

Transplantation of adrenal medullary tissue to striatum in parkinsonism. First clinical trials. *J Neurosurg*, **62**, 169–73

Bankiewicz KS, Plunkett RJ, Kopin IJ, Jacobowitz DM, London WT, and Oldfield EH (1988) Transient behavioral recovery in hemiparkinsonian primates after adrenal medullary allografts. *Prog Brain Res*, **78**, 543–9

Bankiewicz KS, Plunkett RJ, Jacobowitz DM, Porzio L, di Prozio U, London WT *et al.* (1990) The effect of fetal mesencephalon implants on primate MPTP-induced parkinsonism. Histochemical and behavioral studies. *J Neurosurg*, **72**, 231–44

Barbeau A, Roy M, Cloutier T, Plasse L, and Paris S (1986) Environment and genetic factors in the etiology of Parkinson's disease. *Adv Neurol*, **45**, 299–306

Barker CF and Billingham RE (1977) Immunologically privileged sites. *Adv Immunol*, **25**, 1–54

Bing G, Notter MFD, Hansen JT, and Gash DM (1988) Comparison of adrenal medullary, carotid body and PC12 cell grafts in 6-OHDA lesioned rats. *Brain Res Bull*, **20**, 399–406

Björklund A and Stenevi U (1979) Reconstruction of the nigrostriatal pathway by intracerebral nigral transplants. *Brain Research*, **177**, 555–60

Blunt SB, Jenner P, and Marsden CD (1991) The effect of chronic L-DOPA treatment on the recovery of motor function in 6-hydroxydopamine-lesioned rats receiving ventral mesencephalic grafts. *Neuroscience*, **40**, 453–64

Bohn MC, Cupit L, Marciano F, and Gash DM (1987) Adrenal medulla grafts enhance recovery of striatal dopaminergic fibers. *Science*, **237**, 913–16

Brundin P and Björklund A (1987) Survival, growth and function of dopaminergic neurons grafted to the brain. *Prog Brain Res*, **71**, 293–308

Brundin P, Strecker RE, Londos E, and Björklund A (1987) Dopamine neurons grafted unilaterally to the nucleus accumbens affect drug-induced circling and locomotion. *Exp Brain Res*, **69**, 183–94

Brundin P, Barbin G, Strecker RE, Isacson O, Prochiantz A, and Björklund A (1988a) Survival and function of dissociated rat dopamine neurones grafted at different developmental stages or after being cultured *in vitro*. *Dev Brain Res*, **39**, 233–43

Brundin P, Strecker RE, Widner H, Clarke DJ, Nilsson OG, Åstedt B *et al.* (1988b) Human fetal dopamine neurons grafted in a rat model of Parkinson's disease: immunological aspects, spontaneous and drug-induced behavior, and dopamine release. *Exp Brain Res*, **70**, 192–208

Brundin P, Widner H, Nilsson OG, Strecker RE, and Björklund A (1989) Intracerebral xenografts of dopamine neurons: the role of immunosuppression and the blood–brain barrier. *Exp Brain Res*, **75**, 195–207

Brundin P, Björklund A, and Lindvall O (1990) Practical aspects of the use of human fetal brain tissue for intracerebral grafting. *Prog Brain Res*. **82**, 707–14

Chalmers RME and Fine A (1991) The influence of L-Dopa on survival and outgrowth of fetal ventral mesencephalic dopaminergic neurons *in vitro* and after intracerebral transplantation. In Lindvall O, Björklund A, and Widner H, eds, *Intracerebral Transplantation in Movement Disorders, Experimental Basis and Clinical Experiences*, Amsterdam, Elsevier, 333–42

Clarke DJ, Dunnett SB, Isacson O, Sirinathsinghji DJS, and Björklund A (1988) Striatal grafts in rats with unilateral neostriatal lesions. I. Ultrastructural evidence of afferent synaptic inputs from the host nigrostriatal pathway. *Neuroscience*, **24**, 791–801

Collier TJ, Redmond DE Jr, Sladek CD, Gallagher MJ, Roth RH, and Sladek JR Jr (1987) Intracerberal grafting and culture of cryopreserved primate dopamine neurons. *Brain Res*, **436**, 363–6

Collier TJ, Sladek CD, Gallagher MJ, Blanchard BC, Daley BF, Foster PN *et al.* (1988) Cryopreservation of fetal rat and non-human primate mesencephalic neurons: viability in culture and neural transplantation. *Prog Brain Res*, **78**, 631–6

Coyle JR and Schwarcz R (1983) The use of excitatory amino acids as selective neurotoxins. In Björklund A and Hökfelt T, eds, *Handbook of Chemical Neuroanatomy*, vol 1, *Methods of Chemical Neuroanatomy*, Amsterdam, Elsevier, 508–27

Cunningham LA, Hansen JT, Short MP, and Bohn MC (1991) The use of genetically altered astrocytes to provide nerve growth factor to adrenal chromaffin cells grafted into the striatum. *Brain Res*, **561**, 192–202

Deckel AW, Robinson RG, Coyle JT, and Sanberg PR (1983) Reversal of long-term locomotor abnormalities in the kainic acid model of Huntington's disease by day 18 fetal striatal implants. *Eur J Pharmacol*, **93**, 287–8

Deckel AW, Moran TH, and Robertson RG (1986) Behavioral recovery following kainic acid lesions and fetal implants of the striatum occurs independent of dopaminergic mechanisms. *Brain Res*, **363**, 383–5

Decombe R, Rivot JP, Aunis D, Abrous N, Peschanski M, and Herman JP (1990) Importance of catecholamine release for the functional action of intrastriatal implants of adrenal medullary cells: pharmacological analysis and *in vivo* electrochemistry. *Exp Neurol*, **107**, 143–53

Divac I, Markowitsch HJ, and Pritzel M (1978) Behavioural and anatomical consequences of small intrastriatal injections of kainic acid in the rat. *Brain Res*, **151**, 523–32
Dohan FC, Robertson JT, Feler C, Schweitzer J, Hall C, and Robertson JH (1988) Autopsy findings in a Parkinson's disease patient treated with adrenal medullary to caudate nucleus transplant. *Soc Neurosc Abstracts*, **7**, 4
Dubach M and German DC (1990) Extensive survival of chromaffin cells in adrenal medulla 'ribbon' grafts in the monkey neostriatum. *Exp Neurol*, **110**, 167–80
Dunnett SB, and Annett LE (1991) Nigral transplants in primate models of parkinsonism. In Lindvall O, Björklund A, and Widner H, eds, *Intracerebral Transplantation in Movement Disorders, Experimental Basis and Clinical Experiences*, Amsterdam, Elsevier, 27–50
Dunnett SB and Iversen SD (1981) Learning impairments following selective kainic acid-induced lesions within the neostriatum of rats. *Behav Brain Res*, **2**, 189–209
Dunnett SB and Iversen SD (1982) Neurotoxic lesions of ventrolateral but not anteromedial neostriatum in rats impair differential reinforcement of low rates (DRL) performance. *Behav Brain Res*, **6**, 213–26
Dunnett SB, Björklund A, Stenevi U, and Iversen SD (1981) Grafts of embryonic substantia nigra reinnervating the ventrolateral striatum ameliorate sensorimotor impairments and akinesia in rats with 6-OHDA lesions of the nigrostriatal pathway. *Brain Res*, **229**, 209–17
Dunnett SB, Björklund A, Schmidt RH, Stenevi U, and Iversen SD (1983) Intracerebral grafting of neuronal cell suspensions. IV. Behavioural recovery in rats with unilateral 6-OHDA lesions following implantation of nigral cell suspensions in different forebrain sites. *Acta Physiol Scand*, **522**, (suppl), 29–37
Dunnett SB, Wishaw IQ, Rogers DC, and Jones GH (1987) Dopamine-rich grafts ameliorate whole body motor asymmetry and sensory neglect but not independent limb use in rats with 6-hydroxydopamine lesions. *Brain Res*, **415**, 63–78
Dunnett SB, Isacson O, Sirinathsinghji DHS, Clarke DJ, and Björklund A (1988) Striatal grafts in rats with unilateral neostriatal lesions. III. Recovery from dopamine dependent motor asymmetry and deficits in skilled paw reaching. *Neuroscience*, **24**, 813–20
Fazzini E, Dwork AJ, Blum C, Burke R, Cote L, Goodman RR *et al.* (1991) Stereotaxic implantation of autologous adrenal medulla into caudate nucleus in four patients with Parkinsonism. One-year follow-up. *Arch Neurol*, **48**, 813–20
Ferrari G, Minozzi M-C, Toffano G, Leon A, and Skaper SD (1989) Basic fibroblast growth factor promotes the survival and development of mesencephalic neurons in culture. *Dev Biol*, **133**, 140–7
Fine A, Hunt SP, Oertel WH, Nomoto M, Chong PN, Bond A *et al.* (1988) Transplantation of embryonic marmoset dopaminergic neurons to the corpus striatum of marmosets rendered parkinsonian by 1-methyl-4-phenyl-1,2,3,6-tetrahydropyridine. *Prog Brain Res*, **78**, 479–89
Finger S and Dunnett SB (1989) Nimodipine enhances growth and vascularization of neural grafts. *Exp Neurol*, **104**, 1–9
Finsen BR, Sørensen T, Gonzalez B, Castellano B and Zimmer J (1991) Immunological reactions to neural grafts in the central nervous system. *Restor Neurol Neurosci*, **2**, 271–82
Fisher LJ, Jinnah HA, Kale LC, Higgins GA, and Gage FH (1991) Survival and function of intrastriatally grafted primary fibroblasts genetically modified to produce L-dopa. *Neuron*, **6**, 371–80
Forno LS and Langston JW (1989) Adrenal medullary transplant to the brain for Parkinson's disease. Neuropathology of an unsuccessful case. *J Neuropathol Exp Neurol*, **48** (suppl), 116
Franco-Bourland RE, Madrazo I, Drucker-Colin R, Torres C, Alvarez F, Carvey P *et al.* (1988) Biochemical analyses of lumbar and ventricular CSF from parkinsonians before and after adrenomedullary autotransplantation to the caudate nucleus. *Neurosci Abstracts*, **5**, 10
Freed CR, Richards JB, Hutt CJ, Kriek EH, and Reite ML (1988) Rejection of fetal substantia nigra allografts in monkeys with MPTP-induced Parkinson's syndrome. *Soc Neurosc Abstracts*, **7**, 7
Freed CR, Breeze RE, Rosenberg NL, Schneck SA, Wells TH, Barrett JN *et al.* (1990) Transplantation of human fetal dopamine cells for Parkinson's disease. *Arch Neurol*, **47**, 505–12
Freed CR, Breeze RE, Rosenberg NL, Schneck SA, Kriek E, Qi J-X *et al.* (1992) Survival of implanted fetal dopamine cells and neurologic improvement 12 to 46 months after transplantation for Parkinson's disease. *N Engl J Med*, **327**, 1549–55
Goetz CG, Olanow CW, Koller WC, Penn RD, Cahill D, Morantz R *et al.* (1989) Multicenter study of autologous adrenal medullary transplantation to the corpus striatum in patients with advanced Parkinson's disease. *N Engl J Med*, **320**, 337–41
Goetz CG, Stebbins GT III, Klawans HL, Koller WC, Grossman RG, Bakay RAE *et al.* (1990a) United Parkinson Foundation neurotransplantation registry multicenter US and Canadian data base. Presurgical and 12 month follow-up. *Prog Brain Res*, **82**, 611–17
Goetz CG, Tanner CM, Penn RD, Stebbins GT III, Gilley DW, Shannon KM *et al.* (1990b) Adrenal medullary transplant to the striatum with advanced Parkinson's disease: 1-year motor and psychomotor data. *Neurology*, **40**, 273–6
Goetz CG, Stebbins GT III, Klawans HL, Koller WC, Grossman RG, Bakay FAE *et al.* and the United

Parkinson Foundation Neural Transplantation Registry (1991) United Parkinson Foundation Neurotransplantation Registry on adrenal medullary transplants: presurgical, and 1- and 2-year follow-up. *Neurology*, **41**, 1719–22

Graham DG, Tiffany SM, Bell WR Jr, and Guthknecht WF (1978) Autoxidation versus covalent binding of quinones as the mechanism of toxicity of dopamine, 6-hydroxydopamine and related compounds toward C 1300 neuroblastoma cells *in vitro*. *Mol Pharmacol*, **14**, 644–53

Graybiel AM, Liu FC, and Dunnett SB (1989) Intrastriatal grafts derived from fetal striatal primordia. I. Phenotopy and modular organization. *J Neurosci*, **9**, 3250–71

Guttman M, Burns RS, Martin WRW, Peppard RF, Adam MJ, Ruth TJ *et al.* (1989) PET studies of Parkinsonian patients treated with autologous adrenal implants. *Can J Neurol Sci*, **16**, 305–9

Hantraye P, Riche D, Maziere M, and Isacson O (1990) A primate model of Huntington's disease: behavioral and anatomical studies of unilateral excitotoxic lesions of the caudate-putamen in the baboon. *Exp Neurol*, **108**, 91–104

Henderson BTH, Clough CG, Hughes RC, Hitchcock ER, and Kenny BG (1991) Implantation of human fetal ventral mesencephalon to the right caudate nucleus in advanced Parkinson's disease. *Arch Neurol*, **48**, 822–7

Hirsch EC, Duyckaerts C, Javoy-Agid F, Hauw J-J, and Agid Y (1990) Does adrenal graft enhance recovery of dopaminergic neurons in Parkinson's disease? *Ann Neurol*, **27**, 676–82

Horellou P, Marlier L, Privat A, and Mallet J (1990) Behavioural effect of engineered cells that synthesize L-dopa or dopamine after grafting into the rat neostriatum. *Eur J Neurosc*, **2**, 116–19

Hurtig H, Joyce J, Sladek JR Jr, and Trojanowski JQ (1989) Postmortem analysis of adrenal-medulla-to-caudate autograft in a patient with Parkinson's disease. *Ann Neurol*, **25**, 607–14

Hyman C, Hofer M, Barde Y-A, Juhasz M, Yancopoulos GD, Squinto SP *et al.* (1991) BDNF is a neurotrophic factor for dopaminergic neurons of the substantia nigra. *Nature*, **350**, 230–2

Isacson O, Brundin P, Kelly PAT, Gage FH, and Björklund A (1984) Functional neuronal replacement by grafted striatal neurones in the ibotenic acid-lesioned striatum. *Nature*, **311**, 458–60

Isacson O, Brundin P, Gage FH, and Björklund A (1985) Neural grafting in a rat model of Huntington's disease: progressive neurochemical changes after neostriatal ibotenate lesions and striatal tissue grafting. *Neuroscience*, **16**, 799–817

Isacson O, Dunnett SB, and Björklund A (1986) Graft-induced behavioural recovery in an animal model of Huntington's chorea. *Proc Natl Acad Sci USA*, **83**, 2728–32

Isacson O, Dawbarn D, Brundin P, Gage FH, Emson PC, and Björklund A (1987) Neural grafting in a rat model of Huntington's disease: striosomal-like organization of striatal grafts as revealed by immunocytochemistry and receptor autoradiography. *Neuroscience*, **22**, 481–97

Isacson O, Riche D, Hantraye P, Sofroniew MV, and Maziere M (1989) A primate model of Huntington's disease: cross-species implantation of striatal precursor cells to the excitotoxically lesioned baboon caudate-putamen. *Exp Brain Res*, **75**, 213–20

Isacson O, Hantraye P, Riche D, Schumacher JM, and Maziere M (1991) The relationship between symptoms and functional anatomy in the chronic neurodegenerative diseases: from pharmacological to biological replacement therapy in Huntington's disease. In Lindvall O, Björklund A, and Widner H, eds, *Intracerebral Transplantation in Movement Disorders, Experimental Basis and Clinical Experiences*. Amsterdam, Elsevier, 245–58

Jankovic J, Grossman R, Goodman C, Pirozzolo F, Schneider L, Zhu Z *et al.* (1989) Clinical, biochemical, and neuropathologic findings following transplantation of adrenal medulla to the caudate nucleus for treatment of Parkinson's disease. *Neurology*, **39**, 1227–34

Jiao S, Zhang W, Cao J, Zhang Z, Wang H, Ding M *et al.* (1988) Study of adrenal medullary tissue transplantation to striatum in parkinsonism. *Prog Brain Res*, **78**, 575–80

Jiao S-S, Ding Y-J, Zhang W-C, Cao J-K, Zhang G-F, Zhang Z-M *et al.* (1989) Adrenal medullary autografts in patients with Parkinson's disease. *N Engl J Med*, **321**, 324–5

Kelly PJ, Ahlskog JE, van Neerden JA, Carmichael SW, Stoddard SL, and Bell GN (1989) Adrenal medullary autograft transplantation into the striatum of patients with Parkinson's disease. *Mayo Clin Prod*, **64**, 282–90

Knüsel B, Michel PP, Schwaber JS, and Hefti F (1990) Selective and nonselective stimulation of central cholinergic and dopaminergic development in vitro by nerve growth factor, basic fibroblast growth factor, epidermal growth factor, insulin and the insulin-like growth factors I and II. *J Neurosci*, **10**, 558–70

Knüsel B, Winslow JW, Rosenthal A, Burton LE, Seid DP, Nikolics K *et al.* (1991) Promotion of central cholinergic and dopaminergic neuron differentiation by brain-derived neurotrophic factor but not neurotrophin 3. *Proc Natl Acad Sci USA*, **88**, 961–5

Kordower JH, Fiandaca MS, Notter MFD, Hansen JT, and Gash DM (1990) NFG-like trophic support from peripheral nerve for grafted rhesus adrenal chromaffin cells. *J Neurosurg*, **73**, 418–28

Kordower JH, Cochran E, Penn RD, and Goetz CG (1991) Putative chromaffin cell survival and enhanced host-derived TH-fiber innervation following a functional adrenal medulla autograft for Parkinson's disease. *Ann Neurol*, **29**, 405–12

Landau WM (1990) Artificial intelligence: the brain transplant cure for parkinsonism. *Neurology*, **40**, 733–40

Langston JW, Irwin I, Langston EB, and Forno L (1984) 1-methyl-4-phenylpyridinium ion (MPP+): identification of a metabolite of MPTP, a toxin selective to the substantia nigra. *Neurosci Lett*, **48**, 87–92

Langston JW, Widner H, Brooks D, Fahn S, Freeman T, Goetz CG *et al.* (1992) Core assessment program for intracerebral transplantations (CAPIT). *Movement Disorders*, **7**, 1–13

Leenders KL, Frackowiak R, Quinn N, and Marsden CD (1986a) Brain energy metabolism and dopaminergic function in Huntington's disease measured *in vivo* using positron emission tomography. *Movement Disorders*, **1**, 69–77

Leenders KL, Palmer AJ, Quinn N, Clark JC, Firnau G, Garnett ES *et al.* (1986b) Brain dopamine metabolism in patients with Parkinson's disease measured with positron emission tomography. *J Neurol Neurosurg Psychiatry*, **49**, 853–60

Lindvall O, Backlund E-O, Farde L, Sedvall G, Freedman R, Hoffer B *et al.* (1987a) Transplantation in Parkinson's disease: two cases of adrenal medullary grafts to the putamen. *Ann Neurol*, **22**, 457–68

Lindvall O, Dunnett SB, Brundin P, and Björklund A (1987b) Transplantation of catecholamine-producing cells to the basal ganglia in Parkinson's disease: experimental and clinical studies. In Rose FC, eds, *Parkinson's Disease: Clinical and Experimental Advances*, London, John Libbey, 189–206

Lindvall O, Rehncrona S, Brundin P, Gustavii B, Åstedt B, Widner H *et al.* (1989) Human fetal dopamine neurons grafted into the striatum in two patients with severe Parkinson's disease: a detailed account of methodology and a 6 month follow-up. *Arch Neurol*, **46**, 615–31

Lindvall O, Brundin P, Widner H, Rehncrona S, Gustavii B, Frackowiak R *et al.* (1990a) Grafts of fetal dopamine neurons survive and improve motor function in Parkinson's disease. *Science*, **247**, 574–7

Lindvall O, Rehncrona S, Brundin P, Gustavii B, Åstedt B, Widner H *et al.* (1990b) Neural transplantation in Parkinson's disease: the Swedish experience. *Prog Brain Res*, **82**, 729–34

Lindvall O, Widner H, Rehncrona S, Brundin P, Odin P, Gustavii B *et al.* (1992) Transplantation of fetal dopamine neurons in Parkinson's disease: one-year clinical and neurophysiological observations in two patients with putaminal implants. *Ann Neurol*, **31**, 155–65

Lindvall O, Sawle G, Widner H, Rothwell JC, Björklund A, Brundin P *et al.* (1993) Evidence for long term survival and function of dopaminergic grafts in progressive Parkinson's disease. *Ann Neurol*, (in press)

Liu F-C, Graybiel AM, Dunnett SB, and Baughman RW (1990) Intrastriatal grafts derived from fetal striatal primordia: II Compartmental alignment of cholinergic and dopaminergic systems. *J Comp Neurol*, **295**, 1–15

Liu FC, Dunnett SB, Robertson HA, and Graybiel AM (1991) Intrastriatal grafts derived from fetal striatal primordia: III Induction of modular patterns of Fis-like immunoreactivity by cocaine. *Exp Brain Res*, **85**, 501–6

López-Lozano JJ, Bravo G, Brera B, Uria J, D'Argallo J, Salmean J *et al.* (1991b) Can an analogy be drawn between the clinical evolution of Parkinson's patients who undergo autoimplantation of adrenal medulla and those of fetal ventral mesencephalon transplant recipients? In Lindvall O, Björklund A, and Widner H, eds, *Intracerebral Transplantation in Movement Disorders, Experimental Basis and Clinical Experiences*, Amsterdam, Elsevier, 87–98

López-Lozano JJ, Bravo G, Abascal J and the Clinica Puerta de Hierro Neural Transplantation Group (1991a) Grafting of perfused adrenal medullary tissue into the caudate nucleus of patients with Parkinson's disease. *J Neurosurg*, **75**, 234–43

López-Lozano JJ, Bravo G, Abascal J, Brera B, Santos H, Gomez-Angulo C, and CHP Neural Transplantation Group (1992) Co-transplantation of peripheral nerve and adrenal medulla in Parkinson's disease. *Lancet*, **339**, 430

Madrazo I, Drucker-Colin R, Diaz V, Martinez-Mata J, Torres C, and Becerril JJ (1987) Open microsurgical autograft of adrenal medulla to the right caudate nucleus in two patients with intractable Parkinson's disease. *N Engl J Med*, **316**, 831–4

Madrazo I, Franco-Bourland R, Aguilera M, and Ostrosky-Solis F (1989) Hispanic registry of graft procedures for Parkinson's disease. *Lancet*, **ii**, 751–2

Madrazo I, Drucker-Colin R, Torres C, Ostrosky-Solis F, Franco-Bourland R, Aguilera M *et al.* (1990a) Long term changes in Parkinson's disease patients with adrenal medullary autografts to the caudate nucleus. In Bunney WE Jr, Hippius H, Lackman FG, and Schmauss M, eds, *Proceedings of the XVIth C.I.N.P. Congress*, Berlin, Springer, 118–32

Madrazo I, Franco-Bourland R, Ostrosky-Solis F, Aguilera M, Cuevas C, Alvarez F *et al.* (1990b) Neural transplantation (auto-adrenal, fetal nigral, and fetal adrenal) in Parkinson's disease. The Mexican experience. *Prog Brain Res*, **82**, 593–602

Madrazo I, Franco-Bourland R, Ostrosky-Solis F, Aguilera M, Cuevas C, Zamorano, C *et al.* (1990c)

Fetal homotransplants (ventral mesencephalon and adrenal tissue) to the striatum of Parkinsonian subjects. *Arch Neurol*, **47**, 1281–5

Madrazo I, Franco-Bourland R, Aguilera M, Ostrosky-Solis F, Cuevas C, Castrejon H *et al.* (1991) Fetal ventral mesencephalon brain homotransplantation in Parkinson's Disease: the Mexican Experience. In Lindvall O, Björklund A and Widner H, eds, *Intracerebral Transplantation in Movement Disorders*, Amsterdam, Elsevier, 123–9

Mandel RJ, Brundin P, and Björklund A (1990) The importance of graft placement and task complexity for transplant-induced recovery of simple and complex sensorimotor deficits in dopamine denerated rats. *Eur J Neurosci*, **2**, 888–94

Mandel RJ, Wictorin K, Cenci MA, and Björklund A (1992) Fos expression in intrastriatal grafts: regulation by host dopaminergic afferents. *Brain Res*, **583**, 207–15

Mason ST and Fibiger HC (1978) Kainic acid lesions of the straitum: behavioural sequelae similar to Huntington's chorea. *Brain Res*, **155**, 313–29

Mason DW, Charlton HM, Jones AJ, Lavy CB, Puklavec M, and Simmonds J (1986) The fate of allogeneic and xenogeneic neuronal tissue transplanted into the third ventricle of rodents. *Neuroscience*, **19**, 685–94

Medawar PB (1948) Immunity to homologous grafted skin. III. The fate of skin homografts transplanted to the brain, to subcutaneous tissue, and to the anterior chamber of the eye. *Br J Exp Pathol*, **29**, 58–69

Molina H, Quinones R, Alvarez L, Galarraga J, Piedra J, Suarez C *et al.* (1991) Transplantation of human fetal mesencephalic tissue in caudate nucleus as treatment for Parkinson's disease: the Cuban experience. In Lindvall O, Björklund A, and Widner H, eds, *Intracerebral Transplantation in Movement Disorders, Experimental Basis and Clinical Experiences*, Amsterdam, Elsevier, 99–110

Nakai M, Itakura T, Kamei I, Nakai K, Naka Y, Imai H *et al.* (1990) Autologous transplantation of the superior cervical ganglion into the brain of parkinsonian monkeys. *J Neurosurg*, **72**, 92–5

Nicholas MK and Arnason BGW (1989) Immunological considerations in transplantation to the central nervous system. In Seil, FJ, ed, *Frontiers in Clinical Neuroscience, vol 6. Neural Regeneration and Transplantation*, New York, Alan Liss, 239–84

Nikkhah G, Odin P, Smits A, Tingström A, Othberg A, Brundin P *et al.* (1993) Platelet-derived growth factor promotes survival of rat and human mesencephalic dopaminergic neurons in culture. *Exp Brain Res*, **92**, 516–23

Norman AB, Giordano M, and Sanberg PR (1989) Fetal striatal tissue grafts into excitotoxin-lesioned striatum: pharmacological and behavioural aspects. *Pharmacol Biochem Behav*, **34**, 139–47

Olanow CW, Koller W, Goetz CG, Stebbins GT, Cahill DW, Gauger LL *et al.* (1990) Autologous transplantation of adrenal medulla in Parkinson's disease. *Arch Neurol*, **47**, 1286–9

Olney JW (1989) Excitatory amino acids and neuropsychiatric disorders. *Biol Psychiatry*, **26**, 505–25

Olson L, Backlund E-O, Ebendal T, Freedman R, Hamberger B, Hanson P *et al.* (1991) Intraputaminal infusion of nerve growth factor to support adrenal medullary autografts in Parkinson's disease. One-year follow-up of first clinical trial. *Arch Neurol*, **48**, 373–81

Otto D and Unsicker K (1990) Basic FGF reverses chemical and morphological deficits in the nigrostriatal system of MPTP treated mice. *J Neurosci*, **10**, 1912–21

Penn RD, Goetz CG, Tanner CM, Klawans HL, Shannon KM, Comella CL *et al.* (1988) The adrenal medullary transplant operation for Parkinson's disease: clinical observations in five patients. *Neurosurgery*, **22**, 999–1004

Perlow MJ, Freed WJ, Hoffer BJ, Seiger Å, Olson L, and Wyatt RJ (1979) Brain grafts reduce motor abnormalities produced by destruction of nigrostriatal dopamine system. *Science*, **204**, 643–7

Peterson DI, Price ML, and Small CS (1989) Autopsy findings in a patient who had an adrenal-to-brain transplant for Parkinson's disease. *Neurology*, **39**, 235–8

Pezzoli G, Silani V, Motti E, and Ferrante C (1988) Clinical and biochemical follow-up after adrenal medulla autograft in Parkinson's disease. In *9th International Symposium on Parkinson's Disease*, 33

Pezzoli G, Motti E, Zecchinelli A, Ferrante C, Silani V, Falini A *et al.* (1990) Adrenal medulla autograft in 3 parkinsonian patients: results using two different approaches. *Prog Brain Res*, **82**, 677–82

Pritzel M, Isacson O, Wiklund L, and Björklund A (1986) Afferent and efferent connections of striatal grafts implanted into the ibotenic acid lesioned neostriatum in adult rats. *Exp Brain Res*, **65**, 112–26

Redmond DE Jr, Naftolin F, Collier TJ, Leranth C, Robbins RJ, Sladek CD *et al.* (1988) Cryopreservation, culture, and transplantation of human fetal mesencephalic tissue into monkeys. *Science*, **242**, 768–71

Redmond DE Jr, Spencer D, Naftolin F, Leranth C, Robbins RJ, Vollmer TL *et al.* (1989) Cryopreserved human fetal neural tissue remains viable 4 months after transplantation into human caudate nucleus. *Soc Neurosci Abstracts*, **54**, 2

Robbins RJ, Torres-Aleman I, Leranth C, Bradberry CW, Deutch AY, Welsh S *et al.* (1990) Cryopreservation of human brain tissue. *Exp Neurol*, **107**, 208–13

Rutherford A, Garcia-Munoz M, Dunnett SB, and Arbuthnott GW (1987) Electrophysiological demonstration of host cortical inputs into striatal grafts. *Neurosci Lett*, **83**, 275–81

Sanberg PR, Giordano M, Henault MA, Nash DR, Ragozzino ME, and Hagermayer-Houser SH (1989) Intraparenchymal striatal transplants required for maintenance of behavioural recovery in an animal model of Huntington's disease. *J Neural Transpl*, **1**, 23–31

Sauer H and Brundin P (1991) Effects of cool storage on survival and function of intrastriatal ventral mesencephalic grafts. *Restor Neurol Neurosci*, **2**, 123–35

Sauer H, Fischer W, Nikkhah G, Weigand SJ, Brundin P, Lindsay RM, and Björklund A (1993) Brain-derived neurotrophic factor enhances function rather than the survival of intrastriatal dopamine cell-rich grafts. *Brain Res* (in press)

Sauer H, Frodl EM, Kupsch A, ten Bruggencate G, and Oertel WH (1992b) Cryopreservation, survival and function of intrastriatal fetal mesencephalic grafts in a rat model of Parkinson's disease. *Exp Brain Res*, **90**, 54–62

Sawle GV, Bloomfield PM, Björklund A, Brooks DJ, Brundin P, Leenders KL *et al.* (1992) Transplantation of fetal dopamine neurons in Parkinson's disease: PET [^{18}F]6-L-fluorodopa studies in two patients with putaminal implants. *Ann Neurol*, **31**, 166–73

Schumacher JM, Short MP, Hyman BT, Breakefield XO and Isacson O (1991) Intracerbal implantation of nerve growth factor-producing fibroblasts protects striatum against neurotoxic levels of excitatory amino acids. *Neuroscience*, **45**, 561–70

Seiger A (1985) Preparation of immature central nervous system regions for transplantation. In Björklund A and Stenevi U eds, *Neural Grafting in the Mammalian CNS*, Amsterdam, Elsevier, 71–7

Shoulson I and The Parkinson Study Group (1989) Effect of deprenyl on the progression of disability in early Parkinson's disease. *N Engl J Med*, **321**, 1364–71

Sirinathsinghji, DJS, Dunnett SB, Isacson O, Clarke DJ, Kendrick K, and Björklund A (1988) Striatal grafts in rats with unilateral neostriatal lesions. II. *In vivo* monitoring of GABA release in globus pallidus and substantia nigra. *Neuroscience*, **24**, 803–11

Sirinathsinghji DJS, Morris BJ, Wisden W, Northrop A, Hunt SP, and Dunnett SB (1990) Gene expression in striatal grafts – I. Cellular localization of neurotransmitter mRNAs. *Neuroscience*, **34**, 675–86

Sladek JR Jr, Redmond DE Jr, Collier TJ, Blount JP, Elsworth JD, Taylor JR *et al.* (1988) Fetal dopamine neural grafts: extended reversal of methylphenyltetrahydropyridine-induced parkinsonism in monkeys. *Prog Brain Res*, **78**, 497–506

Sofroniew MV, Isacson O, and Björklund A (1986) Cortical grafts prevent atrophy of cholinergic basal nucleus neurons induced by excitotoxic cortical damage. *Brain Res*, **378**, 409–15

Spencer DD, Robbins RJ, Naftolin F, Marek KL, Vollmer T, Leranth C *et al.* (1992) Unilateral transplantation of human fetal mesencephalic tissue into the caudate nucleus of patients with Parkinson's disease. *N Engl J Med*, **327**, 1541–8

Steece-Collier K, Yurek DM, Collier TJ, and Sladek JR Jr (1991) Neuropharmacological interactions of levodopa and dopamine grafts: possible impaired development and function of grafted embryonic neurons. In Lindvall O, Björklund A, and Widner, H, eds, *Intracerebral Transplantation in Movement Disorders, Experimental Basis and Clinical Expericnces*, Amsterdam, Elsevier, 325–31

Steinbusch HW, Vermeulen RJ, and Tonnaer JA (1990) Basic fibroblast growth factor enhances survival and sprouting of fetal dopaminergic cells implanted in the denervated rat caudate-putamen: preliminary observations. *Prog Brain Res*, **82**, 81–6

Strecker RE, Miao R, and Loring JF (1989) Survival and function of aggregate cultures of rat fetal dopamine neurons grafted in a rat model of Parkinson's disease. *Exp Brain Res*, **76**, 315–22

Strömberg I, Herrera-Marschitz M, Ungerstedt U, Ebendal T, and Olson L (1985) Chronic implants of chromaffin tissue into the dopamine-denervated striatum. Effects of NGF on graft survival, fiber growth and rotational behavior. *Exp Brain Res*, **60**, 335–49

Takeuchi J, Tabeke Y, Sakakura T, Hara Y, Yasuda T, and Imai T (1990) Adrenal medulla transplantation into the putamen in Parkinson's disease. *Neurosurgery*, **26**, 499–503

Tanner CM, Watts RL, Bakay RAE, and Petruk KC (1989) Adrenal medullary autografts in patients with Parkinson's disease. *N Engl J Med*, **321**, 325

Tetrud JW and Langston JW (1989) The effect of deprenyl (selegiline) on the natural history of Parkinson's disease. *Science*, **245**, 519–22

Tulipan N, Huang S, Whetsell WO, and Allen GS (1986) Neonatal striatal grafts prevent lethal syndrome produced by bilateral intrastriatal injection of kainic acid. *Brain Res*, **377**, 163–7

Tyce GM, Ahlskog JE, Carmichael SW, Chritton SL, Stoddard SL, van Heerden JA *et al.* (1989) Catecholamines in CSF, plasma, and tissue after autologous transplantation of adrenal medulla to the brain in patients with Parkinson's disease. *J Lab Clin Med*, **114**, 185–92

Weiner WJ and Lang AE (1989) *Movement Disorders: A Comprehensive Survey*, New York, Futura

Wictorin K and Björklund A (1989) Connectivity of striatal grafts implanted into the ibotenic acid lesioned striatum. II. Cortical afferents. *Neuroscience*, **30**, 297–311

Wictorin K, Lagenaur CF, Lund RD, and Björklund A (1991) Efferent projections to the host brain from intrastriatal striatal mouse-to-rat grafts: time-course and tissue-type specificity as revealed by a mouse specific neuronal marker. *Eur J Neurosci*, **3**, 86–101

Wictorin K, Isacson O, Fischer W, Nothias F, Peschanski M, and Björklund A (1988) Connectivity of striatal grafts implanted into the ibotenic acid-lesioned striatum. I. Subcortical afferents. *Neuroscience*, **27**, 547–62

Wictorin K, Clarke DJ, Bolam JP, and Björklund A (1989a) Host corticostriatal fibres establish synaptic connections with grafted striatal neurons in the ibotenic acid lesioned striatum. *Eur J Neurosci*, **1**, 189–95

Wictorin K, Ouimet CC, and Björklund A (1989b) Intrinsic organization and connectivity of intrastriatal striatal transplants in rats as revealed by DARPP-32 immunohistochemistry: specificity of connections with the lesioned host brain. *Eur J Neurosci*, **1**, 690–701

Wictorin K, Simerley RB, Isacson O, Swanson L, and Björklund (1989c) Connectivity of striatal grafts implanted into the ibotenic acid lesioned striatum. III. Efferent projecting graft neurons and their relation to host efferents within the grafts. *Neuroscience*, **30**, 313–30

Wictorin K, Brundin P, Gustavii B, Lindvall O, and Björklund A (1990) Reformation of long axon pathways in adult rat central nervous system by human forebrain neuroblasts. *Nature*, **347**, 556–8

Wictorin K, Brundin P, Sauer H, Lindvall O, and Björklund A (1992) Long distance directed axonal growth from human dopaminergic mesencephalic neuroblasts implanted along the nigrostriatal pathway in 6-hydroxydopamine lesioned adult rats. *J Comp Neurol*, **323**, 475–94

Widner H and Brundin P (1988) Immunological aspects of grafting in the mammalian central nervous system. A review and speculative synthesis. *Brain Res Rev*, **13**, 287–324

Widner H, Brundin P, Björklund A, and Möller E (1989a) Survival and immunogenicity of dissociated allogeneic fetal neural dopamine-rich grafts implanted into the brains of adult mice. *Exp Brain Res*, **76**, 187–97

Widner H, Brundin P, Björklund A, and Möller E (1989b) Survival and immunogenicity of fetal allogeneic neural grafts implanted into the adult brains of mice and rats. *Restor Neurol Neurosci* (suppl. 1), 13

Widner H, Brundin P, and Lindvall O (1990) Clinical trials with allogeneic fetal neural grafts in Parkinson's disease: theoretical and practical immunological aspects. In Johansson BB, Owman Ch, and Widner H, eds, *Pathophysiology of the Blood–Brain Barrier*, Amsterdam, Elsevier, 593–608

Widner H, Tetrud J, Rehncrona S, Snow B, Brundin P, Gustavii B *et al.* (1992) Bilateral fetal mesencephalic grafting in two patients with parkinsonism induced by 1-methyl-4-phenyl-1,2,3,6-tetrahydropyridine (MPTP). *N Engl J Med*, **327**, 1556–63

Wilson CJ, Emson P, and Feler C (1987) Electrophysiological evidence for the formation of a corticostriatal pathway in neostriatal tissue grafts. *Soc Neurosci Abstracts*, **13**, 11

Wolff JA, Fisher LJ, Xu L, Jinnah HA, Langlais PJ, Iuvone PM *et al.* (1989) Grafting fibroblasts genetically modified to produce L-dopa in a rat model of Parkinson's disease. *Proc Natl Acad Sci USA*, **86**, 9011–14

Xu ZC, Wilson CJ, and Emson PC (1989) Restoration of the corticostriatal projection in rat neostriatal grafts: electron microscopic analysis. *Neuroscience*, **29**, 539–50

Xu ZC, Wilson CJ, and Emson PC (1990) Restoration of thalamostriatal projections in rat neostriatal grafts: an electron microscopic analysis. *J Comp Neurol*, **303**, 2–14

Xu ZC, Wilson CJ, and Emson PC (1991) Synaptic potentials evoked in spiny neurons in rat neostriatal grafts by cortical and thalamic stimulation. *J Neurophysiol*, **65**, 477–93

13
Multiple system atrophy

Niall Quinn

INTRODUCTION

Multiple system atrophy (MSA) is a term introduced in 1969 by Graham and Oppenheimer. It refers to a disease characterized clinically by any combination of parkinsonian, autonomic, pyramidal or cerebellar symptoms and signs, and pathologically by cell loss and gliosis in some or all of the following structures: putamen, caudate, globus pallidus, substantia nigra, locus coeruleus, inferior olives, pontine nuclei, cerebellar Purkinje cells, and the intermediolateral cell columns and Onuf's nucleus of the spinal cord. It is perhaps unfortunate that their index case of MSA was clinically slightly atypical for the disorder as a whole, in that parkinsonian features were absent in life, as some degree of clinical parkinsonism is present before death in about 90% of cases of MSA. However nigra, putamen and globus pallidus were all pathologically, if subclinically, affected. Unfortunately, some other authors then seized upon MSA as an umbrella term for all sorts of degenerative conditions involving the basal ganglia and/or brainstem/cerebellar or other structures, so that the term was in danger of losing its currency. As will be emphasized later, the term MSA should be restricted to a particular combination of clinical and pathological features. Other cases in which clinical and/or pathological features point to involvement of multiple systems in the brain either have their own designations (e.g. Huntington's disease, Pick's disease) or should alternatively be labelled multisystem degenerations, but *not* MSA. Moreover, I propose that the term MSA should be restricted to subjects with sporadic disease, a usage more restricted than that originally proposed by Graham and Oppenheimer, who were happy to include both sporadic and familial cases.

HISTORY

I have dealt with some of the key historical markers in the development of the concept of MSA in some detail elsewhere (Quinn, 1989a). Cases of MSA have been described under the rubrics of olivopontocerebellar atrophy (OPCA), idiopathic orthostatic hypotension (IOH) or progressive autonomic failure, Shy–Drager syndrome (SDS) and striatonigral degeneration (SND). However, not all cases described as examples of these disorders necessarily had MSA. Moreover the most common circumstance has been for cases of MSA to be misdiagnosed as idiopathic Parkinson's disease (IPD).

All concerned with research in IPD will be familiar with the common requirement (due, it seems, to the dictates of non-parametric statistics) that a minimum of 6 patients be studied. They will also have had the experience of discovering before (or after) publication that at least 1 of these patients did not have IPD, perhaps the only point in favour of the inordinately long delay from submission to publication in most journals (and books!) today. In this context, James Parkinson's (1817) description of his index case I, upon whom much of the classical description of paralysis agitans is based, merits close scrutiny. He was the only patient that Parkinson was able to follow to death. 'A man rather more than fifty years of age' who had gradually developed tremor and fatigue. Then, 'as the disease proceeds . . . the utmost care is necessary to prevent frequent falls. Towards its last stage . . . words are now scarcely intelligible . . . food is with difficulty retained in the mouth until masticated; and then as difficultly swallowed. The chin is almost immoveably bent down upon the sternum. The power of articulation is lost. The urine and faeces are passed involuntarily'. It is at least possible that the patient upon whom most of the classic description of Parkinson's disease was based had MSA. There was, of course, no pathology in this case, so we shall never know.

Berciano, in his comprehensive 1982 review, considered the cases of Pierret (1871) and Schultze (1887) to be the first examples of pathologically confirmed OPCA. However, I feel it would be misleading to place either of them within the rubric of MSA. Pierret's case developed cerebellar ataxia and dysarthria at the age of 4, and died aged 68. The pathological appearances would be more in keeping with dysgenesis than degeneration. Schultze (1887) reported an alcoholic man who developed cerebellar symptoms, increased knee jerks (Babinski first described his response in 1896), diabetes insipidus and a wasted tongue at age 39, dying at age 43. Although there was atrophy of olives, pons and cerebellum, nigra and basal ganglia were not mentioned. Royet and Collet (1893) described a man who developed cerebellar and pyramidal signs and incontinence of urine from age 48, dying at age 55. However, there was no parkinsonism, and despite OPCA the state of nigra and striatum was not mentioned. Although Dejerine and Thomas (1900) were the first to record, *en passant*, clinical evidence of parkinsonism in OPCA, they did not emphasize it as such; nor did they mention the state of the nigra and striatum in their autopsied case, save for a cursory mention, in the conclusion, of the 'relative integrity of the central grey matter'. However, one should also note that it was only in 1919 that Trétiakoff focused attention on nigral pathology in parkinsonism.

The case of von Stauffenberg (1918), diagnosed in life as OPCA, was really the first to associate cerebellar, autonomic and parkinsonian features in life with identified pathological lesions not only of olives, pons and cerebellum, but also of basal ganglia pigmentation and atrophy of putamen, with additional cell loss in caudate and globus pallidus (nigra was not mentioned). Six years later, von Fleischhacker (1924) described the first case of predominant parkinsonism showing the pathology of MSA (the patient had been diagnosed in life by Oppenheim as paralysis agitans).

In 1960 Shy and Drager reported two men with a complex picture incorporating not only parkinsonism and autonomic failure but also incoordination and pyramidal features. Unfortunately the term SDS has been used so variably by different authors that it, too, has been in danger of losing its original currency. The *syndrome* Shy and Drager described was *not* Parkinson's disease, or even parkinsonism, with autonomic failure. It comprised additional signs incompatible with PD, and its pathological substrate (in their one autopsied case) was that of MSA.

If Shy and Drager's intended meaning was erroneously widened by others, the reverse is true of Adams *et al.*'s description of striatonigral degeneration (SND). Their 1961 abstract (van der Eecken *et al.*, 1961) might suggest that they were describing pure parkinsonism due to a pure lesion of nigra and striatum. However, close scrutiny of the 4 sporadic cases described between their two full papers (Adams *et al.*, 1961, 1964) reveals that varying admixtures of pyramidal and cerebellar features and autonomic failure, together with pathological findings of OPCA, were also present.

It is important to note that all of these reports antedated the introduction of levodopa for the treatment of Parkinson's disease in 1967, and to recall that overall a poor, atypical, waning or absent response to treatment is often the single most helpful early diagnostic clue that one is not dealing with IPD (see the section on treatment and management, below).

After the paper by Graham and Oppenheimer (1969) introducing the term MSA to cover many examples of OPCA, SDS and SND, the next major landmark was Bannister and Oppenheimer's 1972 review of 16 cases of 'degenerative diseases of the nervous system associated with autonomic failure'. They stressed that, among other causes, autonomic failure could be due to Lewy body pathology (with, $n=2$, or without, $n=3$, parkinsonism) or to MSA with other (cerebellar or pyramidal) neurological signs with ($n=8$) or without ($n=3$) parkinsonism. This view of the neurological spectrum of MSA was necessarily limited by reviewing only 12 cases, all with prominent autonomic failure. A feature which emerges from a much larger review of the literature (see below) is that in one fifth of cases of pathologically proven MSA, in life only parkinsonism with (11%) or without (10%) autonomic failure has been recorded, and it is these cases that are the most difficult to diagnose correctly in life. Close attention to possible evidence of autonomic failure might, however, shift a number of cases from the first of these categories to the second.

DIAGNOSIS – CLINICAL AND PATHOLOGICAL

Pathological diagnostic criteria

Gray *et al.* (1988) advanced pathological diagnostic criteria for MSA derived from those of Oppenheimer (1983). They defined it as a primary degeneration of the nervous system, sporadic, and with onset in middle life, characterised by cell loss and gliosis in a selection (at least three) of the following structures: striatum pigmented brainstem nuclei (substantia nigra and locus coeruleus), pontine nuclei and middle cerebellar peduncles, cerebellar Purkinje cells, inferior olives and dorsal vagal nuclei.

However, I would now accept for a dignosis of MSA cell loss and gliosis in only two structures (which could be different brainstem nuclei), provided characteristic inclusions (see below) are also present. Thus, we have recently encountered two patients with MSA (Wenning *et al.*, in press) whose brains showed cell loss only in nigra and locus coeruleus, but contained widespread oligodendroglial cytoplasmic inclusions. When parkinsonism is clinically present, substantia nigra always, and striatum almost always, shows cell loss and gliosis.

The striatal lesion may sometimes only be evident on glial fibrillary acidic protein (GFAP) staining and, when present, the changes in putamen (which begin dorsolaterally in its posterior two-thirds and, with increasing severity, extend in a dorsal to ventral and posterior to anterior direction) are more severe than those in the external segment of globus pallidus, which in turn is more severely affected than its internal segment and than the caudate nucleus (Fearnley and Lees, 1990). The lesion in substantia nigra compacta is maximal in the ventrolateral cell group, which is even more selectively involved in IPD.

In addition, now that the clinical picture in pathologically proven cases of MSA has become sufficiently characterized, the clinical course and features should, for certain diagnosis, also fall within the known range for the disorder.

Thus, patients with other causes of parkinsonism or pseudoparkinsonism such as hydrocephalus, multi-infarct states or Binswanger's disease with parkinsonism–ataxia or lower-body parkinsonism would not qualify for a clinical diagnosis of MSA. Occasional cases of MSA may, however, be shown at autopsy to have a second, coincidental, pathology.

Duvoisin (1989) found that only 24 of 34 (71%) 'recognised leading authorities on Parkinson's disease in 10 countries' agree with the statement: 'Although Lewy bodies may occur in other conditions, if there are no Lewy bodies, it isn't Parkinson's disease'. My own view, shared with others in the UK and encouraged by the meticulous work of Gibb and Lees (1988), is that the brain of a patient with IPD must contain Lewy bodies in substantia nigra. However, the converse is not true. Thus, not all brains containing Lewy bodies necessarily come from patients who had clinical IPD in life. Crucially, the finding of cell loss and Lewy bodies in brainstem pigmented nuclei of a patient who exhibited clinical parkinsonism during life does not exclude other causes of parkinsonism such as MSA. Striatum, olives, pons and cerebellum should therefore *always* be examined using GFAP staining in any case of parkinsonism. The presence of oligodendroglial and intraneuronal cytoplasmic inclusions (see below) would now also be considered a *sine qua non* for a pathological diagnosis of MSA. Although commonly affected, the intermediolateral cell columns are often not available for examination. Nevertheless, predominant cell loss in intermediolateral cell columns can reasonably be included in the proposed modified pathological diagnostic criteria set out in Table 13.1. The neuropathology of MSA is the subject of excellent reviews by Oppenheimer (1983) and Daniel (1992).

Clinical diagnostic criteria

In 1989 I proposed provisional clinical diagnostic criteria for MSA (Quinn, 1989a). An updated and slightly revised version is set out in Table 13.2. This schema has certain theoretical drawbacks. For example, it does not include a separate category for those cases (who would reasonably be called 'mixed') in which parkinsonism and cerebellar features assume equal prominence, and patients may progress in the course of their disease from one category to the other. Nevertheless, I have personally found it a convenient and reliable way of diagnosing patients. Moreover, out of many cases seen, all 15 of those I have personally assessed in life as clinically probable MSA according to this schema, and who have also come to postmortem, have then had MSA pathologically confirmed. However, a diagnosis of possible MSA is considerably less secure. Theoretically, one might object that it makes no allowance for cases of

Table 13.1 Pathological diagnostic criteria

*Histological**
Cell loss and gliosis in at least two of the following structures:

Striatum (posterior putamen maximally affected) }
Substantia nigra } one or other is almost invariably involved
Locus coeruleus
Pontine nuclei and/or middle cerebellar peduncles
Cerebellar Purkinje cells
Inferior olives
Intermediolateral cell columns,

together with:

Cytological
Typical oligodendroglial inclusions should be present on Bielschowsky silver or anti-ubiquitin staining

Note:
1. GFAP (glial fibrillary acidic protein) staining should be used to detect gliosis
2. Clinical features should be within the range found in multiple systm atrophy
3. No other cause for the pathology can be found

*Derived from Oppenheimer (1983) and Gray *et al.* (1988).

Table 13.2 Multiple system atrophy: proposed clinical diagnostic criteria

Striatonigral type (predominantly parkinsonism)		Olivopontocerebellar type (predominantly cerebellar)
Sporadic adult-onset non poorly levodopa-responsive parkinsonism*	Possible	Sporadic adult-onset cerebellar syndrome with parkinsonism
Above**, plus severe symptomatic autonomic failure*** or cerebellar signs or pyramidal signs or pathological sphincter electromyogram	Probable	Sporadic adult-onset cerebellar syndrome* (with or without parkinsonism or pyramidal signs), plus severe symptomatic autonomic failure*** or pathological sphincter electromyogram
Postmortem confirmed	Definite	Postmortem confirmed

*Without *DSM-III* dementia, generalized tendon areflexia, prominent supranuclear palsy for downgaze or other identifiable cause.
**Moderate or good, but often waning, response to levodopa may occur, in which case multiple atypical features need to be present.
***Postural syncope and/or urinary incontinence or retention not due to other causes.
Sporadic: no other case of MSA among first- or second-degree relatives.
Adult-onset: onset age 30 years or above.
Modified from Quinn (1989a), with permission.

MSA who, in life, show neither parkinsonism nor cerebellar signs. However, as will be seen later, of 188 cases of pathologically proven MSA there was not a single case where pure autonomic failure (PAF), a pure cerebellar or a pure pyramidal syndrome persisted in isolation until death, and only 1 case (0.5%) had not developed either cerebellar or parkinsonian features, or both, during life. However, the first case of MSA manifesting until death solely as PAF has recently been reported (Mochizuki *et al.*, 1992 – case 4). This is of course not to deny that patients can present with an isolated syndrome – just that other features are highly likely to appear as time passes. It is important to recognize that some cases initially show a dramatic response to levodopa. A diagnosis of probable MSA may still be made in them if enough other atypical features are present. For example, when 1 of my patients died after 3 years of levodopa treatment, she was still responding objectively by more than 50%, with fluctuations and dyskinesias, but had developed frequent falls, urinary incontinence (with abnormal sphincter electromyogram), respiratory stridor, postural hypotension and cerebellar atrophy on computed tomography (CT) scan.

Some explanation of the clinical exclusion criteria is needed. Onset should be age 30 years or more (there is no typical, pathologically proven sporadic case recorded with younger onset). There should be no family history of MSA although by chance about 10% of patients will have a relative with IPD. The rationale for excluding inherited adult-onset ataxias is not only their inherited nature, but also the fact that they generally start younger, survive much longer, and may have additional clinical features such as chorea, dementia, optic atrophy, pigmentary retinopathy, prominent ophthalmoplegia, areflexia or cataracts, and that parkinsonism and autonomic failure are less common (Berciano, 1982). They also lack the characteristic cellular inclusions (see later).

Dementia is not a feature of MSA, although the condition does not protect against developing coincidental Alzheimer's disease (Trotter, 1973; Neumann, 1977; Kosaka *et al.*, 1981). In my experience the scenario of the demented parkinsonian with autonomic failure (and often antecollis) most frequently occurs in Lewy body disease (Burkhardt *et al.*, 1988). However, subjects with MSA show more impairment that IPD patients on tests sensitive to frontal lobe dysfunction (Robbins *et al.*, 1992), a divergence that must presumably relate to the differing pathology of the two conditions. In this context, it is interesting to note that in MSA glial cytoplasmic inclusions can be found not only in basal ganglia but also in premotor and primary motor cortex and in the paracentral gyrus, and neuronal cytoplasmic inclusions may be seen in motor fields of cerebral cortex.

Once one has dismissed IPD and other clinical 'look-alikes' such as arteriosclerotic pseudoparkinsonism, the patients most likely to be misdiagnosed as MSA (and vice versa) are those with the Steele–Richardson–Olszewski (SRO) disease, and some with corticobasal degeneration (CBD). Sometimes severe oculomotor pareses (often accompanied by depressed or absent tendon reflexes, and sometimes by cataracts, muscle cramps, head titubation and facial weakness) may be seen in unusual cases of apparently sporadic (Guillain, 1937; Guillain *et al.*, 1942), but more commonly autosomal dominant, OPCA (Wadia and Swami, 1971; Koeppen and Hans, 1976; Wadia, 1984), but not in MSA.

Sustained nystagmus, incompatible with IPD, is seen in a minority of MSA subjects. Using electro-oculographic recordings, Rascol *et al.* (1991) have shown a pathological degree of square wave jerks in virtually all subjects with clinically diagnosed SRO, a majority of those with MSA, and a minority of those with apparent IPD. Ocular dysmetria or markedly impaired smooth pursuit and vestibulo-ocular reflex suppression may be seen in MSA (T. Anderson, personal communication). Limitation of upgaze and convergence can both occur, as in IPD. However, a prominent horizontal or downgaze palsy is an exclusion criterion for a clinical diagnosis of MSA, although a mild degree of gaze limitation is sometimes seen. The early case of SRO, before the downgaze palsy has appeared, can be misdiagnosed as MSA, but other features such as neck extension, marked palilalia, a growling dysarthria, and the later appearance of a downgaze palsy, should ultimately lead to a correct diagnosis. Though rare, those cases of SRO who never display a downgaze palsy in life remain a particular diagnostic problem.

CBD can also cause a levodopa-unresponsive akinetic–rigid syndrome. This condition classically presents grossly unilaterally (but so may MSA), often with stimulus-sensitive myoclonus (so may MSA, but this is usually initially more focal in CBD), and often with the gradual development of a supranuclear gaze palsy (leading to confusion with SRO). The usual marked limb apraxia is diagnostically helpful, but can sometimes be hard to differentiate from a very severe degree of akinesia.

Unexplained optic atrophy and retinitis pigmentosa, although sometimes seen in familial OPCA, are not part of MSA. I would now add unexplained generalised tendon areflexia as an exclusion criterion; enough evidence has accumulated to justify such cases being separated off (see above). Chorea or ballism, in the absence of drug therapy, is not a feature of classical MSA. The question of dopaminergic responsiveness is clearly of great importance in diagnosis, and will be considered under the section on treatment and management, below.

Other clinical pointers

Apart from the important cerebellar, pyramidal and autonomic features considered earlier, other 'soft' clinical features, always considered as only part of an overall picture, may raise suspicions that a patient's parkinsonism is atypical, or even help point towards MSA. Among these are early instability and falls, rapid progression, severe hypophonic dysarthria, pain unrelieved by levodopa, disproportionate antecollis (Quinn, 1989b), a recent past history of hypertension (often supine) giving way to erect normo- or hypotension, the presence of contractures, and dusky discoloration and/or coldness of the extremities not due to drugs, or Raynaud's phenomenon, which may be provoked by ergot drugs. Excessive snoring at night, and vocal cord abductor palsy leading to nocturnal and sometimes daytime stridor, may occur, and the latter is highly suggestive of MSA. Occasional deep involuntary sighs may occur. Pseudobulbar crying spells may be evident in some patients; more commonly this frequent phenomenon may only be elicited by direct questioning. Depression can also certainly occur in MSA, but its nature and frequency have never been formally studied.

CLINICAL AND PROGNOSTIC FEATURES IN PATHOLOGICALLY PROVEN CASES

In an exhaustive (but not quite comprehensive) review of pathologically proven cases of MSA from the world literature, I have tabulated 231 cases for which sex was known (135 males, 96 females – ratio 1.4 : 1), 232 cases for which age at death was known, and 213 cases for which age at onset, and survival from onset to death, were known (reference list available from author on request). The pathological data given have often not been as complete as one would ideally like, and the reports antedate the discovery of oligodendroglial inclusions. However, they relate to adult-onset

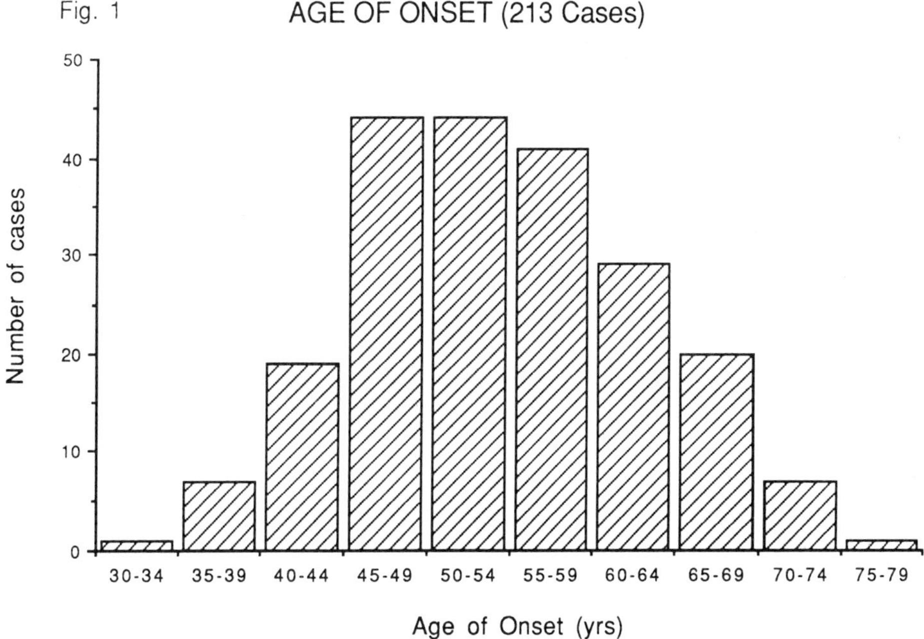

Figure 13.1 Bar histograms showing age at disease onset in 213 cases of pathologically confirmed MSA.

sporadic cases with striatonigral and/or olivopontocerebellar degeneration at autopsy, and fit into a recurring clinical and pathological theme.

When one considers age of onset (median 53 years; Fig. 13.1) it is apparent that incidence rates climb to a maximum between the ages of 45 and 59, and then decline. Some 92.5% of cases begin between the ages of 40 and 69. Less than 4% begin between 30 and 39, and the same proportion between 70 and 79 years. The youngest recorded onset is at age 31 (the next youngest being at age 35), and the oldest is at age 78 (the next oldest being age 73). This striking pattern could of course be due to sampling artefact. However, if real, it suggests that parkinsonism with autonomic failure beginning at age 70 or older is more likely to be due to IPD. It also raises the possibility that individuals may run into, and then out of, a 'window' of peak susceptibility to the disease. Could the switching on, and later off, of 'age-related genes' conceivably play a role in this phenomenon?

The age of death of 232 pathologically proven cases is shown in Figure 13.2. The numbers of cases in each quintile in which incidental Lewy bodies were also found in brainstem are within the range expected for a control population.

Survival from first symptom or sign to death in 217 published cases for which this information is available is set out in Figure 13.3. The median is 5–6 (range 1–14) years, but there are at least two reasons why this almost certainly paints an excessively gloomy picture. Firstly, when the diagnosis has not been considered in life, closer enquiry about autonomic symptoms, which are often the first indication of the disease, would frequently have lengthened the total length of history. Indeed, writing from the perspective of an autonomic research unit, Polinsky and Nee (1988) found

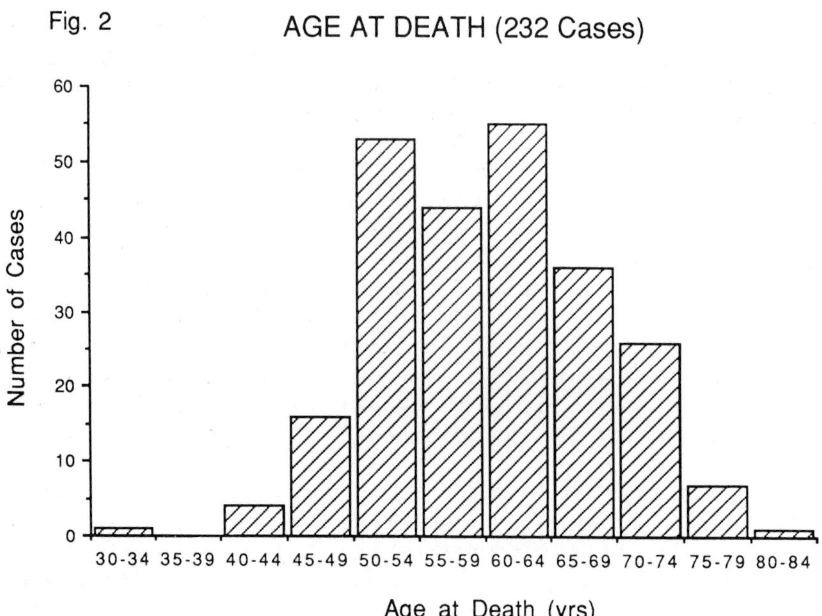

Figure 13.2 Bar histograms showing age at death in 232 cases of pathologically confirmed MSA.

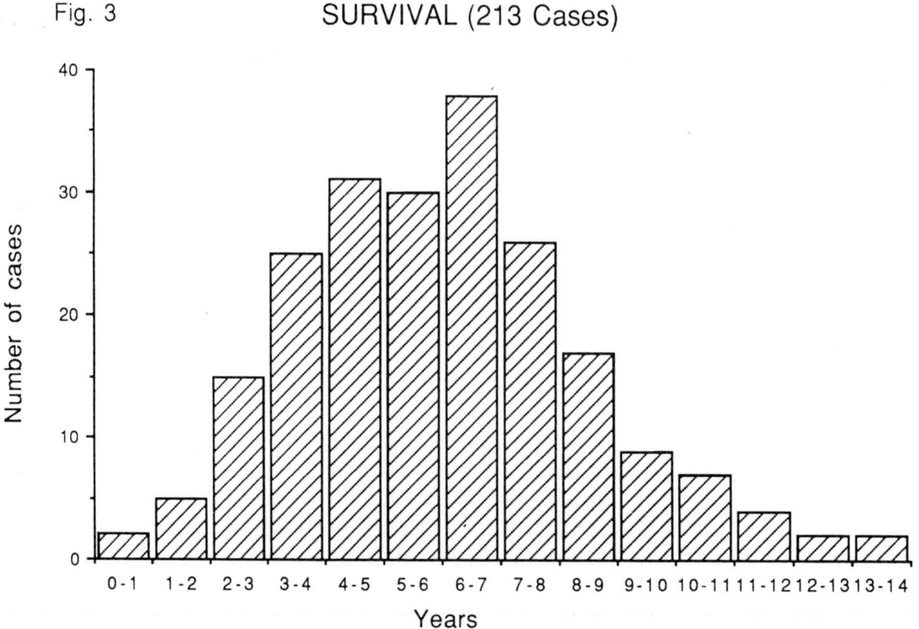

Figure 13.3 Bar histograms showing survival from recorded disease onset to death in 213 cases of pathologically confirmed MSA. Note that this gives an inordinately gloomy prognosis, and that two clinical series (see text) have given median survivals of 8.3 and 9.5 years respectively.

that among 46 deceased patients with a *clinical* diagnosis of MSA, the illness lasted 8.3 ± 0.5 years. In 75% of their patients with clinical MSA, autonomic symptoms had appeared 4.1 ± 0.5 years before the onset of neurological symptoms. In the remaining 25%, neurological symptoms preceded autonomic ones by 2.1 ± 0.3 years. Secondly, a group of deceased cases who have come to postmortem is not necessarily representative of the course of a population of living patients, still less predictive of the prognosis for an individual patient. Nevertheless, there can be no doubt that MSA significantly shortens life, all the more so because it usually strikes people in middle, rather than old, age.

Our figures for the 35 cases of MSA in the UK Parkinson's Disease Society Brain Bank as of July 1992 (Quinn *et al.*, 1993) differ slightly from those in the literature, with median age of onset 55 years, age at death 63 years, and median survival 7.3 years. Moreover, in our own series of 100 cases followed clinically (Wenning *et al.*, 1993) median age at onset was 53 years, age at death among the 42 deceased cases was 65 years, and median survival (by Kaplan-Meier analysis) for the whole aeries is 9.5 years.

Table 13.3 sets out the varying combinations of parkinsonism, cerebellar and pyramidal signs, and autonomic failure recorded as appearing prior to death in 188 pathologically proven cases of MSA for which adequate clinical information was available. The figures for autonomic failure may well be an underestimate due to failure systematically to enquire about potency, sphincter dysfunction and postural faintness. Similarly, it may be difficult in the patient with advanced parkinsonism confidently to ascribe severe dysarthria and postural instability to cerebellar dysfunction, and vice versa (Quinn and Marsden, in press). The existence of the

Table 13.3 Presence of parkinsonism, cerebellar or pyramidal signs and autonomic failure among 188 cases of pathologically proven multiple system atrophy in which details on presence or absence of each of these four features during life were available

Parkinsonism	Cerebellar signs	Pyramidal signs	Autonomic failure	*n*	%
+	+	+	+	53	28
+	–	+	+	33	18
+	–	–	+	21	11
+	+	–	+	21	11
+	–	–	–	19	10
–	+	+	+	11	6
+	–	+	–	10	5
–	+	–	+	6	3
+	+	+	–	5	3
+	+	–	–	5	3
–	+	+	–	3	2
–	–	+	+	1	0.5
–	+	–	–		
–	–	+	–	0	0.0
–	–	–	+		

Note:
1. Overall, parkinsonism was recorded in 89% (i.e. not present during life in only 11%), autonomic failure in 78%, pyramidal signs in 61% and cerebellar signs in 55%.
2. Although 10% of cases had isolated parkinsomism, there were no cases in which an isolated cerebellar or pyramidal syndrome, or pure autonomic failure, remained the only clinical feature until death.

striatal foot response can also confuse the issue of whether there are pyramidal, as well as extrapyramidal, signs. The commonest terminal picture, in 28% of cases, was a 'full house'. Next, at 18%, came the combination of parkinsonism with pyramidal signs and autonomic failure. Some 11% had parkinsonism with autonomic failure and cerebellar signs, 11% parkinsonism with autonomic failure, and 10% pure parkinsonism (thus, 21% had parkinsonism without additional neurology). Other combinations occurred with frequencies of 0.5–6%. Overall, parkinsonism was noted in 89%, autonomic failure in 78%, pyramidal signs in 61% and cerebellar signs in 55%. Thus, in only 11% was parkinsonism not present during life. Among the 167 cases with parkinsonism during life, 40 (24%) had no additional pyramidal or cerebellar signs.

LUMPING VERSUS SPLITTING

The notion that nosologically one is either a lumper or a splitter is perhaps nonsensical (Fig. 13.4), since the two activities are complementary. Lumping is a necessary prelude to splitting, which in turn sculpts a new, but smaller, lump. This can in turn be analysed to see if it has clinical, pathological and genetic coherence, or whether further splitting can be justified. This remodelling process has traditionally underpinned the classification of neurological disease. In the coming years the techniques of molecular genetics will reveal what kind of a job we have made of classifying inherited conditions (Rosenberg, 1990).

In the context of MSA, it makes sense clinically (younger onset, longer duration, etc.) and genetically to separate familial OPCA from sporadic cases, and to include the latter, together with SND and 'true' SDS under the umbrella term MSA. However, does the resultant lump comprise one or more disease entities? After splitting off those cases with areflexia that are often atypical in so many other ways (and also pathologically often have posterior column involvement), one is left with the case

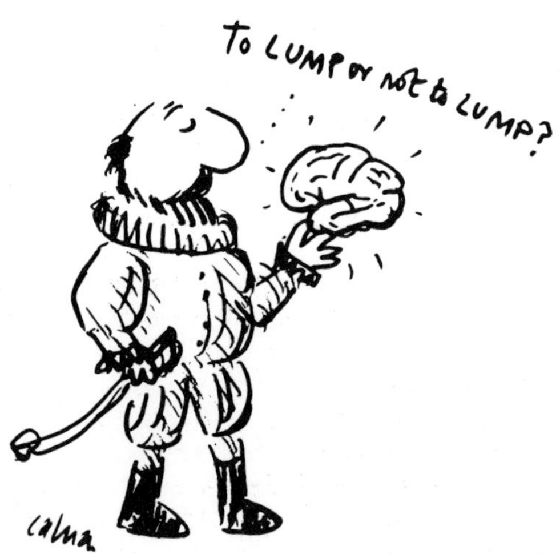

Figure 13.4 Lumping versus splitting.

material described above, which possesses at least a certain homogeneity. However, does the patient whose illness begins at age 78 have the same disease as the one affected from age 31, and do patients dying within 2 years have the same disease that killed others after 13 years? There may be more splitting yet to be done.

Independent and convincing evidence of a subcellular feature common to, and specific for, brains with MSA has been provided. Papp *et al.* (1989) found glial cytoplasmic inclusions in all of 11 brains from patients with sporadic MSA (all with parkinsonism, 9 with cerebellar and 3 with pyramidal signs, and 8 with autonomic failure). These inclusions were not found in any of 284 other brains from patients with other neurological diseases, including Parkinson's disease ($n=61$) and SRO disease ($n=5$). Nakazato *et al.* (1990) examined the brains of 6 sporadic and 2 hereditary cases of OPCA. Other than sex, age and disease duration, no other clinical details were given. 'Oligodendroglial microtubular tangles' were found in all of the sporadic cases. They were also apparently found in 1 of the 2 hereditary cases, but were completely absent in the other case of 'hereditary' OPCA and in 14 other hereditary OPCA cases reported by other authors. Kato *et al.* (1991) found glial inclusions in 18 cases of sporadic OPCA. Costa *et al.* (1992) found oligodendroglial inclusions in 9 cases of sporadic MSA, but not in 1 case of dominantly inherited OPCA, and Dr Susan Daniel (personal communication) has found then, when fixation was adequate, in all of 35 cases of MSA in the UK Parkinson's Disease Society Brain Bank.

In addition Kato *et al.* (1990), Papp and Lantos (1992) and Costa *et al.* (1992) have described neuronal as well as glial intracytoplasmic inclusions, in the same MSA brains, that are also not found in hereditary OPCA or in neurological controls.

THE EPIDEMIOLOGY OF MSA

There exist no reliable figures for the population prevalence of MSA. One obstacle has been the absence of agreed clinical diagnostic criteria. Even with the diagnostic criteria proposed above, such a study presents special difficulties. Firstly, the identification of cases of MSA demands a greater degree of sophistication and experience on the part of the clinical investigator than simply recognizing whether parkinsonism is, or is not, present. Secondly, if one assumes, say, that the prevalence rate may be anything from 5 to 15 per 100 000, then small numbers will lead to greater sampling error. Finally, since the quality of response to levodopa is a major diagnostic clue, it is very difficult, and often impossible, to diagnose MSA in untreated patients, unless there are also clear cerebellar or pyramidal signs.

As has been noted earlier, postmortem studies are more likely to reflect diagnostic certainty, but are necessarily selective. Thus, atypical cases of parkinsonism are likely to be preferably recruited, and patients with rapidly progressive disease and a poor prognosis are more likely than those with benign, long-duration disease to find their way into a brain bank, especially during its early years. Even if all cases of parkinsonism ended up in a brain bank, the proportion of brains therein showing MSA would be more a reflection of the relative *incidence*, rather than the prevalence, of MSA because of its worse prognosis. Accepting all these drawbacks, it is nevertheless instructive to examine the 'necroepidemiology' of MSA. In 1963 Tygstrup and Nørholm autopsied 12 patients who had died 1 week to 4 years after a stereotactic operation for parkinsonism. Only 5 brains contained Lewy bodies, and two of the remaining 7 probably had MSA. In 1973 Takei and Mirra found MSA in 7 (8%) of 89 brains of patients with parkinsonism in life. Dr Kutt Jellinger (personal communication) found MSA in 11% of 110 brains of parkinsonians examined between 1957 and 1970, and 3.6% of 490 brains examined between 1971 and 1987 (thus 5% of 600 brains from 1957 to 1987). Fearnley and Lees (1990) reported that 22% of the first 73 brains in the UK Parkinson's Disease Society Brain Bank showed MSA. Rajput *et al.* (1991) found MSA in 22% of 59 brains of patients with parkinsonism examined since 1968.

These data suggest that MSA could account for anything from 3.6 to 22% of incident cases of parkinsonism. A mean figure derived from all the above series is 8.2% (68/833). Thus the incidence of MSA may be considerably, and its prevalence slightly greater than that of Huntington's disease. The proportion of cases of parkinsonism incident between the ages of 45 and 59, and prevalent between the ages of 50 and 64 years, who have MSA may also be greater than suggested by the above figures. There is a pressing need for prospective population-based studies of the epidemiology of MSA, with pathological follow-up.

INVESTIGATIONS

Despite group differences in studies of plasma catecholamines, in the individual patient neither these nor other conventional cardiovascular autonomic function tests, taken in isolation, can yet reliably distinguish between autonomic failure due to Lewy body disease and that due to MSA. Nevertheless, the demonstration of abnormalities may add weight to other evidence suggesting MSA. For further details concerning autonomic failure in this condition the reader is referred to Bannister and Mathias (1992).

CT brain scan may be normal thoughout much of the course of the disease, or can show any combination of cerebellar, brainstem (Staal *et al.*, 1990; Fulham *et al.*, 1991) and even cerebral atrophy. It cannot delineate striatal pathology in MSA.

Drayer *et al.* (1986) found that magnetic resonance imaging (MRI) scanning using a 1.5 T magnet and T2-weighted images revealed abnormal putaminal signal (thought by many to reflect iron content) in many, but not all, of their patients with 'atypical parkinsonism'. However Stern *et al.* (1989) showed that a minority of patients with apparently typical IPD may show similar findings. Because of this overlap, MRI scanning has hitherto not been considered sufficiently reliable in the individual case to determine the presence of striatal pathology. Recently, Olanow (1992) has presented further evidence of a good correlation between putaminal hypointensity in *de novo* parkinsonians and their subsequent response to treatment and evolution into atypical parkinsonism. However, it is not yet clear to what degree abnormal striatal images in such patients necessarily relate to MSA as opposed to other conditions. The correlation of MRI images with clinicopathological findings (O'Brien *et al.*, 1990) is important to clarify these matters. At present 1.5 T MRI (for those who have access to it) remains but one of a battery of non-specific tests in which abnormal results help to sway the balance of diagnostic probability.

Positron emission tomography (PET) scanning has been undertaken in patients with a clinical diagnosis of MSA in several centres. In studies at the Hammersmith Medical Research Council Cyclotron Unit, ^{10}F-fluorodopa uptake into putamen has been reduced to the same degree as in IPD. However, in about half of MSA subjects caudate uptake has also been markedly, but less, diminished, in contrast to only moderate reduction in IPD (Brooks *et al.*, 1990). This presumably reflects more extensive nigral pathology involving projections to caudate. In view of the generally poor response of MSA subjects to treatment with both pre- and postsynaptic dopaminergic drugs, and of the fact that putamen often bears the brunt of the pathological process, one might expect to find a dramatic reduction in putaminal ^{11}C-raclopride binding sites. Whilst ^{11}C-raclopride PET may indeed show a striking reduction in striatal binding in early untreated MSA relative to IPD (Sawle *et al.*, 1993), and ^{123}I-iodobenzamide SPECT scanning may also be useful in assessing striatal dopamine receptors in *de novo* parkinsonians (Herrlinger *et al.*, 1992; Schelosky *et al.*, 1992; Schwarz *et al.*, 1992), the diminution in striatal ^{11}C-raclopride binding in MSA relative to levodopa-treated patients with IPD may be more modest (Brooks *et al.*, 1990). Much of the reason for the inefficacy of treatment therefore lies downstream of the cell bodies that bear most of the dopamine receptors. Indeed, recent PET studies suggest that the use of ^{11}C-diprenorphine (Burn *et al.*, 1993), ^{18}F-fluorodeoxyglucose (Eidelberg *et al.*, 1993) and ^{11}C-SCH 23390 (Shinotoh *et al.*, 1993) as markers of striatal pathology may help differentiate between MSA and IPD in some patients.

In general, the results of routine neurophysiological examinations are normal, or sometimes mildly abnormal (Cohen *et al.*, 1987) in MSA patients, and are not helpful in diagnosis unless they turn up a very abnormal result incompatible with the diagnosis. However, two particular investigations can be of considerable help. The first is the use of electro-oculographic recordings, mentioned earlier. The second, and most useful of all, is the external urethral or rectal sphincter electromyogram (EMG; Eardley *et al.*, 1989). Part of the reason for the urinary incontinence that may occur in MSA is the frequent dropout of neurons in Onuf's nucleus, a column of specialized anterior horn cells running from S2 to S4 whose axons supply the striated muscle of the external urethral and rectal sphincters. As in analogous situations elsewhere, this loss of anterior horn cells causes remaining axons to sprout, so that many then supply more than their usual complement of muscle fibres. The EMG correlates of this denervation and reinnervation are increased amplitude, polyphasia and long duration of individual motor units. False-positive results may occur after transabdominal (but not usually transurethral) prostatectomy and other pelvic operations, and interpretation needs to be cautious in multiparous women, or those with a traumatic obstetric history. Otherwise, however, a clearly abnormal result in the appropriate clinical context is very highly suggestive of MSA. However, some patients have a normal result, and such a finding in the presence of severe urinary symptoms in some patients with pathologically proven MSA serves to remind us that lesions elsewhere also contribute to their bladder problems.

Despite all the investigative tools at our disposal, as yet there is no test that has 100% specificity and sensitivity, so that the diagnosis of MSA is still essentially clinical.

TREATMENT AND MANAGEMENT

There is no specific treatment for the cerebellar and pyramidal features of the disease. Such medical treatment as exists is largely directed towards mitigating the extrapyramidal and autonomic features.

Because their striatum is intact, patients with IPD always respond adequately to treatment with an adequate dose of levodopa given for an adequate period of time.

Failure to do so excludes IPD, but the converse does not necessarily hold – some subjects with other disorders causing parkinsonism, including MSA, may show such a response, at least in the initial stages. However, what constitutes adequate? A subjective response of less than 50% would cast doubt on a diagnosis of IPD. Although most patients with IPD will respond within days or weeks, lack of response should only be definitively pronounced after 3 months of treatment. Although most IPD subjects will respond to 3 intermediate-strength capsules (Madopar 125) or tablets (Sinemet 10/ or 25/100) per day, and one should begin to suspect lack of response at Madopar 250 or Sinemet 25/250 t.d.s., I would only consider a patient definitely non-levodopa-responsive to a dose of 6 × Madopar 250 or Sinemet 25/250 per day (although I have even heard Stanley Fahn advocate 8 tablets per day). Unfortunately, some patients are intolerant to levodopa, and may only be able to cope with much lower doses, or not at all, even with extra inhibitor and the addition of domperidone. This may be more common among patients with MSA than among those with IPD.

The bald statement that patients with MSA are non- or poorly levodopa-responsive is misleading. In our experience about two thirds show no response at all, or a poor response which is often only apparent when the drug is withdrawn. The remaining third show either a moderate or good response, with about a tenth showing an excellent response within the range expected in IPD. However, what response there is usually declines over the course of the first 1 or 2 years of treatment. The dopaminergic response in MSA has also been reviewed elsewhere (Hughes *et al.*, 1992; Lees, 1992; Parati *et al.*, 1993).

Hand-in-hand with this poor or waning levodopa-responsiveness, the obvious mobile choreodystonic levodopa-induced involuntary movements of the limbs seen in IPDA patients of equivalent age are usually mild or absent in MSA, although they can certainly be seen in a minority of cases (Lang *et al.*, 1986). In contrast, dyskinesias in MSA often predominate in, or are largely restricted to, the neck or face, and often take the form of more sustained dystonic spasms. Unilateral facial dystonic spasms (Quinn, 1992) are particularly suggestive of MSA.

It is exceptional for a patient with MSA, after levodopa has been well-tolerated to an adequate dose with no response, subsequently to show a substantial response to bromocriptine or any other postsynaptic agonist. The (pathologically proven) case of van Leeuwen and Perquin (1988) derived temporary benefit from bromocriptine only after levodopa, which also caused clinical improvement, had been stopped because of side-effects. Similarly, acute challenges with subcutaneous apomorphine give essentially the same result (usually negative, occasionally positive) as single oral doses of, or sustained treatment with, levodopa (Oertel *et al.*, 1989; Hughes *et al.*, 1990). This, together with the PET data, indicates that the parkinsonian syndrome of MSA is not due simply either to the nigral lesion or to the loss of postsynaptic dopamine receptors. In spite of these observations, there is nothing to be lost by trying agonists in such patients, although the chances of additional benefit are small.

Some patients with MSA derive some degree of useful benefit from anticholinergics (if not contraindicated by sphincter problems). I have also found that amantadine is sometimes of considerably more benefit than levodopa, presumably due to actions at downstream sites within the basal ganglia, perhaps via NMDA receptor antagonism. A possible role for selegiline as either symptomatic or potentially disease-modifying treatment remains essentially unexplored, but I have not noted any obvious benefit in my own patients when given this drug.

Postural hypotension is frequently unmasked or worsened when MSA patients are given dopaminergic drugs, thus limiting their dosage or even precluding their use. However, although disabling postural faintness does occur in a minority of subjects, in most it is not a major feature. When troublesome, it can often be alleviated by progressively introducing elastic support stockings or tights (intensely disliked by most patients), head-up tilt of the bed at night (an adequate tilt is rarely achieved) and increasing salt intake, then if necessary adding fludrocortisone at night.

Male impotence can be partially circumvented by the use of intracavernosal papaverine injections or penile implants. Urinary symptoms are due to a complex mixture of central and peripheral nervous problems, sometimes superimposed on prostatic hypertrophy in males, and perineal laxity and uterine descent in females. Peripherally acting anticholinergic drugs may help incontinence, but often at the expense of promoting retention, when they may have to be stopped. If the main problem is sphincter laxity, the use of a urethral sheath in males may be indicated. However, if a large postmicturition residue is present, or retention occurs, then an indwelling catheter or, preferably (if hand function permits), intermittent self-catheterization may be needed. Anticholinergics, if beneficial to the parkinsonism, can then be restarted. Sometimes sleep is disrupted because of a large diuresis at night. The administration of DDAVP on retiring to bed may also reverse this pattern. Expert uroneurological advice and the services of a continence adviser are invaluable.

The fixed and disproportionate antecollis frequently seen in the later stages of the disease is difficult to manage. I have found braces, mechanical supports and botulinum toxin injections uniformly disappointing. One patient has derived functional benefit from the prescription of prismatic spectacles as used in ankylosing spondylitis (Kelly and Storey, 1989). I have not explored cervical fusion in any of my patients.

The management of respiratory stridor in MSA poses particular practical and ethical problems. On the one hand, stridor, even without desaturation, may be a harbinger of sudden death, often at night – Munschauer *et al.* (1990) therefore proposed that the presence of mild obstruction during sleep should prompt early tracheostomy. However, although few would question considering the use of tracheostomy (or the alternative procedures of anchoring one vocal cord in abduction or of a laser cricoarytenoidectomy), to relieve distressing daytime stridor, it is debatable whether preventing sudden death at night is necessarily a kindness if the patient is otherwise severely affected by MSA. Clearly the situation is different when stridor occurs early in the disease. Indeed, it may even be the presenting feature (Kew *et al.*, 1990).

A number of patients who have died after adrenal autografts, or after fetal nigral cell grafting, for supposed IPD have had MSA (Redmond *et al.*, 1990). There may ultimately be a therapeutic role for neural grafting in MSA, but fetal striatal, or combined nigral and striatal, rather than adrenal or nigral, cell grafts would seem most worth investigating.

Unfortunately, even if successful, grafting is unlikely ever to cure or arrest MSA. Because of the progressive nature and wide extent of the disease, the best hope for future patients with MSA lies in a systematic approach to defining the histological (Kanazawa *et al.*, 1985; Goto *et al.*, 1989; Fearnley and Lees, 1990), cytological (Papp *et al.*, 1989; Kato and Nakamura, 1990; Nakazato *et al.*, 1990; Costa *et al.*, 1992; Daniel, 1992; Papp and Lantos, 1992; Abe *et al.*, 1992), biochemical (Quik *et al.*, 1979; Spokes *et al.*, 1979; Kanazawa *et al.*, 1985; Kwak, 1985), and immunocytochemical (Kwak, 1985; Goto *et al.*, 1989, 1990; Goto and Hirano, 1990; Sakamoto *et al.*, 1992; Mochiazuki *et al.*, 1992) features that link the diseased cells, and distinguish them from others unaffected by the disease process. One gene responsible for inherited spinocerebellar ataxia type 1 has already been discovered (Orr *et al.*, 1993) and others will certainly follow (Rosenberg, 1990; Young and Duckett, 1990), allowing the principles of reverse genetics to be used to elucidate molecular pathology in these disorders. Hopefully this may indicate possible mechanisms for disease modification in these conditions, but whether these will be applicable to MSA cannot at present be predicted. Whilst waiting for these breakthroughs, a fruitful area of research will be to establish in what areas the cellular and subcellular pathology of MSA matches or differs from that of inherited OPCA.

Meanwhile, people will continue to suffer from this malignant and distressing condition, often deriving minimal benefit from strictly medical treatment. It is therefore all the more important that they have maximum access to speech, occupational and physiotherapists, social workers, wheelchair clinics and continence advisers. Until we can effectively treat or prevent it, MSA will continue to present neurologists with another major challenge – that of providing the rapport, empathy, trust and compassion necessary to support patients and family in the face of progressive and incurable disease.

This chapter is dedicated to the memory of Dr David Oppenheimer in recognition of his original insights into the disease, and in gratitude for helpful discussions and correspondence on the subject.

Acknowledgements

I gratefully acknowledge the help of Drs Berciano, Castro-Caldas, Gershanik, Kanazawa and Serdaru in tracking down obscure references; of Drs Meierkord, Straathof and Ugawa for help with translation from German, Dutch and Japanese respectively; of Miss Tina Holmes for typing the manuscript, and of Mr Mel Calman for drawing Figure 13.4. Our own recent work on MSA has been supported by a grant from the United Kingdom Parkinson's Disease Society.

References

Abe H, Yagishata S, Amano N, Iwabuchi A, Hasegawa K, and Kowa K (1992) Argyrophilic glial intracytoplasmic inclusions in multiple system atrophy: immunocytochemical and ultrastructural study. *Arch Neuropath*, **84**, 273–7

Adams RD, van Bogaert L, and van der Eecken H (1961) Dégénérescences nigro-striées et cérébello-nigro-striées. *Psychiatria Neurologia*, **142**, 219–59

Adams RD, van Bogaert L, and van der Eecken H (1964) Striato-nigral degeneration. *J Neuropathol Exp Neurol*, **23**, 584–608

Babinski J (1896) Sur le réflexe cutané plantaire dans certains affections organiques du système nerveux central. *Computes Rendu Hebdomadaires des Séances et Mémoires de la Société Biologique*, **48**, 207–8

Bannister R and Mathias CJ (1992) Clinical features and investigation of the primary autonomic failure syndromes. In Bannister R and Mathias CJ, eds, *A Textbook of Clinical Disorders of the Autonomic Nervous System*, 3rd edn, Oxford, Oxford University Press pp 531–47

Bannister R and Oppenheimer DR (1972) Degenerative diseases of the nervous system associated with autonomic failure. *Brain*, **95**, 457–74

Berciano J (1982) Olivopontocerebellar atrophy. A review of 117 cases. *J Neurol Sci*, **53**, 253–72

Brooks DJ, Ibanez V, Sawle GV, Quinn N, Lees AJ, Mathias CJ *et al.* (1990) Differing patterns of striatal 18-F-Dopa uptake in Parkinson's disease, multiple system atrophy and progressive supranuclear palsy. *Ann Neurol*, **28**, 547–55

Burkhard CR, Filley CM, Kleinschmidt-de Masters BK, de la Monte S, Norenberg MD, and Schnecck

SA (1988) Diffuse Lewy body disease and progressive dementia. *Neurology*, **38**, 1520–8
Cohen J, Low P, Fealey R, Sheps S, and Jiang N-S (1987) Somatic and autonomic function in progressive autonomic failure and multiple system atrophy. *Ann Neurol*, **22**, 692–9
Costa C, Duyckaerts C, Cervera P, and Hauw J-J (1992) Les inclusions oligodendrogliales, un marqueur des atrophies multisystématisées. *Rev Neurol*, **148**, 274–80
Daniel SE (1992) The neuropathology and neurochemistry of multiple system atrophy. In Bannister R and Mathias CJ, eds, *Autonomic Failure: A Textbook of Disorders of the Autonomic Nervous System*, 3rd edn, Oxford, Oxford University Press, 564–85
Dejerine J and Thomas AA (1890) L'atrophie olivo-ponto-cérébelleuse. *Nouv Iconogr Salpêtrière*, **13**, 330–70
Drayer BP, Olanow W, Burger P, Johnson CA, Herfkens R, and Riederer S (1986) Parkinson plus syndrome: diagnosis using high field MR imaging of brain iron. *Radiology*, **159**, 493–8
Duvoisin RC (1989) Is there a Parkinson's disease? In Quinn NP and Jenner PG, eds, *Disorders of Movement: Clinical, Pharmacological and Physiological Aspects*, London, Academic Press, 1–10
Duvoisin RC, Yahr MD, Lieberman J, Antunes J, and Rhee S (1972) The striatal foot. *Trans Am Med Assoc*, **97**, 267
Eardley I, Quinn NP, Fowler CJ, Kirby RS, Parkhouse HM, Marsden CD *et al.* (1989) The value of urethral sphincter electromyography in the differential diagnosis of parkinsonism. *Br J Urol*, **64**, 360–2
Eidelberg D, Takikawa S, Moeller JR, Dhawan V, Redington K, Chaly T *et al.* (1993) Striatal hypometabolism distinguishes striatonigral degeneration from Parkinson's disease. *Ann Neurol*, **33**, 518–27
Fearnley JM and Lees AJ (1990) Striatonigral degeneration: a clinico-pathological study. *Brain*, **113**, 1823–42
Fulham MJ, Dubinsky RM, Polinsky RJ, Brooks RA, Brown RT, Curras MT *et al.* (1991) Computed tomography, magnetic resonance imaging and positron emission tomography with $[^{18}F]$ fluorodeoxyglucose in multiple system atrophy and pure autonomic failure. *Clin Auton Res*, **1**, 27–36
Gibb WRG and Lees AJ (1988) The relevance of the Lewy body to the pathogenesis of idiopathic Parkinson's disease. *J Neurol Neurosurg Psychiatry*, **51**, 745–52
Goto S and Hirano A (1990) Inhomogeneity of the putaminal lesion in striatonigral degeneration. *Acta Neuropathol*, **80**, 204–7
Goto S, Hirano A, and Matsumoto S (1989) Subdivisional involvement of nigrostriatal loop in idiopathic Parkinson's disease and striatonigral degeneration. *Ann Neurol*, **26**, 766–70
Goto S, Hirano A, and Matsumoto S (1990) Metenkephalin immunoreactivity in the basal ganglia in Parkinson's disease and striatonigral degeneration. *Neurology*, **40**, 1051–6
Graham JG and Oppenheimer DR (1969) Orthostatic hypotension and nicotine sensitivy in a case of multiple system atrophy. *J Neurol Neurosurg Psychiatry*, **32**, 28–34
Gray F, Vincent D, Hauw J-J (1988) Quantitative study of lateral horn cells in 15 cases of multiple system atrophy. *Acta Neuropathologica*, **75**, 513–18
Guillain G (1937) Sur une affection non héréditaire du système nerveux caractérisée par un syndrome cérébelleux progressif avec abolition des réflexes tendineus des membres. *Ann Méd*, **42**, 102–18
Guillain G, Bertrand I, and Godet-Guillain J (1942) Examen anatomopathologique d'un cas de syndrome cérébelleux progressif non-héréditaire avec abolition des réflexes tendineux des membres. *Rev Neurol*, **74**, 330–3
Herrlinger K, Wagner-Manslau C, Ceballos-Baumann AO, and Weindl A (1992) 123-I-iodobenzamide – SPECT dopamine D_2 receptor imaging in normals, patients with Parkinson's disease and other akinetic-rigid syndromes. *Movement Disorders*, **7** (suppl 1), 146
Hughes AJ, Lees AJ, and Stern GM (1990) Apomorphine test to predict dopaminergic responsiveness in parkinsonian syndromes. *Lancet*, **ii**, 32–4
Hughes AJ, Colosimo C, Kleedorfer B, Daniel SE, and Lees AJ (1992) The dopaminergic response in multiple system atrophy. *J Neurol Neurosurg Psychiatry*, **55**, 1009–13
Kanazawa I, Kwak S, Sasaki H, Mizusawa H, Muramoto O, Yoshizawa K *et al.* (1985) Studies on neurotransmitter markers and neuronal cell density in olivopontocerebellar atrophy and cortical cerebellar atrophy. *J Neurol Sci*, **71**, 193–208
Kato S and Nakamura H (1990) Cytoplasmic argyrophilic inclusions in neurons of pontine nuclei in patients with olivopontocerebellar atrophy: immunohistochemical and ultrastructural studies. *Acta Neuropathol*, **79**, 584–94
Kato S, Nakamura H, Hirano A, Ito H, Llena JF, and Yen S-H (1991) Argyrophilic ubiquitinated cytoplasmic inclusions of Leu-7-positive glial cells in olivopontocerebellar atrophy (multiple system atrophy). *Acta Neuropathol*, **82**, 488–93
Kelly SP and Storey JK (1989) Mobility spectacles for ankylosing spondylitis. *Br Med J*, **298**, 1704
Kew J, Gross M, and Chapman P (1990) Shy–Drager syndrome presenting as isolated paralysis of vocal cord abductors. *Br Med J*, **300**, 1441

Koeppen AH and Hans MB (1976) Supranuclear ophthalmoplegia in olivopontocerebellar degeneration. *Neurology*, **26**, 764–8

Kosaka H, Iizuka R, Mizutani Y, Kondo T, and Nagatsu T (1981) Striatonigral degeneration combined with Alzheimer's disease. *Acta Neuropathol*, **54**, 253–6

Kwak S (1985) Biochemical analysis of transmitters in the brains of multiple system atrophy. *No Shinkei*, **37**, 691–4

Lang AE, Birnbaum A, Blair RDG, and Kierans C (1986) Levodopa dose-related fluctuations in presumed olivopontocerebellar atrophy. *Movement Disorders*, **1**, 93–102

Lees AJ (1992) The treatment of multiple system atrophy. In Bannister R and Mathias CJ, eds, *Autonomic Failure. A Textbook of Clinical Disorders of the Autonomic Nervous System*, 3rd edn, Oxford, Oxford University Press, 646–55

Mochizuki A, Mizusawa H, Ohkoshi N, Yoshizawa K, Komatsuzaki Y, Inoue K, and Kanazawa I (1992) Argentophilic intracytoplasmic inclusions in multiple system atrophy. *J Neurol*, **239**, 311–16

Munschauer FE, Loh L, Bannister R, and Newsom-Davis J (1990) Abnormal respiration and sudden death during sleep in multiple system atrophy with autonomic failure. *Neurology*, **40**, 677–9

Nakazato Y, Yamazaki H, Hirato J, Ishida Y, and Yamaguchi H (1990) Oligodendroglial microtubular tangles in olivopontocerebellar atrophy. *J Neuropathol Exp Neurol*, **49**, 521–30

Neumann M A (1977) Pontocerebellar atrophy combined with vestibular-reticular degeneration. *J Neuropathol Exp Neurol*, **36**, 321–37

Obeso JA, Rodriguez ME, Artieda J, Grandas F, Vaamonde J, Tuñón T *et al.* (1989) Focal reflex myoclonus: a useful sign in the differential diagnosis of parkinsonism. *Ann Neurol*, **26**, 164–5

O'Brien C, Sung JH, McGeachie RE, and Lee MC (1990) Striatonigral degeneration: clinical, MRI and pathologic correlation. *Neurology*, **40**, 710–11

Oertel WH, Gasser T, Ippisch R, Trenkwalder C, and Poewe W (1989) Apomorphine test for dopaminergic responsiveness. *Lancet*, **1**, 1262–3

Olanow CW (1992) Magnetic resonance imaging in parkinsonism. *Neurol Clin*, **10**, 405–20

Oppenheimer D (1983) Neuropathology of progressive autonomic failure. In Bannister R, ed, *Autonomic Failure. A Textbook of Clinical Disorders of the Autonomic Nervous System*. Oxford, Oxford University Press, 267–83

Orr HT, Chung M, Banfi S *et al.* (1993) Expansion of an unstable trinucleotide CAG repeat in spinocerebellar ataxia type 1. *Nature Genetics*, **4**, 221–6

Papp MI and Lantos PL (1992) Accumulation of tubular structures in oligodendroglial and neuronal cells as the basic alteration in multiple system atrophy. *J Neurol Sci*, **107**, 172–82

Papp MI, Kahn JE, and Lantos PL (1989) Glial cytoplasmic inclusions in the CNS of patients with multiple system atrophy (striatonigral degeneration, olivopontocerebellar atrophy and Shy–Drager syndrome). *J Neurol Sci*, **94**, 79–100

Parati EA, Fetoni V, Geminiani GC, Soliveri P, Giovannini P, Testa D *et al.* (1993) Response to L-dopa in multiple system atrophy. *Clinical Neuropharmacol*, **16**, 139–44

Parkinson J (1817) *An Assay on the Shaking Palsy*, London, Sherwood, Neely and Jones

Pierret M (1871) Note sur un cas d'atrophie périphérique du cervelet avec lésion concomitante des olives bulbaires. *Arch Physiol Normale Pathol*, **72**, 765–70

Polinsky RJ and Nee LE (1988) Autonomic failure: nosology, clinical evaluation and prognosis. *Ann Neurol*, **26**, 121

Quik M, Spokes EG, Mackay AVP, and Bannister R (1979) Alterations in [^{3}H] spiperone binding in human caudate nucleus, substantia nigra and frontal cortex in the Shy–Drager syndrome and Parkinson's disease. *J Neurol Sci*, **43**, 429–37

Quinn N (1989a) Multiple system atrophy – the nature of the beast. *J Neurol Neurosurg Psychiatry*, (suppl), 78–89

Quinn N (1989b) Disproportionate antecollis in multiple system atrophy. *Lancet*, **i**, 844

Quinn N (1992) Unilateral facial dystonia in multiple system atrophy. *Movement Disorders*, **7**, (suppl 1), 79

Quinn NP, Wenning GK, Magalhães M, Daniel S, and Lees A (1993) A clinico-pathological study of multiple system atrophy. *Neurology* (suppl 2), A179

Quinn NP and Marsden CD. The motor disorder of multiple system atrophy. *J Neurol Neurosurg Psychiatry*, (in press)

Rajput AH, Rozdilsky B, and Rajput A (1991) Accuracy of clinical diagnosis in parkinsonism – a prospective study. *Can J Neurol Sci*, **18**, 275–8

Rascol O, Sabatini U, Simonetta-Moreau M, Montastruc J-L, Rascol A, and Clanet M (1991) Square wave jerks in parkinsonian syndromes. *J Neurol Neurosurg Psychiatry*, **54**, 599–602

Redmond DE, Leranth C, Spencer DD, Robbins R, Vollmer T, Kim JH *et al.* (1990) Fetal neural graft survival. *Lancet*, **ii**, 820–2

Robbins TW, James M, Lange KW, Owen AM, Quinn NP, and Marsden CD (1992) Cognitive performance in multiple system atrophy. *Brain*, **115**, 271–91

Rosenberg RN (1990) Autosomal dominant cerebellar phenotypes: the genotype will settle the issue. *Neurology*, **40**, 1329–31

Royet H and Collet J (1893) Sur une lésion systématisée du cervelet et de ses dépendences bulbo-protubérantielles. *Arch Neurol (Paris)*, **26**, 353–74

Sakamoto S, Goto S, Ito H, and Hirano (1992) Striosomal organization of substance P-like immunoreactivity in parkinsonian patients. *Neurology*, **42**, 1071–5

Sawle GV, Playford ED, Brooks DJ, Quinn N and Frackowiak RSJ (1993) Asymmetrical pre-synaptic and post-synaptic changes to the striatal dopamine projection in dopa naive parkinsonism: diagnostic implications of the D_2 receptor status. *Brain*, **116**, 853–67

Schelosky L, Hierholzer J, Cordes M, and Poewe W (1992) Correlation of clinical response in apomorphine test with D-2 receptor status as demonstrated by 123-I IBZM-SPECT. *Movement Disorders*, **7**, (suppl 1), 146

Schultze V (1887) Ueber einen Fall von Kleinhirnschwund mit Degenerationen im verlangerten Marke und im Ruckenmarke (wahrsheinlich in Folge von Alkolismus). *Virchows Arch Pathol Anat Physiol Klin Med*, **108**, 331–43

Schwarz J, Tatsch K, Arnold G, Gasser T, Trenkwalder C, Kirsch CM *et al.* (1992) 123 I-iodobenzamide-SPECT predicts dopaminergic responsiveness in patients with de novo parkinsonism. *Neurology*, **42**, 556–61

Shinotoh H, Inoue O, Hirayama K, Aotsuka A, Asahina M, Shrara T *et al.* (1993) Dopamine D1 receptors in Parkinson's disease and striatonigral degeneration: a positron emission tomography study. *J Neurol Neurosurg Psychiatry*, **56**, 467–72

Shy GM and Drager GA (1960) A neurologic syndrome associated with orthostatic hypotension. *Arch Neurol*, **2**, 511–27

Spokes EG, Bannister R, and Oppenheimer DR (1979) Multiple system atrophy with autonomic failure – clinical, histological and neurochemical observations on four cases. *J Neurol Sci*, **43**, 59–82

Staal A, Meerwaldt JD, van Dongen KK, Mulder PGH, and Busch HFM (1990) Non-familial degenerative disease and atrophy of brainstem and cerebellum. Clinical and CT data in 47 patients. *J Neurol Sci*, **95**, 259–69

Stern MB, Braffman BH, Skolnick BE, Hurtig HI, and Grossman RI (1989) Magnetic resonance imaging in Parkinson's disease and parkinsonian syndromes. *Neurology*, **39**, 1524–6

Takei Y and Mirra SS (1973) Striato-nigral degeneration: a form of multiple system atrophy with clinical parkinsonism. In Zimmerman HM, ed, *Progress in Neuropathology*, vol 2, New York, Grune and Stratton, 217–51

Trétiakoff MC (1919) Contribution à l'étude de l'anatomie pathologique du Locus niger de Soemmering. Thesis, University of Paris

Trotter JL (1973) Striato-nigral degeneration, Alzheimer's disease, and inflammatory changes. *Neurology*, **23**, 1211–16

Tygstrup I and Nørholm T (1963) Neuropathological findings in 12 patients operated for parkinsonism. *Acta Neurol Scand*, **39** (suppl 4), 188–95

van der Eecken H, Adams RD, and van Bogaert L (1960) Striopallidal-nigral degeneration. A hitherto undescribed lesion in paralysis agitans. *J Neuropathol Exp Neurol*, **19**, 159–61

van Leeuwen RB and Perquin WVM (1988) Bromocriptine therapy in striatonigral degeneration. *J Neurol Neurosurg Psychiatry*, **51**, 592

von Fleischhacker H (1924) Afamiliare chronisch progressive Erkrankung der mittleren lebensalters vom Pseudesklerosetyp. *Z Gesamte Neurol Psychiatrie*, **91**, 1–22

von Stauffenberg (1918) Zur kenntnis des extrapyramidalen motorischen systems und mitteilung eines falles von sog "Atrophie olivo-pontocérébelleuse". *Z Gesamte Neurol Psychiatrie*, **39**, 1–55

Wadia NH (1984) A variety of olivopontocerebellar atrophy distingued by slow eye movements and peripheral neuropathy. *Adv Neurol*, **41**, 149–77

Wadia NH and Swami RK (1971) A new form of heredofamilial spinocerebellar degeneration with slow eye movements (nine families). *Brain*, **94**, 359–74

Wenning GK, Magalhães M, Quinn NP (1993) Multiple system atrophy: clinical features and natural history of 94 cases. *Neurology*, **43**, (suppl 2), A349

Wenning GK, Quinn N, Magalhães M, Mathias C, and Daniel SE "Minimal change" multiple system atrophy. *Movement Disorders*, (in press)

Young JD and Duckett DP (1990) Familial cerebellar ataxia and possible cosegregation with an inversion in chromosome 4. *J Neurol Neurosurg Psychiatry*, **53**, 441–2

14
Corticobasal ganglionic degeneration

Ray L. Watts, Suzanne S. Mirra and E. P. Richardson Jr

INTRODUCTION AND HISTORICAL PERSPECTIVE

Corticobasal ganglionic degeneration (CBGD) is a clinically and pathologically distinctive neurodegenerative disease which has emerged as a defined subset of the Parkinson-plus disorders (akinetic–rigid syndromes with other clinical features which are not characteristic of Parkinson disease, e.g. corticospinal tract signs, supranuclear gaze palsy, cerebellar ataxia, etc.). CBGD usually presents as parkinsonism unresponsive to levodopa with signs of cortical dysfunction appearing relatively early in the course of the illness.

This disorder was first described in 1967 and 1968 by Rebeiz *et al.* as 'corticodentatonigral degeneration with neuronal achromasia'. The authors noted that the illness in their 3 patients was clinically and pathologically so unusual as to be unlike anything that they had seen personally or encountered in the literature. Because of its rarity, or underrecognition, no subsequent reports of this disorder appeared until 1985 when Watts and colleagues reported their experience with 6 patients at the Massachusetts General Hospital diagnosed on clinical grounds, 1 of whom had undergone confirmatory postmortem examination and was subsequently reported in detail in Case Records of the Massachusetts General Hospital (1985).

In 1988 Riley and Lang described 6 cases from Toronto, 1 with pathological confirmation. By this time the disorder began to be more generally recognized worldwide, and additional reports have appeared subsequently (Gibb *et al.*, 1988; Eidelberg *et al.*, 1991; LeWitt *et al.*, 1989; Sawle *et al.*, 1989; Watts *et al.*, 1989; Blin *et al.*, 1990; Lippa *et al.*, 1990b; Paulus and Selim, 1990; Thompson *et al.*, 1990; Sawle *et al.*, 1991). The most comprehensive reports are those of Gibb *et al.* (1989), who describe the clinical and pathological features of 3 cases seen in London, and Riley *et al.* (1990), who amplified their earlier report (Riley and Lang, 1988) and added a second autopsied case. The report of Greene *et al.* (1990) includes a video tape of several clinical examinations over time of a patient in whom eventual postmortem confirmation of CBGD was obtained. The distinguishing clinical and neuropathological features of CBGD have become more sharply focused, but more well-studied clinical cases with pathological confirmation are needed.

We will herein review current knowledge of the clinical, laboratory and pathological features of CBGD based upon our experience and the extant literature.

Review of the first reported cases

Rebeiz *et al.* (1967, 1968) described 3 patients who exhibited a unique pattern of progressive motor impairment in later life. The disorder was characterized by slow, awkward volitional limb movements hampered further by tremor and dystonic posturing. Each of the 3 patients had impairment beginning and continuing to be most prominent in the left limbs; stiffness, clumsiness and 'numbness' or 'deadness' were the initial symptoms. The insidious progression included gait impairment, with particular difficulty in initiating steps, marked limb rigidity, loss of dexterity, impaired position and other sensory function of the left limbs, and interference with attempted movements from involuntary synkinesia of the contralateral limbs. Although motor impairment progressed, intellectual function remained relatively intact. The illness terminated in death 6–8 years after onset as a result of continuing motor disability.

The pathological findings in all 3 were distinctive, with an unusual pattern of frontoparietal neuronal loss. The asymmetrical presentation of signs and symptoms correlated with asymmetrical atrophy in the contralateral frontal and parietal cortex in 2 of the 3 cases. The atrophic cortex showed extensive neuronal loss, with gliosis. Some of the pyramidal neurons, mainly in the third and fifth layers, had an unusual swollen, hyaline appearance. Except for faint eosinophilia, their cytoplasm failed to take up most stains. Affected neurons often had eccentric nuclei, and some contained cytoplasmic vacuoles. There was marked to complete loss of Nissl substance in the swollen neurons. The cytoplasm of swollen neurons displayed only a few minute eosinophilic granules and small amounts of lipofuscin. Because of the lack of staining, the authors termed these *achromatic* neurons.

These striking pathological findings were not accompanied by features typical of other neurodegenerative conditions, such as Pick bodies, neurofibrillary tangles, senile plaques, or Lewy bodies. The topography of neuronal dropout in the cortex coincided with sites in the distribution of the achromatic neurons, being mostly in the frontal, Rolandic and parietal regions. Although these abnormalities were also found elsewhere in cerebral cortex, they were absent in the hippocampal formation, occipital cortex, and inferior and medial temporal cortex. Considerable loss of pigmented neurons in the substantia nigra was evident in all 3 cases. The medial portion of the subthalamic nucleus also showed gliosis and swollen neurons. In 2 cases, there were similar neuronal changes in the dentate and roof nuclei of the cerebellum; the cerebellar cortex, however, was spared. In 1 case swollen pale neurons were found in the oculomotor nucleus. Evidence of secondary corticospinal tract degeneration was present in 2 of the 3 cases. In each case, the general autopsy, including examination of the circulatory system as well as other organ systems, gave no clues concerning the pathogenesis of the unusual neuropathological findings.

Illustrative case

The additional case from the Massachusetts General Hospital with pathological confirmation of CBGD was presented in 1985 (Case Records of the Massachusetts General Hospital, 1985; Watts *et al.*, 1985) and provides a good example of a 'typical' case of CBGD diagnosed during life with subsequent postmortem confirmation.

CLINICAL FINDINGS

In his 60th year, a right-handed accountant and violist noted insidiously progressive stiffness of the proximal right arm. A year later right arm rigidity was worse, dexterity was impaired and there was a rapid irregular action tremor, preventing him from musical performance. His right leg also became stiff, and impaired balance resulted in several falls. In the third year of the illness, his speech was slurred and sentences were shorter and less complex. He was no longer able to work with his advancing disabilities. By the fourth year the right arm and leg were rigid, and stiffness, incoordination and tremor had spread to the left arm. He was unable to walk without assistance.

Examination at age 65 revealed full orientation and a reasonably good grasp of current events. The patient spoke hesitantly in short sentences, often eliminating articles. There was a startled quality to his facial expression, with widely opened eyes and wrinkled forehead. Spontaneous blink frequency was decreased, and blepharospasm occurred if the eyes were approached. Ocular movements were full, but with saccadic breakdown of smooth pursuit. The right upper limb was adducted at the shoulder, flexed at the elbow, and pronated at the forearm, with fingers curled into a fist. There was intense rigidity in the arm, with minimal voluntary movement. The right leg was rigidly extended, but the foot was flexed and inverted. Movement of the left upper limb was very slow and limited to 90° of abduction. He was incapable of individual finger movements with the left hand, but he could grasp a built-up fork and feed himself clumsily. There was an intense grasp reflex in the left hand and he could not use the left arm to demonstrate how to salute, use a comb or toothbrush, or wave goodbye. Postural and directed movements of the left arm were often interrupted by a large-amplitude, irregular tremor. There was no tremor at rest or dysmetria. Sensory examination was normal except for reduced sensation in the left median nerve distribution. Myotatic reflexes were not increased. The left plantar response was extensor, but the right foot and toe did not move in response to plantar stimulation. Fasciculations were seen in many muscle groups of the upper and lower limbs.

The family history was negative for any similar disorder, and there was no history of encephalitis. Laboratory analyses of blood, urine and cerebrospinal fluid (CSF) were normal. Microscopic examination of a biopsy specimen of the right sural nerve showed morphometric and ultrastructural changes consistent with segmental demyelination and mild Wallerian degeneration. White blood cell aryl-sulphatase A and urinary sulphatide values were normal. Cranial computed tomographic (CT) scan revealed peri-Rolandic cortical atrophy, and attenuation of the white matter beneath the left central sulcus (Fig. 14.1). Magnetic resonance imaging (MRI) revealed no additional abnormalities. Electrophysiological tremor testing documented an 8–10 Hz action/postural tremor. Electromyography (EMG) and nerve conduction studies demonstrated a sensorimotor peripheral neuropathy, and tibial nerve somatosensory evoked potential (SSEP) testing showed delayed peripheral and borderline normal central conduction. Pattern shift visual evoked potentials (VEP) revealed prolonged P100 latencies bilaterally. Brain stem auditory evoked potentials (BAEP) and median nerve SSEPs were normal.

Therapeutic trials of carbidopa/levodopa, bromocriptine, benztropine, trihexiphenidyl, clonazepam, baclofen, propranolol, clonidine and methysergide were without benefit. Tremor and anxiety were mitigated with diazepam therapy. He died in the sixth year of his illness.

PATHOLOGICAL FINDINGS

Neuropathological examination revealed moderate generalized cortical atrophy, with severe asymmetrical atrophy of gyri adjacent to the central sulci, worse on the left. Histological abnormalities, too, were most severe in the pre- and postcentral gyri. There was neuronal loss and reactive gliosis in all layers, most severe in layers III and V (Fig. 14.2B). Very few large pyramidal neurons remained in layer V, and no Betz cells were identified in the sections examined. In the subjacent white matter, there was extensive loss of myelinated axons and gliosis. Changes that were histologically similar though less severe were found in the premotor, anterior cingulate, inferior parietal, insular and anterior temporal regions. Occasional neuritic plaques were noted in layers I–III, but there were no neurofibrillary tangles seen. In areas of intermediate histological severity, such as the premotor cortex, many medium-sized to large pyramidal neurons were swollen, with indistinct nuclei and pale cytoplasm that stained poorly with basic dyes (achromasia) or reduced silver techniques

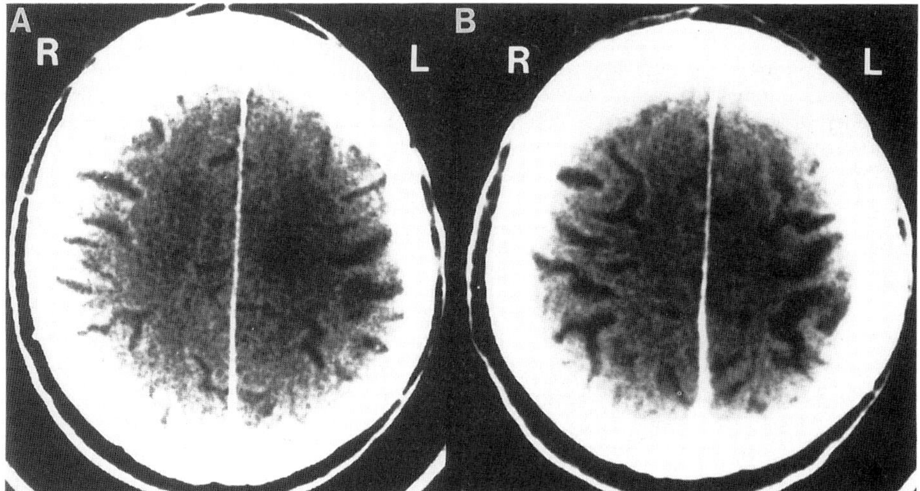

Figure 14.1 Cranial computed tomography images from the autopsied case of Watts *et al.* (1985), in the fifth year of illness (see Illustrative case in the text). (A and B) There is asymmetrical (left greater than right) frontoparietal cortical atrophy, most prominent in the peri-Rolandic regions. Note the attenuation of subcortical white matter underlying the central sulcus in A.

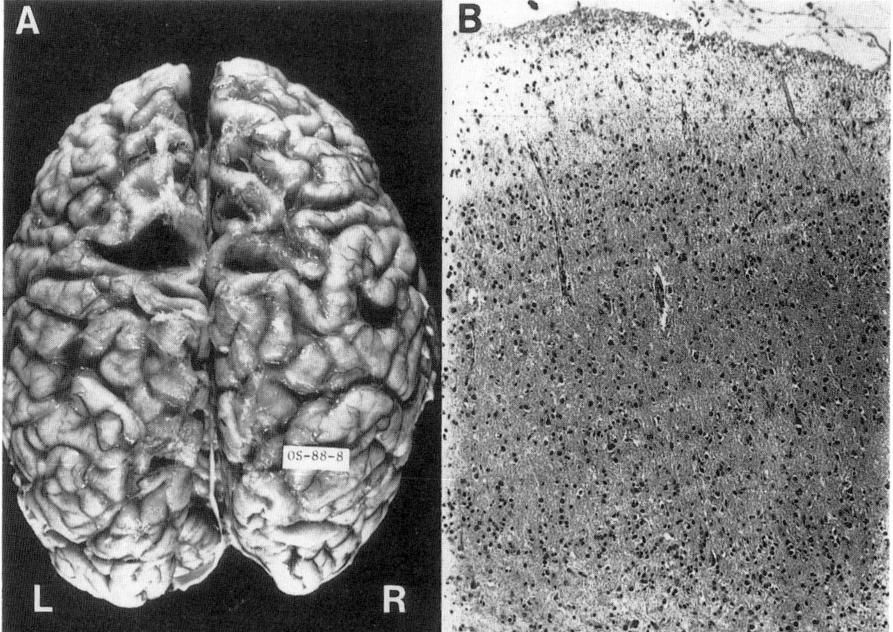

Figure 14.2 (A) Gross inspection of the brain from a 75-year-old man with corticobasal ganglionic degeneration (CBGD; Watts *et al.*, 1989) reveals marked asymmetrical frontoparietal cortical atrophy, left more than right. The atrophy is most evident in the left peri-Rolandic region where sulci are gaping. (B) Photomicrograph of the left precentral gyrus (area 4) from a 66-year-old man with CBGD (Watts *et al.*, 1985), demonstrating the loss of the normal laminar cytoarchitectural pattern (see Illustrative case in the text). There is severe neuronal loss and gliosis but no ballooned neurons are observed. LHE, 120 ×.

(compare Fig. 14.3). There was neuronal loss and gliosis in the substantia nigra bilaterally, but no Lewy bodies were seen. No histological abnormalities were present in the striatum, globus pallidus, substantia innominata, amygdala, hypothalamus, tegmental nuclei of the brainstem, cerebellum, including the dentate nucleus, or spinal cord. There were decreased numbers of myelinated axons with reactive gliosis in the cerebral peduncles, more pronounced on the left, consistent with Wallerian degeneration. The peripheral nerves revealed loss of myelinated fibres, and there were typical denervation changes in skeletal muscles.

CLINICAL FEATURES (Table 14.1)

Both sexes are affected by this disorder. The disease makes its appearance in mid to late adult life, with symptoms usually beginning after age 60, and the onset is insidious. The occurrence appears to be sporadic, since, with the possible exception of case 2 of Rebeiz *et al.* (1968), family histories of affected patients are negative for any type of similar disorder. Ethnic backgrounds are mixed. No associated history of toxic or infectious exposure has been found.

The core clinical picture of CBGD consists of an asymmetrical extrapyramidal syndrome of the akinetic–rigid type, with or without tremor, beginning insidiously on one side and then gradually extending to the contralateral limbs within 1 to several years of onset. Postural instability, loss of facial expression, speech impairment and other signs of midline or generalized motor impairment of extrapyramidal type also develop within 1 or more years. Signs of cortical dysfunction are evident within 1–3 years of onset, with apraxia and cortical sensory loss being especially prominent. Many patients exhibit the 'alien hand/limb' phenomenon, and this may be striking. In the early stages cognition is remarkably intact, but variable degrees of intellectual,

Table 14.1 Clinical features

Major
Akinetic–rigid parkinsonian syndrome (loss of dexterity, slowness of movement, increased muscle tone, postural/gait disturbance, hypomimia, hypophonic dysarthria)
Cortical signs (apraxia – limb, orobuccolingual, oculomotor; cortical sensory disturbance – astereognosis, decreased graphaesthesia, double simultaneous tactile extinction; dysphasia – especially paraphasic errors; extensor plantar responses and other corticospinal tract signs)
Dystonia (especially flexion dystonia of upper limb(s) – distal greater than proximal)
Action/postural tremor (rapid, irregular, jerky)
Myoclonus
'Alien hand/limb' phenomenon
Minor
Choreoathetotic involuntary movements
Supranuclear gaze abnormalities (saccades affected more than smooth pursuit)
Intellectual impairment/dementia (cognition remarkably well-preserved until late in the course)
Frontal 'release' signs (grasps, brisk facial and palmomental reflexes)
Cerebellar signs
Blepharospasm

memory and language impairment may slowly develop. As voluntary limb movement becomes progressively slower and clumsier, many patients develop a characteristic dystonic posture with the hand and forearm flexed and arm adducted. The illness generally progresses to a state of rigid immobility after 5–7 years, and the patients usually die from aspiration pneumonia and sepsis.

A very important early clinical clue that one is confronted with a Parkinson-plus disorder and not idiopathic Parkinson's disease is the lack of beneficial response to levodopa therapy. Other clinical features which are commonly seen are: (1) an irregular, jerky action/postural tremor; (2) myoclonus; (3) corticospinal signs (hyperreflexia and Babinski sign(s)); (4) supranuclear gaze abnormalities; (5) choreoathetotic involuntary movements; (6) blepharospasm; and (7) frontal 'release' signs (Table 14.1). The tremor differs from the typical rest or postural tremor seen with Parkinson's disease; it is a more rapid (6–8 Hz), irregular and jerky action/postural tremor, and myoclonus is often superimposed in advanced stages.

The myoclonus is focal, at least initially, and tends to be present to a greater extent in the most affected limb(s). Myoclonus, like tremor, is best seen during action or maintenance of a posture; it is also stimulus-sensitive in many cases. Eventually most patients exhibit signs of corticospinal dysfunction, with extensor plantar responses and hyperreflexia. The differentiation of spasticity from rigidity in these patients is clinically very difficult, but the loss of voluntary movement is almost certainly related in part to degeneration of primary and secondary motor cortical regions which contribute to the corticospinal tract.

Eye movement abnormalities are common in CBGD. In the early stages of disease smooth pursuit eye movements may be slow and exhibit saccadic breakdown, but the range of movement is generally full (except for upgaze in elderly patients). As the illness progresses, patients gradually lose the ability to make rapid saccades to verbal command, and they may have further impairment of pursuit eye movements. Oculocephalic reflexes are preserved, and even accentuated, as the eye movement abnormalities worsen – indicating the supranuclear nature of the gaze palsy (Gibb *et al.*, 1989). Spontaneous onset of choreoathetotic involuntary movements involving the limb and facial muscles may be seen, as well as blepharospasm and other focal dystonias. In fairly advanced stages, frontal 'release' signs (grasp, glabellar and exaggerated facial and palmomental reflexes) may become prominent. Speech becomes slow and monotonous, and paraphasic errors and dysphasia may evolve. In the most advanced stages, patients may become anarthric.

LABORATORY STUDIES

Routine laboratory studies of blood, urine and CSF are normal, including copper and ceruloplasmin levels. Heavy metal toxic screens of urine have been negative. Watts *et al.* (1985) found that CSF levels of somatostatin were significantly decreased in all 3 patients assayed, 2 of whom had autopsy confirmation of CBGD.

Radiographic evaluation with brain CT scans and MRI may be normal in the early stages, but as the disease progresses a pattern of asymmetrical frontoparietal cortical atrophy (greatest contralateral to the most severely affected limbs; see Fig. 14.1), or bilateral cortical atrophy, evolves. As the atrophy becomes more prominent, abnormal signal attentuation is seen in the underlying subcortical white matter (see Fig. 14.1A). Serial evaluation of CT or MRI scans over time at 6–12-month intervals is generally more useful than one isolated scan.

Electrophysiological studies can be useful in the evaluation of patients with CBGD. Electroencephalography (EEG) is usually normal when symptoms first emerge, but as the disease progresses the EEG may reveal asymmetrical slowing (most prominent over the cerebral hemisphere contralateral to the most affected limbs). When correlated with asymmetrical radiographic changes in a similar distribution and a typical clinical picture of CBGD, this laboratory finding further supports the diagnosis. In late stages the EEG usually shows bilateral slowing, so the time reference of the EEG in the evaluation of an individual patient can be very important. Electrophysiological tremor/movement studies, employing accelerometric and EMG recording techniques, indicate that the tremor present with CBGD is clearly different from the classic parkinsonian 'rest' or postural tremor. It is more rapid (typically 6–8 Hz) and is most evident during action, and the amplitude may vary, giving it a more irregular appearance. Myoclonus may be recorded using similar techniques of examination, and provocative manoeuvres such as action of a limb, startle or tactile stimulation help to bring it out. Thompson *et al.* (1990) and Carella *et al.* (1991) found that myoclonus was not preceded by a cortical discharge and reported that central motor conduction was normal. Results of evoked potential (EP) studies have been mixed. SSEP studies may yield poorly formed or absent thalamocortical potentials, and latencies have been normal or minimally prolonged. We, Thompson and coworkers (1990) and Carella and colleagues (1991) have not found enlargement of the secondary component of the cortical potential, as can be seen with cortical reflex myoclonus or epilepsia partialis continua. Pattern shift visual EP studies have been normal in most patients, but one of our pathologically confirmed cases had prolonged P100 latencies bilaterally. BAEP studies have been normal in our experience. Routine EMG/nerve conduction studies have turned up occasional focal or generalized neuropathies in a few patients, but no clear-cut pattern has emerged, and these are usually subclinical or do not contribute significantly to overall disability.

Positron emission tomography (PET) findings in CBGD patients have been reported from several institutions (Watts *et al.*, 1985, 1989; Riley and Lang, 1988; Eidelberg *et al.*, 1991; Sawle *et al.*, 1989, 1991; Blin *et al.*, 1990; Riley *et al.*, 1990). Two general approaches have been taken, and these have given similar patterns of results; (1) studies of cerebral metabolism (oxygen or glucose) and blood flow; and (2) assessment of fluorodopa uptake into the striatum (evaluating the integrity of the nigrostriatal dopaminergic system). Several groups have found abnormalities of cerebral metabolism with a corresponding reduction of cerebral blood flow (CBF): (1) decreased oxygen metabolism in the frontoparietal (Watts *et al.*, 1985, 1989) and medial frontal, parietal and temporal cortical regions (Sawle *et al.*, 1989, 1991), most prominently in the cerebral hemisphere contralateral to the most affected limbs; (2) decreased glucose metabolism (fluorodeoxyglucose) in the parietal cortex and thalamus, in an asymmetrical distribution with the greatest decrease contralateral to the most affected limbs (as with oxygen metabolism and CBF; Eidelberg *et al.*, 1991; Blin *et al.*, 1990); and (3) decreased fluorodopa uptake in the striatum, indicative of dysfunction of the nigrostriatal dopaminergic system (Riley and Lang, 1988; Sawle *et al.*, 1989, 1991; Riley *et al.*, 1990). The general patterns of these *in vivo* metabolic abnormalities conform to the known pattern of neuronal degeneration in CBGD, indicating that PET studies may help differentiate this disorder from other types of Parkinson-plus or motor system degeneration syndromes. The number of cases of CBGD studied by PET is still small, however, so that further correlative studies, especially with pathological confirmation, are needed.

NEUROPATHOLOGY

The principal neuropathological abnormalities in CBGD are: (1) a distinctive pattern of asymmetric atrophy of the cerebral cortex involving mainly the frontoparietal and Rolandic regions, with relative sparing of the temporal and occipital regions, associated with neuronal swelling and achromasia of variable numbers of the pyramidal neurons; (2) loss of melanin-containing neurons, with gliosis, in the pars compacta of the substantia nigra, but generally no typical Lewy bodies; and (3) variable neuronal loss and gliosis of other subcortical, brainstem and cerebellar grey matter (Table 14.2). Neuronal swelling may also occur at these sites. Corresponding to the neuronal loss in the frontoparietal cortex, there typically is asymmetrical secondary degeneration of the corticospinal (pyramidal) tracts, especially on the side related to the most severe cortical atrophy.

The atrophy of the cortex is generally recognizable on gross inspection of the brain (Fig. 14.2A); it characteristically is more pronounced on the side contralateral to the most severely affected limbs. This asymmetry can be correlated with the findings on CT, MRI, EEG and PET studies. On microscopic examination, the cortical atrophy

Table 14.2 Neuropathological features

Macroscopic
Frontoparietal cerebral cortical atrophy–asymmetrical, prominent around central sulcus
Enlargement of lateral ventricles
Reduction of cerebral white matter, cerebral peduncles (asymmetrical) and corpus callosum
Pallor of substantia nigra
Microscopic
Neuronal loss, gliosis and swollen, ballooned achromatic neurons in cerebral cortex – especially frontoparietal (immunoreactive with neurofilament protein antibodies; intermediate filaments by electron microscopy)
Disorganization of laminar pattern of cerebral cortex in regions of heavy neuronal loss
Abnormal cerebral white matter – swollen axons, demyelination of axons, spongiform appearance of neuropil in regions of heavy neuronal loss
Pigmented nerve cell loss and gliosis in substantia nigra
Variable neuronal loss and gliosis in subthalamic nucleus, globus pallidus, corpus striatum, red nucleus, claustrum, thalamus, dentate and cerebellar roof nuclei, and scattered brainstem nuclei (swollen, achromatic neurons occasionally found)
Immunocytochemical
Positive reaction of swollen, achromatic cortical neurons and axons with antibodies to 160/200 kDa neurofilament proteins
Positive reaction of nigral neurons containing 'corticobasal inclusions' with monoclonal antineurofilament antibody RT97
Negative reaction with antibodies to glial fibrillary acid protein and tau (microtubule-associated) proteins
Electron microscopic
Swollen, achromatic neurons and occasional swollen axons filled with aggregates of 10 nm filaments

is associated with marked neuronal loss, disruption of the normal cytoarchitecture and extensive fibrillary gliosis. In some regions, layers III and V appear to be most severely affected. The loss of cortical tissue can be so extensive, however, as to result in gross thinning, and a spongy, loose-textured appearance of the neuropil.

The distinctive neuronal abnormality that is typical for CBGD is, as already indicated, cytoplasmic swelling (giving a somewhat rounded contour to the cell), and loss of typical staining properties of the neuronal cytoplasm so that it appears markedly pale and homogeneous with common histological staining methods, such as haematoxylin and eosin (which brings out a faint eosinophilia), cresyl violet (Nissl method), silver impregnation techniques, and periodic acid–Schiff. The nucleus is often eccentric, and the cytoplasm at times contains scattered vacuoles of varying size (Fig. 14.3). The cortical neurons so affected are medium-sized to large pyramidal cells. They are most frequent in the regions of the cortex that are moderately (rather than most severely) involved, but they can be seen in isolation in relatively intact regions. They also can be found in the subcortical nuclei and even, at times, in the brainstem and cerebellar nuclei. Immunocytochemical (ICC) staining of these abnormal neurons is positive with antibodies to 160/200 kDa phosphorylated neurofilament proteins (Wang *et al.*, 1991; Smith *et al.*, 1992), ubiquitin (Smith *et al.*, 1992), Alz 50 (Smith *et al.*, 1992), alpha beta crystallin (Lowe *et al.*, 1992) but usually negative with antibodies to tau (a microtubule-associated protein) and/or glial fibrillary acidic protein (GFAP; Gibb *et al.*, 1989; Watts *et al.*, 1989; Smith *et al.*, 1992). Ultrastructural examination reveals that the cytoplasm of the swollen pale neurons is filled with aggregates of 10 nm intermediate filaments (see Fig. 14.3E; Watts *et al.*, 1989). Some axons show similar aggregates.

The white matter immediately underlying the atrophic cortex shows variable rarefaction that may be striking. Silver stain reveals variable axonal loss, with some of the remaining disordered axons displaying irregular thickenings. In most cases, neuronal degeneration in the substantia nigra is recognizable grossly as pallor of the pars compacta. Histologically, the loss of pigmented neurons usually is severe and is accompanied by marked gliosis (Rebeiz *et al.*, 1968; Watts *et al.*, 1985, 1989; Gibb *et al.*, 1989; Greene *et al.*, 1990; Riley *et al.*, 1990), In some cases, the neuronal loss is most severe in the lateral and mid-portions of the substantia nigra, with relative sparing in the medial part (Rebeiz *et al.*, 1968). Unlike Parkinson's disease or diffuse Lewy body disease, Lewy bodies are only rarely (and possibly only incidentally) seen in CBGD. Gibb and co-workers (1989) described round or oval inclusions in the substantia nigra, variable in size (up to 25 μm) and weakly basophilic with a faint fibrillary appearance; these 'corticobasal inclusions' stained positively with RT 97, a monoclonal antineurofilament antibody that recognizes 210 K neurofilament epitopes and also labels neurofibrillary tangles. Whether or not these structures are truly distinct from changes in other ballooned neurons warrants further study.

Other brain regions are involved to varying degrees in CBGD. The claustrum, amygdala, striatum and pallidum, subthalamic nucleus, red nucleus, and thalamus (particularly the lateral nuclei) in the forebrain, various nuclei in the brainstem (locus ceruleus, midbrain tegmentum, raphe nuclei, oculomotor nuclei), and the dentate and roof nuclei of the cerebellum may show neuronal swelling with achromasia and gliosis (Rebeiz *et al.*, 1968; Case Records of the Massachusetts General Hospital, 1985; Watts *et al.*, 1985, 1989; Gibbs *et al.*, 1989; Greene *et al.*, 1990; Riley *et al.*, 1990). The degenerative changes in these subcortical structures, however, are always less severe than those in the cerebral cortex. The nucleus basalis of Meynert has been found to be unremarkable except for a few swollen pale neurons (Gibb *et al.*, 1989).

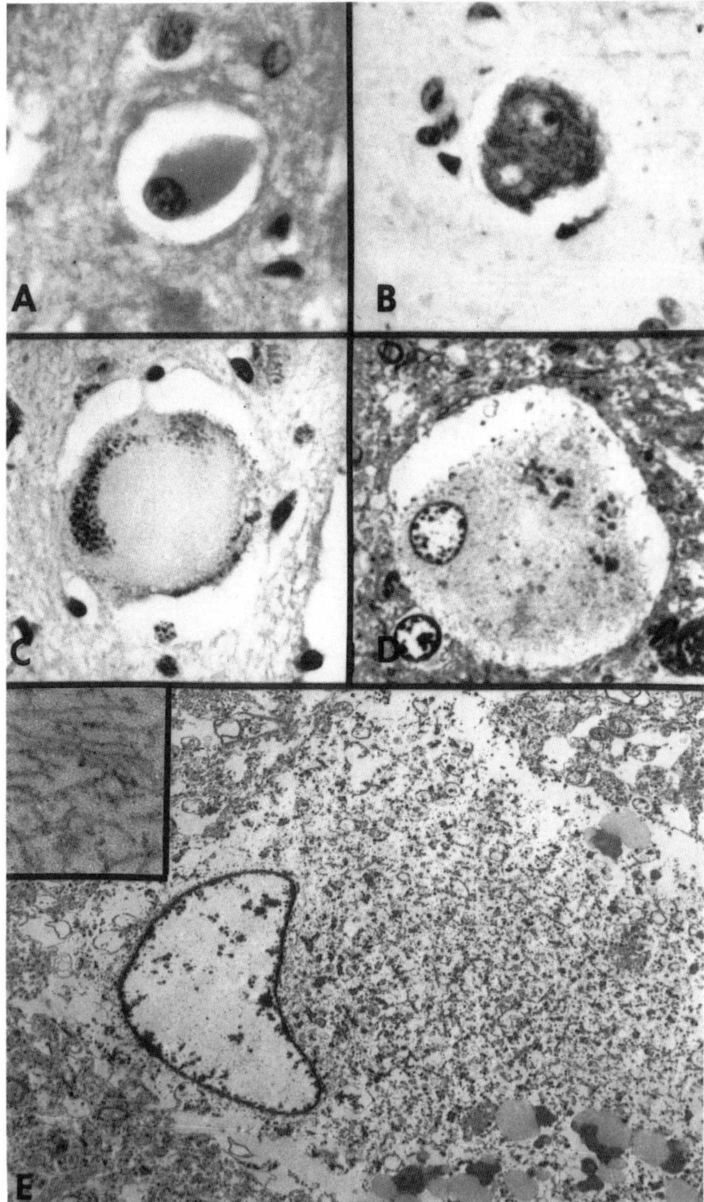

Figure 14.3 Swollen achromatic neurons from the prefrontal cortex of a 75-year-old man with corticobasal ganglionic degeneration (Watts *et al.*, 1989). (A) A cortical neuron shows an eccentric nucleus and swollen eosinophilic cytoplasm. Haematoxylin and eosin ×200. (B) The cytoplasm of a swollen neuron is labelled with antibodies to phosphorylated epitopes of 200 kDa neurofilament protein. Peroxidase ×400. (C) Nissl substance is dispersed to the periphery of a swollen cell body. Cresyl violet ×1000. (D) Swollen neuron shows eccentric nucleus and peripheral cytoplasmic lipofuscin on plastic semithin section. Toluidine blue ×1000. (E) Electron micrograph of a swollen achromatic neuron demonstrates an eccentric nucleus. The cytoplasm displays disordered filaments and lipofuscin. ×4200. Inset: Higher magnification reveals intermediate filaments approximately 10 nm in diameter. ×37 700.

DIFFERENTIAL DIAGNOSIS

The pattern of deficits presented by CBGD is sufficiently distinctive that, when fully developed, the syndrome generally would not be misdiagnosed as Parkinson's disease. The best early clues that allow one to distinguish this disorder from idiopathic Parkinson's disease are: (1) the lack of beneficial response to levodopa or dopamine agonists; and (2) signs of cortical dysfunction, most notably apraxia, cortical sensory impairment, or an extensor plantar response.

The differential diagnosis consists of the nosologically distinct extrapyramidal syndromes associated with basal ganglionic and cortical degeneration that present as a Parkinson-plus syndrome. Disorders with similar presentations include progressive supranuclear palsy (Steele *et al.*, 1964), striatonigral degeneration (Adams *et al.*, 1964; Takei and Mirra, 1973), multisystem atrophy (including olivopontocerebellar atrophy; Spokes *et al.*, 1979; see Chapter 13), Parkinson's disease with associated Alzheimer disease, atypical variants of Pick disease (Akelaitis, 1944; Tissot *et al.*, 1975; Cole *et al.*, 1979), the dementia–Parkinson–amyotrophic lateral sclerosis complex (Hirano *et al.*, 1961a,b), Wilson's disease (Wilson, 1912), Huntington's disease (especially the rigid form usually seen in juveniles; Bruyn, 1967), variants of Azorean disease (Nakano *et al.*, 1972; Woods and Schaumburg, 1975; Romanul *et al.*, 1977; Sachdev *et al.*, 1982) and familial progressive basal ganglia, corticobulbar and corticospinal systems degeneration (Morin *et al.*, 1980; Boustany *et al.*, 1984), all of which differ in many clinical and pathological respects. Some cases of CBGD, however, may show overlapping clinical and pathological features with other disorders (Paulus and Selim, 1990).

PATHOPHYSIOLOGY

In order to correlate the clinical signs and symptoms with the known neuropathological abnormalities, the predilection for involvement of the primary and secondary motor and somatic sensory cortical areas and closely related regions of association cortex merits attention. It is known from animal and human studies that these brain regions are intimately related to the planning and execution of voluntary limb movement, somaesthesia, the control of muscle tone and posture, and the control of saccadic eye movements, all of which can be abnormal in CBGD (Mountcastle *et al.*, 1975; Bruce and Goldberg, 1984; Wise, 1985; Alexander *et al.*, 1986). Dysfunction of the parietal cortex alone may result in apraxia, cortical sensory impairment, and pseudoathetosis (Gomez *et al.*, 1985).

The symptoms of rigidity, bradykinesia and loss of dexterity may be related to loss of neurons in the substantia nigra. An alternative possibility is involvement of the supplementary motor cortex and related areas. In monkeys it has been shown that the supplementary motor cortex receives a major pallidothalamic system input, thus serving as a major motor cortical receiving area for basal ganglia output related to motor function (Schell and Strick, 1984). The flexed and abducted posture of the upper limbs seen late in the illness is similar to the decorticate posture of primates that have lesions of large areas of frontal cortex and underlying white matter.

Pursuit eye movements are usually intact early, but most develop saccadic breakdown, implicating affection of supranuclear oculomotor control centres. Voluntary saccades to verbal command are lost late, indicative most likely of involvement of the frontal eye fields (area 8 of Brodmann; Bruce and Goldberg,

1984), but possibly also due to disease of the substantia nigra. Hikosaka and Wurtz (1983) demonstrated a role for the pars reticulata of the substantia nigra in the non-sensory control of saccadic eye movements in animals. While CBGD and progressive supranuclear palsy (PSP) both result in supranuclear gaze abnormalities, in PSP it is more severe earlier in the course of illness.

THERAPY

Pharmacotherapy has generally been ineffective. There is little or no beneficial response to levodopa/carbidopa, L-tyrosine or dopamine agonists (bromocriptine, pergolide); indeed, this is a characteristic feature. Clonazepam has been the most beneficial agent for action tremor and myoclonus. Baclofen may improve rigidity and tremor also, but to a lesser degree. Anticholinergics have not been beneficial, and they have been tolerated poorly. Dopamine antagonsists, such as haloperidol, have been used sparingly and have not been helpful. Propanolol may benefit the action tremor early in the course in some, but later its effectiveness wanes, particularly as the tremor becomes myoclonic. Trials of ethanol, physostigmine, methysergide, diphenhydramine and clonidine have produced no improvement.

Other aspects of patient care, not involving pharmacotherapy, can be of special importance for these patients. Physiotherapy is very helpful for maintenance of mobility and prevention of contractures. Pain related to dystonic posturing can be lessened by maintenance of good range of motion, and occasionally splinting can be helpful. Occupational therapy can help patients maintain some degree of functional independence by providing specially made devices such as eating utensils with large handles. Speech therapy may offer practical hints and exercises to optimize speech function and guard against aspiration secondary to swallowing difficulty. Over time, most patients develop severe dysphagia and require percutaneous feeding gastrostomy tube placement. This assists with maintenance of nutrition with a reduced risk of aspiration. The decision to place a gastrostomy in a patient with a chronically progressive neurodegenerative disease must be handled on an individual basis. Good home care assistance can help prolong the time a patient can remain at home before requiring domiciliary/nursing home placement.

DISCUSSION

Based on the current evidence, CBGD appears to be a distinctive nosological entity. When fully developed and observed over time, the clinical presentation is sufficiently characteristic to allow correct diagnosis during life with a relatively high probability. Additional studies, including CT and MRI, electrophysiology, PET and CSF neurotransmitter studies, while not diagnostic, can provide supportive data. The ultimate confirmation however still rests with the neuropathological examination.

Indeed, perhaps clues to the nosological classification of CBGD can be found in its neuropathological manifestations. Of all the neurodegenerative disorders, CBGD may have the most in common with Pick's disease. Striking, often asymmetrical cortical atrophy, albeit typically frontal-temporal, and nigral degeneration, occur in Pick's disease (Tomlinson and Corsellis, 1984). The predominant clinical presentation of these Pick disease cases, however, is one of dementia and personality change.

Pick cells, virtually identical to the swollen achromatic neurons of CBGD, are frequently seen in Pick's disease (Constantinidis *et al.*, 1974) and are also immunoreactive with antibodies to neurofilament proteins (Probst *et al.*, 1983). In contrast, the argyrophilic Pick body, although also neurofilament protein-positive (Probst *et al.*, 1983), shares antigenic determinants with the microtubule-associated protein, tau (Pollock *et al.*, 1986; Murayama *et al.*, 1990), as well as ubiquitin (Murayama *et al.*, 1990), and has a different fine structure (Munoz-Garcia and Ludwin, 1984).

Other conditions have been described in which swollen achromatic neurons are a prominent feature. The brain of a 7-week-old baby with profound psychomotor retardation displayed numerous Pick cells in a diffuse cortical distribution (De Leon *et al.*, 1986). Clark and colleagues observed frontal cortical degeneration and prominent swollen achromatic neurons, but no Pick bodies, in 2 patients with dementia (Clark *et al.*, 1986). In contrast with CBGD, these patients presented primarily with progressive dementia and lacked motor signs. As similar achromatic cells have been described in Creutzfeldt–Jakob disease (Beck and Daniel, 1979; Nakazato *et al.*, 1990), the possibility of transmissibility has been considered (Clark *et al.*, 1986). Lippa and co-workers (1990) described a 64-year-old man with dementia, temporal atrophy, and ballooned neurons in the basis pontis.

The cytoskeletal pathology in CBGD is exemplified by the aberrant localization of phosphorylated neurofilament proteins in the cytoplasm of the swollen neurons. Although present within central nervous system axons, phosphorylated neurofilament proteins do not normally occur within neuronal cell bodies (Cork *et al.*, 1988a). However, cytoplasmic aggregates of phosphorylated neurofilament proteins have been observed in a variety of human and animal disorders (Cork *et al.*, 1988a; Manetto *et al.*, 1988). In Alzheimer's disease and in aged bears, neurofibrillary tangles contain epitopes of phosphorylated neurofilaments (Sternberger *et al.*, 1985; Cork *et al.*, 1986, 1988b), as do the Lewy bodies of Parkinson's disease (Forno *et al.*, 1986). Swollen cortical neurons in Creutzfeldt–Jakob disease also exhibit these changes (Nakazato *et al.*, 1990). Experimental intoxication with B, B′-iminodiproprionitrile (Cork *et al.*, 1986b) and aluminium (Bizzi and Gambetti, 1986; Troncosco *et al.*, 1986) produces accumulation of perikaryal phosphorylated neurofilaments. The co-localization of alpha beta crystallin in ballooned neurons in several neurodegenerative diseases (Kato *et al.*, 1992; Lowe *et al.*, 1992) suggested to Lowe and co-workers the possible involvement of alpha beta crystallin in aggregation and remodelling of neurofilaments in disease.

CBGD may be linked to other neurological disorders in humans and animals affecting motor neurons which similarly contain abnormal aggregates of phosphorylated neurofilaments. Chromatolytic lower motor neurons and proximal swollen axons from patients with amyotrophic lateral sclerosis contain clusters of neurofilaments (Chou, 1979; Hirano, 1982; Hirano *et al.*, 1989) which are atypically phosphorylated (Manetto *et al.*, 1988). Similarly, ballooned neurons in multiple sites, including anterior horn in Werdnig–Hoffmann disease, were stained with antiphosphorylated neurofilament antibodies (Kato and Hirano, 1990; Murayama *et al.*, 1991), as well as neurons of extraocular muscle nuclei by antiubiquitin (Kato and Hirano, 1990). Motor neurons in hereditary canine spinal muscular atrophy, shaker calves, rabbit and pig motor neuron disease, swayback of lambs and kids, and zebra myelopathy all contain epitopes of phosphorylated neurofilament protein in cell bodies (Cork *et al.*, 1988a). Ballooned neurons positive for phosphorylated neurofilament epitopes have also been observed in a patient with progressive supranuclear palsy and olivary hypertrophy (Giaconne *et al.*, 1988). The concomitant vacuolization of the cytoplasm of the achromatic neurons in CBGD (Rebeiz *et al.*, 1968) is recapitulated in ballooned neurons in humans in various conditions (Dickson *et al.*, 1986) and in motor disorders in mice (Andrews, 1975).

Some evidence suggests that axonal damage may be fundamental to the changes of CBGD and other conditions with achromatic neurons. Phosphorylated neurofilaments accumulate in neurons exhibiting central chromatolysis following experimental axonal injury (Drager and Hofbauer, 1984; Goldstein *et al.*, 1987; Rosenfeld *et al.*, 1987), although Wang and co-workers did not obtain immunostaining with monoclonal phosphorylated neurofilament antibodies of neurons with central chromatolysis secondary to axonal injury (Wang *et al.*, 1991). Hall and co-workers, however, found that microtubule destabilization and neurofilament phosphorylation precede dendritic sprouting after experimental axotomy of lamprey central neurons (Hall *et al.*, 1991). When coupled with the observed axonal pathology in the subcortical white matter in some cases of CBGD, this raises the question as to whether or not the primary changes in CBGD are axonal. Indeed, such a mechanism has been proposed in Pick's disease (Onari and Spatz, 1926) as well as in other disorders having ballooned neurons (Dickson *et al.*, 1986). Together, these findings lend credence to Gajdusek's hypothesis that impaired axoplasmic transport of neurofilaments may be a common factor in many neurodegenerative disorders (Gajdusek, 1985), and perhaps also in CBGD.

Therapy has been of minimal benefit, and this can best be ascribed to the multisystem degenerative nature and predominance of cortical involvement in the disease. CSF neurotransmitter and metabolite studies, while limited thus far, provide some corroborative evidence for this concept. CSF somatostatin values were significantly low (in the range of values seen with Alzheimer's disease) in all 3 patients studied, indicative of severe degeneration of cerebral cortex (Watts *et al.*, 1985, 1989). We have measured CSF levels of homovanillic acid (a dopamine metabolite) in these patients and find significant reductions in some, though not all, cases (R.L. Watts and J.H. Growdon, unpublished observations). Hence, the homovanillic acid abnormality is not as consistent as the somatostatin abnormality, perhaps indicating that at a given stage of disease the cortical degeneration is as bad as or worse than that in the substantia nigra.

Despite all therapeutic efforts, the illness is relentlessly progressive, leading to rigid immobility within 3–5 years and death within 5–10 years. Identification of *in vivo* biological markers (to improve diagnostic accuracy), development of better therapeutic strategies and extension of our fundamental knowledge of the cellular and molecular defect(s) are high priorities for future studies.

Acknowledgements

We are indebted to the many neurologists and other physicians who have referred patients for investigation: at Massachusetts General Hospital – Robert R. Young, John H. Growdon, Roger Williams, C. Miller Fisher, Raymond D. Adams; at Emory University – Charles Epstein and Robert F. Kibler; at Duke University – Albert Heyman and James Villier (Charlotte); in Virginia, Jon D. Dorman and Della C. Williams. Special thanks to our collaborators: M. Flint Beal and John H. Growdon (CSF studies); E. Clarke Haley and Robert Ackerman (PET studies). This work was supported in part by the Emory University Parkinson Research Fund and Center for Age-Related Neurological Diseases. Suzanne S. Mirra's work is supported by a Veterans Affairs Merit Award and National Institutes of Health (Bethesda, MD) grant AG06790 and AG10130.

References

Adams RD, Van Bogaert L, and van der Eecken H (1964) Striatonigral degeneration. *J Neuropathol Exp Neurol*, **23**, 584–608

Alexander GE, DeLong MR and Strick PL (1986) Parallel organization of functionally segregated circuits linking basal ganglia and cortex. In Cowan WM, ed, *Annual Review of Neuroscience*, vol 9, 357–81

Andrews JM (1975) The fine structure of the cervical spinal cord, ventral root and brachial plexus in the Wobbler (wr) mouse. *J Neuropathol Exp Neurol*, **34**, 12–27

Beck E and Daniel PM (1979) Kuru and Creutzfeldt-Jakob disease: neuropathological lesions and their significance. In Prusiner SB, Hadlow WJ, eds, *Slow Transmissible Diseases of the Nervous System*, vol 1. *Clinical, Epidemiological, Genetic and Pathological Aspects of the Spongiform Encephalopathies*. New York, Academic Press, 253–70

Bizzi A and Gambetti P (1986) Phosphorylation of neurofilaments is altered in aluminum intoxication. *Acta Neuropathol (Berl)*, **71**, 154–8

Blin J, Vidailhet M, Bonnet AM, Dubois B, Pillon B, Syrota A *et al.* (1990) PET study in cortico-basal degeneration. *Movement Disorders*, **5** (suppl 1), 19

Boustany RM, Tyler KL, Kolodny EH, and Adams RD (1984) A new familial progressive degeneration of the basal ganglia, corticobulbar, and corticospinal systems. *Neurology*, **34** (suppl 1), 149

Bruce CJ and Goldberg ME (1984) Physiology of the frontal eye fields. *Trends Neurosci*, **7**, 436–41

Bruyn GW (1967) The Westphal variant and juvenile type of Huntington's chorea. In Barbeau A and Brunette JR, eds, *Progress in Neurogenetics*, Amsterdam, Excerpta Medica Foundation, 666–73

Carella F, Scaioli V, Franceschetti S, Girotti F, Giovannini P, Ciano C *et al.* (1991) Focal reflex myoclonus in corticobasal degeneration. *Funct Neurol*, **6**, 165–70

Case Records of the Massachusetts General Hospital (Case 38) (1985). *N Engl J Med*, **313**, 739–48 (case of corticonigral degeneration with neuronal achromasia)

Chou SM (1979) Pathognomy of intraneuronal inclusions in amyotrophic lateral sclerosis. In Tsuboki T, Toyokura Y, eds, *Amyotrophic Lateral Sclerosis*, Baltimore, University Park Press, 135–76

Clark AW, Manz HJ, White CL, Lehmann J, Miller D, and Coyle JT (1986) Cortical degeneration with swollen chromatolytic neurons: its relationship to Pick's disease. *J Neuropathol Exp Neurol*, **45**, 268–84

Cole M, Wright D, and Banker BQ (1979) Familial aphasia due to Pick's disease. *Ann Neurol*, **6**, 158

Constantinidis J, Richard J, and Tissot R (1974) Pick's disease. Histological and clinical correlations. *Eur Neurol*, **11**, 208–17

Cork LC, Sternberger NH, Sternberger LA, Casanova MF, Struble RG, and Price DL (1986a) Phosphorylated neurofilament antigens in neurofibrillary tangles in Alzheimer's disease. *J Neuropathol Exp Neurol*, **64**, 253–8

Cork LC, Troncoso JC, Griffin JW *et al.* (1986b) Immunocytochemical studies of neurofilamentous changes in neurons. In *X International Congress of Neuropathology*, Abstracts, September 7–12, 1986, Stockholm, Sweden, Stockholm: Gotab 217

Cork LC, Troncoso JC, Klavano GG, Johnson ES, Sternberger LA, Sternberger NH *et al.* (1988a) Neurofilamentous abnormalities in motor neurons in spontaneously occurring animal disorders. *J Neuropathol Exp Neurol*, **47**, 420–31

Cork LC, Powers RE, Selkoe DJ, Davies P, Geyer JJ, and Price DL (1988b) Neurofibrillary tangles and senile plaques in aged bears. *J Neuropathol Exp Neurol*, **47**, 629–41

De Leon GA, Breningstall G, and Zaeri N (1986) Congenital Pick cell encephalopathy: a distinct disorder characterized by diffuse formation of Pick cells in the cerebral cortex. *Acta Neuropathol (Berl)*, **70**, 235–42

Dickson DW, Yen SH, Suzuki KI, Davies P, Gargia JH, and Hirano A (1986) Ballooned neurons in select neurodegenerative diseases contain phosphorylated neurofilament epitopes. *Acta Neuropathol*, **71**, 216–33

Drager UC and Hofbauer A (1984) Antibodies to heavy neurofilament subunit detect a subpopulation of damaged ganglion cells in retina. *Nature*, **309**, 624–6

Eidelberg D, Dhawan V, Moeller JR, Sidtis JJ, Ginos JZ, Strother SC *et al.* (1991) The metabolic landscape of corticobasal ganglionic degeneration: regional asymmetries studied with positron emission tomography. *J Neurol Neurosurg Psychiatry*, **54**, 856–62

Forno LS, Sternberger LA, Sternberger NH, Strefling AM, Swanson K, and Eng LF (1986) Reaction of Lewy bodies with antibodies to phosphorylated and nonphosphorylated neurofilaments. *Neurosci Lett*, **64**, 253–8

Gajdusek DC (1985) Hypothesis: interference with axonal transport of neurofilaments as a common pathogenetic mechanism in certain diseases of the central nervous system. *N Engl J Med*, **312**, 714–19

Giaccone G, Tagliavini F, Street JS, Ghetti B, and Bugiani O (1988) Progressive supranuclear palsy with hypertrophy of the olives. An immunocytochemical study of the cytoskeleton of argyrophilic neurons. *Acta Neuropathol*, **77**, 14–20

Gibb WRG, Luthert PJ, and Marsden CD (1988) Clinical and pathological features of corticobasal degeneration. In *9th International Symposium on Parkinson Disease Abstracts*, Jerusalem, Israel, 83

Gibb WRG, Luthert PJ, and Marsden CD (1989) Corticobasal degeneration. *Brain*, **112**, 1171–92

Goldstein ME, Cooper HS, Bruce J, Carden MJ, Lee VM, and Schlaepfer WW (1987) Phosphorylation of neurofilament proteins and chromatolysis following transection of rat sciatic nerve. *J Neurosci*, **7**, 1586–94

Gomez C, Cruz-Rodriguez RF, Horenstein S, and Chung HD (1985) Movement disorders may result

Gomez C, Cruz-Rodriguez RF, Horenstein S, and Chung HD (1985) Movement disorders may result from parietal lobe lesions. *Ann Neurol*, **18**, 148

Greene PE, Fahn S, Lang AE, Watts RL, Eidelberg D, and Powers J (1990) Progressive unilateral rigidity, bradykinesia, tremulousness, and apraxia, leading to fixed postural deformity of the involved limb (What Is It? Case 1, 1990 – Cortical-Basal Ganglionic Degeneration). *Movement Disorders*, **5**, 341–51

Hall GF, Lee VM-Y, and Kosik KS (1991) Microtubule destabilization and neurofilament phosphorylation precede dendritic sprouting after close axotomy of lamprey central neurons. *Proc Natl Acad Sci USA*, **88**, 5016–20

Hikosaka O and Wurtz RH (1983) *J Neurophysiol*, **49**, 1230–53

Hirano A (1982) Aspects of the ultrastructure of amyotrophic lateral sclerosis. In Rowland LP, ed, *Human Motor Neuron Diseases. Advances in Neuroloty*, vol 36, New York, Raven Press, 75–88

Hirano A, Malamud M, and Kurland LT (1961a) Parkinsonism-dementia complex on the Island of Guam. II. Pathological features. *Brain*, **84**, 662–79

Hirano A, Kurland LT, Krooth RS *et al.* (1961b) Parkinsonism-dementia complex, an endemic disease on the Island of Guam: I. Clinical features. *Brain*, **84**, 642–61

Hirano A, Donnenfeld H, Sasaki S, and Nakano J (1984) Fine structure observations of neurofilamentous changes in amyotrophic lateral sclerosis. *J Neuropathol Exp Neurol*, **43**, 461–70

Kato S and Hirano A (1990) Ubiquitin and phosphorylated neurofilament epitopes in ballooned neurons of the extraocular muscle nuclei in a case of Werdnig Hoffman disease. *Acta Neuropathol*, **80**, 334–7

Kato S, Hirano A, Umahara T, Kato M, Hertz F, and Ohama E (1992) Comparative immunohistochemical study on the expression of alpha B crystallin, ubiquitin and stress-response protein 27 in ballooned neurons in various disorders. *Neuropathol Appl Neurobiol*, **18**, 335–40

LeWitt P, Friedman J, Nutt J *et al.* (1989) Progressive rigidity with apraxia: the variety of clinical and pathological features. *Neurology*, **39** (suppl 1), 140

Lippa CF, Smith TW, and Fontneay N (1990a) Corticonigral degeneration with neuronal achromasia. A clinicopathologic study of two cases. *J Neurol Sci*, **98**, 301–10

Lippa CF, Smith TW, and DeGirolami U (1990b) Lobar atrophy with pontine neuronal chromatolysis ("ballooned" neurons). *Human Pathol*, **21**, 1076–9

Lowe J, Errington DR, Lennox G, Pike I, Spendlove I, Landon M *et al.* (1992) Ballooned neurons in several neurodegenerative diseases and stroke contain alpha B crystallin. *Neuropathol Appl Neurobiol*, **18**, 341–50

Manetto V, Sternberger NH, Perry G, Sternberger LA, and Gambetti P (1988) Phosphorylation of neurofilaments is altered in amyotrophic lateral sclerosis. *J Neuropathol Exp Neurol*, **47**, 642–53

Morin P, Lechevalier B, and Bianco C (1980) Atrophie cérébelleuse et lésions pallido-luyso-nigriques avec corps de Lewy. *Rev Neurol (Paris)*, **136**, 381–90

Mountcastle VB, Lynch JC, Georgopoulos A, Sakata H, and Acuna C (1975) Posterior parietal association cortex of the monkey: command functions for operation within extrapersonal space. *J Neurophysiol*, **38**, 871–908

Munoz-Garcia D and Ludwin SK (1984) Classic and generalized variants of Pick's disease: a clinicopathological, ultrastructural, and immunocytochemical comparative study. *Ann Neurol*, **16**, 467–80

Murayama S, Mori H, Ihara Y, and Tomonaga M (1990) Immunocytochemical and ultrastructural studies of Pick's disease. *Ann Neurol*, **27**, 394–405

Murayama S, Bouldin TW, and Suzuki K (1991) Immunocytochemical and ultrastructural studies of Werdnig–Hoffman disease. *Acta Neuropathol*, **81**, 408–17

Nakano KK, Dawson DM, and Spence A (1972) Machado disease. A hereditary ataxia in Portuguese emigrants to Massachusetts. *Neurology*, **22**, 49–55

Nakazato Y, Hirato J, Ishida Y, Hoshi S, Hasegawa M, and Fukuda T (1990a) Swollen cortical neurons in Creutzfeldt–Jakob disease contain a phosphorylated neurofilament epitope. *J Neuropathol Exp Neurol*, **49**, 197–205

Onari K and Spatz H (1926) Anatomische Beiträge zur Lehre von der Pickschen umschreibenen Grosshirnrinden-Atrophie ("Picksche Krankheit"). *Z Gesamte Neurol Psychiatrie*, **101**, 470–511

Paulus W and Selim M (1990) Corticonigral degeneration with neuronal achromasia and basal neurofibrillary tangles. *Acta Neuropathol*, **81**, 89–94

Pollock NJ, Mirra SS, Binder LI, Hansen LA, and Wood JG (1986) Filamentous aggregates in Pick's disease, progressive supranuclear palsy, and Alzheimer's disease share antigenic determinants with microtubule-associated protein, tau. *Lancet*, **2**, 1211

Probst A, Anderton BH, Ulrich J, Kohler R, Kahn J, and Heitz PU (1983) Pick's disease: an immunocytochemical study of neuronal changes: monoclonal antibodies show that Pick bodies share antigenic determinants with neurofibrillary tangles and neurofilaments. *Acta Neuropathol* (*Berl*), **60**, 175–82

Rebeiz JJ, Kolodny EH, and Richardson EP (1967) Corticodentatonigral degeneration with neuronal achromasia: a progressive disorder of late adult life. *Trans Am Neurol Assoc*, **92**, 23–6

Rebeiz JJ, Kolodny EH, and Richardson EP (1968) Corticodentatonigral degeneration with neuronal achromasia. *Arch Neurol*, **18**, 20–33

Riley DE and Lang AE (1988) Corticobasal ganglionic degeneration (CBGD): further observations on six additional cases. *Neurology*, **38** (suppl 1), 360

Riley DE, Lang AE, Lewis A, Resch L, Ashby P, Hornykiewicz O *et al.* (1990) Cortical-basal ganglionic degeneration. *Neurology*, **40**, 1203–12

Romanul FCA, Fowler HL, Radvany J, Feldman RG, and Feingold M (1977) Azorean disease of the nervous system. *N Engl J Med*, **296**, 1505–8

Rosenfeld J, Dorman ME, Griffin JW, Sternberger LA, Sternberger NH, and Price DL (1987) Distribution of neurofilament antigens after axonal injury. *J Neuropathol Exp Neurol*, **46**, 269–82

Sachdev HS, Forno LS, and Kane CA (1982) Joseph disease: a multisystem degenerative disorder of the nervous system. *Neurology*, **32**, 192–5

Sawle GV, Brooks DJ, Thompson PD, Marsden CD, and Frackowiak RSJ (1989) PET studies on the dopaminergic system and regional cortical metabolism in corticobasal degeneration. *Neurology*, **39** (suppl 1), 163

Sawle GV, Brooks DJ, Marsden CD, and Frackowiak RS (1991) Corticobasal degeneration. A unique pattern of regional cortical oxygen hypometabolism and striatal fluorodopa uptake demonstrated by positron emission tomography. *Brain*, **114**, 541–56

Schell GR and Strick PL (1984) The origin of thalamic inputs to the arcuate premotor and supplementary motor areas. *J Neurosci*, **4**, 539–60

Smith TW, Lippa CF, and De Girolami U (1992) Immunocytochemical study of ballooned neurons in cortical degeneration with neuronal achromasia. *Clin Neuropathol*, **11**, 28–35

Spokes EGS, Bannister R, and Oppenheimer DR (1979) Multiple system atrophy with autonomic failure. *J Neurol Sci*, **43**, 59–82

Steele JC, Richardson JC, and Olszewski J (1964) Progressive supranuclear palsy. *Arch Neurol*, **10**, 333–58

Sternberger NH, Sternberger LA, and Ulrich J (1985) Aberrant neurofilament phosophorylation in Alzheimer disease. *Proc Natl Acad Sci USA*, **82**, 4274–6

Takei Y and Mirra SS (1973) Striatonigral degeneration: a form of multiple system atrophy with clinical parkinsonism. *Prog Neuropathol*, **2**, 217–51

Thompson PD, Day BL, Rothwell JC, and Marsden CD (1990) Clinical and electrophysiological findings in corticobasal degeneration. *Movement Disorders*, **5** (suppl 1), 43

Tissot R, Constantinidis J, and Richard J (1975) *La Maladie de Pick*, Paris, Masson

Tomlinson BE and Corsellis JAN (1984) Ageing and the dementias. In Adams JH, Corsellis JAN, Duchen LW, eds, *Greenfield's Neuropathology*, 4th edn, New York, John Wiley, 988

Troncoso JC, Sternberger NH, Sternberger LA, Hoffman PN, and Price DL (1986) Immunocytochemical studies of neurofilament antigens in the neurofibrillary pathology induced by aluminum. *Brain Res*, **364**, 295–300

Wang LN, Kowall NW, and Richardson EP (1991) Phosphorylated neurofilament epitopes in the achromasic neurons of corticonigral degeneration. *Clin Med J*, **104**, 1011–17

Watts RL, William RS, Growdon JH *et al.* (1985) Corticobasal ganglionic degeneration. *Neurology*, **35** (suppl 1), 178

Watts RL, Mirra SS, Young RR *et al.* (1989) Corticobasal ganglionic degeneration (CBGD) with neuronal achromasia: clinical-pathological study of two cases. *Neurology*, **39** (suppl 1), 140

Wilson SAK (1912) Lenticular degeneration. *Brain*, **34**, 295–321

Wise SP (1985) The primate premotor cortex: past, present, and preparatory. In Cowan WM, ed, *Annual Review of Neuroscience*, vol 8, Palo Alto, CA, Annual Reviews, 1–19

Woods BT and Schaumburg HH (1975) Nigrospinodentatal degeneration with nuclear ophthalmoplegia. In Vinken PJ and Bruyn GW, eds, *Handbook of Clinical Neurology*, vol 22, Amsterdam, North-Holland, 157–76

Part III

Dyskinesias

15
Problems in the dyskinesias

Stanley Fahn and C. David Marsden

In *Movement Disorders 1* (1982), we chose the management of Huntington's disease (Ira Shoulson), myoclonus (with Mark Hallett), and tardive dyskinesia (Angus McKay, and Chris Goetz and Harold Klawans), along with surgical approaches to several of the dyskinesias. In *Movement Disorders 2* (1987) it was the turn of dystonia (anatomy and pathophysiology, John Rothwell and Jose Obeso; classification and investigation, with Donald Calne; and treatment), tics (neurology, Joe Jankovic; psychopathology, Mike Trimble and Mary Robertson), and essential tremor (pathophysiology, Bob Lee; pharmacology, Les Findley). Thus, previous volumes over the past decade have covered the major categories of dyskinesias. We will discuss further advances in each of these fields here.

In *Movement Disorders 3*, we have chosen to highlight rare categories of dyskinesias, including paroxysmal, epileptic (with David Fish) and psychogenic movement disorders, as well as odd tremors (with Lesley Findley and Lynn Cleeves). We asked Joe Jankovic to review the complex problem of stereotypies, Philip Thompson the topic of stiff people, Peter Brown the concept of spinal myoclonus, and Mark Hallett and J. Matsumoto the startle syndromes; there have been advances in each of these areas. One of the major therapeutic advances undoubtedly has been the exploitation of botulinum toxin therapy, so this is highlighted (with Paul Greene, Mitchell Brin and Andrew Blitzer).

Anyone working at a movement disorder clinic is only too aware of the large range of odd dyskinesias that occur. There is still ignorance of the variety of ways in which dysfunction of the nervous system can generate abnormal movement. New syndromes regularly are being described, and their clinical features and pathophysiology are being explored and updated. Many of these bizarre conditions, rare as they may be, are inherited. Understanding may well come from their molecular genetics. Collection of informative, large-core families remains a clinical priority. This is a worldwide endeavour, for the best clues may come from remote areas. We would encourage all those with access to such informative clinical material to make best use of the opportunities.

Among advances in dyskinesias since the last volume, and not specifically covered by a chapter in this one, is the discovery of the locus for a gene – known as DYT1 – causing idiopathic torsion dystonia. In both the Ashkenazi Jewish and in some non-Jewish families, dystonia has definitely been found to be inherited as an autosomal dominant with incomplete penetrance (Bressman *et al.*, 1989), with the DYT1 gene located at chromosome 9q34 (Ozelius *et al.*, 1989; Kramer *et al.*, 1990). Allelic association has been found in the Ashkenazi Jewish patients with dystonia, even those young-onset individuals without a positive family history (Ozelius *et al.*, 1992), so that presymptomatic and prenatal genetic counselling is now possible (de Leon *et al.*, 1989). There has been uncertainty as to whether essential tremor is a part of the spectrum of idiopathic torsion dystonia. Conway *et al.* (1993) performed linkage analysis in 15 families with essential tremor containing 60 definitely affected individuals. They used dinucleotide repeat polymorphisms at the ASS locus and the Abelson locus (ABL) on chromosome 9q34, and found that this DYT1 locus is not linked to the families with essential tremor.

X-linked recessive dystonia–parkinsonism, which occurs in Filipino males (and locally referred to as *lubag*) has also been studied with molecular genetics. The abnormal gene has been reported to be near the centromere on the X chromosome at Xq13 (Wilhelmsen *et al.*, 1991; Kupke *et al.*, 1992; Graeber *et al.*, 1992). A single patient known to have this disorder has been autopsied, and the pathology shows patches of gliosis in the striatum (Waters *et al.*, 1993), identical to the pathology reported in an earlier case of dystonia from California, who happened to be a Filipino man (Altrocchi and Forno, 1983; Walters *et al.*, 1993), and therefore very likely another case of this disorder, and in a non-Filipino dystonic boy from England (Gibb *et al.*, 1992). Thus, there now has been elucidated the striatal pathology of one type of 'atypical' dystonia, a type that clinically appears distinct from classical idiopathic torsion dystonia.

Another familial disease related to dystonia has been recognized, namely alcohol-responsive myoclonic dystonia (Kurlan *et al.*, 1988; Quinn *et al.*, 1988; Kyllerman *et al.*, 1990). Inherited as an autosomal dominant trait, it is characterized by the onset of myoclonic jerks and/or dystonia in the first two decades of life, and a relatively benign course. The jerks are often brief and fast, usually affect the upper body, and respond dramatically to alcohol. Sometimes the myoclonus is oscillatory, and tremor may be present. Torticollis, axial dystonia, arm dystonia and occasionally leg dystonia occur, usually but not always with myoclonus. Another large family with this or a related condition has been described as hereditary essential myoclonus (Fahn and Sjaastad, 1991). Myoclonus, sensitive to alcohol, dominated the clinical expression of the genetic abnormality in this family, but some affected members also had mild dystonia. This illustrates an area of diagnostic uncertainty. The latter authors have taken the view that 'if myoclonus is the predominant clinical phenomenology, even if some affected members also have features of dystonia, the disorder should be labelled as essential myoclonus'. There are, of course, a number of earlier reports of hereditary essential myoclonus in the literature, and some of families described as benign hereditary chorea may have had a similar condition. Genetic linkage studies are in progress to identify the gene or genes responsible for these conditions, which will clarify the situation.

There have been advances in understanding the peripheral physiology of the dystonias. Patients with cranial and cervical dystonias have enhanced excitability of brainstem interneurons responsible for the blink reflex. The size of the R2 component and the rate of its recovery after a prior conditioning shock to the supraorbital nerve are considerably enhanced (Berardelli *et al.*, 1985; Tolosa *et al.*, 1988). This result has also been found in patients with generalized idiopathic dystonia without any blepharospasm, but not in patients with focal arm dystonia (Nakashima *et al.*, 1990). This abnormality is interpreted as due to excessive drive, perhaps from the basal ganglia, on the polysynaptic pathways in the lateral reticular formation of the brainstem responsible for the late component of the blink reflex. In limb dystonia, there is an abnormality of the normal reciprocal inhibition between agonist and antagonist. The second longer phase of reciprocal inhibition is much reduced or even absent in affected limbs in dystonia (Nakashima *et al.*, 1989a). This has been interpreted as evidence for reduced presynaptic inhibition of muscle afferent input to the inhibitory interneurons as a result of defective descending motor control. Another example of abnormal brainstem interneuronal excitability is the finding of reduced exteroceptive inhibition of electromyographic activity in the sternomastoid muscle following a supraorbital nerve stimulus in spasmodic torticollis (Nakashima *et al.*, 1989b). The picture that emerges from all these physiological studies is that the brainstem and spinal interneuronal machinery are functioning abnormally in dystonia. Presumably this is due to defective basal ganglia control either via direct descending pathways or via their output to premotor cortical regions.

The treatment of the focal dystonias has been revolutionized by the use of botulinum toxin injections, but the management of more widespread segmental, multifocal or generalized dystonia remains difficult. Botulinum toxin can be used to relieve some local disabling manifestations, but drug therapy is the mainstay of treatment. The recognition of the clinical spectrum of dopa-responsive dystonia has shown this to be an important 'curable' condition (Segawa *et al.*, 1976; Nygaard *et al.*, 1988). Any child or adolescent presenting with dystonia, particularly of the legs and gait must have an adequate trial of levodopa therapy first. Those with this condition respond dramatically to small doses, and maintain smooth uncomplicated benefit (Nygaard *et al.*, 1991). It is now appreciated that some affected individuals with this condition, inherited as an autosomal dominant trait, may present in adult life with parkinsonism (Nygaard *et al.*, 1992). ^{18}F-dopa positron emission tomography scans show normal or near-normal uptake into caudate and putamen in both those with onset in childhood and adult life (Sawle *et al.*, 1991; Nygaard *et al.*, 1992). The implication is that the condition is due to failure of synthesis of dopamine proximal to dopa decarboxylation, but the gene for tyrosine hydroxylase has been excluded (Fletcher *et al.*, 1989).

If levodopa fails, the next most effective drug treatment for widespread dystonia is high-dose anticholinergic therapy, usually with trihexyphenidyl (Artane; Greene *et al.*, 1988). A good response can be expected in 40–50% of cases, especially in those who commence therapy in the first 5 years of their illness. Unfortunately, unwanted side-effects often limit dosage, but the response can be considerable. That anticholinergic treatment can produce chorea in those with dystonia has been recognized (Nomoto *et al.*, 1987).

If levodopa and high-dose anticholinergic therapy fails, what to do next? Baclofen probably is the third drug of choice (Greene *et al.*, 1988; Greene and Fahn, 1992). Around 10–20% of patients may benefit. Clonazepam and dopamine antagonists (especially tetrabenazine) also may help a minority.

A number of other new observations on dystonia are worthy of comment. The first attempt at estimating the population incidence and prevalence of the dystonias in Rochester, Minnesota (Nutt *et al.*, 1988) has shown what we have long believed, namely that these are common conditions. Although the numbers were small, the prevalence of generalized dystonia (34 per million) and focal dystonias (295 per million) greatly exceeds that of muscular dystrophy (60 per million) and amyotrophic lateral sclerosis (64 per million) in the same population, and allowing for undiagnosed cases approaches that of multiple sclerosis.

The pathology of the idiopathic dystonias remains a mystery. A few more cases with pathological examination of the brain have been reported. For example, no significant abnormalities were found in 3 patients with cranial dystonia, although a fourth case had an angioma in the dorsal pons (Gibb *et al.*, 1988). Unfortunately, the number of brains available for study from patients with dystonia remains small, and every attempt should be made to obtain such material.

New variants of focal dyskinesias have been described, for example 'belly dancer's dyskinesia of the abdomen' (Iliceto *et al.*, 1990), 'Golfer's cramp' or the 'yips' has joined the list of occupational cramps (Sachdev, 1992), which appear to afflict an increasing range of musicians, sports enthusiasts, and others. A range of movement disorders also now is recognized in Rett's syndrome (Fitzgerald *et al.*, 1990).

Dystonic tics have been increasingly recognized in Tourette's syndrome. Indeed, around 50% of patients with this disease manifest one or more dystonic tics as part of their illness (Jankovic and Stone, 1991). They must be distinguished from the tardive dystonia that can occur in those treated with long-term neuroleptic therapy (Singh and Jankovic, 1988). The treatment of Tourette's syndrome remains difficult, the problem being to weigh up the long-term risks of dopamine antagonist drugs against their benefit for the tics. However, the use of newer antidepressant drugs affecting serotonin mechanisms to control the obsessive-compulsive components of the illness is gaining favour. In desperation, neurosurgical anterior cingulotomy may be of value in reducing disastrous or self-destructive obsessive-compulsive behaviour resistant to medication (Kurlan *et al.*, 1990).

In the field of tremor, some advances in understanding the pathophysiology of essential tremor have been made, and an excellent monograph on the subject has been published (Elble and Koller, 1990). Positron emission tomographic studies have implicated abnormalities of cerebellar activity, bilaterally and even at rest (Colebatch *et al.*, 1990; Jenkins *et al.*, 1993), and there are hints of overactivity of the inferior olive (Dubinsky and Hallett, 1987). An abnormality of timing of compensatory stabilizing muscle bursts on movement or in response to displacements has been identified (Britton *et al.*, 1993), which may be responsible for the tremor oscillations, and could be due to cerebellar dysfunction.

The whole field of essential tremor has been compounded by the problem of definition. Many have referred to any postural tremor of the arms as an essential tremor, but this would include such tremors due to dystonia or Parkinson's disease. A recent study of the clinical phenotype of hereditary essential tremor (Bain *et al.*, unpublished observations) found no evidence of dystonia or Parkinson's disease in 131 relatives, examined personally, of 20 index cases. Nor were there any examples of isolated focal tremors of the face, jaw, tongue, neck, trunk or legs. Many examples of such isolated focal tremors, sometimes familial, have been described as examples of focal essential tremors, with the implication that they are due to the genetic abnormality responsible for hereditary essential tremor, but this seems unlikely to be the case. Many of them may turn out to be manifestations of focal dystonia, or other conditions such as primary orthostatic tremor (Britton *et al.*, 1991). A recent ^{18}F-dopa positron emission tomographic study (Brooks *et al.*, 1992) has shown that most isolated focal leg tremors, at rest, and some sporadic postural arm tremors are likely to be due to Parkinson's disease.

True hereditary essential tremor appears to be a relatively distinct condition, inherited as a single autosomal dominant trait, with complete penetrance by the age of 65 years. All exhibit postural arm tremor, which may spread to the legs, neck, voice, jaw, tongue and face.

It has long been known that a lesion of the ventrolateral nucleus of the thalamus (Vim) can relieve contralateral limb tremor of all types. Relief of parkinsonian tremor and essential tremor has also been reported with electrical stimulation of this nucleus (Blond *et al.*, 1992). Further assessment of this procedure is awaited with interest.

The persistent movement disorders induced by drugs that block dopamine receptors, e.g. typical antipsychotic agents, consist of a variety of different abnormal movements. Since *Movement Disorders* 2, two other syndromes, tardive myoclonus (Little and Jankovic, 1987; Tominaga *et al.*, 1987) and tardive tremor (Stacy and Jankovic, 1992) have been added to those of classical tardive dyskinesia (or orobuccolingual dyskinesia), tardive dystonia, tardive akathisia and withdrawal emergent syndrome. The management of these various tardive syndromes remains difficult. The best chance of recovery, albeit often after months or years, is to stop the offending neuroleptic drug. However, often this is not an option in those with chronic schizophrenia. A switch from conventional neuroleptics to the new agent clozapine, which causes a very low incidence of extrapyramidal side-effects, would seem the best tactic. However, the small risks of agranulocytosis and marrow depression with clozapine have meant that there are major practical monitoring constraints to its use.

Anticholinergic drugs may help some with tardive dystonia, but worsen tardive orobuccolingual dyskinesias. Dopamine depletors such as reserpine and tetrabenazine are most likely to help tardive akathisia (Burke *et al.*, 1989).

Finally, after 10 years of intensive effort, the gene mutation responsible for Huntington's disease has been identified (Huntington's Disease Collaborative Research Group, 1993). As a result, mutation analysis will now allow a test for the disease that is both accurate and specific. The abnormality, as in a number of other dominantly inherited neurological diseases (mytonic dystrophy, one type of dominant ataxia, X-linked bulbospinal neuronopathy, and fragile X syndrome), is an unstable trinucleotide repeat (CAG) on the short arm of chromosome 4 in Huntington's disease. The longer the repeat sequence, the earlier the age of onset. The next exciting discovery will be to determine the functional malfunction of the product of this gene, now known as huntingtin.

References

Altrocchi PH and Forno LS (1983) Spontaneous oral-facial dyskinesia: neuropathology of a case. *Neurology*, **33**, 802–5

Bain PG, Findley LJ, Thompson PD, Gresty M, Rothwell JC, Harding AE and Marsden CD (1993) A study of hereditary essential tremor. Submitted to *Brain*

Berardelli A, Rothwell JC, Day BL, and Marsden CD (1985) Pathophysiology of blepharospasm and oromandibular dystonia. *Brain*, **108**, 593–609

Blond S, Caparros-Lefebvre D, Parker F, Assaker R, Petit H, Guieu J-D *et al.* (1992) Control of tremor and involuntary movement disorders by chronic stereotactic stimulation of the ventral intermediate thalamic nucleus. *J Neurosurg*, **77**, 62–8

Bressman SB, de Leon, Brin MF, Risch N, Burke RE, Greene PE *et al.* (1989) Idiopathic torsion dystonia among Ashkenazi Jews: evidence for autosomal dominant inheritance. *Ann Neurol*, **26**, 612–20

Britton TC, Thompson PD, Van der Kamp W, Rothwell JC, Day BL, and Marsden CD (1991) Primary orthostatic tremor: further observations in five cases. *J Neurol*, **239**, 209–17

Britton TC, Thompson PD, Day BL, Rothwell JC, Findley LJ, and Marsden CD (1992) Resetting of postural tremors in the wrist with mechanical stretches in Parkinson's disease, essential tremor, and normal subjects mimicking tremor. *Ann Neurol*, **31**, 507–14

Britton TC, Thompson PD, Day BL, Rothwell JC, Findley LJ, and Marsden CD (1993) Rapid wrist movements in patients with essential tremor: The critical role of the second agonist burst. *Brain*, (in press)

Brooks DJ, Playford ED, Ibanez V, Sawle GV, Thompson PD, Findley LJ *et al.* (1992) Isolated tremor and disruption of the nigrostriatal dopaminergic system: an ^{18}F-dopa PET study. *Neurology*, **42**, 1554–60

Burke RE, Kang UJ, Jankovic J, Miller LG, and Fahn S (1989) Tardive akathisia: an analysis of clinical features and response to open therapeutic trials. *Movement Disorders*, **4**, 157–75

Conway D, Bain PG, Warner TT, Davis MB, Findley LJ, Thompson PD, Marsden CD, and Harding AE (1993) Linkage analysis with chromosome-9 markers in hereditary essential tremor. *Movement Disorders*, **8**, 374–6

Colebatch JG, Findley LJ, Frackowiak RSJ, Marsden CD, and Brooks DJ (1990) Preliminary report: activation of the cerebellum in essential tremor. *Lancet*, **336**, 1028–30

de Leon D, Brin M, Murphy P, Bressman S, Ozelius I, Cardon N, Reich S, Breakefield XO, and Fahn S (1991) Genetic counselling for idiopathic torsion dystonia: first use of DNA based carrier detection in Ashkenazic Jews. *Movement Disorders*, **6**, 273–4

Dubinsky R and Hallett M (1987) Glucose hypermetabolism of the inferior olive in patients with essential tremor. *Ann Neurol*, **22**, 118

Elble RJ and Koller WC (1990) *Tremor*, Baltimore, The John Hopkins University Press

Fahn S and Sjaastad O (1991) Hereditary essential myoclonus in a large Norwegian family. *Movement Disorders*, **6**, 237–47

Fitzgerald PM, Jankovic J, and Percy AK (1990) Rett syndrome and associated movement disorders. *Movement Disorders*, **5**, 195–202

Fletcher NA, Holt IJ, Harding AE, Nygaard TG, Mallet J, and Marsden CD (1989) Tyrosine hydroxylase and levodopa responsive dystonia. *J Neurol Neurosurg Psychiatry*, **52**, 112–14

Gibb WRG, Lees AJ, and Marsden CD (1988) Pathological report of four patients presenting with cranial dystonias. *Movement Disorders*, **3**, 211–21

Gibb WRG, Kilford L, and Marsden CD (1992) Severe generalised dystonia associated with a mosaic pattern of striatal gliosis. *Movement Disorders*, **7**, 217–23

Graeber MB, Kupke KG, and Muller U (1992) Delineation of the dystonia parkinsonism syndrome locus in Xq13. *Proc Natl Acad Sci USA*, **89**, 8245–8

Greene PE and Fahn S (1992) Baclofen in the treatment of idiopathic dystonia in children. *Movement Disorders*, **7**, 48–52

Greene P, Shale H, and Fahn S (1988) Analysis of open-label trials in torsion dystonia using high dosages of anticholinergics and other drugs. *Movement Disorders*, **3**, 46–60

Huntington's Disease Collaborative Research Group (1993) A novel gene containing a trinucleotide repeat that is expanded and unstable in Huntington's disease chromosomes. *Cell*, **72**, 971–83

Iliceto G, Thompson PD, Day BL, Rothwell JC, Lees AJ, and Marsden CD (1990) Diaphragmatic flutter, the moving umbilicus syndrome, and "belly dancer's" dyskinesia. *Movement Disorders*, **5**, 1522

Jankovic J and Stone L (1991) Dystonic tics in patients with Tourette's syndrome. *Movement Disorders*, **6**, 248–52

Jenkins IH, Bain PG, Colebatch JG, Thompson PD, Findley LJ, Frackowiak RSJ *et al.* (1993) A PET study of essential tremor: evidence for overactivity of cerebellar connections. *Ann Neurol*, **34**, 82–90

Kramer PL, Ozelius L, de Leon D, Risch N, Brin MF, Bressman SB *et al.* (1990) Dystonia gene in Ashkenazi Jewish population located on chromosome 9q32–34. *Ann Neurol*, **27**, 114–20

Kupke KG, Graeber MB, and Muller U (1992) Dystonia-parkinsonism syndrome (XDP) locus – flanking markers in Xq12–q21.1. *Am J Hum Genet*, **50**, 808–15

Kurlan R, Behr J, Medved L, and Shoulson I (1988) Myoclonus and dystonia: a family study. In Fahn S, Marsden CD, and Calne DB, eds, *Advances in Neurology*, vol 50, *Dystonia 2*, New York, Raven Press, 385–9

Kurlan R, Kersun J, Ballantine HT, and Caine ED (1990) Neurosurgical treatment of severe obsessive-compulsive disorder associated with Tourette's syndrome. *Movement Disorders*, **5**, 152–5

Kyllerman M, Forsgren L, Sanner G, Holmgren G, Wahlstrom J, and Drugge U (1990) Alcohol-responsive myoclonic dystonia in a large family: dominant inheritance and phenotypic variation. *Movement Disorders*, **5**, 270–9

Little JT and Jankovic J (1987) Tardive myoclonus. *Movement Disorders*, **2**, 307–11

Nakashima K, Rothwell JC, Day BL, Thompson PD, Shannon K, and Marsden CD (1989a) Reciprocal inhibition between forearm muscles in patients with writer's cramp and other occupational cramps, symptomatic hemidystonia and hemiparesis due to stroke. *Brain*, **112**, 681–97

Nakashima K, Thompson PD, Rothwell JC, Day BL, Stell R, and Marsden CD (1989b) An exteroceptive reflex in the sternocleidomastoid muscle produced by electrical stimulation of the supraorbital nerve in normal subjects and patients with spasmodic torticollis. *Neurology*, **39**, 1354–8

Nakashima K, Rothwell JC, Thompson PD, Day BL, Berardelli A, Agostino R *et al.* (1990) The blink reflex in patients with idiopathic torsion dystonia. *Arch Neurol*, **47**, 413–16

Nomoto M, Thompson PD, Sheehy MP, Quinn NP, and Marsden CD (1987) Anticholinergic-induced chorea in the treatment of focal dystonia. *Movement Disorders*, **2**, 53–6

Nutt JG, Muenter MD, Aronson A, Kurland LT, and Melton LJ (1988) Epidemiology of focal and generalized dystonia in Rochester, Minnesota. *Movement Disorders*, **3**, 188–94

Nygaard TG, Marsden CD, and Duvoisin RC (1988) Dopa-responsive dystonia. In Fahn S, Marsden CD, and Calne DBD, eds, *Dystonia 2. Advances in Neurology*, vol 50, New York, Raven Press, 377–84

Nygaard TG, Marsden CD, and Fahn S (1991) Dopa-responsive dystonia: long-term treatment response and prognosis. *Neurology*, **41**, 174–81

Nygaard TG, Takahashi H, Heiman GA, Snow BJ, Fahn S, and Calne DB (1992) Long-term treatment response and fluorodopa positron emission tomography scanning of parkinsonism in a family with dopa-responsive dystonia. *Ann Neurol*, **32**, 603–8

Ozelius L, Kramer PL, Moskowitz CB, Kwiatkowski DJ, Brin MF, Schuback DE *et al.* (1989) Human gene for tosion dystonia located on chromosome 9q32–34. *Neuron*, **2**, 1427–34

Ozelius LJ, Kramer PL, de Leon D, Risch N, Bressman SB, Schuback DE *et al.* (1992) Strong allelic association between torsion dystonia gene (DYT1) and loci on chromosome 9q34 in Ashkenazi Jews. *Am J Hum Genet*, **50**, 619–28

Quinn NP, Rothwell JC, Thompson PD, and Marsden CD (1988) Hereditary myoclonic dystonia, hereditary torsion dystonia and hereditary essential myoclonus: an area of confusion. In Fahn S, Marsden CD, and Calne DB, eds, *Advances in Neurology*, vol 50, *Dystonia 2*, New York, Raven Press, 391–401

Sachdev P (1992) Golfer's cramp: clinical characteristics and evidence against it being an anxiety disorder. *Movement Disorders*, **7**, 326–32

Sawle GV, Leenders KL, Brooks DJ, Harwood G, Lees AJ, Frackowiak RSJ, and Marsden CD *et al.* (1991) Dopa-responsive dystonia: [^{18}F]dopa positron emission tomography. *Ann Neurol*, **30**, 24–30

Segawa M, Hosaka A, Miyagawa F, Numura F, Imai H (1976) Hereditary progressive dystonia with marked diurnal fluctuation. In Eldridge R and Fahn S, eds, *Advances in Neurology*, vol 14, New York Raven Press, 215–33

Singh SK and Jankovic J (1988) Tardive dystonia in patients with Tourette's syndrome. *Movement Disorders*, **3**, 274–80

Stacy M and Jankovic J (1992) Tardive tremor. *Movement Disorders*, **7**, 53–7

Tolosa E, Montserrat L, and Bayes A (1988) Blink reflex studies in focal dystonias: enhanced excitability of brainstem interneurons in cranial dystonia and spasmodic torticollis. *Movement Disorders*, **3**, 61–9

Tominaga H, Fukuzako H, Izumi K, Koja T, Fukuda T, Fujh H *et al.* (1987) Tardive myoclonus. *Lancet*, **322**

Waters CH, Faust PL, Powers J, Vinters H, Moskowitz C, Nygaard T, Hunt AL, and Fahn S (1993) Neuropathology of lubag (X-linked dystonia parkinsonism). *Movement Disorders*, **8**, 387–90

Wilhelmsen KC, Weeks DE, Nygaard TG, Moskowitz CB, Rosales RL, dela Paz DC *et al.* (1991) Genetic mapping of "lubag" (X-linked dystonia-parkinsonism) in a Filipino kindred to the pericentromeric region of the X chromosome. *Ann Neurol*, **29**, 124–31

16
The paroxysmal dyskinesias

Stanley Fahn

INTRODUCTION

The overwhelming majority of patients with hyperkinetic movement disorders have symptoms that are continuous or continual (e.g. chorea, dystonia, tardive dyskinesia), except for relief with sleep, and with some variation in intensity during periods of stress and relaxation, or other factors such as voluntary movements (e.g. action dystonia, intention myoclonus, intention tremor) or maintaining certain postures (e.g. essential tremor). Some dyskinesias (Table 16.1), however, are characterized as occurring intermittently, such as myoclonus (Fahn *et al.*, 1986; Hallett *et al.*, 1987) and startle syndromes (Andermann and Andermann, 1986) that can be triggered by a variety of stimuli. Perhaps the commonest dyskinesias occurring intermittently are tics, which are suppressible to varying degrees (Koller and Biary, 1989). Although tics and myoclonic jerks, since they commonly occur out of a normal background, could possibly be considered as paroxysmal, this term is usually reserved for an entirely different set of hyperkinetic movement disorders, which is the topic of this chapter. The term paroxysmal dyskinesia has been applied to these disorders.

The common neurological paroxysmal disorders are epilepsy and migraine. Movement disorders that appear 'out of the blue' and are transient and recurring are uncommon, and often present to the clinician as confusing diagnostic problems.

Table 16.1 Classical movement disorders that usually appear in bursts or with specific actions, but are not considered paroxysmal dyskinesias. The movements usually occur so frequently that they are not distinguished with a paroxysmal label

Action dystonia
Action myoclonus
Action and intention tremor
Arrhythmic myoclonus
Hyperekplexia
Periodic movements in sleep
Restless legs syndrome
Sandifer's syndrome
Tics

Not uncommonly, the history provided by the patient does not convey the information that the episodes of abnormal movements occur at intermittent intervals, and the clinician must consider the possibility that he/she is dealing with a paroxysmal dyskinesia, and thereby ask the appropriate questions that can lead to the proper diagnosis. To confound the problem, the pathophysiology of paroxysmal dyskinesias is not understood, their classification is still incomplete and evolving, and treatment for many of them is often unsuccessful.

DEFINITIONS: PAROXYSMAL, EPISODIC AND PERIODIC

It is not clear how the label *paroxysmal* became the accepted terminology applied to this group of dyskinesias. Why not the terms episodic or periodic? According to *Dorland's Medical Dictionary* a paroxysm is defined as: (1) a sudden recurrence of intensification of symptoms; and (2) a spasm or seizure. A similar definition is given by *Webster's Third International Dictionary*.

The term *periodic* is defined by both *Dorland's* and *Webster's* as recurring at regular intervals of time. *Episodic* is not listed in *Dorland's*; *Webster's* defines episodic as occurring, appearing, or changing at usual, irregular intervals.

Since the paroxysmal dyskinesias do not recur at regular intervals, the term periodic would not be appropriate. Despite this, in neurology this term is used for the condition of familial periodic paralysis (Rowland, 1989) and familial periodic ataxia (Vighetto *et al.*, 1988), even though muscle weakness and ataxia in these disorders, respectively, do not occur at regular intervals. Some authors (Griggs *et al.*, 1978) have used the term paroxysmal ataxia in preference to periodic ataxia, and others the term episodic ataxia (Zasorin *et al.*, 1983).

According to the dictionary definitions, either paroxysmal or episodic would be appropriate terms for the dyskinesias under discussion here. By common usage, and with few exceptions (Margolin and Marsden, 1982), paroxysmal has been chosen in preference over episodic for this purpose. The term has been utilized to indicate that the symptoms occur suddenly out of a background of normal motor behaviour. It does not define the frequency, severity, duration, aggravating factors or type of dyskinesia of the attack. These features vary, and are important in the current nosology and classification of the paroxysmal dyskinesias.

HISTORICAL ASPECTS

In this review of historical highlights, it is important to point out that many papers on paroxysmal dyskinesias were reported in the Japanese literature in the 1960s, and I have not reviewed them. Fortunately, a review of paroxysmal dyskinesia referring to many of these Japanese papers is available in English by Hishikawa *et al.* (1973), and I have relied on this for information.

Earliest descriptions: reported as epilepsy (Table 16.2)

Although Gowers (1885) is often credited with the first report of movement-induced seizures, it is not clear that his cases actually represent paroxysmal dyskinesia. One of his patients was a boy whose attack lasted 15 seconds, but he was said to be

Table 16.2 Some of the earliest reports of paroxysmal choreoathetosis/dystonia reported as seizures

Authors	*Case no.*	*Sex*	*Age at onset*	*Aetiology*	*FH*	*Sensory triggers*	*Abnormal aura*	*Movements**	*Treatment*
Gowers (1885)	1	M	Boy	Probably idiopathic	?	Movement	0		
	2	F	11	Probably idiopathic	?	Movement	0		
Sterling (1924)	10			Epidemic encephalitis					
Wimmer (1925)	1	M	Boy	Probably idiopathic				Athetoid	
Spiller (1927)	1	F	62	Probably secondary	0	Movement	+		
	2	F	46	Probably vascular	0	Passive, active movement	+		
Wilson (1930)	1	M	5	Probably idiopathic	?	Excitement	+	Torsion	
Pitha (1938)	1	M	6	Idiopathic	0	Movement	+		Anticonvulsants

+ = Present or yes; 0 = absent or no; ? = no information given.
FH = Family history of similar attacks.
*Chorea, athetosis or other movements present in addition to sustained muscle contractions (dystonia).

unconscious during his initial attack. Later, he remained awake during the attacks. Another patient was a girl whose attacks started at the age of 11 and occurred on suddenly arising after prolonged sitting. But at least one of her attacks was said to be associated with a terrified expression, flushed facies and dilated pupils. These, perhaps, more closely resemble pilomotor seizures described by Brody *et al.* (1960). Subsequent to Gowers, a number of reports of 'movement-induced seizures' have appeared in the literature. Many of these reports have been published under the designation of reflex epilepsy and tonic seizures induced by movement. But, unlike most motor convulsions, there was no alteration in the state of consciousness. Moreover, some of these reports had more than tonic contraction, namely sustained twisting, athetosis and chorea. These characteristics are today referred to as paroxysmal dystonia and paroxysmal choreoathetosis, rather than convulsive seizures. Even the presence of choreoathetosis did not lead the earliest interpreters of these brief attacks to conclude they were a movement disorder, but considered them as a form of epilepsy, with the cerebral site of these 'seizures' being in the basal ganglia or in the subcortical region.

Sterling (1924) used the term extrapyramidal epilepsy to describe a series of patients with encephalitis lethargica who had brief or prolonged (up to 6 hours) painful sustained spasms that occurred intermittently. Consciousness was unimpaired. He used the term tetanoid to depict the postures of the hands and feet. Years later, Lance (1963) questioned the use of the term extrapyramidal epilepsy because of the long duration of some of the attacks, as well as the origin of the attacks.

Wimmer (1925) used the term striatal epilepsy to describe a boy who had attacks of torticollis and unilateral tonic limb spasms, lasting a few seconds without loss of consciousness. Because these attacks subsequently became one of athetoid or torsion spasms, Wimmer labelled them as striatal epilepsy, based on a previous report by

Stertz (cited in Wilson, 1930) who described a postencephalitic patient who had developed seizures and then dystonia, with postmortem evidence of lesions in the striatum.

After the report of Gowers, the next report of movement-induced paroxysmal movements appears to be that of Spiller in 1927. Spiller described 2 patients with brief tonic spasms brought on by voluntary movement of the involved limbs, and in 1 of them, also by passive manipulation. The contractions were paintul and accompanied by sensations of heat or burning. No autopsy was performed. Spiller preferred the term subcortical epilepsy rather than striatal epilepsy because of the pain associated with the attacks. Wilson (1930) described a 5-year-old boy who had brief attacks of unilateral torsion and tonic spasm that lasted up to 3 minutes and were precipitated by fright or excitement. There was no loss of consciousness. The attacks could be preceded by pain. Wilson considered this to be reflex tonic epilepsy and thought it also to be subcortical in origin.

In more recent times, the concept that these attacks of tonic, often twisting, contractions without loss of consciousness are uncommon seizure disorders has continued. For example, Lishman *et al.* (1962) described 7 patients with tonic and athetoid spasms induced by movement while remaining conscious. Abnormal sensations of numbness, vibration and tightness, but not pain, were noted in the affected limbs before the attacks. These authors considered that the movement-induced attacks were a form of reflex epilepsy and discussed other idiopathic cases in the literature (Pitha, 1938; Michaux and Granier, 1945). Two years after the paper by Lishman *et al.*, these authors reported an additional 5 cases of movement-induced 'seizures' (Whitty *et al.*, 1964), and Burger *et al.* (1972) described 2 patients with this label. Japanese neurologists, e.g. Fukuyama and Okada, (1967) and others (see review by Hishikawa *et al.*, 1973) have also referred to these as some form of epilepsy. It would appear that today these movement-induced involuntary movements would be considered paroxysmal choreoathetosis/dystonia rather than convulsive movements of the reflex epilepsy type.

Not all attacks of tonic spasms are induced by movement. Lance (1963) reported 8 patients with attacks of tonic (dystonic) spasms, some with choreoathetosis, usually affecting only one side of the body, and often preceded by pain or tingling. Two patients had secondary attacks (static encephalopathy and multiple sclerosis). One was idiopathic and sporadic, and the remaining 5 were members of the same family. The attacks lasted less than 1 minute in 2 patients, 2–5 minutes in the patient with multiple sclerosis, and 5–60 minutes in the 5 familial cases. He labelled these attacks as tonic seizures. These attacks were not precipitated by movement. The familial cases were aggravated by excitement and fatigue. No electroencephalogram (EEG) abnormality was recorded between attacks. Years later, Lance (1977) recognized them as paroxysmal dystonic choreoathetosis (PDC).

Differentiation of the attacks between cortical seizures and paroxysmal dyskinesias is sometimes difficult. Clouding of consciousness, if it occurs, would point to a seizure disorder. This is exemplified by the case reported by Falconer *et al.* (1963) of a man who had focal seizures induced by movement, lasting for 10–20 seconds. There was clouding of consciousness with severe attacks, but not with mild attacks. The patient underwent a craniotomy and had a cicatrix removed from the involved hemisphere, which resulted in a cessation of further attacks. Lishman *et al.* (1962) refer to the report by Strauss (1940) of an individual with a movement-induced Jacksonian march as another example of movement-induced epilepsy. However, this case does not justify the other reports of cases without a Jacksonian march as being examples of epilepsy, because the presence of the march is so distinctive and specific that it would clearly be an example of a cortical-induced seizure.

All the above authors writing either about reflex epilepsy (movement-induced spasms) or about brief tonic or athetoid spasms without loss of consciousness (but not movement-induced) considered these attacks to be related to epilepsy. Nevertheless, by 1966 and 1967, when papers bearing the title of paroxysmal choreoathetosis began regularly to appear (Stevens 1966; Kertesz, 1967; Mushet and Dreifuss, 1967), particularly those cases induced by movements, there were still occasional papers referring the condition to a seizure disorder (Downzenko and Zielinsky, 1966; De Bolt, 1967), and some authors linked paroxysmal dyskinesias and seizures (Hudgins and Corbin, 1966).

Reported as a paroxysmal disorder of involuntary movements

In 1940, a new concept was introduced by Mount and Reback, that of labelling attacks of tonic spasms plus choreic and athetotic movements as a paroxysmal type of movement disorder. They described a 23-year-old man who had 'spells' since infancy, both large and small. Both types were preceded by a sensory aura of tightness in parts of the body or by a feeling of tiredness. The movements involved the arms and legs, and were usually a combination of sustained twisted posturing and chorea and athetosis. The small attacks lasted from 5 to 10 minutes. Longer attacks were considered large and also involved the neck (retrocollis), the eyes (upward gaze), face (ipsilateral to the limbs, if the limb involvement was unilateral), and speech. These large attacks lasted for as long as 2 hours, and the movements were considered to resemble those seen in Huntington's disease. There was never a loss of consciousness or clonic convulsive movements, biting of the tongue or loss of sphincter control. Drinking alcohol, coffee, tea or cola would usually bring out an attack. Fatigue, smoking and concentrating were other precepitating factors. The attacks would clear more rapidly if the patient lay down and would be aborted by asleep. He had an average of one large and two small attacks a day. Between attacks, the neurological examination was normal. Phenytoin and phenobarbitone were without effect, and scopolamine was the only drug found to reduce the frequency, severity and duration of the attacks. The family history revealed 27 other members who had similar attacks, with the pedigree showing autosomal dominant inheritance with what appears to be complete penetrance. Mount and Reback called this disorder familial paroxysmal choreoathetosis.

The paper by Mount and Reback has become the seminal paper in the field of paroxysmal dyskinesias. Following its publication, most of the reports in the literature referenced it over the next five decades. However, the next report of a large family with similar attacks of muscle spasms did not refer to it. In 1961 Forssman described a family with autosomal dominant inheritance in which there were attacks lasting from 4 minutes to 3 hours. The attacks were induced by cold, mental tension, irritation, fatigue, lack of sleep, alcohol and caffeine. The attacks consisted of sustained muscle contractions, usually of a twisting nature. The onset of symptoms was in early childhood in most of the affected members. The attack might begin with tonic spasm in one hand, spread up the arm, to the other arm, both legs, then cranial muscles, including tongue, so that the patient could not speak in a severe attack. Clonic spasms could appear at the height of the attack. The onset would often be preceded by a 'tugging' sensation in the affected body part. Forssman considered the disorder to be a new entity, possibly related somehow to myotonia and paramyotonia. He ruled out these conditions because they are not triggered by alcohol. He did not consider it a form of epilepsy since there was no alteration of consciousness, although the patient had been considered an epileptic by other neurologists.

The next large family described was in 1963 by Lance. Like Forssman (1961), Lance also did not relate this to nor reference Mount and Reback's report, nor did he mention the report by Forssman. In fact, Lance considered his patients to have a form of epilepsy, similar to the concept of Spiller (1927), Wilson (1930), and Lishman *et al.* (1962). Later, in 1977, Lance was to write one of the definitive papers in this field, containing a useful classification scheme, in which he relates his family to those of Mount and Reback (1940), Forssman (1961) and Richards and Barnett (1968).

In 1941, the year following Mount and Reback's paper, Smith and Heersema reported 3 similar cases (2 of them familial) seen at the Mayo Clinic which they labelled as periodic dystonia. The ages at onset were 7, 8 and 14. These authors thought that their cases were similar to the family of Mount and Reback. Their first patient was described as being able to induce the involuntary movements by shaking a leg. In reporting a family with 3 members affected by brief attacks of torsion movements of the torso and choreoathetosis of the limbs precipitated by initiation of sudden movement seen at the Mayo Clinic, Hudgins and Corbin (1966) also provided a follow-up report of the 3 individuals reported by Smith and Heersema (1941). From a review of the Mayo Clinic records, Hudgins and Corbon recognized that the initiation of movement was the principal factor in the provocation of the daily dystonic attacks in the 3 cases reported by Smith and Heersema. Thus, it appears that the first report of paroxysmal kinesigenic choreoathetosis/dystonia was that of Smith and Heersema, although these authors did not particularly recognize this phenomenon as a critical factor.

Although there were reports of patients whose paroxysmal dyskinesias were induced by sudden movement, they were not particularly denoted by any special terminology until 1967, when Kertesz introduced the label *paroxysmal kinesigenic choreoathetosis* (PKC). This label has developed into a most useful and widely accepted designation since the kinesigenic feature has proven to be so characteristic. Kinesigenicity has an important place in the classification of the paroxysmal dyskinesias, although, as will be pointed out below, the PKC designation can be applied to some select patients who do not have the dyskinesias triggered by sudden movement (or startle).

Kertesz reported 10 new cases of paroxysmal dyskinesia and reviewed the literature. Among the important features of his paper, Kertesz differentiated the kinesigenic variety (induced by sudden movement) from that described by Mount and Reback, by Forssman, and by Lance, which were not aggravated by movement but by alcohol, caffeine and fatigue. (It should be noted that Kertesz differentiated the kinesigenic type from that reported by Mount and Reback (1940) and by Lance (1963), but he failed to mention the paper by Forssman (1961).)

Williams and Stevens (1963), Stevens (1966), and Rosen (1964), who described kinesigenic cases, had adopted the term paroxysmal choreoathetosis as proposed by Mount and Reback. There were a large number of additional kinesigenic cases reported after the introduction of the kinesigenic terminology by Kertesz (1967).

After the paper by Lance, Weber (1967) reported a family of 4 affected members with non-kinesigenic paroxysmal dystonia and used the term familial paroxysmal dystonia. Richards and Barnett (1968) reported the next big family with the same type of paroxysmal dyskinesia as Mount and Reback's case, and thought that Lance's family (1963) represented a variant since there were only tonic spasms and no movements in that family. The family of Richards and Barnett consisted of 9 affected members with the trait inherited in an autosomal dominant pattern. They emphasized the non-kinesigenic nature of the attacks and felt that a wide array of terms could describe the attacks, depending on the severity of each one. They considered that the terms rigidity, tremor, dystonia, torsions spasm, athetosis, chorea, and hemiballism could all be used for such movements, often blending into each other. To emphasize the postural and increased tone, they added dystonic to the label. They recommended avoiding the term epilepsy until the pathophysiology is better known. Richards and Barnett coined the term *paroxysmal dystonic choreoathetosis* (PDC), which was later adopted by Lance in 1977, and which today is the most commonly used term for those paroxysmal dyskinesias not induced by sudden movement. The terms paroxysmal non-kinesigenic choreoathetosis or paroxysmal dystonia are sometimes used instead of PDC (Bressman *et al.*, 1988).

Although phenytoin was recognized earlier as a very useful agent for paroxysmal kinesigenic choreoathetosis/dystonia, carbamazepine was later found to be as useful and was introduced as a treatment by Kato and Araki (1969). This drug currently appears to be the one most commonly used for this disorder.

The original cases reported as paroxysmal dyskinesias were idiopathic and usually familial. It was not long before symptomatic cases began to be reported in which the attacks of movements were reported as a paroxysmal dyskinesia: perinatal encephalopathy (Rosen, 1964), encephalitis (Mushet and Dreifuss, 1967) and head injury (Whitty *et al.*, 1964; Robin, 1977). However, earlier reports of symptomatic paroxysmal non-kinesigenic dyskinesias had been described as a manifestation of multiple sclerosis, but considered as a form of epilepsy (Matthews, 1958; Joynt and Green, 1962; Verheul and Tyssen, 1990) and of idiopathic hypoparathyroidism (Arden, 1953). Many other aetiologies have been reported since the earlier cases in the 1950s and 1960s (see below).

Perhaps the most recent enlightening paper in this field is that of Lance (1977). Lance: (1) discovered Forssman's paper (1961); (2) placed together as one syndrome the families reported by Mount and Reback (1940), Forssman (1961), Richards and Barnett (1968) and himself (1963), bringing them all in under the term familial PDC, which has a duration of attacks from 5 minutes to 4 hours; (3) expanded the description of his own previously reported family (1963) that he now classified as having this disorder instead of a seizure disorder as he originally had reported it; (4) added another family of paroxysmal dyskinesia who had attacks induced by continuous exercise and not sudden movement that affected the legs and with a duration between 5 and 30 minutes; (5) classified the paroxysmal dyskinesias into three groups separated primarily by duration of action (prolonged, intermediate and brief attacks) and secondarily by precipitating factors; (6) reported the therapeutic response to clonazepam in some patients with the prolonged attacks; (7) mentioned normal autopsy findings in 2 individuals with the prolonged attacks; (8) summarized the literature to that date; (9) mentioned that the Forssman and Lance families with the prolonged attacks had dystonic postures without choreoathetosis while the Mount and Reback and the Richards and Barnett families had choreoathetosis; (10) described that over time those with sustained spasms can eventually develop writhing movements, thereby linking these phenotypes together; and (11) commented that in all types of paroxysmal dyskinesias males are more affected than females.

The next historical advances were the recognition that: (1) idiopathic PDC can occur sporadically and not just in families (Bressman *et al.*, 1988); and (2) sporadic PDC is often psychogenic in origin (Bressman *et al.*, 1988; Fahn and Williams, 1988).

Before closing this discussion, it should be noted that a recent argument has been raised by Martinelli and Gabellini (1991) that a description of PKC was made in 1884, but their description of the original communication is not convincing.

Paroxysmal hypnogenic dyskinesia

Horner and Jackson (1969) described two families in which several members of the family had attacks of involuntary movement that occurred during sleep. These appear to be the first cases of hypnogenic paroxysmal dyskinesia reported. Family W is of particular interest because some affected members had classical paroxysmal kinesigenic dyskinesia, some hypnogenic, and others a combination. Case 3 in this family began with the hypnogenic variety at age 8. By age 11, daytime attacks also occurred, sometimes triggered by sudden movement. Gradually the hypnogenic episodes disappeared, leaving him with kinesigenic dyskinesia that responded to anticonvulsants. Lugaresi and his colleagues (Lugaresi and Cirignotta, 1981; Lugaresi *et al.*, 1986) independently rediscovered and eventually popularized the syndrome of hypnogenic paroxysmal dyskinesias.

Lugaresi and Cirignotta (1981) described 5 patients with onset of hypnogenic dystonia at ages 5, 7, 26, 30 and 40. The attacks occurred almost every night during sleep, with the onset occurring in stages 2–4 of sleep. The attacks lasted 15–45 seconds, and several attacks can occur in the same night. The attacks can awaken the patient who may even emit a cry. The movements appear to to be a mixture of dystonia, athetosis and some more rapid flinging movements. The EEG is normal during sleep and while awake. Carbamazepine is effective therapy. In their next paper Lugaresi *et al.* (1986) described the movements as choreoathetosis and ballism in addition to dystonia. Maccario and Lustman (1990) emphasized that tachycardia is a characteristic occurrence during these episodes.

In addition to the above short-duration attacks, long-duration hypnogenic attacks were reported by Lugaresi *et al.* (1986). Such long-duration attacks occur in a minority of individuals with hypnogenic paroxysmal dyskinesia. These longer attacks last from 2 to 50 minutes and do not respond to medication, including anticonvulsants, tricyclics, benzodiazepines and antipsychotics.

The disorder was originally described in non-familial cases, but has since been reported to occur in 3 members of a family (Lee *et al.*, 1985). Other sporadic cases have since been reported (Rajna *et al.*, 1983; Crowell and Anders, 1985; Godbout *et al.*, 1985; Tartara *et al.*, 1988), including a case with a concurrent reflex dystonic reaction provoked by stimulation of the right foot (Lehkuniec *et al.*, 1988). Besides the paper by Horner and Jackson mentioned above, another link with PKC is suggested by the report of Morley (1970) who described a father as having hypnogenic dyskinetic attacks while his son had PKC. Both individuals responded to phenytoin.

There has long been considerable speculation as to whether the short-duration hypnogenic attacks could be a manifestation of epilepsy since they respond so well to anticonvulsants. The lack of abnormal EEG findings during the attack were against this concept. Tinuper *et al.* (1990) described 3 patients with this disorder who had EEG evidence for frontal lobe seizures as a cause of these attacks. Sellal *et al.* (1991) and Meierkord *et al.* (1992) studied a series of patients with hypnogenic dystonia and have concluded that these represent seizure disorders, particularly of frontal lobe epilepsy. It appears that the short-lasting attacks could be either seizures or more akin to the paroxysmal dyskinesias. See Chapter 17 for a full discussion of this issue.

Recently, Montagna *et al.* (1990) described paroxysmal arousals during sleep. These can occur frequently and may be associated with complex movements.

Transient paroxysmal dystonia/torticollis in infancy

Snyder (1969) introduced a new type of paroxysmal dyskinesia that he called paroxysmal torticollis in infancy. He described 12 cases of intermittent head tilting in young infants. The age at onset was between 2 and 8 months of age, except for 3 cases whose first attacks occurred at 14, 17 and 30 months. The attacks would occur about two to three times a month and last from 10 minutes to 14 days, usually 2–3 days. The head would tilt to either side and often rotate slightly to the opposite side. There is no distress unless a parent attempts to straighten the head, upon which the baby cries. In some cases the head-tilting is associated with vomiting, pallor and agitation for a short period. The infant is normal between attacks, and the attacks disappear after months or years, usually around age 2 or 3 years. Subsequently, a number of similar cases have been described (Gourley, 1971; Sanner and Bergstrom, 1979; Bratt and Menelaus, 1992), including familial cases (Lipson and Robertson, 1978). Sanner and Bergstrom (1979) reported a patient whose father had a similar condition in early infancy, indicating that this disorder is hereditary.

The clinical picture of paroxysmal torticollis in infancy that has evolved is that the trunk can also be involved with lateral curvature concave to the same side as the head tilting, and the ipsilateral leg can be flexed. Onset can be as early as the first months of life and recur every couple of weeks until they disappear before the age of 2 years. Each attack can last a couple of hours to a couple of weeks. In between attacks the child is normal. The main differential diagnosis is a posterior fossa tumor and Sandifer's syndrome (Menkes and Ament, 1988).

In 1988, the clinical spectrum expanded with the report by Angelini *et al.* under the title of 'transient paroxysmal dystonia in infancy'. They described 9 patients who had onset of paroxysmal dyskinesias between 3 and 5 months of age, except for 1 with an onset at 1 month. Three had a history of perinatal brain damage; 9 did not. The attacks consisted of opisthotonus, increased muscle tone with twisting of the limbs, and, in 3, with neck and trunk twisting, thereby linking this with paroxysmal torticollis in infancy. The attacks last several minutes, with a maximum of 2 hours in 1 patient. They would occur from several attacks per day to once a month. Remission occurred between the ages of 8 to 22 months, with 2 not yet having reached a remission.

Dunn (1988) described an infant with head-turning and posturing of the right arm lasting 45 minutes to 18 hours. There were 6 attacks from age 26 months to age 40 months. The author did not mention the possible diagnosis of paroxysmal torticollis in infancy, and made a diagnosis of PDC. One should consider the possibility that PDC may occur in infancy and disappear over several months. If so, then the paroxysmal torticollis in infancy of Snyder and the paroxysmal dystonia in infancy of Angelini may represent the lowest age spectrum of PDC, and a benign form of the disorder.

This disorder should not be confused by the syndrome referred to as benign paroxysmal tonic upgaze of childhood (Ouvrier and Billson, 1988; Deonna *et al.*, 1990; Echenne and Rivier, 1992), which is a sustained tonic conjugate upward deviation of the eyes beginning in infancy, and eventually disappearing in childhood. Ataxia may be present. They lessen in the morning hours and disappear with sleep.

Acetazolamide is not effective. Perhaps the tonic upgaze with diurnal fluctuations would be a better term than paroxysmal. Another paroxysmal ocular disorder was recently described in brain-damaged infants, known as paroxysmal ocular downward deviation (Yokochi, 1991). The ocular displacement was accompanied by closure of the upper eyelids, and the episode would last seconds.

Paroxysmal ataxias and tremor

Intermittent ataxia has been reported with metabolic defects such as Hartnup disease (Baron *et al.*, 1956), pyruvate decarboxylase deficiency (Lonsdale *et al.*, 1969; Blass *et al.*, 1970, 1971) and maple syrup urine disease (Dancis *et al.*, 1967). Fever often triggers the attacks of ataxia. In 1 case with pyruvate decarboxylase deficiency (Blass *et al.*, 1971), choreoathetosis tended to accompany the chorea. Paroxysmal ataxia and dysarthria have also been reported to occur in multiple sclerosis (Andermann *et al.*, 1959; Espir *et al.*, 1966; DeCastro and Campbell, 1967; Miley and Forster, 1974; Gorard and Gibberd, 1989), which, as remarked above, is a disorder that also can cause paroxysmal choreoathetosis/dystonia. The attacks of paroxysmal ataxia due to multiple sclerosis last seconds, much shorter than the attacks described below. They also can respond to carbamazepine.

In 1946, Parker described 6 patients in 4 families with idiopathic familial paroxysmal ataxia, which he labelled as periodic ataxia. The age at onset ranged from 21 to 32 years. The attacks affected gait and speech and lasted from 30 seconds to 30 minutes. There could be several attacks per day, or there could be interval-free periods of several weeks. Vestibular symptoms occurred in some of the patients. Progressive cerebellar ataxia developed in some members.

In 1963, Farmer and Mustian (1963) reported another family with idiopathic paroxysmal ataxia. The major clinical differences from Parker's cases were the high frequency of accompanying vestibular symptoms of vertigo, diplopia and oscillopsia, and the lack of speech involvement. They labelled their family as vestibulocerebellar ataxia. The age at onset ranged from 23 to 42 years. The attacks ranged from a few minutes to 2 months. The brief episodes may occur daily, but free intervals could last a year or more. Some affected members also developed progressive ataxia.

Hill and Sherman (1986) described another family, but with onset in childhood in many of those affected, and no development of progressive ataxia. Another family of childhood onset and benign course was described by White (1969). All the families showed inheritance as autosomal dominant.

An important advance was the discovery by Griggs *et al.* (1978) that acetazolamide can effectively prevent attacks. These authors showed this benefit in one kindred with familial paroxysmal ataxia. Donat and Auger (1979) the following year had similar results in another kindred. Fahn (1983, 1984) reported a woman who had paroxysmal tremor, both intention and resting, associated with ataxia and postural instability during the attack: acetazolamide eliminated the attacks. Factor *et al.* (1991) reported an infant who had 3 attacks of coarse tremor and an orofacial dyskinesia that resembled that seen with tardive dyskinesia. Each attack lasted several hours, before spontaneously clearing. Tetrahydrobiopterin, the cofactor for the enzymes tyrosine hydroxylase and phenylalanine hydroxylase, was reduced. The child responded to levodopa.

Mayeux and Fahn (1982) reported a patient with PDC in a background of hereditary ataxia. Onset of PDC was at age 10; onset of ataxia was age 19. During an attack, which lasted 10 minutes to 4 hours, there was also an accompanying increase of ataxia. Initially there was an 8-month response to acetazolamide. After the drug was no longer effective, the patient's PDC responded to clonazepam. It is possible that this patient might be a link between familial PDC and paroxysmal ataxia.

Several other reports of acetazolamide-responsive familial paroxysmal ataxia have been reported (Aimard *et al.*, 1983; Zasorin *et al.*, 1983; Koller and Bahamon-Dussan, 1987). Although computed tomography (CT) has been normal, magnetic resonance imaging (MRI) studies have revealed selective atrophy in the anterior cerebellar vermis (Vighetto *et al.*, 1988).

Families with a combination of periodic ataxia and persistent, continuous electrical activity in several muscles, reported as either myokymia (Van Dyke *et al.*, 1975; Hanson *et al.*, 1977; Gancher and Nutt, 1986; Brunt and Van Weerden, 1990) or as neuromyotonia (Vaamonde *et al.*, 1991), have been described. Description of the attacks, which are of brief duration and are sometimes preceded by sudden movement, include dyskinetic movements and sustained posturing, as well as ataxia, dysarthria and vertigo.

Gancher and Nutt (1986) classified the hereditary episodic ataxias into three syndromes. The first group are those with attacks of ataxia (with or without interictal nystagmus, and with or without persistent ataxia), responding to acetazolamide or amphetamines. The attacks are precipitated by exercise, fatigue, stress and occasionally by carbohydrate or alcohol ingestion. In addition to ataxia, the attacks are accompanied by vertigo, headache, nausea and malaise. The attacks last for several hours or until the patient falls asleep. In recent years additional families have been reported with these features (Baloh and Winder, 1991; Bain *et al.*, 1991; Hawkes, 1992). The siblings reported by Bain *et al.* (1991) had persistent diplopia due to superior oblique paresis as part of the syndrome. Using [^{31}P] nuclear magnetic resonance spectroscopy, Bain and his colleagues (1992) found the pH levels in the cerebellum to be increased in untreated subjects with acetazolamide-responsive paroxysmal ataxia; the pH dropped to normal with treatment.

The second group is associated with persistent myokymia or neuromyotonia. Attacks are precipitated by fatigue, excitement, stress and physical trauma, but the family reported by Vaamonde *et al.* (1991) had attacks triggered by sudden movement. There is no dizziness or vertigo. The attacks last 2 minutes or less. Acetazolamide and anticonvulsants are ineffective.

The third group is that in which the attacks are induced by sudden movement, i.e. kinesigenic. Typical PKC can occur in some members of the family. The attacks of ataxia last minutes to hours, while the PKC lasts seconds. The disorder can resolve with time. Acetazolamide appears to be ineffective, but phenytoin is effective for both the kinesigenic ataxia and the PKC.

A recent case was reported in which a young girl had attacks of ataxia associated with fevers and accompanied by vertical supranuclear ophthalmoplegia (Nightingale and Barton, 1991). The ataxia and eye findings can last days.

Miscellaneous paroxysmal disorders

Two patients with posttraumatic periodic, rhythmical movements of the tongue were reported by Keane (1984). The attacks occurred about every 20 seconds and each attack lasted 10 seconds. They consisted of undulations at 3 per second. Eventually, the movements diminished.

Table 16.3 Clinical features of non-epileptic paroxysmal movements seen in children

Symptoms	*n*
Head movements	3
Eye movements	12
Staring	7
Mouth movements	7
Respiratory	2
Tonic posturing	13
Tremors	6
Myoclonus	2
Other	7

From Donat and Wright (1990).

Other paroxysmal dyskinesias should be mentioned, but will not be discussed further. These are Sandifer's syndrome (prolonged head-tilting in children following eating, due to gastro-oesophageal reflux; see review by Menkes and Ament (1988)), hyperekplexia (excessive startle syndrome with complex movements; see review by Andermann and Andermann, (1986)), shuddering attacks in children (Holmes and Russman, 1986), stereotypy (Duchowny *et al.*, 1988) and paroxysmal bursts of myoclonus and tics. Classically, stereotypy, myoclonus and tics are each recognized as a specific class of movement disorders and they characteristically present as paroxysmal bursts of their type of movement. As a result, their discussion should be separated from those conditions labelled as paroxysmal. Donat and Wright (1990) recently reviewed non-epileptic paroxysmal movements seen in children. Of 31 children with such clinical attacks, 18 had more than one type of movement during an attack, and 6 had more than one type of attack. The types of movements encountered are listed in Table 16.3.

The description of each of these types were not provided so it is difficult to recognize how each fits into the classification scheme provided here. One wonders if a number of these represent tics. For example, paroxysmal eye movements are common in tics (Frankel and Cummings, 1984). It seems likely that those labelled by Donat and Wright as tonic posturing could be one of the types of paroxysmal dyskinesias reviewed here.

In this review, paroxysmal hypnogenic dyskinesias, paroxysmal dystonia/torticollis in infancy, paroxysmal ataxias, and the miscellaneous disorders mentioned in this section will not be further discussed. Hereafter, this review will discuss only the classical paroxysmal dyskinesias of PKC, PDC and the intermediate form associated with prolonged exercise. Both the idiopathic and symptomatic forms will be discussed.

CLASSIFICATION OF THE PAROXYSMAL DYSKINESIAS

Paroxysmal dystonia/choreoathetosis

As pointed out by Lance (1977), the best method to classify the paroxysmal dyskinesias is by the duration of the attacks – short, intermediate and long-lasting. However, historically, the introduction of the term kinesigenic by Kertesz (1967) has been so well-accepted that this is the standard term commonly used. Since all kinesigenic cases are also associated with short attacks of dyskinesias, it seems reasonable to accept the term in the classification scheme, although some cases with short-duration attacks are not necessarily induced by sudden movement (or startle, see below).

1. *Kinesigenic (paroxysmal kinesigenic choreoathetosis; PKC)*
   Duration: seconds to 5 minutes
   Triggers: sudden movement, startle, hyperventilation
   precipitant: stress
   Treatment: sensitive to anticonvulsants

   Aetiology
      Idiopathic – familial, sporadic
      Symptomatic

   Note: the effectiveness of anticonvulsants correlates with the brief duration of the paroxysms, rather than their being triggered by sudden movement

2. *Non-kinesigenic (paroxysmal dystonic choreoathetosis; PDC)*
   Duration: 2 minutes to 4 hours
   Trigger: none known
   Precipitant: stress, alcohol, caffeine, excitement, fatigue
   Treatment: not sensitive to anticonvulsants

   Aetiology:
      Idiopathic – familial, sporadic
      Symptomatic
      Psychogenic

3. *Intermediate form (intermediate PDC)*
   Duration: 3–30 minutes
   Precipitant: continued exertion

   Aetiology
      Idiopathic – familial, sporadic
      Symptomatic
      Psychogenic

4. *Hypnogenic paroxysmal dyskinesia*
   Brief attacks (some may be seizures)
   Prolonged attacks

5. *Benign paroxysmal dystonia/torticollis in infancy*

6. *Miscellaneous*

Paroxysmal ataxia and tremor

1. *Without myokymia/neuromyotonia*
   Duration: hours
   Precipitant: exercise, fatigue, stress, alcohol
   Treatment: sensitive to acetazolamide
   Other features: vertigo, oscillopsia, headache, nausea, malaise, interictal nystagmus, may develop persistent ataxia

2. *With myokymia/neuromyotonia*
   Duration: brief; <2 minutes
   Precipitant: exercise, fatigue, stress, trauma; also reported as triggered by sudden movement
   Treatment: not sensitive to acetazolamide
   Other feature: persistent myokymia/neuromyotonia
3. *Kinesigenic*
   Duration: minutes to hours
   Triggers: sudden movement or startle
   Treatment: ataxia not sensitive to acetazolamide, sensitive to anticonvulsants
   Other features: may be accompanied by PKC

Hyperekplexia

Sandifer's syndrome

Shuddering attacks

Stereotypies

PAROXYSMAL KINESIGENIC CHOREOATHETOSIS

Clinical features

The attacks of PKC consist of any combination of dystonic postures, chorea, athetosis and ballism. They can be unilateral – always on one side or on either side – or bilateral. Unilateral episodes can be followed by a bilateral one. The attacks are brief, usually only seconds, but rarely can last up to 5 minutes. They are precipitated by a sudden movement or a startle, usually after the patient has been sitting quietly for some time. The attacks can be severe enough to cause a patient to fall down. There can be as many as 100 attacks per day. After an attack, there is usually a short refractory period before another attack can take place. Speech can sometimes be affected, with inability to speak due to dystonia, but there is never any alteration of consciousness. The attacks can sometimes be aborted if the patient stops moving or warms up slowly. Very often patients report variable sensations at the beginning of the paroxysms. These can consist of paraesthesias, a feeling of stiffness, crawling sensations or a tense feeling.

Equivalent to PKC are equally brief attacks that are not precipitated by sudden movement or startle. Because the duration and therapeutic response are the same as PKC, I am listing these under the PKC rubric, rather than developing an entirely new category. Often these few-seconds attacks can be triggered by hyperventilation.

A patient with typical brief dyskinesias occurring many times a day, preceded by paraesthesias, and responding to anticonvulsants, but not induced by sudden movement was reported as case 4 by Kinast *et al.* (1980). Although technically not PKC because sudden movements did not trigger any attacks, the clinical feature otherwise resemble the attacks seen in PKC. As mentioned above, this type of paroxysmal dyskinesia is placed in this category of PKC. Since the attacks of PDC are usually so prolonged and because they don't ordinarily respond to anticonvulsants, this case does not fit into the PDC category. Further discussion on this classification of these brief attacks as symptomatic PKC is dealt with below.

Table 16.4 Laterality of attacks of paroxysmal kinesigenic choreoathetosis

Laterality of attacks	*n*
Unilateral – one side only	25
Unilateral – either side	12
Unilateral and bilateral	11
Bilateral only	22
Not stated	3
Total	73

From Plant (1983)

Plant (1983) emphasized the focal and unilateral nature of PKC in many patients. Table 16.4 summarizes the 73 cases of PKC in the literature reviewed by him.

Idiopathic PKC

The aetiology of most case reports of PKC have been idiopathic, and predominantly hereditary, with inheritance being autosomal dominant. For some unexplained reason males are more often affected than females by a ratio of 3.75:1 (75 males and 20 females reported in Tables 16.2 and 16.5). Age at onset shows a wide range, usually in childhood between the ages of 6 and 16, but can range from 6 months to 40 years. The mean age at onset is 12; the median, 12. Familial cases may be more common among the Japanese (Kishimoto, 1957; Fukuyama and Okada, 1967; Kato and Araki, 1969) and Chinese (Jung *et al*., 1973). There is one report of PKC developing in a patient who had essential tremor (Nair *et al*., 1991). EEGs are generally normal, and CT scans are also normal (Goodenough *et al*., 1978; Kinast *et al*., 1980; Suber and Riley, 1980; Bortolotti and Schoenhuber, 1983; Lou, 1989) with a few exceptions, such as the case reported by Watson and Scott (1979) with suggested brainstem atrophy, and the one by Gilroy (1982) with an ill-defined unilateral hemispheric lesion. However, Hirata *et al*. (1991) demonstrated an abnormal EEG with rhythmic 5 Hz discharges over the entire scalp during episodes of PKC, raising the possibility that the PKC may have an epileptogenic basis.

The attacks tend to diminish with age. Fortunately, PKC responds dramatically to anticonvulsants. The early literature indicates that phenytoin was the most popular, followed by phenobarbitone and primidone. Recently, carbamazepine appears to be the drug most commonly used. Valproate has also been effective (Suber and Riley, 1980). There is one report of response to levodopa (Loong and Ong, 1973), but another reports lack of effect by this drug (Garello *et al*., 1983). Analogously, there is one report of 3 patients with PKC worsening with haloperidol (Przuntek and Monninger, 1983), but Garello *et al*. (1983) reported no effect from this drug (as well as levodopa) in 2 brothers. The calcium channel blocker flunarizine, which is also a neuroleptic, was effective in a 7-year-old girl, who did not respond to carbamazepine or methylphenidate (Lou, 1989).

Homan *et al*. (1980) reported that children with PKC need doses of phenytoin that are similar to that used to treat epilepsy, while adults can respond to lower doses. These authors also describe a patient who may have had interictal chorea (however, described as fidgety) and suggested that this might represent a possible link to benign hereditary chorea. However, the fidgetiness described may not have been chorea. On the other hand, these authors supported their notion with the report by Bird *et al.* (1978) in which a women had anxiety-induced dystonia/choreoathetosis and random, adventitious small jerky movements when she does not have an attack (first reported by Perez-Borja *et al.*, 1967); her daughter had delayed milestones and persistent choreoathetosis. However, it seems likely that the daughter's choreoathetosis is not idiopathic but secondary, so it seems that paroxysmal dyskinesias and hereditary benign chorea should not be linked together on the basis of a couple of these cases.

The pathophysiology of PKC is still unclear, and its relationship with epilepsy remains speculative. Because movement-induced seizures can occur (for example, the case of Falconer *et al.*, 1963) and because PKC responds dramatically to anticonvulsants, these are not sufficient reasons to consider PKC a form of epilepsy. The retention of consciousness and lack of postictal phenomena, as well as the presence of dystonia and choreoathetosis, should be sufficient to disqualify PKC from the epilepsies. Franssen *et al.* (1983) investigated the contingent negative variation (CNV) in 1 patient. CNV is a slow cerebral potential that follows a warning stimulus which prepares the subject to expect an imperative stimulus requiring a decision or motor response. The slow negative wave component of the CNV was more pronounced compared to control subjects. It returned to normal after phenytoin treatment.

The differential diagnosis of PKC is focal epilepsy, tetany, hyperekplexia and hysteria, as noted in the misdiagnosis of the case reported by Waller (1977). The clinical features are so distinctive, particularly if triggered by sudden movement, that there is little likelihood for not diagnosing the condition correctly once one is aware of its existence. However, the non-kinesigenic, brief attacks of hemidystonia, often precipitated by hyperventilation and controlled with anticonvulsants may be a sign of epilepsy (Kotagal *et al.*, 1989; Newton *et al.*, 1992). So each case of such suspected non-kinesigenic PKC needs to be evaluated for a convulsive disorder.

In addition to the cases of PKC described in the historical highlights and above, there have been a number of other reports that should be cited to make the review complete (Zacchetti *et al.*, 1983; Boel and Casaer, 1984; Lang, 1984).

There have been reports of 2 autopsies in PKC. Case 4 of Kertesz (1967) died, apparently by suicide, and a postmorten examination revealed no clear-cut abnormality in brain, just the presence of some melanin pigment in macrophages in the locus coeruleus. Stevens (1966) had earlier reported the postmortem findings of 1 of his patients, which was also essentially normal, showing only a slight asymmetry of the substantia nigra.

Table 16.5 summarizes the reports of idiopathic PKC.

Symptomatic PKC (Table 16.6)

The overwhelming majority of reported cases of PKC are idiopathic or familial in aetiology. Many cases of symptomatic PKC have been reported, however, the most common being associated with multiple sclerosis and head injury. Although most of the paroxysmal dyskinesias associated with multiple sclerosis are not triggered by sudden movement, not uncommonly a patient with multiple sclerosis will manifest typical PKC (Matthews, 1958). In fact, the presenting symptom of multiple sclerosis

Table 16.5 Reports of idiopathic paroxysmal kinesigenic choreoathetosis/dystonia (PKC)

Authors	*Case no.*	*Sex*	*Age at onset*	*Aetiology*	*FH*	*Triggers*	*Sensory aura*	*Treatment*
Smith and	1	M	8	Idiopathic	+	Sudden movement	0	
Heersema	2	M	14	Idiopathic	0	?	+	
(1941)	3	M	7	Idiopathic	+	Movement	+	
Michaux and Granier (1945)	1	F	6	Idiopathic	0	Sudden movement	+	Anticonvulsants
Pryles *et al.*	1	M	8	Idiopathic	+	?	+	PHY, AMPH
(1952)	2	M	13	Idiopathic	+	?	+	Anticonvulsants
Kishimoto	1	M	8	Idiopathic	+	Sudden movement	0	
(1957)	2	M	12	Idiopathic	+	Sudden movement	0	
	3	M	9	Idiopathic	+	Sudden movement	?	Barbiturate
	4	M	9	Idiopathic	+	Sudden movement	0	
Lishman *et al.*	1	M	3	Idiopathic	0	Sudden movement	+	Anticonvulsants
(1962)	2	M	5	Idiopathic	0	Sudden movement	?	Anticonvulsants
	3	M	14	Idiopathic	0	Sudden movement	+	Anticonvulsants
	4	M	20	Idiopathic	0	Exercise	0	
	5	M	7	Idiopathic	0	Sudden movement	0	Anticonvulsants
	6	M	15	Idiopathic	0	Sudden movement	+	PHY
	7	M	11	Idiopathic	0	Sudden movement	+	PHY
Williams and Stevens (1963)	1	F	1	Idiopathic	?	Sudden movement	+	PHY
Whitty *et al.*	1	M	13	Idiopathic	0	Sudden movement	+	Anticonvulsants
(1964)	2	M	12	Idiopathic	0	Sudden movement surprise	0	Anticonvulsants
	4	M	<18	Idiopathic	+	Sudden movement	0	Anticonvulsants
	5	M	8	Idiopathic	+	Sudden movement	0	Phenobarbitone
Hudgins and	1	M	5	Idiopathic	+	Sudden movement	0	Anticonvulsants
Corbin (1966)	2	F	11	Idiopathic	+	Movement, stress	+	Anticonvulsants
	3	F	13	Idiopathic	+	Movement	?	Remission
Stevens	1	Same case as reported by Williams and Stevens (1963)						
(1966)	2	M	14	Idiopathic	0	Sudden movement	?	Anticonvulsants
	3	M	33	Idiopathic	0	Sudden movement	?	PHY
	4	M	child	Idiopathic	+	Sudden movement	+	
Dowzenko and Zielinsky (1966)	1	F	18	Idiopathic	0	Sudden movement	+	PHY
Kertesz	1	F	9	Idiopathic	+	Sudden movement	+	PHY
(1967)	2	M	14	Idiopathic	+	Sudden movement	+	
	3	F	13	Idiopathic	0	Sudden movement	+	Remission
	4	M	10	Idiopathic	0	Movement	+	
	5	M	12	Idiopathic	+	Sudden movement	+	Anticonvulsants
	6	M	10	Idiopathic	+	Sudden movement	+	Remission
	7	M	15	Idiopathic	+	?	+	Anticonvulsants
	8	M	10	Idiopathic	+	Sudden movement	+	Anticonvulsants
	9	F	8	Idiopathic	+	Sudden movement	+	Anticonvulsants
	10	F	15	Idiopathic	0	Sudden movement	+	PHY
Perez-Borja *et al.* (1967)	2	F	6	Idiopathic	0	Sudden movement	0	Anticonvulsants
DeBolt	1	M	?	Idiopathic	?	Sudden movement	?	PHY
(1967)	2	M	?	Idiopathic	?	Sudden movement	?	PHY

Table 16.5 (continued)

Authors	Case no.	Sex	Age at onset	Aetiology	FH	Triggers	Sensory aura	Treatment
Kato and Araki (1969)	1	F	8	Idiopathic	+	Sudden movement	+	Carbamazepine
Horner and Jackson (1969)	1	M	7	Idiopathic	+	Sudden movement hyperventilation	+	
	2	M	23	Idiopathic	+	During sleep	0	PHY, phenobarbitone
	3	M	8	Idiopathic	+	During sleep, later daytime sudden movement	+	As case 2
Tassinari and Fine (1969)	1	M	11	Idiopathic	0	Sudden movement	+	PHY
Morley (1970)	1	M	2	Idiopathic	0	Sudden movement	+	Carbamazepine
	2	M	20	Idiopathic	+	Hypogenic	0	PHY
	3	M	13	Idiopathic	+	Sudden movement	+	PHY
Burger *et al.* (1972)	1	M	15	Idiopathic	0	Movement	0	PHY
	2	M	12	Idiopathic	0	Sudden movement	0	PHY, phenobarbitone
Jung *et al.* (1973)	1	M	8	Idiopathic	+	Sudden movement vigorous activity	+	PHY, phenobarbitone
	2	M	15	Idiopathic	+	Sudden movement	+	Anticonvulsants
	3	M	16	Idiopathic	0	Vigorous activity	+	PHY
	4	M	16	Idiopathic	0	Sudden movement	?	PHY
Loong and Ong (1973)	1	M	19	Idiopathic	0	Sudden movement	?	PHY, L-dopa
Waller (1977)	1	F	8	Idiopathic	0	Sudden movement	+	PHY
Goodenough *et al.* (1978)	1	M	2	Idiopathic	0	Sudden movement	+	PHY
	2	M	14	Idiopathic	0	Sudden movement	0	PHY
	3	M	16	Idiopathic	0	Sudden movement	0	PHY
Watson and Scott (1979)	1	M	14	Idiopathic versus brainstem atrophy	0	Sudden movement	0	
Kinast *et al.* (1980)	1	M	11	Idiopathic	0	Sudden movement	0	PHY
	3	M	16	Idiopathic	0	Sudden movement	0	PHY
	5	M	17	Idiopathic	0	Sudden movement	+	PHY
Homan *et al.* (1980)	1	M	2	Idiopathic	+	Sudden movement	0	PHY
	2	F	4	Idiopathic	0	Sudden movement	+	PHY
	3	F	7	Idiopathic	+	Sudden movement	0	PHY
	4	M	12	Idiopathic	+	Sudden movement, ethanol	0	PHY
	5	M	8	Idiopathic	0	Sudden movement	+	PHY
Suber and Riley (1980)	1	F	5	Idiopathic	+	Sudden movement	0	Valproate
Przuntek and Monninger (1983)	1	F	?	Idiopathic	?	Sudden movement	?	Carbamazepine
	2	M	?	Idiopathic	?	Sudden movement	?	Carbamazepine
	3	F	?	Idiopathic	?	Sudden movement	?	Carbamazepine
Zacchetti *et al.* (1983)	1	M	13	Idiopathic	?	Sudden movement	+	PHY

Table 16.5 (continued)

Table 16.5 (continued)

Authors	*Case no.*	*Sex*	*Age at onset*	*Aetiology*	*FH*	*Triggers*	*Sensory aura*	*Treatment*
Garello *et al.* (1983)	1	M	4	Idiopathic	+	Sudden movement	+	Phenobarbitone
	2	M	6	Idiopathic	+	Sudden movement	+	Phenobarbitone
Franssen *et al.* (1983)	1	M	17	Idiopathic	0	Sudden movement	0	
Bortolotti and Schoenhuber (1983)	1	M	13	Idiopathic	+	Sudden movement	0	Carbamazepine
	2	M	40	Idiopathic	+	Sudden movement	0	Remission
Plant (1983)	1	M	6	Idiopathic	+	Sudden movement	0	PHY
	2	M	14	Idiopathic	+	Sudden movement	+	PHY
	3	M	15	Idiopathic	0	Sudden movement	0	PHY
	4	M	11	Idiopathic	0	Sudden movement	0	PHY
Boel and Casaer (1984)	1	M	10	Idiopathic	+	Sudden movement	+	PHY
Lang (1984)	1	F	22	Idiopathic	0	Sudden movement	0	
Nardocci *et al.* (1989)	1	M	10	Idiopathic	+	Sudden movement	0	
Lou (1989)	1	F	2	Idiopathic	0	Sudden movement	0	Flunarizine
Hirata *et al.* (1991)	1	M	13	Idiopathic	0	Sudden movement	0	PHY, clonazepam
Nair *et al.* (1991)	1	M	21	Idiopathic	0	Sudden movement	0	

+ = Present or yes; 0 = absent or no; ? = no information given.
FH = Family history of similar attacks.
AMPH = Amphetamine; PHY = phenytoin.

Table 16.6 Reports of symptomatic paroxysmal kinesigenic choreoathetosis/dystonia

Authors	*Case no.*	*Sex*	*Age at onset*	*Aetiology*	*FH*	*Triggers*	*Sensory aura*	*Treatment*
Arden (1953)	1	M	13	Hypoparathyroidism	0	Sudden movement	0	Calciferol
Matthews (1958)	1	F	48	Multiple sclerosis	0	Sudden movement	+	Phenobarbitone
	2	F	27	Multiple sclerosis	0	Sudden movement	0	
	4	F	42	Multiple sclerosis	0	Sudden movement	+	Phenytoin
Whitty *et al.* (1964)	3	M	13	Head injury	0	Sudden movement	+	Anticonvulsants
Rosen (1964)	1	M	12	Perinatal hypoxia	0	Movement, startle plus body contact	0	Antimuscarinic, antihistaminic
Tabaee-Zadeh *et al.* (1972)	1	M	19	Hypoparathyroidism	0	Vigorous activity	0	Calciferol
Robin (1977)	1	M	33	Head injury	0	Sudden movement	+	Phenobarbitone
Kinast *et al.* (1980)	2	M	5	Hemiatrophy	0	Anticipation of movement	0	Phenytoin
Gilroy (1982)	1	M	5	Unknown	0	Sudden movement	0	Carbamazepine

Table 16.6 (continued)

Authors	*Case no.*	*Sex*	*Age at onset*	*Aetiology*	*FH*	*Triggers*	*Sensory aura*	*Treatment*
Huffstutter and Myers (1983)	2	F	4	Infant hemiplegia	0	Sudden touch	+	Anticonvulsants
Berger *et al.* (1984)	1	M	27	Multiple sclerosis	0	Sudden movement	+	Phenytoin
	4	F	24	Multiple sclerosis	0	Sudden movement	0	Remission
	5	M	16	Multiple sclerosis	0	Sudden movement	+	Phenytoin
Drake *et al.* (1986)	1	M	22	Head injury	0	Sudden movement	0	Phenobarbitone
	2	M	30	Head injury	0	Sudden movement	0	Lorazepam
Adam and Orinda (1986)	1	F	56	Progressive supranuclear palsy	0	Sudden movement	0	Carbamazepine
Merchut and Brumlik (1986)	1	F	33	Putaminal infarct	0	Sudden movement	+	Carbamazepine
Richardson *et al.* (1987)	1	M	18	Head injury	0	Sudden movement	0	Carbamazepine
Barabas and Tucker (1988)	1	M	12	Hypoparathyroidism	0	Sudden movement	0	Calciferol
Camac *et al.* (1990)	1	F	53	Thalamic infarct	0	Sudden movement	+	Phenytoin
George *et al.* (1990)	1	M	33	Head trauma	0	Touch	0	Diazepam
Verheul and Tyssen (1990)	1	F	28	Multiple sclerosis	0	Hyperventilation	0	Carbamazepine
Roos *et al.* (1991)	1	F	35	Multiple sclerosis	0	Emotion, movement, speaking, writing	0	Phenytoin
Fuh *et al.* (1991)	1	F	52	Stroke	0		+	Diazepam
Burguera *et al.* (1991)	1	M	26	Multiple sclerosis	0	Hyperventilation, writing, standing	+	Carbamazepine
Sethi *et al.* (1992)	1	F	30	Multiple sclerosis	0	Sudden movement hyperventilation	+	Acetazolamide
	2	M	44	Multiple sclerosis	0	Hyperventilation	0	Acetazolamide
	3	F	36	Multiple sclerosis	0	Hyperventilation	+	Acetazolamide + carbamazepine

+ = Present or yes; 0 = absent or no; ? = no information given.
FH = Family history of similar attacks.

can be paroxysmal kinesigenic dyskinesias as in the case reported by Roos *et al.* (1991); these attacks were associated with a lesion in the caudate nucleus and responded to phenytoin. Three of the 8 patients reported by Berger *et al.* (1984) with paroxysmal dyskinesia associated with multiple sclerosis had the attacks induced by sudden movement; they were relieved with anticonvulsants.

As mentioned above, attacks lasting seconds are sometimes induced not by sudden movement, but by hyperventilation. These also usually respond to anticonvulsants, such as carbamazepine, and are also seen in multiple sclerosis (Verheul and Tyssen,

1990; Sethi *et al.*, 1992). I have also encountered a patient with attacks lasting seconds, induced by hyperventilation and without being induced by sudden movement, following a mild cerebral ischaemic episode, that also responded to carbamazepine. These pharmacological responses suggest that the briefness of the attack is the more important element than is the sudden movement to distinguish the classification of the paroxysmal dyskinesias. Sethi *et al.* (1992) reported success in treating 3 patients with paroxysmal dystonia (not induced by movement, but triggered by hyperventilation and lasting many seconds) with acetazolamide with or without a combination of carbamazepine. The case of PKC with multiple sclerosis reported by Burguera *et al.* (1991) had a lesion in the left thalamus demonstrated by MRI. The PKC was the presenting symptom, as in other cases of demyelinating disease.

Case 3 of Whitty *et al.* (1964) was a 13-year-old boy with onset 9 months after mild head trauma. Robin (1977) reported a 33-year-old man with severe head injury who developed PKC 8 months later. Two of the 3 cases of posttraumatic paroxysmal dyskinesias reported by Drake *et al.* (1986) had the movements induced by sudden movement of the affected body part. Another posttraumatic case was reported by Richardson *et al.* (1987). These posttraumatic cases of PKC responded to anticonvulsants, similar to idiopathic PKC. Attacks of dystonia lasting several seconds and induced by tactile stimulation were reported secondary to a head injury; they disappeared within 2 months without treatment (George *et al.*, 1990). Another case of tactile-induced dyskinesias was reported by Nijssen and Tijssen (1992) as a result of a thalamic infarct.

Rosen (1964) appears to have been the first to report a case of PKC associated with perinatal hypoxic encephalopathy, with the onset beginning at age 12. This boy's attacks were usually triggered by a combination of startle and body contact. Mushet and Dreifuss (1967) described a 9-year-old boy who developed brief attacks of athetosis and dystonia. They usually occurred when he was startled, but also could occur following sudden movement. At age 6 months he had a febrile illness, retrospectively thought to be encephalitis. He had considerable motor regression and was not able to walk, nor did he gain syntactical speech. His dyskinetic attacks were not suppressed by anticonvulsants, but did respond to anticholinergics.

Idiopathic hypoparathyroidism with basal ganglia calcifications associated with PKC was first reported by Arden (1953). Subsequent cases were reported (Tabaee-Zadeh *et al.*, 1982; Barabas and Tucker, 1988). Calciferol was effective in controlling these attacks. The case reported by Soffer *et al.* (1977) was not noted to have the attacks induced by sudden movement, but the briefness of the attack resembles PKC.

Case 2 of the 5 cases described by Kinast *et al.* (1980) had attacks of left hemidystonia lasting 1 minute and occurring up to 50 times a day. The major precipitating factor was not sudden movement, but stress and the anticipation of movement (also reported in 1 patient by Franssen *et al.*, 1983). Technically, like their case 4 described above, this patient does not fulfil the criterion of attacks induced by sudden movement. This is another example, because of the brief duration, the frequency of the attacks, and their response to phenytoin that otherwise resembles PKC, and again points out why such non-kinesigenic cases are placed under the PKC rubric in our classification scheme. Examination of this boy revealed left-sided hemiatrophy and hyperreflexia, with a normal CT scan. Because the hemiatrophy syndrome can be associated with a delayed-onset movement disorder (Buchmann *et al.*, 1988), it seems reasonable to consider it an aetiological factor in this particular case.

Gilroy (1982) reported a 32-year-old man with an abnormal right hemisphere on CT scan who had multiple daily brief attacks of left hemidystonia present since the age of 5 that were typical of PKC. The speculation is that the PKC was secondary to pathology in the involved hemisphere. An arteriogram and cortical biopsy did not shed further light on the pathology.

With the advent of MRI, more cases of PKC have been reported as a result of cerebral infarcts – with putaminal infarct (Merchut and Brumlik, 1986), thalamic infarct (Camac *et al.*, 1990; Nijssen and Tijssen, 1992), and infarct probably in the cortex (Fuh *et al.*, 1991). As mentioned above, the case of Nijssen and Tijssen (1992) had attacks stimulated by touch of the affected limb. PKC has also been reported to occur in a patient with progressive supranuclear palsy (Adam and Orinda, 1986), basal ganglia calcifications with or without hypoparathyroidism (Arden, 1953), and hyperglycaemia in the presence of a lenticular vascular malformation (Vincent, 1986). The attacks secondary to infarcts (Merchut and Brumlik, 1986; Fuh *et al.*, 1991) or to multiple sclerosis (Sethi *et al.*, 1992) can be painful tonic spasms.

An unusual case was reported by Sunohara *et al.* (1984) of a 61-year-old man who had an infarct in the right posterolateral ventral thamalus and subsequently developed action-induced rhythmical dystonia, triggered by any type of voluntary movement, including speaking. This type of triggered dyskinesia is usually called overflow dystonia, and it is typical in cerebral palsy and also commonly occurs in many patients with idiopathic torsion dystonia, although not usually to as extreme a degree as described in this patient. Administration of 5-hydroxytryptophan and clonazepam abolished the dyskinesia.

Table 16.6 summarizes the reports of symptomatic PKC.

PAROXYSMAL NON-KINESIGENIC DYSTONIC CHOREOATHETOSIS

Clinical features

Like PKC, the attacks of PDC consist of any combination of dystonic postures, chorea, athetosis and ballism. They can be unilateral – always on one side or on either side – or bilateral. Unilateral episodes can be followed by a bilateral one. They can affect a single region of the body or be generalized. Involvement of the neck can be a combination of torticollis and head tremor (Hughes *et al.*, 1991). The major distinctions from PKC are the longer duration of each attack, the smaller frequency of the attacks, and a host of different precipitants of the attacks. The attacks last minutes to hours, sometimes longer than a day. Usually they range from 5 minutes to 4 hours. They are precipitated by consuming alcohol, coffee or tea, and also by psychological stress or excitement, and by fatigue. There are usually no more than three attacks per day, and often attacks may be months apart. The attacks can be severe enough to cause a patient to fall down. Speech is often affected, with inability to speak due to dystonia, but there is never any alteration of consciousness. The attacks can sometimes be aborted if the patient goes to sleep. As with PKC, very often patients report variable sensations at the beginning of the paroxysms. These can consist of paraesthesias, a feeling of stiffness, crawling sensations or a tense feeling.

A form of PDC, known as intermediate PDC, is triggered only by prolonged exercise and not the other precipitants. This was first described by Lance (1977) and subsequently reported in another family by Plant *et al.* (1984) and in a sporadic case by Nardocci *et al.* (1989). This form will be discussed separately.

Idiopathic PDC

The initial reports of PDC were familial (Mount and Reback, 1940; Forssman, 1961; Lance, 1963; Weber, 1967; Richards and Barnett, 1968; Horner and Jackson, 1969; Tibbles and Barnes, 1980; Walker, 1981; Mayeux and Fahn, 1982; Przuntek and Monninger, 1983; Jacome and Risko, 1984), with hereditary transmission being autosomal dominant. In 1980 Kinast *et al.* (1980) (case 4) and in 1981 Dunn each described a child with PDC without a positive family history. Since then Bressman *et al.* (1988) described 7 sporadic cases of PDC, and Nardocci *et al.* (1989) added another one. The familial cases of idiopathic PDC still greatly outnumber sporadic cases according to the reports in the literature. However, the sporadic cases are much more difficult to diagnose, and they have the difficulty of the need to be differentiated from a pyschogenic aetiology (Bressman *et al.*, 1988; Fahn and Williams, 1988). Based on the experience of Bressman and her colleagues (1988), the sporadic form may actually be more common than the familial form, but is just rarely reported.

For some unexplained reason males are slightly more often affected than females by a ratio of 1.4 : 1 (39 males and 28 females reported in the reviewed English literature; Table 16.7). Age at onset shows a wide range, usually in childhood between the ages of 6 and 16, but can range from 2 months to 40 years. The mean age at onset is 12; the median, 12. CT scans are normal (Mayeux and Fahn, 1982; Jacome and Risko, 1984).

The EEGs are generally normal, but the case of Jacome and Risko (1984) may be of interest. The patient had unilateral PDC, and had normal interictal EEGs. Photic stimulation at low frequencies induced paroxysmal lateralized epileptiform discharges from the contralateral hemisphere. From this the authors suggest that the disorder may have some epileptogenic basis.

Sleep aborts the episodes in one family that had myokymia in addition to the PDC (Byrne *et al.*, 1991). The presence of myokymia links this particular family to several with paroxysmal ataxia, in which myokymia is a feature (Van Dyke *et al.*, 1975; Vaamonde *et al.*, 1991).

A family reported by Kurlan *et al.* (1987) had some atypical features for classical PDC. The long-duration attacks were painful dystonic spasms that were not precipitated by alcohol, caffeine or excitement, but could follow exposure to cold or heat or result from exertional cramping. Other members of the family had only exertional cramping without PDC. The authors suggested that exertional cramping may be a *forme fruste* of PDC. It is also possible that the PDC in this family may fall into the category of the intermediate form of paroxysmal dyskinesia that was reported by Lance (1977) and Plant *et al.* (1984). Also unusual was the presence of some fixed dystonia, which had not been reported previously. Bressman *et al.* (1988) also described some sporadic cases of PDC who had some interictal dystonia.

Lance (1977) mentioned that autopsies performed on 2 patients with PDC revealed no pathology. His case II.4 had normal macroscopic findings. His case IV.2 died of crib death; macroscopic and microscopic findings were normal.

The attacks may diminish spontaneously with age (Lance, 1977; Kinast *et al.*, 1980; Bressman *et al.*, 1988). Unfortunately, most patients have persistence of their attacks and they are difficult to treat. As a general rule, PDC does not respond to the same type of anticonvulsants that so effectively treat PKC. An occasional patient will respond to such agents as carbamazepine and valproate. Clonazepam, as introduced for PDC by Lance (1977), appears to be the most successful agent, for both idiopathic PDC and symptomatic PDC. A number of other drugs have been tried, sometimes with success. These include antimuscarinics (Mount and Reback, 1940), chlordiazepoxide (Perez-Borja *et al.*, 1967; Walker, 1981), and acetazolamide (Mayeux and Fahn, 1982; Bressman *et al.*, 1988), oxazepam and other benzodiazepines (Kurlan and Shoulson, 1983; Kurlan *et al.*, 1987) and L-tryptophan (Kurlan *et al.*, 1987).

Kurlan and Shoulson (1983) treated 1 patient with familial PDC on alternate-day oxazepam. He had marked benefit from diazepam but only for 4 weeks. Clonazepam and oxazepam gave relief for 2–3 weeks each. Eventually the patient was placed on a regimen of 40 mg oxazepam given on alternate days. The concept was that the benzodiazepine receptors became desensitized on daily doses. Alternate-day administration prevented this desensitization.

Trials of the dopamine receptor antagonist haloperidol were carried out by Przuntek and Monninger (1983) and Coulter and Donofrio (1980) with benefit. In the obverse, Przuntek and Monninger (1983) found that levodopa worsened 1 patient.

In contrast to idiopathic PKC which is so distinctive, the major difficulty in the diagnosis of idiopathic PDC is to differentiate it from a psychogenic movement disorder, particularly in sporadic cases. The problem is that the disappearance of the movements with placebo or psychotherapy could be coincidental since the attacks disappear spontaneously. However, if the paroxysms are frequent and the attacks are prolonged, then repeated trials with placebo can be informative. If such trials consistently produce remissions, then one can be convinced that the diagnosis is a psychogenic disorder (see Chapter 18).

Table 16.7 summarizes the reports of idiopathic PDC.

Symptomatic PDC (Table 16.8)

The overwhelming majority of reported cases of PDC are idiopathic or familial in aetiology. A number of symptomatic PKC have been reported, however, the most common being associated with multiple sclerosis (Matthews, 1958; Joynt and Green, 1962; Lance, 1963; Berger *et al.*, 1984; Verheul and Tyssen, 1990; Sethi *et al.*, 1992), perinatal encephalopathy (Lance, 1963; Erickson and Chun, 1987; Bressman *et al.*, 1988), and psychogenic (Bressman *et al.*, 1988; Fahn and Williams, 1988). In multiple sclerosis, the paroxysmal movements may be only ocular, lasting several minutes (MacLean and Sassin, 1973).

Other causes of PDC are encephalitis (Mushet and Dreifuss, 1967; Bressman *et al.*, 1988), cystinuria (Cavanagh *et al.*, 1974), hypoparathyroidism (Soffer *et al.*, 1977; Yamamoto and Kawazawa, 1987), basal gangiia calcifications without altered serum calcium (Micheli *et al.*, 1986), thyrotoxicosis (Fischbeck and Layzer, 1979), transient ischaemic attacks (Margolin and Marsden, 1982; Bennett and Fox, 1989), infantile hemiplegia (Huffstutter and Myers, 1983), head injury (Perlmutter and Raichle, 1984; Drake *et al.*, 1986), hypoglycaemia (Newman and Kinkel, 1984; Winer *et al.*, 1990), acquired immune deficiency syndrome (AIDS; Nath *et al.*, 1987), diabetes (Haan *et al.*, 1988), anoxia (Bressman *et al.*, 1988) and brain tumour (Bressman *et al.*, 1988). The patient with AIDS (Nath *et al.*, 1987) had two attacks of dystonia, but details are lacking in regard to duration or characteristics of the attacks.

PDC caused by endocrine disorders responds to appropriate treatment. But, in general, treatment is not often effective.

Micheli *et al.* (1987) reported an interesting case of a mentally retarded youth who had received dopamine receptor-blocking drugs since the age of 3. At age 16 he

Table 16.7 Reports of idiopathic paroxysmal non-kinesigenic choreoathetosis/dystonia

Authors	*Case no.*	*Sex*	*Age at onset*	*Aetiology*	*FH*	*Triggers*	*Sensory aura*	*Treatment*
Mount and Reback (1940)	1	M	Infancy	Idiopathic	+	Alcohol, caffeine, fatigue	+	Antimuscarinic
Forssman (1961)	1	M	6	Idiopathic	+	Cold, stress, fatigue, alcohol, lack of sleep	+	
Lance (1963)	3	M	13	Idiopathic	0	Startle	+	
	4	M	22	Idiopathic	+	Relaxed, startle	+	
	5	M	2	Idiopathic	+	Excitement, alcohol, fatigue	+	
	6	F	2	Idiopathic	+	Excitement, fatigue	+	
	7	M	2	Idiopathic	+	Excitement, fatigue	+	
	8	M	9	Idiopathic	+	Excitement, fatigue	+	Anticonvulsants
Weber (1967)	1	M	12	Idiopathic	+	Excitement	+	
	3	M	22	Idiopathic	+	Excitement	+	
	4	F	19	Idiopathic	+	Nervousness	0	
Perez-Borja *et al.* (1967)	1	F	6 months	Idiopathic	0	Anxiety	0	Chlordiazepoxide
		Case 1 reported 11 years later by Bird *et al.* (1978) as familial						
Richards and Barnett (1968)	1	F	Infancy	Idiopathic	+	Stress, caffeine		
	2	F	Child	Idiopathic	+		0	Phenobarbitone
	3	F	Sister of case 2; no details given					
	4	M	Brother of case 2; no details given					
	5	M	Infancy	Idiopathic	+		0	
	6	M	Child	Idiopathic	+	Excitement, fatigue	0	Phenobarbitone
	7	M	Infancy	Idiopathic	+	Alcohol	+	
	8	F	1	Idiopathic	+	Excitement, fatigue	0	
	9	F	2 months	Idiopathic	+		0	
Lance (1977)	First pedigree:							
	I.2	Same as Lance (1963) case 4						
	II.4	Same as Lance (1963) case 5, later developed writing movements						
	II.5	M	?	Idiopathic	+	Alcohol, excitement	?	
	III.2	Same as Lance (1963) case 6; age at onset now listed at 6 weeks of life						Clonazepam
	III.3	M	13	Idiopathic	+	Alcohol, fatigue	+	Clonazepam
	III.4	Same as Lance (1963) case 7						Clonazepam
	III.5	Same as Lance (1963) case 8						
	IV.2	M	2 months	Idiopathic	+	Fatigue	?	
Tibbles and Barnes (1980)	1	M	4	Idiopathic	+	Ethanol, chocolate, caffeine	+	Clonazepam
Kinast *et al.* (1980)	4	M	8	Idiopathic	0	0	+	Carbamazepine
Coulter and Donofrio (1980)	1	M	19	Idiopathic	+	0	0	Haloperidol
	2	F	12	Idiopathic	+	0	0	Haloperidol Carbamazepine
Dunn (1981)	1	M	2	Idiopathic	0	0	0	

Table 16.7 (continued)

Authors	*Case no.*	*Sex*	*Age at onset*	*Aetiology*	*FH*	*Triggers*	*Sensory aura*	*Treatment*
Walker (1981)	1	M	Infancy	Idiopathic	+	Caffeine, alcohol, fatigue, exercise	0	Chlordiazepoxide
	2	F	Infancy	Idiopathic	0	As above	0	As above
Mayeux and Fahn (1982)	1	M	10	Hereditary ataxia	+	0	0	Acetazolamide Clonazepam
Przuntek and Monninger (1983)	4–18	6M 9F	?	Idiopathic Dopa → worse in 1; haloperidol → better in 7	+	Alcohol	+	Valproate
Kurlan and Shoulson (1983)	1	M	20	Idiopathic	+	0	+	Oxazepam
	2	F	24	Idiopathic	+	0	?	Oxazepam
Jacome and Risko (1984)	1	F	Teens	Idiopathic	+	Stress	0	
Kurlan *et al.* (1987)	III.4	F	6	Idiopathic	+	Cold, long exercise	0	Quinine
	IV6	M	15	Idiopathic	+	As above, heat	0	Benzodiazepines L-tryptophan
	V25	F	23	Idiopathic	+	Cold, exertion, long exercise	0	Benzodiazepines L-tryptophan
	(Cases IV6 and V25 were reported by Kurlan and Shoulson, above)							
Bressman *et al.* (1988)	1	F	3	Idiopathic	0	Stress	0	Carbamazepine
	2	M	6	Idiopathic	0	Laughing, etc.	0	Carbamazepine
	3	F	14	Idiopathic	0	Fatigue	0	Acetazolamide
	4	M	18	Idiopathic	0	Alcohol, stress, fatigue, heat	0	Acetazolamide (unsustained)
	5	M	27	Idiopathic	0	Awakening	0	
	6	F	29	Idiopathic	0		0	Remission
	7	F	30	Idiopathic	0	Fatigue, stress	0	Clonazepam
Nardocci *et al.* (1989)	2	M	1	Idiopathic	0	0	0	Clonazepam
Hughes *et al.* (1991)	1	M	16	Idiopathic	0	Tiredness, anxiety, fasting, alcohol, eating	+	
	2	M	20	Idiopathic	0	0	0	
Byrne *et al.* (1991)	III3	M	40	Idiopathic	+	Excitement, tension	+	
	III4	F	10	Idiopathic	+	Tension	+	
	IV1	F	Infancy	Idiopathic	+	Excitement, alcohol	+	
	IV2	M	13	Idiopathic	+	Emotion	?	
	V1	M	14	Idiopathic	+	?	?	

+ = Present or yes; 0 = absent or no; ? = no information given.
FH = Family history of similar attacks.

developed paroxysmal dystonia. The attacks could be precipitated by stress but not by movement, caffeine, cold, fatigue or hyperventilation. The episodes lasted from 30 minutes to 3 hours. They did not respond to anticonvulsants, but were abolished with trihexyphenidyl 20 mg/day. It is possible that the PDC in this youth represents a variant of tardive dystonia (Burke *et al.*, 1982; Kang *et al.*, 1986).

Table 16.8 Reports of symptomatic paroxysmal non-kinesigenic choreoathetosis/dystonia

Authors	*Case no.*	*Sex*	*Age at onset*	*Aetiology*	*FH*	*Triggers*	*Sensory aura*	*Treatment*
Matthews (1958)	3	F	26	Multiple sclerosis	0	0	+	
Joynt and Green (1962)	1	M	19	Multiple sclerosis	0	0	+	Phenytoin
	2	F	39	Multiple sclerosis	0	0	+	Phenytoin
	3	M	29	Multiple sclerosis	0	0	0	Remission
	4	M	31	Multiple sclerosis	0	During sleep	0	Phenytoin
Lance (1963)	1	F	12	Perinatal hypoxia (bouts also occur during sleep)	0	Fright	+	Anticonvulsants
	2	F	47	Multiple sclerosis	0		0	0
Mushet and Dreifuss (1967)	1	M	0.5	Encephalitis	0	Startle, excitement, sudden movement	?	Antimuscarinic
Cavanagh *et al.* (1974)	1	M	4	Cystinuria	+	0	0	
	2	M	4	Cystinuria	+	0	0	
Soffer *et al.* (1977)	1	F	17	Hypoparathyroidism	0	0	0	Vitamin D, Ca^{2+}
Fischbeck and Layzer (1979)	1	F	34	Thyrotoxic	0	0	0	Propylthiouracil
Margolin and Marsden (1982)	1	M	51	Transient ischaemic attacks	0	0	0	
	2	M	61	Transient ischaemic attacks	0	0	0	
	3	M	57	Transient ischaemic attacks	0	0	0	
	4	M	74	Transient ischaemic attacks	0	0	0	
Huffstutter and Meyers (1983)	1	F	4	Infantile hemiplegia	0	0	+	Anticonvulsants
	2	F	4	Infantile hemiplegia	0	Sudden touch	+	Anticonvulsants
Perlmutter and Raichle (1984)	1	M	50	Head injury	0	Stress	0	Phenytoin + trihexyphenidyl
Newman and Kinkel (1984)	1	F	45	Hypoglycaemia	0	0	0	Glucose
Berger *et al.* (1984)	2	F	55	Multiple sclerosis	0	0	+	Chlorazepate
	3	M	45	Multiple sclerosis	0	0	+	Remission
	6	M	17	Multiple sclerosis	0	0	0	Carbamazepine
	7	F	41	Multiple sclerosis	0	Hypogenic	0	Carbamazepine
	8	F	38	Multiple sclerosis	0	0	0	Remission
Sunohara *et al.* (1984)	1	M	61	Stroke	0	Any movement	0 0	Clonazepam + 5-hydroxy-tryptophan
Kawazawa *et al.* (1985)	1	F	38	Hypoparathyroidism	0	Emotion, caffeine, fatigue	0	Vitamin D, Ca^{2+}
translated by Yamamoto and Kawazawa (1987)								
Drake *et al.* (1986)	3	M	18	Head injury	0	0	0	Phenobarbitone

Table 16.8 (continued)

Authors	*Case no.*	*Sex*	*Age at onset*	*Aetiology*	*FH*	*Triggers*	*Sensory aura*	*Treatment*
Micheli *et al.* (1986)	1	F	37	Basal ganglia calcification	0	0	+	Clonazepam
Nath *et al.* (1987)	1	F	32	AIDS	0	0	?	
Erickson and Chun (1987)	1	F	16	Perinatal hypoxia	0	0	0	Phenytoin
	2	M	4	Perinatal hypoxia	0	0	0	Clonazepam
	3	F	15	Perinatal hypoxia	0	Excitement	0	Phenytoin
Micheli *et al.* (1987)	1	M	16	Dopamine blockers	0	Stress	0	Trihexyphenidyl
Haan *et al.* (1988)	1	F	80	Diabetes	0	0	0	
Bressman *et al.* (1988)	1	M	7 months	Perinatal hypoxia	+	Sleep	0	Carbamazepine
	2	F	8	Perinatal hypoxia	0	0	0	
	3	M	12	Perinatal hypoxia	0	0	0	
	4	M	24	Anoxia	0	0	0	
	5	M	28	Encephalitis	0	0	0	Clonazepam
	6	F	39	Ischaemia	0	0	0	
	7	F	61	Meningioma	0	0	0	
Bressman *et al.* (1988)	1	F	11	Psychogenic	0	0	0	Faith
	2	F	16	Psychogenic	0	0	0	Hypnotherapy
	3	M	22	Psychogenic	0	0	0	
	4	F	31	Psycgogenic	0	0	0	
	5	F	32	Psychogenic	0	0	0	
	6	M	32	Psychogenic	0	0	0	
	7	M	34	Psychogenic	0	0	0	Placebo
	8	F	35	Psychogenic	0	0	0	Psychotherapy
	9	F	36	Psychogenic	0	0	0	
	10	F	42	Psychogenic	0	0	0	Placebo
	11	F	49	Psychogenic	0	0	0	Placebo
Bennett and Fox (1989)	1	F	82	Transient ischaemic attacks	0	0	0	Aspirin
Winer *et al.* (1990)	1	F	58	Hypoglycaemia	0	Exercise, fasting	0	
Fahn and Williams (1988)	11	F	25	Psychogenic	0	Walking	0	Psychotherapy
	13	F	30	Psychogenic	0	0	0	Physiotherapy
	14	F	31	Psychogenic	0	0	0	Psychotherapy
	15	M	33	Psychogenic	0	Walking, various sudden stimuli	0	Placebo
	16	F	36	Psychogenic	0	0	0	Placebo
	17	F	36	Psychogenic	0	0	0	Suggestion, psychotherapy
	19	F	41	Psychogenic	0	Walking	0	Suggestion, placebo

+ = Present or yes; 0 = absent or no; ? = no information given.
FH = Family history of similar attacks.

A positron emission tomography study was performed on 1 patient with posttraumatic paroxysmal hemidystonia (Perlmutter and Raichle, 1984). Decreased oxygen metabolism, decreased oxygen extraction, increased blood volume, and increased blood flow in the contralateral basal ganglia were found.

Table 16.8 summarizes the reports of symptomatic PDC.

INTERMEDIATE PAROXYSMAL NON-KINESIGENIC DYSTONIC CHOREOATHETOSIS

Lance (1977) was the first to describe what he called an intermediate form of PDC. It was in a family in which the attacks were briefer than classical PDC, lasting from 5 to 30 minutes, and in which the attacks are precipitated by prolonged exercise and not by cold, heat, stress, alcohol, excitement or anxiety. The spasms affected mainly the legs. A second family was reported by Plant *et al.* (1984). In both families, the inheritance pattern was that of autosomal dominant transmission. A sporadic case was reported by Nardocci *et al.* (1989; case 3). This patient also had interictal chorea without any family history of a similar condition. This patient was the only one who was helped by clonazepam. The family of Plant *et al.* (1984), like Lance's family, derived no benefit from barbiturate, levodopa or clonazepam. Another sporadic case was recently reported (Wali, 1992); this was an 18-year-old man in whom attacks of right hemidystonia lasting about 10 times were precipitated by prolonged running (about 10 minutes) or by cold. The EEG and CT scan were normal, and anticonvulsants were not helpful.

The 7 reported cases (Table 16.9) consisted of 5 women and 2 men. The age at onset ranged from 2 to 20 years, with all but 2 beginning in childhood.

Table 16.9 Reports of intermediate paroxysmal non-kinesigenic choreoathetosis/dystonia (intermediate paroxysmal dystonic choreoathetosis)

Authors	*Case no.*	*Sex*	*Age at onset*	*Aetiology*	*FH*	*Triggers*	*Sensory aura*	*Treatment*
Lance	Second pedigree							
(1977)	I4	M	?	Idiopathic	+	Continuous exertion	0	
	II4	F	20	Idiopathic	+	Continuous exertion	0	
	III1	F	3	Idiopathic	+	Continuous exertion	0	
Plant *et al.* (1984)	1	F	2	Idiopathic	+	Continuous exertion, vibration, passive movement	0	
	2	F	3	Idiopathic	+	Continuous exertion, vibration, passive movement	0	
Nardocci *et al.* (1989)	3	F	2	Idiopathic	0	Continuous exertion	0	
Wali (1992)	1	M	18	Idiopathic	0	Continuous exertion, cold	0	

+ = Present or yes; 0 = absent or no; ? = no information given.
FH = Family history of similar attacks.

Table 16.10 Clinical features of paroxysmal kinesigenic choreoathetosis (PKC) and paroxysmal non-kinesigenic dystonic choreoathetosis (PDC)

Feature	*PKC*	*PDC*	*Intermediate*
Inheritance	Autosomal dominant	Autosomal dominant	Autosomal dominant
Male : female	3.75 : 1	1.4 : 1	2 : 5 (n=7)
Age at onset			
Range	<1–40	<1–30	2–20
Median	12	12	3
Mean	12	12	8
Attacks			
Duration	<5 minutes	2 min–4 hour	5–30 min
Frequency	100/day–1/month	3/day–2/year	1/day–2/month
Trigger	Sudden movement, startle, hyperventilation	Nil	Prolonged exercise, vibration, passive movement, cold
Precipitant	Stress	Alcohol, stress caffeine, fatigue	Stress
Treatment	Anticonvulsants acetazolamide, antimuscarinics	Clonazepam, benzodiazepines	0

Some patients labelled as PKC (e.g. cases 1 and 3 of Jung *et al.*, 1973) and PDC (e.g. the family of Kurlan *et al.*, 1987) have attacks that occur after prolonged exercise. It is possible that such patients may be a variant of intermediate PDC, or represent a combination of it and one of the other paroxysmal dyskinesias. However, if the attacks last only seconds and respond to anticonvulsants, they fit clinically with these features of PKC.

Table 16.10 lists the major distinguishing features of PKC, PDC and intermediate PDC.

MISCELLANY

There are probably a number of other types of paroxysmal dyskinesias that do not fit well into the classification scheme listed above. For example, a case of truncal flexion spasms that persist repeatedly in attacks lasting several hours has been described (Brown *et al.*, 1991). These were considered to be due to spinal origin, presumably involving the propriospinal pathways. I have seen a patient with multiple brief dystonic spasms, lasting seconds, in a woman following cardiac arrhythmias. These attacks have all the clinical features of symptomatic PKC, except that they were not precipitated by sudden movement or startle. Similar to PKC, they responded dramatically to low dosages of carbamazepine. Perhaps the major delimiter in classifying the paroxysmal dyskinesias should not be whether they are kinesigenic or not, but the duration of the attacks.

SUMMARY

The paroxysmal dyskinesias are usually divided into kinesigenic choreoathetosis/dystonia (which are induced by sudden movement and are brief in duration, lasting seconds to 5 minutes) and non-kinesigenic dystonia (which are longer in duration and not induced by sudden movement). The latter group is divided into the classical form (duration 2 minutes to 4 hours, up to 2 days) and intermediate form (duration 5–30 minutes). The classical form is often induced by alcohol, cold, heat, fatigue, caffeine and stress. The intermediate form is induced by prolonged exercise.

The kinesigenic variety ordinarily responds extremely well to a variety of anticonvulsants, whereas these drugs are usually not beneficial in the non-kinesigenic types. The latter are sometimes sensitive to clonazepam, benzodiazepines, acetazolamide, anticholinergics and neuroleptics.

Variants of these disorders are the paroxysmal dyskinesias that occur during sleep (hypnogenic paroxysmal dyskinesias) and the transient paroxysmal dystonias (particularly torticollis) in infants. The relationship of any of these different clinical varieties with each other is not clear.

References

Adam AM and Orinda D (1986) Focal paroxysmal kinesigenic choreoathetosis preceding the development of Steele–Richardson–Olszewski syndrome. *J Neurol Neurosurg Psychiatry*, **49**, 957–68

Aimard G, Vighetto A, Trillet M, Ventre JJ, and Devic M (1983) Ataxie paroxystique familiale sensible a l'acetazolamide. *Rev. Neurol (Paris)*, **139**, 251–7

Andermann F and Andermann E (1986) Excessive startle syndromes: startle disease, jumping, and startle epilepsy. *Adv Neurol*, **43**, 321–38

Andermann F, Cosgrove JBR, Lloyd-Smith D, and Watters AM (1959) Paroxysmal dysarthria and ataxia in multiple sclerosis: a report of 2 unusual cases. *Neurology*, **9**, 211–15

Angelini L, Rumi V, Lamperti E, and Nardocci N (1988) Transient paroxysmal dystonia in infancy. *Neuropediatrics*, **19**, 171–4

Arden F (1953) Idiopathic hypoparathyroidism. *Med J Aust*, **2**, 217–19

Bain PG, Larkin GBR, Calver DM, and O'Brien MD (1991) Persistent superior oblique paresis as a manifestation of familial periodic cerebellar ataxia. *Br J Ophthalmol*, **75**, 619–21

Bain PG, O'Brien MD, Keevil SF, and Porter DA (1992) Familial periodic cerebellar ataxia: a problem of cerebellar intracellular pH homeostasis. *Ann Neurol*, **31**, 147–54

Baloh RW and Winder A (1991) Acetazolamide-responsive vestibulocerebellar syndrome: clinical and oculographic features. *Neurology*, **41**, 429–33

Barabas G and Tucker SM (1988) Idiopathic hypoparathyroidism and paroxysmal dystonic choreoathetosis. *Ann Neurol*, **24**, 585

Baron DN, Dent CE, Harris H, Hart EW, and Jepson JB (1956) Hereditary pellagra-like skin rash with temporary cerebellar ataxia, constant renal amino-aciduria and other bizarre biochemical features. *Lancet*, **2**, 421–8

Bennett DA and Fox JH (1989) Paroxysmal dyskinesias secondary to cerebral vascular disease – reversal with aspirin. *Clin Neuropharmacol*, **12**, 215–16

Berger JR, Sheremata WA, and Melamed E (1984) Paroxysmal dystonia as the initial manifestation of multiple sclerosis. *Arch Neurol*, **41**, 747–50

Bird TD, Carlson CB, and Horning M (1978) Ten year follow-up of paroxysmal choreoathetosis: a sporadic case becomes familial. *Epilepsia*, **19**, 129–32

Blass JP, Avigan J, and Uhlendorf BW (1970) A defect in pyruvate decarboxylase in a child with an intermittent movement disorder. *J Clin Invest*, **49**, 423–32

Blass JP, Kark RAP, and Engel WK (1971) Clinical studies of a patient with pyruvate decarboxylase deficiency. *Arch Neurol*, **25**, 449–60

Boel M and Casaer P (1984) Paroxysmal kinesigenic choreoathetosis. *Neuropediatrics*, **15**, 215–17

Bortolotti P and Schoenhuber R (1983) Paroxysmal kinesigenic choreoathetosis. *Arch Neurol*, **40**, 529

Bourgeois M, Aicardi J, and Goutieres F (1993) Alternating hemiplegia of childhood. *J Pediatr*, **122**, 673–9
Bratt HD and Menelaus MB (1992) Benign paroxysmal torticollis of infancy. *J Bone Joint Surg*, **74**, 449–51
Bressman SB, Fahn S, and Burke RE (1988) Paroxysmal non-kinesigenic dystonia. *Adv Neurol*, **50**, 403–13
Brody IA, Odom GL, and Kunkle EC (1960) Pilomotor seizures: report of a case associated with a cerebral glioma. *Neurology*, **10**, 993–7
Brown P, Thompson PD, Rothwell JC, Day BL, and Marsden CD (1991) Paroxysmal axial spasms of spinal origin. *Movement Disorders*, **6**, 43–8
Brunt ERP and Van Weerden TW (1990) Familial paroxysmal kinesigenic ataxia and continuous myokymia. *Brain*, **113**, 1361–82
Buchman AS, Goetz CG, and Klawans HL (1988) Hemiparkinsonism with hemiatrophy. *Neurology*, **38**, 527–30
Burger LJ, Lopez RI, and Elliott FA (1972) Tonic seizures induced by movement. *Neurology*, **22**, 656–9
Burguera JA, Catala J, and Casanova B (1991) Thalamic demyelination and paroxysmal dystonia in multiple sclerosis. *Movement Disorders*, **6**, 379–81
Burke RE, Fahn S, Jankovic J, Marsden CD, Lang AE, Gollomp S *et al.* (1982) Tardive dystonia: late-onset and persistent dystonia caused by antipsychotic drugs. *Neurology*, **32**, 1335–46
Byrne E, White O, and Cook M (1991) Familial dystonic choreoathetosis with myokymia; a sleep responsive disorder. *J Neurol Neurosurg Psychiatry*, **54**, 1090–2
Camac A, Greene P, and Khandji A (1990) Paroxysmal kinesigenic dystonic choreoathetosis associated with a thalamic infarct. *Movement Disorders*, **5**, 235–8
Cavanagh NP, Bicknell J, and Howard F (1974) Cystinuria with mental retardation and paroxysmal dyskinesia in 2 brothers. *Arch Dis Child*, **49**, 662–4
Coulter DL and Donofrio P (1980) Haloperidol for nonkinesiogenic paroxysmal dyskinesia. *Arch Neurology*, **37**, 325–6
Crowell JA and Anders TF (1985) Hypnogenic paroxysmal dystonia. *J Am Acad Child Psychiatry*, **24**, 353–8
Dancis J, Hutzler J, and Rokkones T (1967) Intermittent branched-chain ketonuria: variant of maple-syrup-urine disease. *N Engl J Med*, **276**, 84–9
DeBolt WL (1967) Movement epilepsy: two case reports with photographs of typical movements. *Bull Los Angeles Neurol Soc*, **32**, 1–5
DeCastro W and Campbell J (1967) Periodic ataxia. *JAMA*, **200**, 892–4
Deonna T, Roulet E, and Meyer HU (1990) Benign paroxysmal tonic upgaze of childhood – a new syndrome. *Neuropediatrics*, **21**, 213–14
Donat JR and Auger R (1979) Familial periodic ataxia. *Arch Neurol*, **36**, 568–9
Donat JF and Wright FS (1990) Episodic symptoms mistaken for seizures in the neurologically impaired child. *Neurology*, **40**, 156–7
Dowzenko A and Zielinsky JJ (1966) Unusual case of epilepsy and akinetic and tonic seizures induced by movement. *Epilepsia*, **7**, 233–7
Dorland's Medical Dictionary (25th ed.) (1976) WB Saunders, Philadelphia
Drake ME Jr, Jackson RD, and Miller CA (1986) Paroxysmal choreoathetosis after head injury. *J Neurol, Neurosurg Psychiatry*, **49**, 837–43
Duchowny MS, Resnick TJ, Deray MJ, and Alvarez LA (1988) Video EEG diagnosis of repetitive behavior in early childhood and its relationship to seizures. *Pediatr Neurol*, **4**, 162–4
Dunn DW (1981) Paroxysmal dystonia. *Am J Dis Child*, **135**, 381–2
Echenne B and Rivier F (1992) Benign paroxysmal tonic upward gaze. *Pediatr Neurol*, **8**, 154–5
Erickson GR and Chun RW (1987) Acquired paroxysmal movement disorders. *Pediatr Neurol*, **3**, 226–9
Espir MLE, Watkins SM, and Smith HV (1966) Paroxysmal dysarthria and other transient neurological disturbances in disseminated sclerosis. *J Neurol, Neurosurg Psychiatry*, **29**, 323–30
Factor SA, Coni RJ, Cowger M, and Rosenblum EL (1991) Paroxysmal tremor and orofacial dyskinesia secondary to a biopterin synthesis defect. *Neurology*, **41**, 930–2
Fahn S (1983) Paroxysmal tremor. *Neurology*, **33** (suppl 2), 131
Fahn S (1984) Atypical tremors, rare tremors, and unclassified tremors. In Findley LJ and Capildeo R, eds, *Movement Disorders: Tremor*, New York, Oxford University, 431–43
Fahn S and Williams DT (1988) Psychogenic dystonia. *Adv Neurol*, **50**, 431–55
Fahn S, Marsden CD, and Van Woert MH (1986) Definition and clinical classification of myoclonus. *Adv Neurol*, **43**, 1–5
Falconer M, Driver M, and Serafetinides E (1963) Seizures induced by movement: report of a case relieved by operation. *J Neurol, Neurosurg Psychiatry*, **26**, 300–7
Farmer TW and Mustian VM (1963) Vestibulocerebellar ataxia. *Arch Neurol*, **8**, 471–80
Fischbeck KH and Layzer RB (1979) Paroxysmal choreoathetosis associated with thyrotoxicosis. *Ann Neurol*, **6**, 453–4
Forssman H (1961) Hereditary disorder characterized by attacks of muscular contractions, induced by

alcohol amongst other factors. *Acta Med Scand*, **170**, 517–33

Frankel M and Cummings JL (1984) Neuro-ophthalmic abnormalities in Tourette's syndrome: functional and anatomic implications. *Neurology*, **34**, 359–61

Franssen H, Fortgens C, Wattendorff AR, and van Woerkom TCAM (1983) Paroxysmal kinesigenic choreoathetosis and abnormal contingent negative variation. A case report. *Arch Neurol*, **40**, 381–5

Fuh JL, Chang DB, Wang SJ, Ju TH, and Liu HC (1991) Painful tonic spasms: an interesting phenomenon in cerebral ischemia. *Acta Neurol Scand*, **84**, 534–6

Fukuyama S and Okada R (1967) Hereditary kinesthetic reflex epilepsy. Report of five families of peculiar seizures induced by sudden movements. *Adv Neurol Sci (Tokyo)*, **11**, 168–97

Gancher ST and Nutt JG (1986) Autosomal dominant episodic ataxia: a heterogeneous syndrome. *Movement Disorders*, **1**, 239–53

Garello L, Ottonello GA, Regesta G, and Tanganelli P (1983) Familial paroxysmal kinesigenic choreoathetosis: report of a pharmacological trial in 2 cases. *Eur Neurol*, **22**, 217–21

George MS, Pickett JB, Kohli H, Allison MA, and Pritchard P (1990) Paroxysmal dystonic reflex choreoathetosis after minor closed head injury. *Lancet*, **336**, 1134–5

Gilroy J (1982) Abnormal computed tomograms in paroxysmal kinesigenic choreoathetosis. *Arch Neurol*, **39**, 779–80

Godbout R, Montplaisir J, and Rouleau I (1985) Hypnogenic paroxysmal dystonia: epilepsy or sleep disorder? A case report. *Clin Electroencephal*, **16**, 136–42

Goodenough DJ, Fariello RG, Annis BL, and Chun RW (1978) Familial and acquired paroxysmal dyskinesias. A proposed classification with delineation of clinical features. *Arch Neurol*, **35**, 827–31

Gorard DA and Gibberd FB (1989) Paroxysmal dysarthria and ataxia-associated MRI abnormality. *J Neurol Neurosurg Psychiatry*, **52**, 1444–5

Gourley IM (1971) Paroxysmal torticollis in infancy. *Can Med Assoc J*, **105**, 504–5

Gowers WR (1885) *Epilepsy and Other Chronic Convulsive Diseases. Their Causes, Symptoms and Treatment*, New York, Dover (Reprint of 1885 edition); 1964, 75–6

Griggs RC, Moxley RT III, Lafrance RA, and McQuillen J (1978) Hereditary paroxysmal ataxia: response to acetazolamide. *Neurology*, **28**, 1259–64

Haan J, Kremer HPH, and Padberg G (1988) Paroxysmal choreoathetosis as presenting symptom of diabetes mellitus. *J Neurol, Neurosurg Psychiatry*, **52**, 133

Hallett M, Marsden CD, and Fahn S (1987) Myoclonus. In *Handbook of Clinical Neurology* (eds Vinken PVJ, Bruyn GU and Klawans HL) *vol 49, Extrapyramidal Disorders*, Amsterdam, Elsevier, 609–25

Hanson PA, Martinez LB, and Cassidy R (1977) Contractures, continuous muscle discharges, and titubation. *Ann Neurol*, **1**, 120–4

Hawkes CH (1992) Familial paroxysmal ataxia: report of a family. *J Neurol Neurosurg Psychiatry*, **55**, 212–13

Hill W and Sherman H (1986) Acute intermittent familial cerebellar ataxia. *Arch Neurol*, **18**, 350–7

Hirata K, Katayama S, Saito T, Ichihashi K, Mukai T, Kayama M *et al.* (1991) Paroxysmal kinesigenic choreoathetosis with abnormal electroencephalogram during attacks. *Epilepsia*, **32**, 492–4

Hishikawa Y, Furuya E, Yamamoto J, and Nan'no H (1973) Dystonic seizures induced by movement. *Arch Psychiatrie Nervenkr*, **217**, 113–38

Holmes GL and Russman BS (1986) Shuddering attacks: evaluation using electroencephalographic frequency modulation radiotelemetry and videotape monitoring. *Am J Dis Child*, **140**, 72–3

Homan RW, Vasko MR, and Blaw M (1980) Phenytoin plasma concentrations in paroxysmal kinesigenic choreoathetosis. *Neurology*, **30**, 673–6

Horner FH and Jackson LC (1969) Familial paroxysmal choreoathetosis. In Barbeau A and Brunette J-R, eds, *Progress in Neuro-Genetics*, Amsterdam, Excerpta Medica Foundation, 745–51

Hudgins RL and Corbin KB (1966) An uncommon seizure disorder: familial paroxysmal choreoathetosis. *Brain*, **89**, 199–204

Huffstutter WM and Myers GJ (1983) Paroxysmal motor dysfunction. *Ala J Med Sci*, **20**, 311–13

Hughes AJ, Lees AJ, and Marsden CD (1991) Paroxysmal dystonic head tremor. *Movement Disorders*, **6**, 85–6

Jacome DE and Risko M (1984) Photic induced-driven PLEDs in paroxysmal dystonic choreoathetosis. *Clin Electroencephalog*, **15**, 151–4

Joynt RJ and Green D (1962) Tonic seizures as a manifestation in multiple sclerosis. *Arch Neurol*, **6**, 293–9

Jung S-S, Chen K-M, and Brody JA (1973) Paroxysmal choreoathetosis: report of Chinese cases. *Neurology*, **23**, 749–55

Kang UJ, Burke RE, and Fahn S (1986) Natural history and treatment of tardive dystonia. *Movement Disorders*, **1**, 193–208

Kato M and Araki S (1969) Paroxysmal kinesigenic choreoathetosis. Report of a case relieved by carbamazepine. *Arch Neurol*, **20**, 508–13

Kawazawa S, Nogaki H, Hara T, Kodama K, and Hirata I (1985) Paroxysmal dystonic choreoathetosis in a case of pesudoidiopathic hypoparathyroidism. Rinsho Shinkeigaku, **25**, 1152–8. Reported by Yamamoto and Kawazawa (1987) *Ann Neurol*, **22**, 556

Keane JR (1984) Galloping tongue: post-traumatic, episodic, rhythmic movements. *Neurology*, **34**, 251–2

Kertesz A (1967) Paroxysmal kinesigenic choreoathetosis. An entity within the paroxysmal choreoathetosis syndrome. Description of 10 cases, including 1 autopsied. *Neurology*, **17**, 680–90

Kinast M, Erenberg G, and Rothner AD (1980) Paroxysmal choreoathetosis: report of five cases and review of the literature. *Pediatrics*, **65**, 74–7

Kishimoto K (1975) A novel case of conditionally responsive extrapyramidal syndrome. In *Annual Report of the Research Institute of Environmental Medicine at Nagoya University*, vol 6, 91–101

Koller W and Bahamon-Dussan J (1987) Hereditary paroxysmal cerebellopathy: responsiveness to acetazolamide. *Clin Neuropharmacol*, **10**, 65–8

Koller WC and Biary NM (1989) Volitional control of involuntary movements. *Movement Disorders*, **4**, 153–6

Kotagal P, Luders H, Morris HH, Dinner DS, Wyllie E, Godoy J *et al.* (1989) Dystonic posturing in complex partial seizures of temporal lobe onset: a new lateralizing sign. *Neurology*, **39**, 196–201

Kurlan R and Shoulson I (1983) Familial paroxysmal dystonic choreoathetosis and response to alternate-day oxazepam therapy. *Ann Neurol*, **13**, 456–7

Kurlan R, Behr J, Medved L, and Shoulson I (1987) Familial paroxysmal dystonic choreoathetosis: a family study. *Movement Disorders*, **2**, 187–92

Lance JW (1963) Sporadic and familial varieties of tonic seizures. *J Neurol Neurosurg Psychiatry*, **26**, 51–9

Lance JW (1977) Familial paroxysmal dystonic choreoathetosis and its differentiation from related syndromes. *Ann Neurol*, **2**, 285–93

Lang AE (1984) Focal paroxysmal kinesigenic choreoathetosis. *J Neurol Neurosurg Psychiatry*, **47**, 1057–60

Lee BI, Lesser RP, Pippenger CE, Morris HH, Luders H, Dinner DS *et al.* (1985) Familial paroxysmal hypnogenic dystonia. *Neurology*, **35**, 1357–60

Lehkuniec E, Micheli F, De Arbelaiz R, Torres M, and Paradiso G (1988) Concurrent hypnogenic and reflex paroxysmal dystonia. *Movement Disorders*, **3**, 290–4

Lipson EH and Robertson WC Jr (1978) Paroxysmal torticollis of infancy: familiar occurrence. *Am J Dis Child*, **132**, 422–3

Lishman WA, Symonds CD, Whitty CW, and Wilson RG (1962) Seizures induced by movement. *Brain*, **85**, 93–108

Lonsdale D, Faulkner WR, Price JW, and Smeby RR (1969) Intermittent cerebellar ataxia associated with hyperpyruvic acidemia, hyperalaninemia, and hyperalaninuria. *Pediatrics*, **43**, 1025–34

Loong SC and Ong YY (1973) Paroxysmal kinesigenic choreoathetosis: report of a case relieved by L-dopa. *J Neurol Neurosurg Psychiatry*, **36**, 921–4

Lou HC (1989) Flunarizine in paroxysmal choreoathetosis. *Neuropediatrics*, **20**, 112

Lugaresi E and Cirignotta F (1981) Hypnogenic paroxysmal dystonia: epileptic seizure or a new syndrome? *Sleep*, **4**, 129–38

Lugaresi E, Cirignotta F, and Montagna P (1986) Nocturnal paroxymal dystonia. *J Neurol, Neurosurg Psychiatry*, **49**, 375–80

Maccario M and Lustman LI (1990) Paroxysmal nocturnal dystonia presenting as excessive daytime somnolence. *Arch Neurol*, **47**, 291–4

MacLean JB and Sassin JF (1973) Paroxysmal vertical ocular dyskinesia. *Arch Neurol*, **29**, 117–19

Margolin DL and Marsden CD (1982) Episodic dyskinesias and transient cerebral ischemia. *Neurology*, **32**, 1379–80

Martinelli P and Gabellini AS (1991) A 19th century description of paroxysmal kinesiogenic choreoathetosis. *J Neurol Neurosurg Psychiatry*, **54**, 475

Matthews WB (1958) Tonic seizures in disseminated sclerosis. *Brain*, **81**, 193–206

Mayeux R and Fahn S (1982) Paroxysmal dystonic choreoathetosis in a patient with familial ataxia. *Neurology*, **32**, 1184–6

Meierkord H, Fish DR, Smith SJM, Scott CA, Shorvon SD, and Marsden CD (1992) Is nocturanl paroxysmal dystonia a form of frontal lobe epilepsy? *Movement Disorders*, **7**, 38–42

Menkes JH and Ament ME (1988) Neurologic disorders of gastroesophageal function. *Adv Neurol*, **49**, 409–16

Merchut MP and Brumlik J (1986) Painful tonic spasms caused by putaminal infarction. *Stroke*, **17**, 1319–21

Michaux M and Granier M (1945) Epilepsie bravais-jacksonienne reflexe: debut crural des crises:

intervention constante dans leur declanchement de contractions musculaires du membre inferieur du meme cote. *Ann Medicopsychol* (*Paris*), **103**, 172–7

Micheli F, Fernandez Pardal MM, Casas Parera I, and Giannaula R (1986) Sporadic paroxysmal dystonic choreoathetosis associated with basal ganglia calcifications. *Ann Neurol*, **20**, 750

Micheli F, Fernandez Pardal M, de Arbelaiz R, Lehkuniec E, and Giannaula R (1987) Paroxysmal dystonia responsive to anticholinergic drugs. *Clin Neuropharmacol*, **10**, 365–9

Miley CE and Forster FM (1974) Paroxysmal signs and symptoms in multiple sclerosis. *Neurology*, **24**, 458–61

Montagna P, Sforza E, Tinuper P, Cirignotta F, and Lugaresi E (1990) Paroxysmal arousals during sleep. *Neurology*, **40**, 1063–6

Morley JB (1970) Movement induced epilepsy: three case reports and comparison with a case of hemiballismus. *Proc Aust Assoc Neurol*, **7**, 19–24

Mount LA and Reback S (1940) Familial paroxysmal choreoathetosis. *Arch Neurol Psychiatry*, **44**, 841–7

Mushet GR and Dreifuss FE (1967) Paroxysmal dyskinesia. A case responsive to benztropine mesylate. *Arch Dis Child*, **42**, 654–6

Nair KR, Bhaskaran R, and Marsden CD (1991) Essential tremor associated with paroxysmal kinesigenic dystonia. *Movement Disorders*, **6**, 92–3

Nardocci N, Lamperti E, Rumi V, and Angelini L (1989) Typical and atypical forms of paroxysmal choreoathetosis. *Dev Med Child Neurol*, **31**, 670–4

Nath A, Jankovic J, and Pettigrew LC (1987) Movement disorders and AIDS. *Neurology*, **37**, 37–41

Newman RP and Kinkel WR (1984) Paroxysmal choreoathetosis due to hypoglycemia. *Arch Neurol*, **41**, 341–2

Newton MR, Berkovic SF, Austin MC, Reutens DC, Mckay WJ, and Bladin PF (1992) Dystonia, clinical lateralization, and regional blood flow changes in temporal lobe seizures. *Neurology*, **42**, 371–7

Nightingale S and Barton ME (1991) Intermittent vertical supranuclear ophthalmoplegia and ataxia. *Movement Disorders*, **6**, 76–8

Nijssen PCG and Tijssen CC (1992) Stimulus-sensitive paroxysmal dyskinesias associated with a thalamic infarct. *Movement Disorders*, **7**, 364–6

Ouvrier RA and Billson MD (1988) Benign paroxysmal tonic upgaze of childhood. *J Child Neurol*, **3**, 177–80

Parker HL (1946) Periodic ataxia. *Mayo Clin Proc*, **38**, 642–5

Perez-Borja C, Tassinari AC, and Swanson AG (1967) Paroxysmal choreoathetosis and seizure induced by movement (reflex epilepsy). *Epilepsia*, **8**, 260–70

Perlmutter JS and Raichle ME (1984) Pure hemidystonia with basal ganglia abnormalities on positron emission tomography. *Ann Neurol*, **15**, 228–33

Pitha V (1938) Epilepsie reflexe. *Rev Neurol* (*Paris*), **70**, 178–81

Plant G (1983) Focal paroxysmal kinesigenic choreoathetosis. *J Neurol Neurosurg Psychiatry*, **46**, 345–8

Plant GT, Williams AC, Earl CJ, and Marsden CD (1984) Familial paroxysmal dystonia induced by exercise. *J Neurol Neurosurg Psychiatry*, **47**, 275–9

Pryles CV, Livington S, and Ford FR (1952) Familial peroxysmal choreoathetosis of Mount and Reback. *Pediatrics*, **8**, 44–7

Przuntek H and Monninger P (1983) Therapeutic aspects of kinesigenic paroxysmal choreoathetosis and familial paroxysmal choreoathetosis of the Mount and Reback type. *J Neurol*, **230**, 163–9

Rajna P, Kundar O, and Halasz P (1983) Vigilance level-dependent tonic seizures: epilepsy or sleep disorder? A case report. *Epilepsia*, **24**, 725–33

Richards RN and Barnett HJ (1968) Paroxysmal dystonic choreoathetosis. A family study and review of the literature. *Neurology*, **18**, 461–9

Richardson JC, Howes JL, Celinski MJ, and Allman RG (1987) Kinesigenic choreoathetosis due to brain injury. *Can J Neurol Sci*, **14**, 626–8

Robin JJ (1977) Paroxysmal choreoathetosis following head injury. *Ann Neurol*, **2**, 447–8

Roos R, Wintzen AR, Vielvoye G, and Polder TW (1991) Paroxysmal kinesiogenic choreoathetosis as presenting symptom of multiple sclerosis. *J Neurol Neurosurg Psychiatry*, **54**, 657–8

Rosen JA (1964) Paroxysmal choreoathetosis. Associated with perinatal hypoxic encephalopathy. *Arch Neurol*, **11**, 385–7

Rowland LP (1989) Familial periodic paralysis. In Rowland LP, ed, *Merritt's Textbook of Neurology*, 8th edn, Philadelphia, Lea & Febiger, 720–4

Sanner G and Bergstrom B (1979) Benign paroxysmal torticollis in infancy. *Acta Paediatr Scand*, **68**, 219–23

Sellal F, Hirsch E, Maquet P, Salmon E, Franck G, Collard M *et al.* (1991) Postures et mouvements anormaux paroxystiques au cours du sommeil: dystonie paroxystique hypnogenique ou epilepsie partielle? (Abnormal paroxysmal movements during sleep: hypnogenic paroxysmal dystonia or focal epilepsy?) *Rev Neurol*, **147**, 121–8

Sethi KD, Hess DC, Huffnagle VH, and Adams RJ (1992) Acetazolamide treatment of paroxysmal dystonia in central demyelinating disease. *Neurology*, **42**, 919–21

Smith LA and Heersema PH (1941) Periodic dystonia. *Staff Meet Mayo Clin*, **16**, 842–6

Snyder CH (1969) Paroxysmal torticollis in infancy. *Am J Dis Child*, **117**, 458–60

Soffer D, Licht A, Yaar I, and Abramsky O (1977) Paroxysmal choreoathetosis as a presenting symptom in idiopathic hypoparathyroidism. *J Neurol Neurosurg Psychiatry*, **40**, 692–4

Spiller WG (1927) Subcortical epilepsy. *Brain*, **50**, 171–87

Sterling W (1924) Le type spasmodique tetanoide et tetaniforme de l'encephalite epidemique remarques sur l'epilepsie "extra-pyramidale". *Rev Neurol (Paris)*, **2**, 484–92

Stevens H (1966) Paroxysmal choreo-athetosis. A form of reflex epilepsy. *Arch Neurol*, **14**, 415–20

Strauss H (1940) Jacksonian seizures of reflex orign. *Arch Neurol Psychiatry*, **44**, 140–52

Suber DA and Riley TL (1980) Valproic acid and normal computerized tomographic scan in kinesigenic familial paroxysmal choreoathetosis. *Arch Neurol*, **37**, 327

Sunohara N, Mukoyama M, Mano Y, and Satoyoshi E (1984) Action-induced rhythmic dystonia: an autopsy case. *Neurology*, **34**, 321–7

Tabaee-Zadeh MJ, Frame B, and Kapphahn K (1972) Kinesiogenic choreoathetosis and idiopathic hypoparathyroidism. *N Engl J Med*, **286**, 762–3

Tartara A, Manni R, and Piccolo G (1988) A long-lasting CBZ controlled case of hypnogenic paroxysmal dystonia. *Ital J Neurol Sci*, **9**, 73–6

Tassinari CA, and Fine RD (1969) Paroxysmal choreoathetosis. *Proc Aust Ass Neurol*, **6**, 71–5

Tibbles JA and Barnes SE (1980) Paroxysmal dystonic choreoathetosis of Mount and Reback. *Pediatrics*, **65**, 149–51

Tinuper P, Cerullo A, Cirignotta F, Cortelli P, Lugaresi E, and Montagna P (1990) Nocturnal paroxysmal dystonia with short-lasting attacks: three cases with evidence for an epileptic frontal lobe origin of seizures. *Epilepsia*, **31**, 549–56

Vaamonde J, Artieda J, and Obeso JA (1991) Hereditary paroxysmal ataxia with neuromyotonia. *Movement Disorders*, **6**, 180–2

Van Dyke DH, Griggs RC, Murphy MJ, and Goldstein MN (1975) Hereditary myokymia and periodic ataxia. *J Neurol Sci*, **25**, 109–18

Verheul GAM and Tyssen CC (1990) Multiple sclerosis occurring with paroxysmal unilateral dystonia. *Movement Disorders*, **5**, 352–3

Vighetto A, Froment JC, Trillet M, and Aimard G (1988) Magnetic resonance imaging in familial paroxysmal ataxia. *Arch Neurol*, **45**, 547–9

Vincent FM (1986) Hyperglycemia-induced hemichoreoathetosis: the presenting manifestation of a vascular malformation of the lenticular nucleus. *Neurosurgery*, **18**, 787–90

Wali GM (1992) Paroxysmal hemidystonia induced by prolonged exercise and cold. *J Neurol Neurosurg Psychiatry*, **55**, 236–7

Walker ES (1981) Familial paroxysmal dystonic choreoathetosis: a neurologic disorder simulating psychiatric illness. *Johns Hopkins Med J*, **148**, 108–13

Waller DA (1977) Paroxysmal kinesigenic choreoathetosis or hysteria? *Am J Psychiatry*, **134**, 1439–40

Watson RT and Scott WR (1979) Paroxysmal kinesigenic choreoathetosis and brain-stem atrophy. *Arch Neurol*, **36**, 522

Weber MB (1967) Familial paroxysmal dystonia. *J Nerv Mental Dis*, **145**, 221–6

Websters's Third International Dictionary (1966) G and C Merriam Co., Springfield, MA

White JC (1969) Familial periodic nystagmus, vertigo, and ataxia. *Arch Neurol*, **20**, 276–80

Whitty CWM, Lishman WA, and FitzGibbon JP (1964) Seizures induced by movement: a form of reflex epilepsy. *Lancet*, **1**, 1403–6

Williams J and Stevens H (1963) Familial paroxysmal chorea-athetosis. *Pediatrics*, **31**, 656–9

Wilson SAK (1930) The Morrison Lectures on nervous semeiology, with special reference to epilepsy. Lecture III. Symptoms indicating increase of neural function. *Br Med J*, **2**, 90–4

Wimmer A (1925) Etudes sur les syndromes extra-pyramidaux: spasm de torsion infantile debutant par crises d'hemispasmes toniques (epilepsie striee). *Rev Neurol (Paris)*, **32**, 281–95

Winer JB, Fish DR, Sawyers D, and Marsden CD (1990) A movement disorder as a presenting feature of recurrent hypoglycaemia. *Movement Disorders*, **5**, 176–7

Yamamoto K and Kawazawa S (1987) Basal ganglion calcification in paroxysmal dystonic choreoathetosis. *Ann Neurol*, **22**, 556

Yokochi K (1991) Paroxysmal ocular downward deviation in neurologically impaired infants. *Pediatr Neurol*, **7**, 426–8

Zacchetti O, Sozzi G, and Zampollo A (1983) Paroxysmal kinesigenic choreoathetosis. Case report. *Ital J Neurol Sci*, **3**, 345–7

Zasorin NL, Baloh RW, and Myers LB (1983) Acetazolamide-responsive episodic ataxia syndrome. *Neurology*, **33**, 1212–14

17
Epilepsy masquerading as a movement disorder

D. R. Fish and C. David Marsden

INTRODUCTION

Epileptic attacks that involve loss of awareness, generalized tonic–clonic activity or other well-recognized seizure patterns present little diagnostic difficulty. However, when these features are absent, and motor phenomena predominate, epilepsy may mimic various movement disorders, leading to diagnostic uncertainties and management difficulties. Furthermore, in precisely such cases the limitations of scalp electroencephalogram (EEG) are the most apparent: only 15–25% of simple partial seizures are associated with scalp EEG changes (Lieb *et al*., 1976; Devinsky *et al*., 1988). In recent years this problem has been exemplified by the difficulties posed by the frontal lobe epilepsies. These may present with bizarre motor attacks, sometimes involving all four limbs, without loss of consciousness and with apparently normal interictal and ictal scalp EEGs.

The overlapping manifestations of epilepsy and movement disorders should not be unexpected given the major pathways connecting cortical areas often involved in seizure generation with the primary and supplementary motor regions, inferior parietal lobule, basal ganglia and brainstem.

Patients presenting with dyskinesias may be divided into three diagnostic categories: nocturnal motor attacks; paroxysmal daytime motor attacks, and persistent dyskinesias. Each of these manifestations may be mimicked by particular forms of epilepsy (Table 17.1).

Awareness of these presentations of epilepsies in the setting of patients referred with movement disorders is important. Consideration will be given to useful diagnostic features which may help in identifying those children and adults whose motor attacks have an epileptic basis. The special diagnostic problems presented by infants with motor attacks will not be discussed in this chapter. To date the possibility of utilizing this overlap to explore the basic mechanisms responsible for dyskinesias has received surprisingly little attention: the similar clinical semiology may suggest either a shared common final pathway of expression or dual involvement at the same or different parts of specific circuits.

Table 17.1 Dyskinesias mimicked by epilepsy

Dyskinesia	*Epilepsy*
Nocturnal motor attacks	Mesial frontal seizures Other partial/generalized seizures
Paroxysmal daytime attacks	Startle/movement-induced motor seizures Mesial frontal seizures Other partial seizures Epileptic drop attacks
Persistent daytime dyskinesias	Epilepsia partialis continua Progressive myoclonic epilepsies Juvenile myoclonic epilepsy Other myoclonic epilepsies*

*It is recognized that any of the myoclonic epilepsies may also present with discrete motor attacks.

NOCTURNAL MOTOR ATTACKS

The range of disorders which may present with nocturnal motor attacks is shown in Table 17.2. The non-epileptic causes will be considered briefly in order to emphasize their distinction from mesial frontal or other seizure disorders.

Two sorts of physiological jerks occur in normal subjects prior to or during sleep. Physiological hypnic jerks are usually of large amplitude, and involve the whole body. They typically occur during presleep wakefulness (Oswald, 1959), rather than during sleep itself. Fragmentary physiological jerks are usually of small amplitude and are limited to the hands or face (De Lisi, 1932). Unlike hypnic jerks, these multifocal twitches occur during stages 1, 2 and rapid eye movement (REM) sleep.

Periodic movements of sleep (PMS) may occur in otherwise healthy adults, particularly in the elderly. They may be associated with a broad range of sleep disorders (e.g. sleep apnoea, narcolepsy; Coleman *et al.*, 1980). PMS are nearly always present in the restless leg syndrome (Lugaresi *et al.*, 1986a), but most patients with PMS do not complain of restless legs. The restless leg syndrome may present in adolescence, as a hereditary condition with autosomal dominant transmission (Walters *et al.*, 1986). However, in patients under the age of 30 years presenting with PMS, particularly with a negative family history, consideration should be given to associated pathology, such as a neuropathy, radiculopathy or spinal cord lesion. The movements are characterized by dorsiflexion of the ankle, fanning of the toes and sometimes flexion of the knee and hip. These are not myoclonic but consist of spasms lasting for 3–5 seconds, and occur at intervals of 15–60 seconds. Their features have been documented by electromyogram (Lugaresi *et al.*, 1986a) and video studies (Smith, 1985). One or both legs may be affected. Rarely there are associated upper limb movements. They usually occur in clusters, lasting for several minutes up to half an hour. They are commonest during light non-REM sleep, but occasional patients also display periodic lower limb movements or other dyskinesias during wakefulness (Hening *et al.*, 1986).

Sleep-walking and night terrors are commonest in children and adolescents, possibly reflecting a disorder of the maturaing arousal mechanisms (Broughton, 1968).

Table 17.2 Causes of nocturnal motor attacks

Mesial frontal seizures
Other partial or generalized seizures
Physiological hypnic jerks
Physiological fragmentary myoclonus
Periodic movements of sleep
Sleep walking/night terrors
REM sleep behaviour disorder
Pathological fragmentary myoclonus
Sleep apnoea
Jactatio capitis/corpora
L-dopa-induced myoclonic attacks

REM = Rapid eye movement.

They arise from slow-wave sleep, and most often occur between 30 and 90 minutes after sleep onset.

Conversely, REM sleep behaviour disorders usually affect the elderly, and may be associated with depression, excess alcohol ingestion, or other central nervous system disorders, particularly if brainstem structures are involved. This condition results from a loss of the normal muscle atonia of REM sleep, and therefore occurs principally during early-morning sleep. The attacks usually involve vocalization and violent or aggressive actions that may reflect 'the acting out of dreams' (Schenck *et al.*, 1987).

Pathological non-REM fragmentary myoclonus differs from physiological fragmentary myoclonus by its severity, occurrence often throughout non-REM sleep (i.e. including stages 3 and 4) but not usually in REM sleep, and association with other sleep disorders (Broughton *et al.*, 1985).

Sleep apnoea may present as nocturnal restlessness, with grunting and flailing movements. Occasionally there may be secondary anoxic seizures. Jactatio capitis/corpora is characterized by nocturnal rocking movements of the head or body (Drake, 1986). These occur during presleep wakefulness and may persist variably into sleep, sometimes associated with vocalizations. Drug-related nocturnal attacks include L-dopa-induced whole-body myoclonic attacks during sleep in patients with Parkinson's disease (Klawans *et al.*, 1975).

The presentation of mesial frontal epilepsy during sleep has been the cause of much confusion. Lugaresi and Cirignota (1981) introduced the term nocturnal paroxysmal dystonia to describe a group of 5 patients with frequent brief motor attacks arising from non-REM sleep. The movements were predominantly dystonic, but could include chorea, myoclonus or ballism. Interictal and ictal scalp EEGs failed to show any epileptiform abnormalities. Subsequent publications from various centres described similar cases (Table 17.3). However, it is likely that this syndrome is due to mesial frontal lobe epilepsy: the clinical and ictal features are indistinguishable from known frontal lobe cases (Meierkord *et al.*, 1992); many of the patients had additional daytime or secondary generalized seizures and often responded favourably to carbamazepine, and occasional patients with similar attacks and normal scalp EEGs subsequently studied with intracranial EEG have been shown to have mesial frontal epileptic activity (Neidermyer and Walker, 1971; Rajna *et al.*, 1983).

The probable involvement of frontal lobe epileptic activity in such attacks has been demonstrated in 2 patients by Lugaresi's group, followed up with scalp EEGs (Tinuper *et al.*, 1990).

Table 17.3 Studies on paroxysmal nocturnal dystonia

Study	*Number of patients*	*Other epileptic seizures*	*Good response to anticonvulsant therapy*	*EEG abnormalities*
Lugaresi and Cirignota (1981)	5	?	?	?
Rajna *et al.* (1983)	1	?	?	1
Godbout *et al.* (1985)	1	?	1	1
Lee *et al.* (1985)	3	0	2	0
Crowell and Anders (1985)	1	0	?	0
Lugaresi *et al.* (1986b)	12	8	All*	0
Lehkuniec *et al.* (1988)	1	0	1	0
Tinuper *et al.* (1990)	3	2	2	2
Meierkord *et al.* (1992)	9	6	5	0

?=Not known.
*All of those tried on carbamazepine responded favourably.
EEG abnormalities refer to interictal or ictal epiletiform discharges.
Adapted from Meierkord *et al.* (1991) with permission.

The dystonic and other motor symptomatology may result from spread of the epileptic activity from the mesial frontal region to the basal ganglia. These two structures have intimate connections (Wall *et al.*, 1951; Kemp and Powell, 1970; Leichnetz and Astruc, 1977; Kuenzle, 1978; Selemon and Goldman-Rakic, 1985), along which seizure propagation has been documented (Walker, 1966). The lack of epileptiform changes on the routine scalp EEG may reflect a deep epileptogenic zone and the technical difficulties of EEG recordings from frontal lobe structures (Quesney *et al.*, 1990a).

Other forms of partial epilepsy or generalized seizures may occur in sleep, although rarely with the frequency of frontal lobe attacks. Usually these other seizure disorders have more easily recognizable epileptic features, such as loss of awareness, automatisms, tonic–clonic seizures or urinary incontinence. Penfield and Jasper (1954) documented jerking in association with spread of seizure activity from the temporal lobe to the inferior central region. Subsequently, Bossi *et al.* (1984) reported the occurrence of motor manifestations including jerking and dystonia in patients with seizures arising in the temporal lobe. However, these were rarely an early feature, and were usually seen late or in association with other ictal clinical behaviour. Furthermore, simultaneous intracranial EEG studies indicated seizure spread, particularly to the frontal and parietal regions. They suggested that motor manifestations were uncommon in temporal lobe epilepsy, and that the variations could reflect different patterns of spread. For example, spread could more readily occur from the superior mesial temporal lobe to the central region, or from inferior structures to more anterior frontal structures, perhaps via the uncinate fasciculus. More recently, Kotagal *et al.* (1989) reported contralateral dystonic posturing in 18 patients with temporal lobe epilepsy. These patients were only studied with surface or subdural electrodes, making it difficult to determine spread to deep structures. Nevertheless, the authors proposed that this could have occurred through direct spread to the basal ganglia, either through the stria terminalis from the amygdala or precommissural portion of the fornix from the hippocampus.

PAROXYSMAL DAYTIME MOTOR ATTACKS

The principal movement disorders presenting with discrete daytime motor attacks are: hyperekplexia, paroxysmal kinesigenic choreoathetosis or paroxysmal dystonic choreoathetosis, and the intermittent ataxias (see Chapter 16). Rarely, multiple sclerosis may present with tonic attacks (Twomey and Espir, 1980). There is indeed a wide range of causes for daytime paroxysmal dyskinesias, some of which are epileptic (Table 17.4).

Startle disease (hyperekplexia) was initially described by Kirstein and Silfverskiod (1958), and subsequently characterized by Suhren *et al.* (1966) and Andermann *et al.* (1980) to involve an exaggerated startle response to unexpected stimuli, sometimes with generalized stiffening, falling and urinary incontinence (presumably secondary to changes in intra-abdominal pressure), without loss of consciousness. It is often inherited with autosomal dominant transmission, although sporadic cases do occur and may be associated with brainstem abnormalities. Hypertonia may be present from infancy, but usually improves with maturity. Patients do not have secondarily generalized convulsions or other clinical features of epilepsy. Scalp EEGs during these attacks have shown variable results: apparent isolated central spikes at the onset may occur, although the cerebral nature of these has been questioned (Markland *et al.*, 1984).

Seizures provoked by unexpected stimuli may occur in patients with epilepsy (Alajuoanine and Gastaut, 1955; Gastaut and Tassinari, 1966; Bancaud *et al.*, 1967, 1975; Nakamura *et al.*, 1975; Gimenez-Roldan and Martin, 1980; Chauvel *et al.*, 1981; Aguilla *et al.*, 1984; Guerrini *et al.*, 1990; Kolbinger *et al.*, 1990). Most of the patients described have gross cerebral damage, often with a congenital hemiparesis, or other neurological disorder (e.g. Down's syndrome, Tay–Sachs). The provoked seizures are usually similar to the patient's spontaneous attacks and therefore may show a variety of clinical forms. However, within this clinical spectrum are cases displaying features similar to hyperekplexia with dystonic posturing or generalized stiffening, falling, sometimes urinary incontinence and preserved consciousness. From the clinical viewpoint the following features help to distinguish such patients from hyperekplexia: the presence of an associated congenital hemiplegia, diplegia or other

Table 17.4 Paroxysmal daytime motor attacks

Startle/movement-induced seizures
Mesial frontal seizures
Other partial epilepsies
Drop attacks*
Hyperekplexia
Paroxysmal kinesigenic choreoathetosis
Paroxysmal dystonic choreoathetosis
Intermittent ataxias
Tonic attacks (e.g. of multiple sclerosis, cord lesions)
Metabolis disorders (e.g. hypoglycaemia)
Transient ischaemic attacks
Drug-induced dyskinesias (e.g. neuroleptic oculogyric crisis)

*See Table 17.5 for epileptic and non-epileptic causes of drop attacks.
Myoclonic disorders are considered together under more persistent dyskinesias.

severe or progressive neurological disorder; asymmetrical posturing or additional epileptic features such as automatisms or clonic activity in the startle-induced attacks; the occurrence of other seizure types, in particular secondary generalized convulsions; the often transient nature of startle sensitivity within the patient's history; and the absence of a family history of startle-induced attacks. Interictal EEGs may show central spikes or other epileptiform abnormalities. Ictal scalp EEG recordings are often obscured by muscle artefact, but may show rhythmic activity (typically at about 10 Hz) or slow or spike and slow-wave activity, following an initial central spike or spike and slow-wave complex (Gastaut and Tassinari, 1966).

Patients with seizures similar to hyperekplexia may have lesions in the supplementary or primary motor areas, or EEG evidence (in some cases from intracranial studies) of mesial frontal or central epilepsy (Bancaud *et al.*, 1967, 1975; Chauvel *et al.*, 1981; Aguglia, 1984). It remains uncertain whether these clinical manifestations are due to seizure propagation to the brainstem activating the same structures involved in hyperekplexia or if the clinical overlap is fortuitous. Additional polygraphic studies are needed in adults with such startle-induced seizures.

Paroxysmal kinesigenic choreoatheotosis or paroxysmal dystonic choreoathetosis represent uncommon involuntary movement disorders (see Chapter 16). Often there is a positive family history, and there may be a favourable response to anticonvulsant medication. Movement-induced epileptic seizures are rare but have been recognized for many years, being described by Gowers (1901). Lishman *et al.* (1962) reported 7 patients, which they classified as movement-induced epilepsy. The attacks usually commenced in childhood. They were characterized by stiffening which could be focal or generalized, and which evolved into choreoathetoid movements, but not clonic movements, and with preserved consciousness. Most of these 7 cases had EEG abnormalities, but some may have been unrecognized cases of paroxysmal kinesigenic choreoathetosis. Subsequently, Falconer *et al.* (1963) reported the case of a 35-year-old man with a 7-year history of frequent (up to 40/day), brief (10–20 seconds) seizures that could occur spontaneously or be precipitated by emotional stress, voluntary contraction of the right thigh or kicking. The attacks were preceded by an increased feeling of tension in the right thigh and followed by stiffening of the right leg, arching of the trunk, abduction of the right shoulder and extension of the elbow. Consciousness usually was preserved. The interictal and spontaneous ictal scalp EEGs were normal. Exposure of the cerebral cortex at operation revealed a small area of cicatrix in the supplementary motor area. Following removal of this scar the patient made a full recovery and became free of attacks. Further cases of movement-induced dystonic or choreiform attacks in association with birth anoxia (Rosen, 1964) or head injuries (Robin, 1977; Drake *et al.*, 1986; Richardson *et al.*, 1987) have been reported. One postbirth anoxia case was associated with epileptiform EEG abnormalities, and one of the post-head-injury cases showed a discrete mid lateral frontal lesion (Richardson *et al.*, 1987). As with startle-induced attacks, the clinical features of attacks classified as a movement disorder and epilepsy show considerable overlap, raising the possibility of a final common pathway, or dual involvement of the neuronal circuits.

Paroxysmal dystonia is not always precipitated by obvious movements. Daytime mesial frontal lobe seizures may be manifest by bilateral or unilateral dystonic posturing affecting the arms, legs and/or trunk with preserved consciousness (Williamson *et al.*, 1985; Morris *et al.*, 1988). Video tape analysis shows the semiology of these attacks to be similar to the nocturnal episodes described above (Meierkord *et al.*, 1991). The diagnosis of such daytime attacks may be suspected because of their frequency, brevity, associated automatisms such as bicycling or kicking leg

Table 17.5 Causes of drop attacks

Epileptic disorders
Lennox–Gastaut syndrome
Frontal lobe epilepsy
Cortical myoclonus
Other partial and generalized epilepsies
Movement disorders
Hyperekplexia
Parkinson's disease
Steele–Richardson–Olszewski syndrome
Multiple system atrophy
Segmental or other subcortical myoclonus
Paroxysmal choreoathetosis
Other disorders
Cardiac
Cerebrovascular
Postural hypotension
Vestibular
Third ventricle tumours
Brainstem/cervical lesions
Lower limb neuromuscular abnormalities
Cataplexy
Psychogenic

movements, vocalizations, or secondary generalization, although again the interictal and ictal scalp EEGs are often normal.

Sudden falls (drop attacks) without reported loss of awareness may occur in a variety of conditions, including both movement disorders and seizure disorders (Table 17.5).

In a survey of 108 patients with drop attacks (defined as a falling spell occurring without warning or postictal symptoms, with immediate righting and without loss of awareness or consciousness), 5% had unequivocal seizures (although the diagnosis was not established in a further 64%; Meisner *et al.*, 1986). Epileptic drop attacks may be tonic, atonic or involve dystonic posturing. They may be due to simple partial seizures, particularly of frontal origin (Pazzaglia *et al.*, 1985). Temporal lobe epilepsy involving falls is usually associated with impairment of consciousness (Jacome, 1989). Generalized epilepsies which include drop attacks are usually associated with impairment of consciousness or additional seizure types, and almost invariably interictal and ictal EEG abnormalities. Particularly important in the younger age group is the Lennox–Gastaut syndrome, characterized by drop attacks, other multiple seizure types and mental deterioration. Sometimes the drop attacks are incomplete, involving a head nod or partial fall. The differentiation of such seizures from non-epileptic head drops was studied in 351 attacks recorded in 24 children using video telemetry (Brunquell *et al.*, 1990). Epileptic drop attacks showed a higher proportion of changes in facial expression and subtle myoclonus of the extremities. Head drops with a faster velocity of descent than return were more often epileptic, whereas recurrent head drops or head bobbing did not occur in the epileptic patients.

Myoclonic disorders may present as drop attacks due to either positive or negative myoclonus. Particular problems arise with the progressive myoclonic epilepsies, where it may be very difficult to differentiate the ataxia from the myoclonus (see below).

PERSISTENT DYSKINESIAS

Most movement disorders are persistent rather than restricted to discrete attacks. In relation to epilepsy the crucial overlap is with cortical myoclonus. Consequently myoclonus will be discussed in this section, recognizing that sometimes the manifestations may be intermittent or more persistent.

Epilepsia partialis continua (EPC) is readily identified when there is rhythmic jerking, with spread to adjacent parts of the body. However, diagnostic difficulties may arise because, unlike simple motor seizures, the movements may become irregular, with at times relatively long intervals between jerks, and variation in the amplitude of movements (Thomas *et al.*, 1977). In the case of distal limb involvement this may lead to a clinical picture manifesting as tremor (Ikeda *et al.*, 1990).

Involvement of the facial muscles, such as the tongue, either with EPC or frequent seizures, may similarly present as a movement disorder (Holtzman *et al.*, 1984; Neufield *et al.*, 1988). Other epileptic facial or head movements, such as ictal automatisms, rarely cause diagnostic difficulty because of associated widespread seizure activity or altered consciousness (Mizrahi, 1988). However, brief automatisms may occur in frontal lobe epilepsy, especially with seizures arising in the dorsolateral convexity (Quesney *et al.*, 1990b), causing possible diagnostic confusion if frequent and not accompanied by other epileptic features.

Restriction of seizure activity to the trunk is rare but may cause particular diagnostic problems. Rosenbaum and Rowan (1990) reported a patient with EPC manifest as unilateral truncal seizures without loss of consciousness, and supported in this instance by EEG abnormalities over the contralateral primary motor region: such activity could mimic spinal myoclonus or other described abdominal dyskinesias (e.g. Iliceto *et al.*, 1990).

Jerking of one side of the body may occur in EPC. It may also be seen as an intermittent manifestation in primary generalized epilepsy (Oller-Daurella, 1985), although the mechanism for this asymmetrical presentation, coexisting with generalized spike and slow-wave activity, is unknown. In such patients the brief alteration of consciousness may not be readily apparent, although the EEG is of clear diagnostic value.

Focal, multifocal or generalized myoclonus may be seen in a variety of primary and secondary epilepsies. It is important to be aware that the myoclonus may precede the occurrence of obvious seizures in several of these conditions, and sometimes it may be the only reported symptom for years. Furthermore, most patients with myoclonus and epilepsy can be categorized into specific diagnostic groups carrying prognostic and therapeutic significance. Those with a primary generalized epilepsy such as absence or juvenile myoclonic seizures responding favourably to sodium valproate and benzodiazepines, and those with fixed or deteriorating encephalopathies, and including the progressive myoclonic epilepsies usually have a worse prognosis and response to treatment. Therefore, for clinical purposes myoclonus should not be accepted as an associated feature of epilepsy of unknown aetiology.

Small isolated jerks, particularly of the face or upper limbs often occur during absence seizures (in association with 3/second spike and slow-wave activity), or there may be very low-amplitude myoclonus of the extremities (Wilkins *et al.*, 1985). These movements are usually of low amplitude: massive myoclonus is not a feature of typical absence seizures. Variant responses to photic stimulation include photomyoclonus (Gastaut and Remond, 1949). This is characterized by eyelid flickering and electromyogram spikes over the anterior head regions, and does not last beyond the stimulus. Although it may also occur in association with a true photoconvulsive response, its incidence in patients with epilepsy is little different from that in the general population (Reilly and Peters, 1973).

Much more prominent myoclonus with massive jerks occurs in juvenile myoclonic epilepsy. The prevalence of this condition is uncertain in the community: it has been reported to account for up to 3–5% of patients with epilepsy (Janz, 1969; Tsuboi, 1977). It is often familial, with about one-quarter of the patients having a family history of epilepsy. Onset is usually around puberty. The myoclonus is usually worse on awakening in the morning, and may be the presenting complaint. Typically the jerks are bilateral, symmetrical and of large amplitude, but may be reported by the patient as appearing asymmetrical or multifocal. The arms are more often affected than the legs, and the face is usually spared (Wolf, 1985). The resting EEG shows generalized spike, or more usually polyspike, and slow discharges. The frequency of the spike and slow wave activity is often faster than 3/second. The myoclonic jerks are usually accompanied by polyspike activity. Photosensitivity has been reported in 30% of these patients, therefore being commoner than in other forms of primary generalized epilepsy (Goosses, 1984).

Multifocal or generalized epilepsy in association with a static or progressive encephalopathy may also present with prominent myoclonus causing diagnostic difficulties. The myoclonus may display a range of distributions: focal, multifocal or generalized. This problem is typified by the progressive myoclonic epilepsies (Table 17.6; Berkovic *et al*., 1986), and progressive myoclonic ataxia where the myoclonus may precede the seizure disorder, and remain the predominant problem. Such patients

Table 17.6 Major causes of progressive myoclonus epilepsy and progressive myoclonic ataxia

Disease	*Age onset (years)*	*Suggestive clinical features*
Unverricht–Lundborg	8–13	Severe myoclonus, dementia absent or mild
Lafora body disease	11–18	Occipital seizures Inexorable dementia
Neuronal ceroid lipofuscinosis		
Late infantile	2.5–4	Severe seizures Rapid regression Fundal changes
Juvenile	4–10	Visual failure Fundal changes
Adult	12–50	
Sialidosis		
Type 1	8–20	Severe myoclonus
Type 2	10–30	Cherry-red spot, dysmorphic
Mitochondrial encephalopathy	5–42	Short stature, deafness

Adapted from Berkovic *et al*. (1986) with permission.

may present with unsteadiness or clumsiness relating either to cerebellar ataxia or frequent myoclonic jerks. The EEG in the progressive myoclonic epilepsies usually shows a slow background with multifocal or generalized epileptiform discharges. Photosensitivity is common, but does not help to distinguish the different disorders.

INVESTIGATION OF SUSPECTED EPILEPTIC DYSKINESIAS

The range of dyskinesias that may be the presentation of epilepsy emphasizes the need for physicians dealing primarily with movement disorders to be aware of such imitations. Investigation of suspected cases needs to take into account the limitations of routine scalp EEG. Seizure generators may be sited in areas that are not readily accessible to scalp recordings such as mesial frontal cortex, cingulate cortex or orbitofrontal cortex. Alternatively, they may be superficial, but too small or inappropriately oriented to be detected on the scalp (e.g. a cortical sulcus within the primary motor strip). Negative interictal and ictal scale EEGs should not deter consideration of an epileptic origin. Repeated scalp EEG studies, including sleep and supraorbital or other appropriate special electrodes (Quesney *et al.*, 1990a; Sutherland *et al.*, 1990), may be helpful to identify such generators.

Patients with nocturnal or daytime paroxysmal attacks may need appropriate prolonged monitoring studies to document these episodes. If the attacks are occurring many times per day or are readily provoked, it may be preferable to use conventional EEG recording equipment (with a video recording as well, if possible). This usually provides more flexibility than commercially available telemetry systems, particularly if combined EEG and surface electromyogram studies are to be undertaken, and the continuous presence of an EEG technician is helpful given the disruption which may occur to electrodes from motor attacks. Attacks occurring less frequently or predominantly at night may require telemetry recordings, although these are usually only worthwhile with attacks occurring at least a few times per week.

The investigation of patients with suspected EPC does not present the difficulty of capturing attacks, but remains problematic. Routine scalp EEGs often fail to reveal epileptic activity, or are obscured by muscle or movement artefact. Often, but not always, EPC will continue at least into early sleep (Thomas *et al.*, 1977), unlike most other dyskinesias which reappear only rarely during overnight recordings (Fish *et al.*, 1991). This may be useful clinically, and should encourage EEG recordings to be undertaken with light sleep. Departmental EEGs may be more readily interpreted if simultaneous electromyogram surface recordings are undertaken in order to correlate the jerks with any EEG changes, which are particularly helpful if the EEG changes precede the movement, thereby excluding artefact. If suitably abrupt surface EMG activity can be recorded, and the required computer facilities are available, back-averaging of the EEG may allow otherwise unidentified cortical correlates of myoclonic jerks to be differentiated from the background noise (Shibasaki *et al.*, 1981). Alternative investigations in EPC include the use of cerebral blood flow or metabolism imaging (e.g. positron emission tomography or single photon emission tomography) which usually show a focal increase in relation to ongoing ictal activity. Conventional imaging with computed tomography or, preferably, magnetic resonance imaging is clearly important to look for underlying structural abnormalities. However, focal gliosis or small anomalies within cortical gyri may produce too little signal change, or occupy too few pixels in each slice to be detected using conventional sequences and planar images. Careful follow-up remains important to exclude progressive pathology.

References

Aguglia U, Tinuper P, and Gastaut H (1984) Startle induced epileptic seizures. *Epilepsia*, **25**, 712–20

Alajouanine T and Gastaut H (1955) La syncinesie-sursaut et l'epilepsie-sursant a declanchment sensoriel ou sensitif inopine. *Rev Neurol (Paris)*, **93**, 29–41

Andermann F, Keene DL, Andermann E, and Quesney LF (1980) Startle disease or hyperekplexia: further delineation of the syndrome. *Brain*, **103**, 985–97

Bancaud J, Talairach J, and Bonis A (1967) Physiopathogenie des epilepsies-sursaut: a propos d'une epilepsie de l'aire motrice supplementaire. *Rev Neurol (Paris)*, **117**, 441–53

Bancaud J, Talairach J, Lamarche M, Bonis A, and Trottier S (1975) Hypotheses neurophysioloques sur l'epilepsie-surtaut chez l'homme. *Rev Neurol (Paris)*, **131**, 559–71

Berkovic SF, Andermann F, Carpenter S, and Wolfe LS (1986) Progressive myoclonus epilepsies: specific causes and diagnosis. *N Engl J Med*, **315**, 209–305

Bossi L, Munari C, Stoffels C, Bonis A, Bacia T, Talairach J *et al.* (1984) Somatomotor manifestations in temporal lobe epilepsy. *Epilepsia*, **25**, 70–6

Broughton R (1968) Sleep disorders: disorders of arousal. *Science*, **158**, 1070–8

Broughton R, Tolentino MA, and Krelina M (1985) Excessive fragmentary myoclonus in nonREM sleep: a report of 38 cases. *Electroenceph Clin Neurophysiol*, **61**, 123–33

Brunquell P, McKeever M, and Russman BS (1990) Differentiation of epileptic and nonepileptic head drops in children. *Epilepsia*, **31**, 401–5

Chauvel P, Liegeois C, and Bancaud J (1981) Analyse neurophysiologique des epilepsies-sursau: resultats preliminaires. In: *Les facteurs declenchment des crises d'epilepsie*, Paris, Journée Médicale, Francais Contre l'Epilepsie, 105–10

Coleman RM, Pollak CP, and Weitzman ED (1980) Periodic movements in sleep (nocturnal myoclonus): relation to sleep disorders. *Ann Neurol*, **8**, 416–21

Crowell JA and Anders TF (1985) Hypnogenic paroxysmal dystonia. *J Am Acad Child Psychiatry*, **24**, 353–8

De Lisi L (1932) Si di un fenomeno motorio constante del somno normale: le myoclonie ipniche fisiologische. *Riv Pat Nerv Ment*, **38**, 481–96

Devinsky O, Kelly K, Porter R, and Theodore WH (1988) Clinical and electroencephalographic features of simple partial seizures. *Neurology*, **38**, 1347–52

Drake ME (1986) Jactatio nocturna after head injury. *Neurology*, **36**, 867–8

Drake ME, Jackson RD, and Miller C (1986) Paroxysmal choreoathetosis following head injury. *J Neurol, Neurosurg Psychiatry*, **49**, 837–8

Falconer MN, Driver MV, and Serafetinides EA (1963) Seizures induced by movement: report of a case relieved by operation. *J Neurol Neurosurg Psychiatry*, **26**, 300–7

Fish DR, Sawyer D, Allen PJ, Lees A, and Marsden CD (1991) The effect of sleep on the dyskinesias of Parkinson's Disease, Huntington's Disease, Gilles de la Tourette syndrome and torsion dystonia. *Arch Neurol*, 1991, **48**, 210–14

Gastaut H and Remond A (1949) L'activation de l'electroencephalogramme dans les affections cerebrales non epileptogenes (vers une neurphysiologie clinique). *Rev Neurol*, **81**, 594–8

Gastaut H and Tassinari CA (1966) Triggering mechanisms in epilepsy: the electroclinical point of view. *Epilepsia*, **7**, 86–138

Gimenez-Roldan S and Martin M (1980) Startle epilepsy complicating Downs' syndrome during aduluthood. *Ann Neurol*, **7**, 78–80

Godbout R, Montplaisir J, and Rouleau I (1985) Hypnogenic paroxysmal dystonia: epilepsy or sleep disorder? A case report. *Clin Electroencephalogr*, **16**, 136–42

Goosses R (1984) *Die Beziehung der Fotosensibitat zu den verschiedenen epilptischen Syndromen*, Thieme, Berlin

Gowers WR (1901) *Epilepsy and other Convulsive Disorders*, Vol 2, Philadelphia, Blakiston

Guerrini R, Genton P, Bureau M, Dravet C, and Roger J (1990) Reflex seizures are frequent in patients with Down syndrome and epilepsy. *Epilepsia*, **31**, 406–17

Hening WA, Waters A, Kavey N, Gidro-Frank S, Cote L and Fahn S (1986) Dyskinesias while awake and periodic movements in sleep in the restless leg syndrome: treatment with opiods. *Neurology*, **36**, 1363–6

Holtzman RNN, Mark MH, Weiner LM, and Minzer L (1984) Linqual epilepsy: a case report of an unusual expression of focal cerebral discharge. *J Neurol, Neurosurg Psychiatry*, **47**, 317–18

Ikeda A, Kakigi R, Funai N, Neshiga R, Kuroda Y, and Shibasaki H (1990) Cortical tremor; a variant of cortical reflex myoclonus. *Neurology*, **40**, 1561–6

Iliceto G, Thompson PD, Day BL, Rothwell JC, Lees AJ, and Marsden CD (1990) Diaphragmatic flutter, the moving umbilicus syndrome, and belly dancer's dyskinesia. *Movement Disorders*, **5**, 15–22

Jacome DE (1989) Temporal lobe syncope: clinical variants. *Clin Electroencephalogr*, **20**, 58–65

Janz D (1969) *Die Epilepsien*, Stuttgart, Thieme

Kemp JM and Powell TP (1970) The cortico-straito projection in the monkey. *Brain*, **93**, 525–46

Kirstein L and Silfverskiod B (1958) A family with emotionally precipitated drop attacks. *Acta Psychiatr Scand*, **33**, 471–6

Klawans HL, Goetz C, and Bergen D (1975) Levodopa induced myoclonus. *Arch Neurol*, **32**, 331–4

Kolbinger HM, Zierz S, Elger CE, and Penin H (1990) Startle induced seizures and their relationship to epilepsy; three case reports. *J Epilepsy*, **3**, 23–7

Kotagal P, Luders H, Morris HH, Dinner DS, Wyllie E, Godoy J *et al.* (1989) Dystonic posturing in complex partial seizures of temporal lobe onset: a new lateralising sign. *Neurology*, **39**, 196–201

Kuenzle H (1978) An autoradiographic analysis of the efferent connections from premotor and adjacent prefrontal regions (areas 6 and 9) in *Macaca fascicularis*. *Brain Behav Evol*, **15**, 185–234

Lee BI, Lesser RP, Pippenger CE, Morris HH, Luders H, Dinner DS *et al.* (1985) Familial paroxysmal hypnogenic dystonia. *Neurology*, **35**, 1357–60

Leichnetz GR and Astruc J (1977) The course of some prefrontal corticofugals to the pallidum, substantia innominata, and amygdaloid complex in monkeys. *Exp Neurol*, **54**, 104–9

Lieb JP, Walsh GO, Babb TL, Walter RD, and Crandall PH (1976) A comparison of EEG seizure patterns recorded with surface and depth electrodes in patients with temporal lobe epilepsy. *Epilepsia*, **17**, 137–60

Lishman WA, Symonds CWM, Whitty CWM, and Willison RG (1962) Seizures induced by movement. *Brain*, **62**, 93–109

Lugaresi E and Cirignota F (1981) Hypnogenic paroxysmal dystonia: epileptic seizure or a new syndrome? *Sleep*, **4**, 129–38

Lugaresi E, Cirignotta F, and Montagna P (1986a) Nocturnal myoclonus and the restless legs syndrome. *Adv Neurol*, **43**, 295–307

Lugaresi E, Cirignotta F, and Montagna P (1986b) Nocturnal paroxysmal dystonia. *J Neurol, Neurosurg Psychiatry*, **49**, 375–80

Markland ON, Garg BP, and Weaver DD (1984) Familial startle disease (hyperekplexia), electrophysiological studies. *Arch Neurol*, **41**, 71–4

Meierkord H, Fish DR, Smith SJM, Scott CA, Shorvon SD, and Marsden CD (1992) Is nocturnal paroxysmal dystonia a form of frontal lobe epilepsy? *Movement Disorders*, **7**, 38–42

Meisner I, Weibers DO, and Swanson JW (1986) The natural history of drop attacks. *Neurology*, **36**, 1029–34

Mizrahi EM (1988) Epileptic facial automatisms and head movements. In Jankovic J and Tolosa E, eds, *Advances in Neurology*. New York, Raven Press, vol 49, 279–87

Morris HH, Dinner DS, Lueders H, Wyllie E, and Kramer R (1988) Supplementary motor seizures: clinical and electroencephalographic findings. *Neurology*, **38**, 1075–82

Nakamura M, Kanai H, and Miyamoto Y (1975) A case of Sturge Weber syndrome with startle epilepsy. *Brain Nerve*, **27**, 325–31

Neidermyer E and Walker AE (1971) Mesial frontal epilepsy. *Electroenceph Clin Neurophysiol*, **31**, 104–5

Neufield MY, Blumen SC, Nisipeanu P, and Korczyn AD (1988) Lingual seizures. *Epilepsia*, **29**, 30–3

Oller-Daurella L (1985) Is there an epilepsy with unilateral seizures? In Dravet C, Bureau M, Dreifuss FE, and Wold P, eds, *Epileptic Syndromes in Infancy, Children and Young Adults*. London, John Libbey Eurotext, 216–21

Oswald I (1959) Sudden body jerks on falling asleep. *Brain*, **82**, 93–103

Pazzaglia P, D'Alessandro R, Ambrosetto G, and Lugaresi E (1985) *Neurology*, **35**, 1725–30

Penfield W and Jasper H (1954) *Epilepsy and the functional anatomy of the human brain*. Boston, Little Brown

Quesney LF, Constain M, Fish DR, and Rasmussen T (1990a) Frontal lobe epilepsy – a field of recent emphasis. *Am J EEG Technol*, **30**, 177–93

Quesney LF, Constain P, Fish D, and Rasmussen T (1990b) The clinical differentiation of seizures arising in the parasagittal and anterolateral dorsal frontal lobe convexisities. *Arch Neurol*, **47**, 677–9

Rajna P, Kundra O, and Halasz P (1983) Vigilance level-dependent tonic seizures: epilepsy or sleep disorder? A case report. *Epilepsia*, **24**, 725–33

Reilly EW and Peters JF (1973) Relationship of some varieties of electroencephalographic photosensitivy to clinical convulsive disorders. *Neurology*, **23**, 1040–57

Richardson JC, Howes JL, Celinski MJ, and Allman RG (1987) Kinesigenic choreoathetosis due to brain injury. *Can J Neurol Sci*, **14**, 626–8

Robin JJ (1977) Paroxysmal choreoathetosis following head injury. *Ann Neurol*, **2**, 447–8

Rosen JA (1964) Paroxysmal choreoathetosis associated with perinatal hypoxic encephalopathy. *Arch Neurol*, **11**, 385–7

Rosenbaum DH and Rowan AJ (1990) Unilateral truncal siezures: frontal origin. *Epilepsia*, **31**, 37–41

Schenck CH, Bundlie SR, Patterson AI, and Mahowald MW (1987) Rapid eye movement sleep behaviour disorder. *JAMA*, **257**, 1786–9

Selemon LD and Goldman-Rakic PS (1985) Longitudinal topography and interdigitation of corticostraital projections in the rhesus monkey. *J Neurosci*, **5**, 776–94

Shibasaki H, Motomura S, Yamashita Y, Shii H, Kuroiwa Y (1981) Periodic synchronous discharge and myoclonus in Creuzfeldt–Jakob disease: diagnostic application of jerk-locked averaging method. *Ann Neurol*, **9**, 150–6

Smith RC (1985) Relationship of RMS (nocturnal myoclonus) and the babinski response. *Sleep*, **8**, 239–43

Suhren O, Bruyn GW, and Tuynman JA (1966) Hyperexplexia. A hereditary startle syndrome. *J Neurol Sci*, **3**, 577–605

Sutherland W, Risinger M, Crandall PH, Becker DP, Baumgartner C, Cahan CD *et al.* (1990) Focal functional anatomy of dorsolateral frontocentral seizures. *Neurology*, **40**, 87–98

Tinuper P, Cerullo A, Cirignotta F, Cortelli P, Lugaresi E and Montagna P (1990) Nocturnal paroxysmal dystonia with short lasting attacks. Three cases with evidence for an epileptic frontal lobe origin of seizures. *Epilepsia*, **31**, 549–56

Thomas J, Reggan J, and Klass D (1977) Epilepsia partialis continua. A review of 32 cases. *Arch Neurol*, **34**, 266–75

Tsuboi T (1977) *Primary Generalised Epilepsy with Sporadic Myoclonias of Myoclonic Petit Mal Type*, Stuttgart, Thieme

Twomey JA and Espir MLE (1980) Paroxysmal symptoms as the first manifestation of multiple sclerosis. *J Neurol, Neurosurg Psychiatry*, **43**, 296–304

Walker EA (1966) Pre-frontal lobe epilepsy. *Int J Neurol*, **5**, 422–9

Wall PD, Glees P, and Fulton JF (1951) Corticofugal connexions of posterior orbital surface in rhesus monkey. *Brain*, **74**, 66–71

Walters A, Hening W, Cote L, and Fahn S (1986) Dominantly inherited restless legs with myoclonus and periodic movements of sleep; a syndrome related to endogenous opiates. *Adv Neurol*, **43**, 309–19

Wilkins DE, Hallett M, and Erba C (1985) Primary generalised epileptic myoclonus; a frequent manifestation of minipolymyoclonus of cortical origin. *J Neurol Neurosurg Psychiatry*, **48**, 506–10

Wolf P (1985) Juvenile myoclonic epilepsy. In Roger J, Dravet C, Bureau M, Dreifuss FE, and Wolf P, eds, *Epileptic Syndromes in Infancy, Childhood and Adolescence*, London, John Libbey Eurotext, 247–58

18
Psychogenic movement disorders

Stanley Fahn

Movement disorder specialists are seeing increasing numbers of patients with movement disorders whose problems are secondary to psychogenic factors. As one may expect, bradykinetic disorders are less likely than hyperkinetic ones to have a psychogenic aetiology. Fixed postures, so-called psychogenic dystonia, account for a sizeable proportion of this group of patients. So, a separate section of this review is devoted to the psychogenic dystonias.

Neurologists usually and appropriately recognize patients with psychogenic movement disorders, but the patients often do not accept this diagnosis and seek other opinions, going from physician to physician, seeking a diagnosis more to their liking. Thus, a strategy is necessary for the best way to inform the patients of the diagnosis. This issue will be discussed in this review. Another common situation is that many physicians do not offer the time-consuming care necessary to restore such patients to normality, preferring instead merely to diagnose the condition and have the referring physician deal with the healing.

An accurate diagnosis of psychogenic movement disorder as against an organic movement disorder is often one of the most difficult there is in this specialty. It is extremely important to be correct in the diagnosis because only then can the appropriate therapy be initiated. The results of an incorrect diagnosis are detrimental. If a patient has a psychogenic disorder that is misdiagnosed, the patient will be given inappropriate and potentially harmful medication and is also denied the proper treatment to overcome the disabling symptoms. If the obverse occurs, that is, if a patient is given a diagnosis of a psychogenic movement disorder when, in fact, he/she suffers from an organic one, again the wrong treatment is given. In this situation, time-consuming and expensive psychotherapy, psychiatric medications and possibly electroconvulsive therapy may be initiated, instead of more appropriate pharmacotherapeutic agents that may provide relief. Moreover, a diagnosis of a psychogenic disorder can create emotional trauma to the patient and his/her family (Cooper, 1976).

Neurological symptoms and signs are a common result of hysteria, and neurologists have long been fascinated with the ability of the brain to be able to produce such clinical expressions on the basis of psychological disturbances. Many great neurologists, such as Charcot and Freud, intensively studied hysterical conversion reactions, using hypnosis as a tool in their investigations and treatment (Goetz, 1987). In their training, neurologists-to-be are taught to differentiate the clinical findings of psychogenic aetiology from those of organic disorders (Gowers, 1893; Oppenheim, 1911a; DeJong, 1958a). However, textbooks in the past would often consider some dyskinesias, recognized today as organic, such as tics, writer's cramp and other occupational cramps, and some other forms of dystonia, as examples of hysteria (DeJong, 1958b).

Although there is a modest neurological literature on psychogenic phenomenology, the literature dealing specifically with psychogenic movement disorders is rather sparse. For example, tremor as the result of a conversion reaction has been long recognized, at least since the days of Gowers (1893), but scientific reports on psychogenic tremor or other movement disorders are rarely described in the literature. Campbell (1979) pointed out that psychogenic tremor is most pronounced when attention is paid to it, and that it disappears when the patient's attention is diverted to another subject or other part of the body. This is a useful distinction in the differential diagnosis of psychogenic tremor, but in my experience withdrawal of attention does not always succeed in making the tremor disappear, so this manoeuvre is often not successful. Therefore, additional findings on examination are often necessary and can be just as helpful in considering the diagnosis of a psychogenic movement disorder; these will be discussed below.

Although the great majority of patients with a psychogenic movement disorder have all their clinical features as a result of only a psychogenic problem, some may have the psychogenic movement disorder on top of an organic movement disorder, as seen in patient 5 in the series of psychogenic dystonias reported by Fahn and Williams (1988) and the cases of Ranawaya *et al.* (1990).

Probably the movement disorders with the highest prevalence rate of a psychogenic origin are the non-familial, idiopathic, non-kinesigenic paroxysmal dyskinesias, as surveyed by Bressman *et al.* (1988). They found that of 18 patients with paroxysmal dystonias, and with no known symptomatic aetiology, 11 were due to psychogenic causes. This respresents 61% of such cases. Their age at onset ranged from 11 to 49 years; 8 of the 11 were female. Thus, unless accompanied by a clear-cut family history, these paroxysmal dystonias are particularly commonly psychogenic, and their diagnosis is extremely difficult to make (Fahn and Williams, 1988) (vida infra).

DEGREE OF CERTAINTY OF THE DIAGNOSIS OF A PSYCHOGENIC MOVEMENT DISORDER

Fahn and Williams (1988) categorized patients into four levels of certainty as to the likelihood of their having a psychogenic movement disorder. These four degrees of certainty are: (1) documented psychogenic disorder; (2) clinically established psychogenic disorder; (3) probable psychogenic disorder; and (4) possible psychogenic movement disorder. This classification has been used by subsequent authors (Koller *et al.*, 1989; Ranawaya *et al.*, 1990). I have incorporated the classification of Fahn and Williams, but expanded somewhat the criteria, taking into account additional observations since their publication.

Documented psychogenic movement disorder

Just being suspicious that the signs and symptoms are psychogenic is insufficient for the diagnosis of documented psychogenic disorder. In order for the disorder to be documented as being psychogenic, the symptoms must be completely relieved by psychotherapy, by the clinician utilizing psychological suggestion including physiotherapy, or by administration of placebos (again with suggestion being a part of this approach), or the patient must be witnessed as being free of symptoms when left alone, supposedly unobserved. This last feature would be a major factor in proving psychogenicity in those who are malingering or have a factitious disorder since such patients would not likely obtain relief of symptoms by manipulations of the examiner. If the signs and symptoms disappear and don't return, that is fairly good evidence that the underlying psychiatric problem has been relieved. But it is not uncommon for the psychogenic movement disorder to return if the patient doesn't obtain complete relief of the psychiatric factors that led to the neurological dysfunction.

A critical issue for using the relief of signs as a criterion for the definition is because most organic movement disorders rarely remit spontaneously and completely except for tics, tardive dyskinesia, infectious (e.g. Sydenham's chorea) and drug-induced reactions, and, rarely, essential myoclonus (Fahn and Sjaastad, 1991). Other organic disorders, such as Parkinson's disease, Huntington's disease, and essential tremor, are persistent and even progressive. Idiopathic torsion dystonia, except for torticollis (Jayne *et al.*, 1984; Friedman and Fahn, 1986; Jahanshahi *et al.*, 1990), rarely totally remits. On occasion, patients with other types of dystonia will show improvement, but this improvement is typically incomplete and temporary (Marsden and Harrison, 1974), although gradual, prolonged, incomplete improvement has been encountered in at least 1 patient (Eldridge *et al.*, 1984).

The degree of remission seen in cases with documented psychogenic movement disorders is usually the dramatic, sudden improvement occurring within a few days with supportive suggestion or placebo treatment. In a few patients with more chronic symptoms, improvement can be more gradual, occurring over weeks to months of 'physiotherapy' which was used as the approach to have the patient relinquish the symptoms in a face-saving manner. Physiotherapy also can have physical benefits for those patients who had developed weakness, spasms or contractures, based on chronic disuse and/or abnormal postures for extended periods, even though they were on a psychogenic basis.

Clinically established psychogenic movement disorder

When the movement disorder is inconsistent over time (the features are different when the patient is observed at subsequent examinations) or is incongruent with a classical movement disorder, one becomes suspicious that the movements are psychogenic. If either inconsistency or incongruity is present, and in addition the patient manifests any of the following, one can feel comfortable in believing that the disorder is psychogenic, and this has been referred to as clinically established psychogenic movement disorder. These additional manifestations are the following:

1. Other neurological signs are present that are definitely psychogenic, e.g. false weakness, false sensory findings and self-inflicted injuries.
2. Multiple somatizations are present.
3. An obvious psychiatric disturbance is present.
4. The movement disorder disappears with distraction.
5. Excessive (appearing deliberate) slowness of movement is present.

It should be noted that the fourth feature listed above by itself is insufficient for a diagnosis of a documented or clinically established psychogenic disorder. This is because some organic movement disorders can be temporarily and voluntarily suppressed (Koller and Biary, 1989). Similarly, akathitic movements and paradoxical dystonia (Fahn, 1989) also tend to disappear with active voluntary movement.

Probable psychogenic movement disorder

This definition contains four categories of patients:

1. Those patients in whom the movements are inconsistent or are incongruent with any classical movement disorder, and there are no other features to provide further support for a diagnosis of psychogenicity.
2. Those patients in whom the movements are consistent and congruent with an organic disorder, and the movements can be made to disappear with distraction, when ordinarily distraction would not be expected to eliminate those movements if they were organic.
3. Those patients in whom the movements are consistent and congruent with an organic disorder, but other neurological signs are present that are definitely psychogenic, e.g. false weakness, false sensory findings, or self-inflicted injuries.
4. Those patients in whom the movements are consistent and congruent with an organic disorder, but multiple somatizations are present.

The last two subdivisions contain psychiatric manifestations that make the clinician highly suspicious that the movement might also be psychogenic, but by themselves they are insufficient to give a higher degree of certainty to the diagnosis of a psychogenic movement disorder.

Possible psychogenic movement disorder

One can be suspicious that the movements are psychogenic if an obvious emotional disturbance is present, but this is not as compelling as the psychiatric features listed above. For the category of a possible psychogenic disorder, the movements would be consistent and congruent for an organic movement disorder.

Degree of certainty of the diagnosis of a psychogenic paroxysmal movement disorder

Paroxysmal movement disorder presents a special and difficult problem. Its natural history characteristically shows prolonged periods of cessation of the abnormal movements, so its disappearance with placebo or by suggestion cannot by itself establish the diagnosis of a psychogenic disorder since the remission could have been coincidental. However, if the paroxysms are frequent and the attacks are prolonged, then repeated trials with placebo can be informative. If such trials consistently produce remissions, then one can be convinced that the diagnosis is a documented psychogenic disorder.

The criteria for clinically established, probable and possible psychogenic movement disorders would be the same for paroxysmal as well as continual movement disorders. It is likely that when there are both a paroxysmal and a continual movement disorder present in the same patient, the aetiology is psychogenic.

DEFINITIONS OF PSYCHIATRIC TERMINOLOGY

Definitions from *DSM-III-R* are used regarding psychogenic movement disorders (American Psychiatric Association, 1980). There are three categories into which patients with psychogenic movement disorder can be subdivided – the somatoform disorders, the factitious disorders and malingering.

Somatoform disorder

A somatoform disorder is one in which the physical symptoms are linked to psychological factors, yet the symptom production is *not under voluntary control.* The two main types of somatoform disorders are conversion disorder and somatization disorder, the latter also being known as hysteria or Briquet's syndrome.

In conversion disorder, psychological factors may be judged to play a primary aetiological role in a variety of ways. This may be suggested by a temporal relationship between the onset or worsening of the symptoms and the presence of an environmental stimulus that activates a psychological conflict or need. Alternatively, the symptom may be noted to free the patient from a noxious activity or encounter. Finally, the symptom may be noted to enable the patient to get support from the environment that otherwise might not be forthcoming.

A somatization disorder involves recurrent and multiple complaints of several years' duration for which medical care has been sought, but which are apparently not due to any physical disorder. The dynamics are presumably the same as those of conversion disorder and the symptoms may emerge from chronic, recurrent, untreated conversion disorder.

Factitious disorder

A factitious disorder is one in which the physical symptoms are *intentionally produced* (hence under voluntary control) due to psychological need. This group includes Münchausen's syndrome. Factitious disorders are due to a mental disorder. They are generally associated with severe dependent, masochistic or antisocial personality disorders.

Malingering

Malingering refers to *voluntarily produced* physical symptoms in pursuit of a goal such as financial compensation, avoidance of school or work, evasion of criminal prosecution or acquisition of drugs. Malingering is not considered to be a mental disorder.

When faced with a patient having a psychogenic movement disorder, it is often not possible with certainty to distinguish among somatoform, factitious and malingering disorders. A patient's volitional intent is often impossible to determine with certainty.

CLUES SUGGESTING THE PRESENCE OF A PSYCHOGENIC MOVEMENT DISORDER

Often there are clues from the history and neurological examination that lead the clinician to suspect a diagnosis of a psychogenic movement disorder. Many of these clues have been enunciated by Fahn and Williams (1988) and by Koller *et al.* (1989). Tables 18.1 and 18.2 list these clues, as well as some additional ones.

The presence of more than one type of dyskinesia is an important clue, because most of the time patients with organic movement disorders present with only a single type. A note of caution is warranted, however. Certain disorders progress to involve more than one type of abnormal movement. For example, Huntington's disease can have chorea, bradykinesia, dystonia and myoclonus (Penney *et al.*, 1990). Neuroacanthocytosis often is manifested by both chorea and tics (Hardie *et al.*, 1991). Some patients with childhood-onset tics may later develop torsion dystonia (Shale *et al.*, 1986; Stone and Jankovic, 1991). Often patients with idiopathic torsion dystonia will have dystonic tremor or rapid movements that resemble myoclonus or chorea (Fahn *et al.*, 1987). Patients with tardive dyskinesia may have a combination of rhythmical orobuccolingual movements plus dystonia and akathitic movements (Fahn, 1984).

The most common type of movements, whether isolated or in the presence of other

Table 18.1 Clues relating to the movements that suggest a psychogenic movement disorder

Abrupt onset
Inconsistent movements (changing characteristics over time)
Incongruous movements and postures (movements don't fit with recognized patterns or with normal physiological patterns)
Presence of additional types of abnormal movements that are not consistent with the basic abnormal movement pattern or are not congruous with a known movement disorder, particularly: Rhythmical shaking Bizarre gait Deliberate slowness in carrying out the requested voluntary movement Bursts of verbal gibberish Excessive startle (bizarre movements in response to sudden, unexpected noise or threatening movement)
Entrainment of the psychogenic tremor to the rate of the requested rapid successive movement the patient is asked to perform
Demonstrating exhaustion and fatigue
Spontaneous remissions
Movements disappear with distraction
Response to placebo, suggestion or psychotherapy
Presence as a paroxysmal disorder
Dystonia beginning as a fixed posture

Table 18.2 Clues relating to other medical observations that suggest a psychogenic movement disorder

False weakness
False sensory complaints
Multiple somatizations or undiagnosed conditions
Self-inflicted injuries
Obvious psychiatric disturbances
Employed in the health profession or in health insurance claims
Presence of secondary gain, including continuing care by a 'devoted' spouse
Litigation or compensation pending

types of movements, in patients with psychogenic movement disorders are shaking movements that can resemble organic tremors or peculiar, atypical tremors. Another note of caution about unusual tremors is that Wilson's disease can also present with unusual tremors (Shale *et al.*, 1987, 1988).

Table 18.1 also lists bizarre gaits as a feature of psychogenicity. After tremors, bizarre gait disorders are the next most common type of unusual movement disorder encountered in patients with mixed features of movements. The psychogenic gait can show posturing, excessive slowness and hesitation. There could be pseudoataxia or careful walking (like walking on ice). The latter resembles the fear-of-falling syndrome, which is discussed in more detail below. There can be sudden buckling of a leg, as if there is weakness (Vecht *et al.*, 1991), but the failure to produce this dipping movement each time the patient steps on the leg would be evidence of inconsistency. Accompanying this bizarre gait would be a variability of impairment and excessive swaying when tested for the Romberg sign, without actually falling.

Another aspect of the presence of abnormal movements is excessive startle that could mimic hyperekplexia, excessive startle syndrome, the jumping Frenchmen of Maine syndrome, or even reflex myoclonus (Andermann and Andermann, 1986). Thompson *et al.* (1992) determined the physiological parameters that are typically seen in patients with psychogenic startles. There is a variable latency to the onset of the jerk; the latencies are greater than those seen in reflex myoclonus of cortical or brainstem origin; the latencies are longer than the fastest voluntary reaction time; there are variable patterns of muscle recruitment within each jerk; and there is significant habituation with repeated stimulation. This last point is probably not specific to psychogenic startle, since organic startles may also show habituation. Noise stimuli can induce other abnormal movements besides startle. Walters and Hening (1992) reported a case with psychogenic tremor following sudden, loud noise; the patient had a posttraumatic stress disorder.

Table 18.1 also indicates that in a patient with psychogenic tremor, when asked to carry out rapid successive movements, such as tapping the index finger on the thumb, the rate of the tremor becomes the same as the rapid successive movements, i.e. the tremor has become entrained. In contrast, an organic tremor is the dominant rate; it will gradually force the voluntary movements to be the same rate as the tremor.

Idiopathic torsion dystonia usually begins with action dystonia (Fahn *et al.*, 1987), but psychogenic dystonia often begins with a fixed posture. The posture may manifest so much rigidity that it is extremely difficult to move the limb about a joint. Often the psychogenic dystonia resembles reflex sympathetic dystrophy because there is accompanying pain and tenderness (Lang and Fahn, 1990; Schwartzman and Kerrigan, 1990). To confuse matters, many cases of psychogenic dystonia of a limb follow a minor trauma to that limb, similar to the pattern of reflex sympathetic dystrophy. On the other hand, organic dystonia of a body part can be preceded by an injury to that body part (Schott, 1985, 1986; Scherokman *et al.*, 1986; Gordon *et al.*, 1990), so the diagnosis can be difficult to distinguish between organic and psychogenic dystonia. The clues in Tables 18.1 and 18.2 should help.

I have been impressed with the frequency of patients with psychogenic movement disorders being employed in some capacity working in the health profession (see Table 18.2). Many are nurses; another large group are employed in the health insurance industry, processing medical claims.

Another clue worth commenting upon is that many of the affected individuals have a devoted spouse, who responds readily to their pressing needs. Some spouses carry a pager so the patient can easily call them while they are at work. Others pamper over the patient, who may even be wheelchair-bound, especially if he/she has psychogenic dystonia.

PSYCHOGENIC DYSTONIA

It is, in some ways, ironic that torsion dystonia can sometimes be due to psychogenic causation. From its earliest beginnings idiopathic torsion dystonia appeared to have been mistaken as a manifestation of a psychiatric disturbance (Schwalbe, 1908). Soon after Schwalbe's description in 1908 (see translation by Truong and Fahn, 1988), however, Oppenheim (1911b) and Flatau and Sterling (1911) set matters right by emphasizing the organic nature of this disorder. Although some early publications on dystonia mentioned the 'functional' nature of the symptoms (Destarac, 1901) or used the label neurosis (Ziehen, 1911), these terms were employed in those days in a manner different from today. 'Functional' referred to a physiological activation of the abnormal movements with voluntary motor activity, which would otherwise disappear when the patient was quiet at rest. Neurosis was a term used to indicate a neurological, rather than a psychiatric, disorder, but one without a structural lesion. Today, it is common for the term functional to be equivalent to psychogenic, and for neurosis not to be used at all in neurology, but to refer to certain types of psychiatric disorders.

Thus, for many decades the organic nature of torsion dystonia was emphasized. Yet, possibly beginning in the 1950s, many patients with various forms of focal, segmental and generalized dystonia began to be misdiagnosed as having a conversion disorder. Among 44 patients with idiopathic dystonia reviewed by Eldridge *et al.* (1969), 23 (52%) had previously been referred for psychiatric treatment (without benefit). Marsden and Harrison (1974) had a similar experience; 43% of their 42 patients were previously diagnosed as suffering from hysteria. Cooper and his colleagues (1976) reviewed their series of 226 patients and found that 56 (25%) had a diagnosis of psychogenic aetiology at some time during their illness. Lesser and Fahn (1978) reviewed the records of 84 patients with idiopathic dystonia seen at Prebsyterian Hospital in New York from 1969 to 1974 and found that in 37 (44%) it had been diagnosed previously that their movement abnormalities were due to an emotional disorder. These 37 patients consisted of 11 with generalized dystonia, 14 with segmental dystonia and 19 with focal dystonia (14 with torticollis, 2 with oromandibular dystonia and 3 with blepharospasm).

Although some authors (Meares, 1971; Tibbets, 1971) suggested that an underlying psychiatric illness may exist in patients with torticollis, others (Zeman and Dyken, 1968; Cockburn, 1971; Riklan *et al.*, 1976) found no differences between dystonic patients and controls in regard to previous psychiatric history and current life adjustment or on psychiatric testing. Similarly, some authors (Crisp and Moldofsky, 1965; Bindman and Tibbets, 1977) considered hand dystonia (writer's cramp, occupational cramp) to be psychogenic. But Sheehy and Marsden (1982) studied 34 patients with writer's or other occupational cramps affecting the hand or arm. All patients underwent assessment by a psychiatric interview technique; these patients compared favourably with a control group, and the investigators concluded that their disorder was not psychiatric in origin. Another recent study involved psychiatric assessment in 20 subjects with focal hand dystonia and also concluded that none had any serious psychopathology (Grafman *et al.*, 1991). Furthermore, patients with writer's cramp do not have increased anxiety (Harrington *et al.*, 1988).

At the time of the first international symposium on dystonia held in 1975, Fahn and Eldridge (1976) noted that no case of proven psychological dystonia had been reported. With the realization that patients with dystonia were being misdiagnosed as a psychiatric disorder, knowledgeable neurologists became sensitive to this problem and since then seemed to avoid a diagnosis of hysterical dystonia. However, at the annual meeting of the American Academy of Neurology in 1983, Fahn *et al.* described 10 patients as having documented psychogenic dystonia. Batshaw *et al.* (1985) had followed a patient who had been misdiagnosed as an organic dystonia and who had had a stereotactic thalamotomy based on that diagnosis; these authors eventually recognized that their patient had psychogenic dystonia and reported her as a case of Münchausen's syndrome. Fahn and Williams (1988) have described 22 cases of documented or clinically established psychogenic dystonia, including a case of a young girl who underwent a stereotaxic thalamotomy.

Psychogenic dystonia is difficult to diagnose since there are no laboratory tests to establish the diagnosis of organic idiopathic dystonia. The clues listed in Tables 18.1 and 18.2 should help alert the clinician to the possibility of a psychogenic aetiology.

Table 18.3 lists the demographics of documented and clinically established cases of psychogenic dystonia seen at our institution. Patients are divided into those with continual dystonia and those with paroxysmal dystonia. Females outnumber males by a ratio of 20 : 2. The age at onset is quite variable. The youngest was at age 8, and the oldest at age 58. Those with paroxysmal dystonia were, as a general rule, older than patients with continual dystonia.

Table 18.3 Demographics of psychogenic dystonia documented and clinically established cases

	Continual	*Paroxysmal*
n	16	6
Gender (F : M)	15 : 1	5 : 1
Age at onset	8, 8, 9, 10, 12, 13, 13, 16, 23, 23, 23, 25, 29, 41, 42, 58	30, 31, 33, 36, 36, 41
Median	19.5	34.5

PSYCHOGENIC NON-DYSTONIC MOVEMENT DISORDERS

Koller *et al.* (1989) diagnosed 24 patients with psychogenic tremors. They described the tremors as complex; usually they were present at rest, with posture and with action. The onset was abrupt, and in all but one the tremors lessened or were abolished with distraction.

Keane (1989) described 60 cases with psychogenic gait abnormality out of 228 patients with psychogenic neurological problems. Among these abnormal gaits were 24 with 'ataxia' (the most common gait abnormality), 9 with trembling, 2 with 'dystonia', 2 with truncal 'myoclonus', and 1 with camptocormia (markedly stooped posture). Among the myriad of associated psychogenic signs were 8 patients with tremor. A knee giving way, with recovery, was seen in 5 patients, and is a feature of a case presented recently as an unknown, unusual movement disorder (Vecht *et al.*, 1991).

According to Keane (1989), this syndrome of fear of falling was referred to as stasobasophobia by Spiller (1933). Fear of falling is a syndrome in which the patient can walk perfectly well if he/she is holding on to someone, but is unable to walk without leaning against the furniture or walls if alone. Sometimes this could be purely due to a psychiatric problem, such as agoraphobia. Most of the patients I have seen with this problem developed the condition after they had fallen, usually from organic causes (such as loss of postural reflexes or ataxia), and now had a marked fear of falling if walking without holding on. One of my patients with essential action myoclonus developed this disorder after suffering several falls, and continued to have fear of falling despite the successful treatment of the myoclonus with clonazepam. The freezing phenomenon (or motor blocks) seen in parkinsonism and the gait in action myoclonus patients are the other major conditions in which the gait also normalizes when the patient holds on to someone.

Table 18.4 lists the types of non-dystonic psychogenic movement disorders I have characterized in 15 patients that were due to documented or clinically established psychogenic aetiology. Another 27 had a classification of probable or possible psychogenicity. None of these patients include those with the fear-of-falling syndrome. Table 18.4 lists the types of movements encountered in these groups. Four patients with documented and established psychogenic disorder had more than one type of movement phenomenology.

Table 18.4 Non-dystonic psychogenic movement disorders

Phenomenology	n	*Documented and established*	*Probable and possible*
Tremor, continual	11	4	7
Tremor, paroxysmal	4	2	2
Parkinsonism	5	2	3
Gait disorder	8	6	2
Myoclonus	2	2	0
Head shakes	2	0	2
Hyperekplexia	2	1	1
Chorea	1	1	0
Hemifacial spasm	2	0	2
Unclassified	9	1	8
Total	46	19	27

Table 18.5 Demographics of non-dystonic psychogenic movement disorders documented and clinically established cases

	Continual	*Paroxysmal*
n	7	8
Gender (F:M)	6:1	5:3
Age at onset	13, 32, 33, 35, 36, 40, 42	26, 33, 36, 36, 41, 51, 66, 73
Median	35	38.5

Table 18.6 Percentage of psychogenic dystonia and non-dystonia patients seen by movement disorder group at Columbia-Presbyterian Medical Center

	Idiopathic dystonia (*n* = 1200)		*Idiopathic non-dystonia* (*n* = 2500)	
	n	%	*n*	%
Documented and established	22	1.8	15	0.6
Probable and possible	17	1.4	25	1.0
All psychogenic	39	3.2	40	1.6

From Table 18.4, it is apparent that shaking movements are the most common type of movement phenomenology encountered clinically in the psychogenic disorders. Such tremors were also encountered in a number of patients in whom the major disability was psychogenic dystonia. Another common type of movement disorder is a bizarre abnormal gait, as indicated in the table. Parkinsonism due to psychogenic causes is uncommon, but does occur (Lang *et al.*, 1992).

Table 18.5 lists the demographics of the 15 documented and clinically established cases of psychogenic movement disorders that are non-dystonic. Patients are divided into those with continual movements and those with paroxysmal movements. Females outnumber males by a ratio of 11 : 4. The age at onset is quite variable. The youngest developed symptoms at age 13, and the oldest at age 73. Those with paroxysmal movements were, as a general rule, older than patients with continual movements.

Psychogenic movement disorders are not common in terms of percentage of patients seen with organic movement disorders. Table 18.6 illustrates this small percentage. Even if the probable and possible psychogenic cases are added into the total number, only 3.2% of what we otherwise diagnose as idiopathic dystonia had a psychogenic aetiology. If we add to the 1200 cases of idiopathic dystonia encountered, the 600 cases of symptomatic dystonia, the percentage due to psychogenic aetiology would be even smaller. In the non-dystonia group, psychogenic aetiology accounts for only 1.6% of the cases.

APPROACHES TO THE PATIENT SUSPECTED TO HAVE A PSYCHOGENIC MOVEMENT DISORDER

The following treatment plan has been developed over the years of attempting to manage patients with psychogenic disorders:

1. Admit the patient to the hospital. Informing the patient on the initial visit in an

outpatient setting usually leads to disbelief and distrust by the patient. He/she will usually never return, will continue to have symptoms and will probably see a number of other physicians looking for an organic diagnosis.

2. Do all necessary and reasonable tests to feel comfortable and secure that an organic basis for the symptoms has not been overlooked. A sleep study with video recording to observe the movements and electroencephalogram monitoring to determine if the patient is asleep may be helpful – it is possible that conversion reactions occur during sleep.
3. The presence of joint contractures does not exclude the diagnosis of a psychogenic movement disorder.
4. Obtain a psychiatric consultation to obtain clues as to the possible psychodynamics underlying the symptoms, to determine if the patient has insight which will be important for eventually informing him/her regarding the nature of the disorder, to conduct hypnosis or amylobarbitone interview, if necessary for obtaining more psychodynamic information, to discuss possible therapeutic approaches, and to establish a rapport between the patient and the psychiatrist for eventual psychotherapy. *The psychiatrist cannot make the diagnosis of a psychogenic movement disorder. That diagnosis can only be made by the neurologist.*
5. Do not underestimate the severity of the underlying psychiatric illness. These patients are prone to committing suicide.
6. Utilize physiotherapy and placebo therapy if necessary to help in documenting the diagnosis, as well as to initiate a treatment regimen. But do not leave the patient on these medications alone, without also informing him/her of the true diagnosis. Patients will not have further trust in the treating physician if they discover placebos for themselves. Placebo infusions can also be used to exacerbate the abnormal movements as well as to relieve them (Levy and Jankovic, 1983; Monday and Jankovic, 1993).
7. Never allow the patients to leave the hospital without being informed of the diagnosis. Discuss the diagnosis with the patient in the presence of the psychiatric consultant, if necessary. Anticipating that the referring physician is in a better position to discuss the diagnosis and manage treatment usually is incorrect.
8. When initially informing the patient about the diagnosis, it is usually helpful to state firmly that he/she has a movement disorder (specifically identify the disorder – dystonia, tremor, etc.) and that 'it is caused by the mind controlling the body. Pent-up emotions need to be expressed, and they do so by producing these abnormal movements'. Explain that such common diseases as hypertension and duodenal ulcer can develop from stress, and that the patient's condition is an analogous situation. This tends to make the psychogenic movement disorder more acceptable to patient and family. Often the patient has a need to belong to a group and will join the local chapter of the lay organization dealing with this disorder.
9. Always be positive and absolute with the patient if you are secure with the diagnosis. Do not convey uncertainty, or else the patient will continue to doubt the diagnosis and fail to respond to therapy. Always give positive reinforcement that the symptoms will progressively improve with time, as the muscles 'are being retrained to move more appropriately'. However, if you are uncertain about the diagnosis, seek another opinion.
10. Try to initiate treatment in the hospital. Use any combination of psychotherapy, positive reinforcement, physiotherapy and placebo therapy. The latter should be used only to establish the diagnosis. Chronic placebo therapy without informing the patient of the correct diagnosis will ultimately fail. Patients who are depressed will usually benefit from psychotherapy or antidepressant medication.

11. Factitious disorders and malingering are usually not benefited. Symptoms will disappear only when the patient is ready to give them up.
12. Somatoform disorders can usually be treated. In some patients, the symptom may return despite the patient being aware that it is due to an emotional problem.

References

American Psychiatric Association (1980) *Diagnostic and Statistical Manual of Mental Disorders*, 3rd edn, Washington, DC

Andermann F and Andermann E (1986) Excessive startle syndromes: startle disease, jumping, and startle epilepsy. *Adv Neurol*, **43**, 321–38

Batshaw ML, Wachtel RC, Deckel AW, Whitehouse PJ, Moses H III, Fochtman LJ *et al.* (1985) Münchausen's syndrome simulating torsion dystonia. *N Engl J Med*, **312**, 1437–9

Bindman E and Tibbets RW (1977) Writer's cramp, a rational approach to treatment? *Br J Psychiatry*, **131**, 143–8

Bressman SB, Fahn S, and Burke RE (1988) Paroxysmal non-kinesigenic dystonia. *Adv Neurol*, **50**, 403–13

Campbell J (1979) The shortest paper. *Neurology*, **29**, 1633

Cockburn JJ (1971) Spasmodic torticollis: a psychogenic condition? *J Psychosom Res*, **15**, 471–7

Cooper IS (1976) *The Victim is Always the Same*, New York, Norton

Cooper IS, Cullinan T, and Riklan M (1976) The natural history of dystonia. *Adv Neurol*, **14**, 157–69

Crisp AH and Moldofsky HA (1965) A psychosomatic study of writer's cramp. *Br J Psychiatry*, **111**, 841–58

DeJong RN (1958a) Examination in cases of suspected hysteria and malingering. In *The Neurological Examination. Incorporating the Fundamentals of Neuroanatomy and Neurophysiology*, 2nd edn, New York, Hoeber-Harper, 931–56

DeJong RN (1958b) Abnormal movements. In *The Neurological Examination. Incorporating the Fundamentals of Neuroanatomy and Neurophysiology*, 2nd edn, New York, Hoeber-Harper, 521–3

Destarac (1901) Torticolis spasmodique et spasmes fonctionnels. *Rev Neurol (Paris)*, **9**, 591–7

Eldridge R, Riklan M, and Cooper IS (1969) The limited role of psychotherapy in torsion dystonia. Experience with 44 cases. *JAMA*, **210**, 705–8

Eldridge R, Ince SE, Chernow B, Milstein S, and Lake CR (1984) Dystonia in 61-year-old identical twins: observations over 45 years. *Ann Neurol*, **16**, 356–8

Fahn S (1984) The tardive dyskinesias. In Matthews WB and Glaser GH, eds, *Recent Advances in Clinical Neurology*, Vol 4, Edinburgh, Churchill Livingstone, 229–60

Fahn S (1989) Clinical variants of idiopathic torsion dystonia. *J Neurol Neurosurg Psychiatry* (Special suppl), 96–100

Fahn S and Eldridge R (1976) Definition of dystonia and classification of the dystonic states. *Adv Neurol*, **14**, 1–5

Fahn S and Sjaastad O (1991) Hereditary essential myoclonus in a large Norwegian family. *Movement Disorders*, **6**, 237–47

Fahn S and Williams DT (1988) Psychogenic dystonia. *Adv Neurol*, **50**, 431–55

Fahn S, Williams D, Reches A, Lesser RP, Jankovic J, and Silberstein SD (1983) Hysterical dystonia, a rare disorder: report of five documented cases. *Neurology*, **33** (suppl 2), 161

Fahn S, Marsden CD, and Calne CB (1987) Classification and investigation of dystonia. In Marsden CD and Fahn S, eds, *Movement Disorders 2*, London, Butterworths, 332–58

Flatau E and Sterling W (1911) Progressive Torsionspasms bie Kindern. *Z Gesamte Neurol Psychiatrie*, **7**, 586–612

Friedman A and Fahn S (1986) Spontaneous remissions in spasmodic torticollis. *Neurology*, **36**, 398–400

Goetz CG (1987) *Charcot, the Clinician: The Tuesday Lessons. Excerpts from Nine Case Presentations on General Neurology Delivered at the Salpetriere Hospital in 1887–88 by Jean-Martin Charcot*, translated with commentary, New York, Raven Press, 102–22 (on hysteria)

Gordon MF, Brin MF, Giladi N, Hunt A, and Fahn S (1990) Dystonia precipitated by peripheral trauma. *Movement Disorders*, **5** (suppl 1), 67

Gowers WR (1893) *A Manual of Diseases of the Nervous System*, vol II, 2nd edn, Philadelphia, Blakiston, 984–1030

Grafman J, Cohen LG, and Hallett M (1991) Is focal hand dystonia associated with psychopathology? *Movement Disorders*, **6**, 29–35

Hardie RJ, Pullon HWH, Harding AE, Owen JS, Pires M, Daniels GL *et al.* (1991) Neuroacanthocytosis – a clinical, haematological and pathological study of 19 cases. *Brain*, **114**, 13–49

Harrington RC, Wieck A, Marks IM, and Marsden CD (1988) Writer's cramp: not associated with anxiety. *Movement Disorders*, **3**, 195–200

Jahanshahi M, Marion M-H, and Marsden CD (1990) Natural history of adult-onset idiopathic torticollis. *Arch Neurol*, **47**, 548–52

Jayne D, Lees AJ, and Stern GM (1984) Remission in spasmodic torticollis. *J Neurol Neurosurg Psychiatry*, **47**, 1236–7

Keane JR (1989) Hysterical gait disorders: 60 cases. *Neurology*, **39**, 586–9

Koller WC and Biary NM (1989) Volitional control of involuntary movements. *Movement Disorders*, **4**, 153–6

Koller W, Lang A, Vetere-Overfield B, Findley L, Cleeves L, Factor S *et al.* (1989) Psychogenic tremors. *Neurology*, **39**, 1094–9

Lang A and Fahn S (1990) Movement disorder of RSD. *Neurology*, **40**, 1476–7

Lang A, Koller W, and Fahn S (1992) Psychogenic parkinsonism (PP). *Movement Disorders*, **7** (suppl 1), 82

Lesser RP and Fahn S (1978) Dystonia: a disorder often misdiagnosed as a conversion reaction. *Am J Psychiatry*, **153**, 349–452

Levy R and Jankovic J (1983) Placebo-induced conversion reaction in a neurobehavioral and EEG study of hysterical aphasia, seizure and coma. *J Abnorm Psychol*, **92**, 243–9

Marsden CD and Harrison MJG (1974) Idiopathic torsion dystonia. *Brain*, **97**, 793–810

Meares R (1971) Features which distinguish groups of spasmodic torticollis. *J Psychosom Res*, **15**, 1–11

Monday K and Jankovic J (1993) Psychogenic myoclonus. *Neurology*, **43**, 349–52

Oppenheim H (1911a) Section on hysteria. In *Textbook of Nervous Diseases for Physicians and Students*, 5th edn, translated by Bruce H, Edinburgh, Otto Schulzle, 1053–111

Oppenheim H (1911b) Uber eine eigenartige Krampfkrankheit des kindlichen und jugendlichen Alters (Dysbasia lordotica progressiva, Dystonia musculorum deformans). *Neurol Centralbl*, **30**, 1090–107

Penney JB, Young AB, Shoulson I, Starosta-Rubenstein S, Snodgrass SR, Sanchez-Ramos J *et al.* (1990) Huntington's disease in Venezuela: 7 years of follow-up on symptomatic and asymptomatic individuals. *Movement Disorders*, **5**, 93–9

Ranawaya R, Riley D, and Lang A (1990) Psychogenic dyskinesias in patients with organic movement disorders. *Movement Disorders*, **5**, 127–33

Riklan M, Cullinan T, and Cooper IS (1976) Psychological studies in dystonia musculorum deformans. *Adv Neurol*, **14**, 189–200

Scherokman B, Husain F, Cuetter A, Jabbari B, and Maniglia E (1986) Peripheral dystonia. *Arch Neurol*, **43**, 830–2

Schott GD (1985) The relation of peripheral trauma and pain to dystonia. *J Neurol Neurosurg Psychiatry*, **48**, 698–701

Schott GD (1986) Mechanisms of causalgia and related clinical conditions. The role of the central nervous and of the sympathic nervous systems. *Brain*, **109**, 717–38

Schwalbe W (1908) Eine eigentumliche tonische Krampfform mit hysterischen Symptomen. Inaug Diss, Berlin, G Schade

Schwartzman RJ and Kerrigan J (1990) The movement disorder of reflex sympathetic dystrophy. *Neurology*, **40**, 57–61

Shale HM, Truong DD, and Fahn S (1986) Tics in patients with other movement disorders. *Neurology*, **36** (suppl 1), 118

Shale HM, Fahn S, Koller WC, and Lang AE (1987) What is it? Case 1-1987: Unusual tremors, bradykinesia, and cerebral lucencies. *Movement Disorders*, **2**, 321–38

Shale HM, Fahn S, Sternlieb I, and Scheinberg IH (1988) Follow-up of "What is it?" Case 1-1987. *Movement Disorders*, **3**, 370

Sheehy MP and Marsden CD (1982) Writer's cramp – a focal dystonia. *Brain*, **105**, 461–80

Spiller WG (1933) Akinesia agera. *Arch Neurol Psychiatry*, **30**, 842–84

Stone LA and Jankovic J (1991) The coexistence of tics and dystonia. *Arch Neurol*, **48**, 862–5

Thompson PD, Colebatch JG, Brown P, Rothwell JC, Day BL, Obeso JA *et al.* (1992) Voluntary stimulus-sensitive jerks and jumps mimicking myoclonus or pathological startle syndromes. *Movement Disorders*, **7**, 257–62

Tibbets RW (1971) Spasmodic torticollis. *J Psychosom Res*, **15**, 461–9

Truong DD and Fahn S (1988) An early description of dystonia: translation of Schwalbe's thesis and information on his life. *Adv Neurol*, **50**, 651–64

Vecht CJ, Meerwaldt JD, Lees AJ, Marsden CD, and Fahn S (1991) Unusual movement disorder, case 1, 1991. Unusual tremor, myoclonus and a limping gait. *Movement Disorders*, **6**, 371–75

Walters AS and Hening WA (1992) Noise-induced psychogenic tremor associated with post-traumatic stress disorder. *Movement Disorders*, **7**, 333–8

Zeman W and Dyken P (1968) Dystonia musculorum deformans. In *Handbook of Clinical Neurology*, (eds PJ Vinken and GU Bruyn), vol 6, Amsterdam, North-Holland, 517–43

Ziehen T (1911) Ein fall von tonischer Torsionsneurose. *Neurol Centralbl*, **30**, 109–10

19
Stiff people

Philip D. Thompson

Muscle stiffness may be the presenting symptom or a common complaint in many disorders affecting the motor system. Diseases of muscle, peripheral nerves, spinal cord, brainstem or basal ganglia can give rise to symptoms of muscle stiffness and spasms or cramps (Table 19.1) which may be accompanied by additional impairment of voluntary movement or difficulty relaxing after voluntary muscle contraction. Within the large differential diagnosis of muscle cramps, spasms and rigidity are many conditions with additional unique clinical features that provide important diagnostic clues (Table 19.2). This applies particularly to metabolic and myotonic myopathies, the parkinsonian or akinetic–rigid syndromes and torsion dystonia. There remains a group of conditions in which muscle stiffness and rigidity are the sole complaints and result from continuous muscle activity without muscle disease or defects in higher motor control. Many of these conditions are rare. In some, the pathology is thought to lie within peripheral motor axons, with or without evidence of a peripheral neuropathy, whilst in others spinal cord disease is thought to be responsible. These conditions must be distinguished from the stiff-man syndrome, a rare disorder which is now thought to have an autoimmune basis although the precise site of pathology is not known. The clinical features of these disorders will be reviewed in this chapter, along with the investigations which help differentiate between them.

STIFF-MAN SYNDROME

Clinical features

The term stiff-man syndrome was first introduced by Moersch and Woltman (1956) to describe the clinical features of 'progressive fluctuating muscular rigidity' and spasm seen in 14 patients at the Mayo Clinic over a period of 32 years. The original case was that of a 49-year-old man who developed episodic tightness of neck muscles which spread to involve muscles of the shoulder and back over a period of 4 years. The sensations of tightness evolved into stiffness of the back, neck, abdomen and thighs. Stiffness of the abdominal muscles was striking and it was described as 'board-like' rigidity. The axial and limb rigidity produced by continuous muscle contraction made voluntary movements and walking slow and awkward.

Table 19.1 Anatomical and pathological classification of syndromes that may present with symptoms of muscle stiffness, spasms, cramps, rigidity or contracture. In many of the disorders listed in this table the anatomical site of the abnormality has been localized by neurophysiology without evidence of pathological change. In these cases the abnormality is presumed to be functional and not structural

Site unknown
Stiff-man syndrome

Cerebral–brainstem
Encephalitis lethargica
Torsion dystonia
Akinetic–rigid syndromes

Spinal cord
Toxins
- Tetanus
- Strychnine poisoning
- Black widow spider bite

Inflammatory myelitis
- Progressive encephalomyelitis with rigidity
- Subacute myoclonic spinal neuronitis
- *Borrelia burgdorferi* infection

Traumatic myelopathy
Spinal cord neoplasm (intrinsic)
Ischaemic myelopathy
Spinal arteriovenous malformation
Cervical spondylotic myelopathy

Peripheral nerve
Neuromyotonia (myokymia with impaired muscle relaxation)
- Idiopathic
- Isaacs syndrome
- Paraneoplastic syndrome
- Hereditary motor and sensory neuropathies
- Inflammatory neuropathies
- Toxic neuropathies
- Radiation plexopathies
- Paroxysmal ataxia and myokymia

Hereditary distal muscle cramps without neuropathy
Schwartz–Jampel syndrome
Tetany (hypocalcaemia, hypomagnesaemia)
Cramps
- Postexertion
- Dehydration/salt depletion
- Pregnancy
- Denervation (motor neuron disease, motor neuropathies)
- Cause unknown

Muscle
Myotonic syndromes
- Myotonic dystrophy
- Myotonia congenita
- Paramytonia congenita

Table 19.1 continued

Muscle continued
Metabolic myopathies
Myophosphorylase deficiency (McArdle's disease)
Phosphofructokinase deficiency
Ca^{2+}-adenosine triphosphatase deficiency (Brody's disease)
Inflammatory myopathies
Polymyositis
Endocrine myopathies
Hypothyroidism
Addison's disease
Congenital myopathies
Stiff-spine syndrome
Emery–Dreifuss muscular dystrophy
Bethlem muscular dystrophy
Other conditions presumed to be muscular in origin
Rippling muscle disease
Rolling muscle disease
Contracture
Bone (ankylosis)
Arthritis
Ankylosing spondylitis
Soft tissue
Volkmann's ischaemic contracture

Superimposed on the muscle rigidity were prolonged and painful muscle spasms which were evoked by voluntary or passive movement. When prolonged the spasms caused him to fall like a 'wooden man'.

The remaining 13 cases described by Moersch and Woltman presented a similar clinical picture. The onset of illness was graudal with symptoms of painful tightness, stiffness, and rigidity of trunk and proximal limb muscles which progressed slowly over many months. Rigidity was most severe in the lumbar and abdominal muscles. Muscles of the face and distal limbs were not affected. Muscle spasms were common early complaints. These varied from minor to severe prolonged spasms of sufficient intensity to throw the patient off his or her feet. Spasms could be precipitated by movement, fright or sudden external stimuli such as a loud noise or eliciting the plantar reflexes. Sphincter function was unimpaired. Tendon reflexes, muscle strength (as best as could be assessed), sensation, coordination and higher mental function were not affected. The duration of illness in 4 of the 14 cases who died during follow-up ranged from 6 to 15 years; in the 7 patients who were alive at the time of their report the illness duration was 2–14 years. No cause for their symptoms was found and no other abnormalities were indentified on investigation, with the exception that 4 of the original 14 patients had diabetes mellitus. Postmortem examination in 1 case, a woman with an illness duration of 10 years who died in diabetic coma, did not reveal any abnormality.

Since the original descriptions, many cases of stiff-man syndrome have been reported from all parts of the world. Symptoms usually begin in the fourth and fifth decades of life. There is also a small number of reports of conditions resembling the

Table 19.2 Summary of major differences between the causes of muscle spasms, rigidity, cramps and contracture

	Myotonia	*Metabolic myopathies*	*Stiff-man syndrome*	*Progressive encephalomyelitis with rigidity*	*Isaacs syndrome (±neuropathy)*	*Tetany/ cramps*	*Contracture*	*Dystonia*
Rigidity	No	No	Yes	Yes	Yes	No	Fixed posture	No
Distribution	Viariable	Variable	Axial	Axial/distal	Distal	Variable	Variable	Variable
Stiffness at rest	No	No	Yes	Yes	Yes	No	Yes	No
Cramps, Spasms								
Muscles affected	All	All	Axial	Axial/distal	Distal	Distal	None	Variable
Exercise induced	Yes	Yes	Yes	Yes	Yes	Yes	No	Yes
Stimulus sensitive	Yes	No	Yes	Yes	Yes	No	No	No
Pain	No	Yes	Yes	Yes	No	Yes	No	No
Contracture	No	Yes	No	No	No	No	Yes	No
Cranial nerves	Normal	Normal	Normal	Affected	Affected	Affected	No	Variable
Weakness, wasting	Yes	Yes	No	Yes	Yes	No	Yes	No
Tendon reflexes	Normal	Normal	Normal	May be absent	May be absent	Normal	Absent	Normal
Sensory loss	No	No	No	Yes	Yes	No	Yes	No
Cerebrospinal fluid	Normal	Normal	Oligoclonal IgG	Oligoclonal IgC Lymphocytes	Normal Oligoclonal IgG*	Normal	Normal	Normal
Autoantibodies	No	No	AntiGAD Endocrine Ab†	AntiGAD Endocine Ab†	Rare AChRAb‡	No	No	No
Electromyography								
At rest	Silent	Silent	CMUA	CMUA	CMUA, CMFA	Normal	Silent	Silent
During spasm/cramp	Myotonic discharges	Silent	Normal units	±Denervation	After-discharges Myokymia ±denervation	Normal units	Silent	Normal units
Spinal anaesthesia	Persists	Cramps persist	Abolishes CMUA	Abolishes CMUA	Activity persists	?	Posture persists	Abolishes
Peripheral block	Persists	Cramps increase	Abolishes CMUA	Abolishes CMUA	Activity persists	Persist	Posture persists	Abolishes
Neuromuscular block	Persists	Cramps persist	Abolishes CMUA	Abolishes CMUA	Activity abolished	Persist	Posture persists	Abolishes
Ischaemia	Persists	Cramps persist	Abolishes CMUA	Abolishes CMUA	Activity enhanced	Increased	Posture persists	Abolishes
Sleep	Persists	Not known	Abolishes CMUA Spasms may persist	Abolishes CMUA	Activity persists	May occur	Posture persists	Abolishes
Nerve conduction velocity	Normal	Normal	Normal	Normal	May be slow	Normal	Normal	Normal
Muscle biopsy	Abnormal	Abnormal	Normal	±Denervation	±Denervation	Normal	Fibrosis	Normal
Treatment	Phenytoin Quinine Procainamide	Nil	Baclofen Diazepam Valproate Clonazepam	Baclofen Diazepam Methylprednisolone	Carbamazepine Phenyloin	?Quinine Calcium	Nil	Benzhexol

CMUA continuous motor unit activity; CMFA continuous muscle fibre activity; GAD glutamic acid decarboxylase; IgG immunoglobulin G; AChRAb anti-acetylcholine receptor antibodies

*Cases of acquired neuromyotonia have recently been described with oligoclonal IgG in cerebrospinal fluid (see text for details).

†Organ specific endocrine antibodies.

‡Anti-acetyl choline receptor antibodies have been reported in a small number of cases with thymoma and CMFA (see text for further details).

Table 19.3 Criteria for the diagnosis of the stiff-man syndrome

Clinical
Gradual onset of aching and tightness of axial muscles
Slow progression; stiffness spreads from axial muscles to limbs (legs > arms)
Persistent contraction of thoracolumbar, paraspinal and abdominal muscles
Abnormal hyperlordotic posture of lumbar spine
Board-like rigidity of abdominal muscles
Rigidity abolished by sleep
Stimulus-sensitive painful muscle spasms
No other abnormal neurological signs
Intellect normal
Cranial muscles rarely (if ever) involved
Neurophysiological
Continuous motor unit activity
EMG activity abolished by sleep, peripheral nerve block, spinal or general anaesthesia
Normal peripheral nerve conduction
Normal motor unit morphology
Other observations that may be helpful but are of uncertain diagnostic specificity
Autoantibodies directed against GABAergic neurons, in particular to GAD
Association with autoimmune endocrine disease

EMG = Electromyogram; GABA = gamma-aminobutyric acid; GAD = glutamic acid decarboxylase.

stiff-man syndrome in younger (Kugelmass, 1961; Klein *et al.*, 1972; Isaacs, 1979; Sander *et al.*, 1979) and older patients (Trethowan *et al.*, 1960). (It is not clear from the case reports of 'congenital stiff-man syndrome', inherited as an autosomal dominant trait (Klein *et al.*, 1972; Sander *et al.*, 1979), whether familial hyperekplexia was excluded.) Overall, males and females appear equally affected, although the sex incidence varies among different series (Gordon *et al.*, 1967; Lorish *et al.*, 1989; Solimena *et al.*, 1990; Blum and Jankovic, 1991).

The following criteria for diagnosis have been modified from the those proposed by Gordon *et al.* (1967) and Lorish *et al.* (1989) which were derived from the observations of Moersch and Woltman (1956; Table 19.3).

1. The illness is of gradual onset and begins with tightness or stiffness of axial (trunk) muscles.
2. It is slowly progressive over periods of up to 28 years (Lorish *et al.*, 1989), during which time stiffness spreads from trunk to proximal limb muscles.
3. Persistent axial muscle contraction, especially of abdominal and thoracolumbar paraspinal muscles, leads to rigidity of these muscles, a characteristic hyperlordosis of the lumbar spine (Fig. 19.1), an abnormal neck posture and restriction in the range of back and hip movement. For example, a common complaint is of difficulty or inability to lean forward to tie shoelaces or put on socks. The exaggerated lumbar lordosis persists when supine at rest. This observation serves to distinguish the lordotic posture in patients with the stiff-man syndrome from that seen in patients with axial torsion dystonia where abnormal postures of the trunk disappear at rest.
4. Muscle spasms superimposed on the rigidity appear early in the illness. Spasms are induced by voluntary movement, and a variety of external stimuli such as sudden unexpected noise, painful stimuli or fright. Spasms may be of sufficient

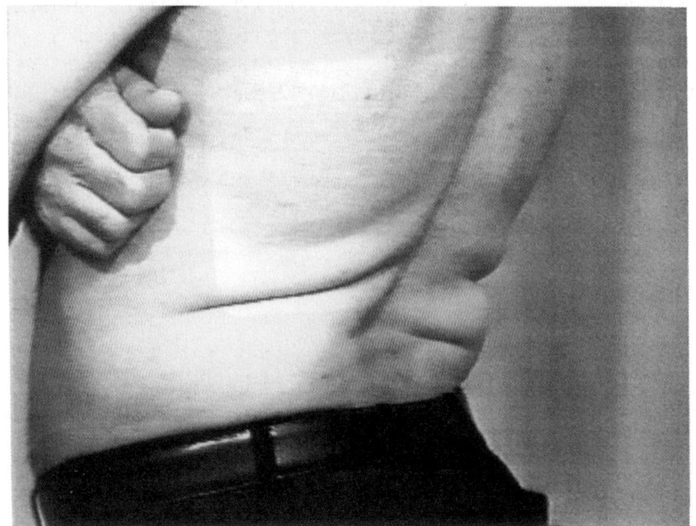

(a)

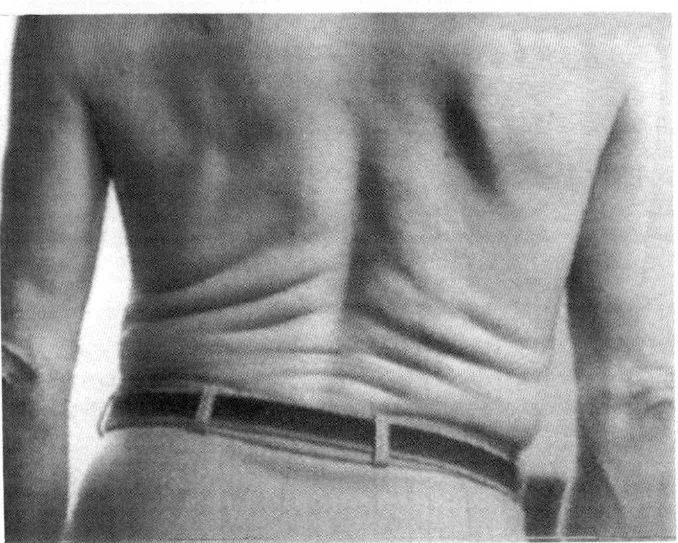

(b)

Figure 19.1 (a and b) Typical posture of an exaggerated lumbar lordosis in 2 patients with the stiff-man syndrome.

intensity to fracture long bones such as the femur or bend the orthopaedic pins inserted to repair them (Asher 1958). The severity of these spasms prompted Asher (1985) to refer to them as 'titanic'. A variety of types of spasms may occur. These are discussed in more detail below. Pain commonly accompanies the spasms and may be severe.

5. The remainder of the neurological examination, including cognitive function, cranial nerve examination, muscle strength, tendon reflexes, sensation and

coordination, is normal. These criteria are important for excluding structural lesions of the spinal cord which may occasionally produce rigidity (alpha rigidity), progressive encephalomyelitis with rigidity, peripheral neuromuscular causes of continuous muscle activity, myotonia or contracture and extrapyramidal diseases presenting as akinetic–rigid syndromes.

6. Electromyography shows continuous motor unit activity despite attempted relaxation, normal motor unit morphology, no signs of denervation; peripheral nerve conduction velocities are normal.

Associated conditions

Insulin-dependent diabetes mellitus is present in one-third to two-thirds of patients (Gordon *et al.*, 1967; Spehlmann and Norcross, 1979; Solimena *et al.*, 1990b). Indeed, diabetic ketoacidosis is a common cause of death in these patients. Other autoimmune endocrine diseases, including thyroid disease, pernicious anaemia and vitiligo, also have been described in association with stiff-man syndrome (Werk *et al.*, 1961; Williams *et al.*, 1988; Harding *et al.*, 1989; Solimena *et al.*, 1990b).

It is of interest that endocrine function also appears to influence symptoms of muscle stiffness and spasm. The level of blood glucose control was reported to alter the degree of stiffness in one patient with diabetes; muscle stiffness deteriorated when blood sugar levels were low (Howard, 1963). Cortisol replacement improved muscle stiffness and spasm in a 42-year-old patient with signs typical of the stiff-man syndrome and postpartum hypopituitarism (George *et al.*, 1984). Symptoms were present before parturition, but were more pronounced when the hypopituitarism became evident.

The incidence of epilepsy in the stiff-man syndrome was estimated to be of the order of 10% (Martinelli *et al.*, 1978), although this has not been confirmed in subsequent reports.

Electrophysiological studies

An important diagnostic criterion is the presence of continuous motor unit activity on electromyography despite attempted relaxation. Continuous motor unit activity may be recorded in many axial muscles and also in leg and proximal arm muscles. This activity is most evident in paraspinal muscles, particularly thoracolumbar, and the rectus abdominis muscles. Agonist and antagonist muscle groups are equally affected. The continuous motor unit activity gives rise to the board-like rigidity of axial muscles and produces the abnormal hyperlordotic posture of the lower trunk. Such activity subsides during sleep, peripheral nerve or spinal nerve root block, spinal anaesthesia and general anaesthesia. These findings indicate a central origin for the abnormal muscle activity. The prominence of rigidity and spasms in axial muscle groups is a universal and striking finding in the stiff-man syndrome. If continuous motor unit discharge is more prominent in distal than paraspinal or abdominal muscles, the diagnosis should be questioned, especially if the typical posture of an exaggerated lumbar lordosis is absent (Lorish *et al.*, 1989). The morphology of the individual motor units is normal and there is no spontaneous activity such as fasciculations, fibrillations or positive sharp waves to suggest denervation. Grouped rhythmic discharges or bizarre high-frequency discharges do not occur. Peripheral nerve motor and sensory conduction velocities are normal.

A central origin for the spasms, rigidity and continuous motor unit activity is suggested by their disappearance after peripheral nerve block and general anaesthesia, and the similarity of the clinical picture to tetanus and strychnine poisoning. A number of sites is possible. Primary enhancement of spinal motoneuron excitability seems unlikely since spinal monosynaptic stretch reflexes and F-waves are normal (Meinck *et al.*, 1984). The excitability of alpha motoneurons, assessed by the ratio of the maximal H-reflex to M-wave size (the H:M ratio) in the soleus muscle has been reported to be normal (Meinck *et al.*, 1984) and, not surprisingly, increased during spontaneous activity (Mamoli *et al.*, 1977). The recovery curve of the soleus H-reflex after a conditioning stimulus has been mormal (Martinelli *et al.*, 1978; Rossi *et al.*, 1988), suggesting that any increase in motoneuron excitability was related to spinal cord inputs other than the Ia afferent system. Heightened gamma motoneuron or fusimotor excitability has been suggested (Olafson *et al.*, 1964; Gordon *et al.*, 1967; Mertens and Ricker, 1968), although there is no conclusive evidence to support or refute this hypothesis. Nevertheless, it appears an unlikely explanation for the rigidity in view of the normal tendon reflexes and proximal and axial distribution of rigidity (Meinck *et al.*, 1984). Defective Renshaw cell function has been proposed but the silent period following a supramaximal peripheral nerve stimulus is normal (Mamoli *et al.*, 1977; Martinelli *et al.*, 1978; Boiardi *et al.*, 1980; Meinck *et al.*, 1984; Rossi *et al.*, 1988). The silent period after a stretch reflex is also normal, distinguishing the rigidity of the stiff-man syndrome from that in tetanus where the silent period can be absent or reduced due to abnormal hyperexcitability of motoneurons (Struppler *et al.*, 1963; Risk *et al.*, 1981). Vibration-induced suppression of the soleus H-reflex was normal in 1 case (Martinelli *et al.*, 1978) and abnormal in 2 (Isaacs, 1979; Rossi *et al.*, 1988), suggesting a disorder of presynaptic inhibition of Ia terminals in the spinal cord. This abnormality of presynaptic reciprocal inhibition was seen in a further case by Gabellini *et al.* (1991). These authors also demonstrated an abnormality of spinal disynaptic reciprocal inhibition between agonist and antagonist muscles, mediated by the Ia spinal inhibitory interneuron. Central sensory and motor conduction was normal in a study of 4 patients (Gabellini *et al.*, 1991).

Abnormal excitability of reflexes mediated by spinal interneuron pathways has been demonstrated by many authors. This may be due to defects within spinal interneuronal networks at a segmental level or in their descending control. This concept is particularly attractive since it would explain the spread of activity from one limb to another and the axial emphasis of the continuous motor unit activity. Isaacs (1979) reported the absence of normal habituation of non-painful polysynaptic reflexes. In a detailed study of a patient with a 20-year history of the stiff-man syndrome, Meinck *et al.* (1984; Meinck and Conrad, 1986) showed abnormal exteroceptive or cutaneomuscular reflexes in the upper and lower limbs. These reflexes were exaggerated, did not habituate and were followed by an increase in the level of tonic electromyographic activity (Fig. 19.2). The exaggerated and non-habituating exteroceptive or cutaneomuscular reflexes in the legs are analogous to flexor withdrawal reflexes. These reflexes occur in response to noxious (and innocuous) stimuli and consist of stereotyped sequences of muscle excitation and inhibition, which are elaborated by polysynaptic spinal pathways and subject to modulation from many supraspinal pathways (Kugelberg *et al.*, 1960; Meinck *et al.*, 1981). One of their main functions is to withdraw the limb from the noxious stimuli. Exaggeration of exteroceptive reflexes in this patient was thought to account for some of the stimulus-induced muscle spasms and jerks. This finding seems to be specific to the stiff-man syndrome. Such abnormalities are not seen in other causes of abnormal

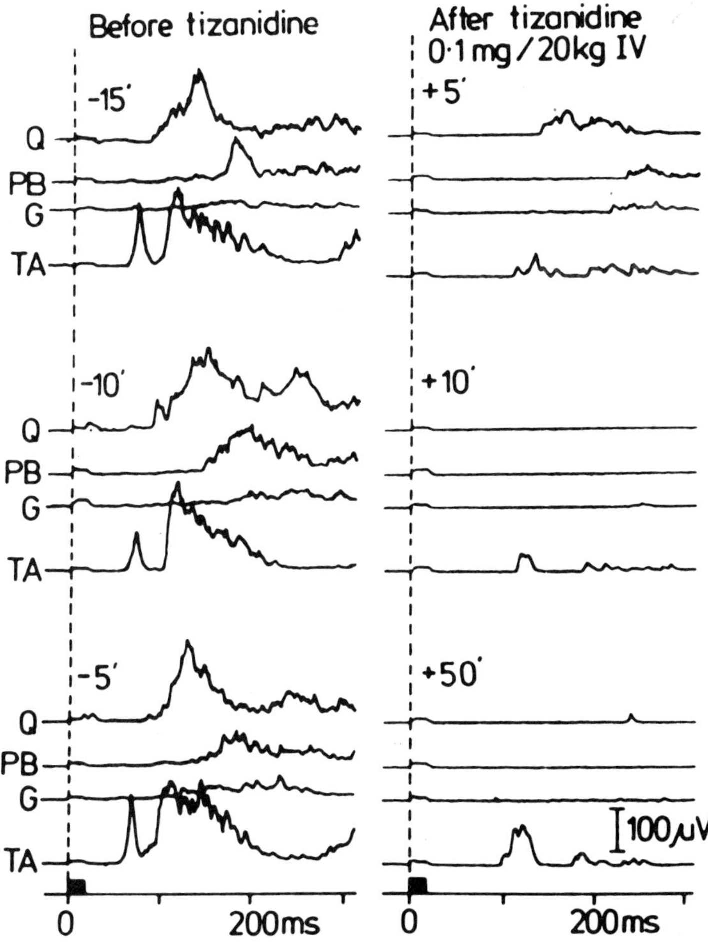

Figure 19.2 Effect of tizanidine (0.1 mg/20 kg intravenously) on cutaneomuscular reflex activity in muscles of the leg (quadriceps femoris, Q; posterior biceps, PB; gastocnemius, G; tibialis anterior, TA) elicited by medial plantar nerve stimulation (pulse train of 400 impulses/second for 20 ms). Stimulus intensity was twice motor threshold and the interstimulus interval was 3 seconds. In the left-hand panel are shown recordings made 15, 10 and 5 minutes before the administration of tizanidine. Reflex activity is abnormally prominent in the proximal leg muscles. Increasing the stimulus intensity and shortening the interstimulus interval led to a progressive reduction in the latency of the tibialis anterior response (from 290 to 38 ms), indicating spatial and temporal facilitation in the pathway mediating this response. Responses 5, 10 and 50 minutes after the infusion of tizanidine are shown in the right-hand panel. Tizanidine greatly reduced the abnormal reflex activity in the leg muscles. This was accompanied by a reduction in muscle tone so that the patient was able to walk freely and lift her arms above her head, having been unable to do this before the infusion. From Meinck *et al.* (1984) with permission.

muscle tone, for example spasticity (Meinck *et al.*, 1984; Meinck and Conrad, 1986). Upper limb reflexes in this patient were slightly different and showed three components (Fig. 19.3). Blink reflexes also were abnormal with bilateral R1 and R3 responses and a lack of the normal habituation of the R2 response. This widespread enhancement of exteroceptive reflexes is best explained by abnormal descending control of segmental interneuronal systems. Pharmacological observations supporting this theory will be discussed below.

Other mechanisms have been reported to contribute to spasms in the stiff-man syndrome. Leigh *et al.* (1980) described a patient with a 10-year history of axial muscle stiffness due to continuous motor unit activity and widespread stereotyped spontaneous and stimulus-induced myoclonus affecting predominantly axial and lower limb muscles. Taps to the mantle region and light touch to perioral skin elicited a generalized myoclonic response. This was thought to originate in the brainstem, but differed from previous descriptions of reticular reflex myoclonus in that conduction 'up the brainstem' was rapid (Leigh *et al.*, 1980). These authors coined the term 'jerking stiff-man' syndrome, to describe the association of prominent jerking with the typical rigidity of the stiff-man syndrome. A similar patient reported by Alberca *et al.* (1982) had a 14-year history of axial and leg stiffness and rigidity that interfered with walking. The abdominal and paraspinal muscles were described as 'wooden'. Violent jerks and spasms occurred in response to a variety of stimuli. Stimulation of the supraorbital nerve elicited a generalized myoclonic jerk with a response latency of about 75 ms in trapezius. The latency of this response is consistent with a pathological exaggeration of the startle response as a further mechanism for the generalized jerks (Boiardi *et al.*, 1980).

Neuropharmacological studies

Evidence for an imbalance in noradrenergic and gamma-aminobutyric acid (GABA) transmitter systems in the brainstem and spinal cord has been discussed by many authors (Guilleminault *et al.*, 1984; Schmidt *et al.*, 1975; Mamoli *et al.*, 1977; Boiardi *et al.*, 1980; Meinck *et al.*, 1984; Meinck and Conrad, 1986). Drugs that increase aminergic (noradrenergic or serotonergic) activity within the central nervous system such as L-dopa (Guilleminault *et al.*, 1973; Isaccs, 1979) or clomipramine (Meinck *et al.*, 1984; Gabellini *et al.*, 1991) increased the severity of spasms, while those that reduce central catecholamine effects such as clonidine (Meinck *et al.*, 1984; Meinck and Conrad, 1986; Gabellini *et al.*, 1991) and tizanidine (Meinck *et al.*, 1984; Meinck and Conrad, 1986) tended to diminish the severity of the spasms (Fig. 19.2). These findings are in agreement with an increase in urinary excretion of 3-methoxy-4-hydroxyphenyl glycol, a metabolite of noradrenaline (Schmidt *et al.*, 1975; Isaacs, 1979), which correlated with muscle tone in one patient (Schmidt *et al.*, 1975), suggesting that central adrenergic mechanisms were important in the production of spasms. However, this finding was not confirmed by Mamoli *et al.* (1977) who could not demonstrate an association between the clinical state and the excretion of noradrenaline metabolites. Diazepam and baclofen improve the spasms and to a lesser extent the rigidity, probably enhancing transmission in GABAergic inhibitory pathways at both supraspinal and spinal levels. Diazepam may also inhibit adrenergic activity within the brainstem (Taylor and Laverty, 1969). As discussed above, alterations in the modulation of many reflex systems may contribute to the rigidity and spasms in the stiff-man syndrome. For example, descending monoaminergic

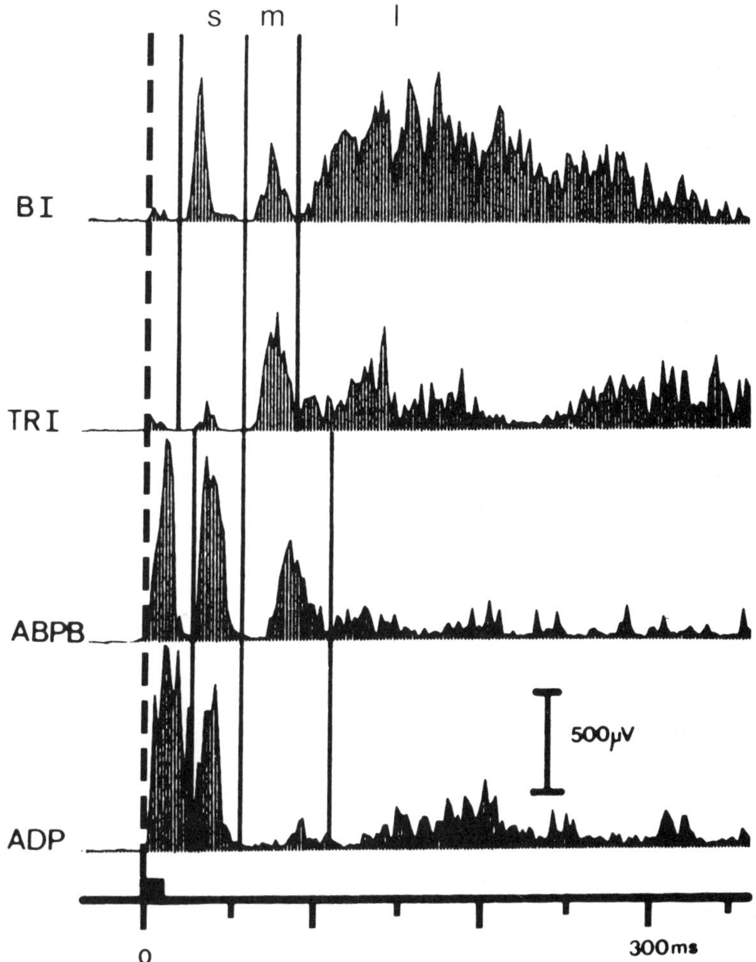

Figure 19.3 Rectified electromyographic responses from upper limb muscles (biceps brachii, BI; triceps, TRI; abductor pollicis brevis, ABPB and adductor pollicis, ADP) illustrating reflexes after median nerve stimulation at the wrist in the stiff-man syndrome. Onset of stimulation is shown by a vertical broken line; stimulus duration is shown by a bar on the time scale. Stimuli were a short train of three 0.1 ms duration rectangular pulses delivered at intervals of 5 ms. The intensity of the stimulus was about 1.5–2 times the motor threshold. Short (s), medium (m) and long (l) latency reflex components are separated by vertical unbroken lines. Eight consecutive reflexes were full-wave rectified and summated. The first component (latency 22–30 ms) was considered to be a spinal reflex since the latency corresponds to that of the F-wave and H-reflex. The medium-latency component (latency 64–72 ms) was considered to correspond to a C-reflex mediated by an transcortical loop. The later long-latency reflex (latency 100–120 ms) was interpreted as a startle response, possibly mediated by a spinoreticulospinal loop. From Meinck and Conrad (1986) with permission.

pathways from the brainstem have inhibitory effects on short-latency spinal flexor reflex afferents and facilitate longer-latency spinal flexor reflex pathways (Schomburg, 1990). However the precise relationship between the various drug effects, the abnormal reflexes and the rigidity remains far from certain.

There is no pharmacological support for the theories that abnormalities of Renshaw cell activity or glycinergic spinal interneuronal inhibitory networks are responsible for the symptoms and signs in the stiff-man syndrome. Anticholinergic or cholinergic drugs which might be expected to interfere with cholinergic transmission at the Renshaw cell have little effect or make symptoms worse (Mamoli *et al.*, 1977; Isaacs, 1979; Menick *et al.*, 1984), while glycine (Schmidt *et al.*, 1975; Mamoli *et al.*, 1977; Isaacs, 1979), an inhibitory transmitter in the spinal cord, and milacemide (Brown *et al.*, 1991a), a glycine precursor, had no effect on symptoms.

Immunological studies

The significance of the association of insulin-dependent diabetes mellitus and the stiff-man syndrome was enhanced by Solimena *et al.* (1988) when they presented evidence for the existence of antibodies directed against glutamic acid decarboxylase (GAD), the GABA-synthesizing enzyme, in a 49-year-old woman with a 10-year history of the stiff-man syndrome and diabetes mellitus. This patient also had antithyroid antibodies, pernicious anaemia with gastric parietal cell antibodies, and an oligoclonal pattern of immunoglobulin G (IgG) in cerebrospinal fluid. The same authors have since found similar antibodies against GABAergic neurons, in a further 33 patients with the stiff-man syndrome (Solimena *et al.*, 1990b). GAD antibodies were detected in the serum and cerebrospinal fluid of 60% of patients with a clinical diagnosis of the stiff-man syndrome (Solimena *et al.*, 1990b). The great majority of these patients also had antibodies directed against pancreatic islet cell antibodies (one-third had insulin-dependent diabetes mellitus) and gastric parietal cells. Thyroid microsomal antibodies were present in one-half and thyroglobulin antibodies were detected in about a third. The autoantigens in both the stiff-man syndrome and insulin-dependent diabetes mellitus have been shown to be GAD, which is present in pancreatic islet cells and some populations of central nervous system neurons (Baekkeskov *et al.*, 1990). The relatively high incidence of insulin-dependent diabetes mellitus in patients with the stiff-man syndrome in contrast to the very low incidence of the stiff-man syndrome in patients with diabetes mellitus may be explained by the rarity of antibodies to GABAergic neurons in diabetes, and the higher anti-GAD antibodies in the stiff-man syndrome (Baekkeskov *et al.*, 1990). Clearly other factors must be involved.

Whether the 40% of patients with a clinical diagnosis of the stiff-man syndrome but undetectable anti-GAD antibodies have the same condition remains to be determined. This observation reinforces the need to establish reliable clinical criteria for the diagnosis of the stiff-man syndrome and to define its range of clinical expression. One reason for seronegativity in some patients may be related to the assay method. Antibodies against GABAergic neurons may be detected in a number of ways. Immunocytochemical techniques show the presence of antibodies in cerebrospinal fluid or serum by staining specific sites in cells, such as Purkinje cells which contain GABAergic neurons. To determine whether the autoantibody is directed against GAD, immunoblotting techniques (Western blotting) are carried out. This will show whether the proteins have similar electrophoretic mobility to an antibody with known anti-GAD activity (sheep antiserum directed against GAD). Finally, autoantibodies may be shown by immunoprecipitation of GAD or a GAD-containing complex. Anti-GAD antibodies were detected by all three methods in the patients reported by Solimena *et al.* (1988, 1990a), but not all cases reported to date exhibit all these immunological characteristics. In a further case described by Solimena *et al.* (1990a) with epilepsy, serological evidence of multiple autoimmune endocrinopathies and antibodies directed against anti-GABAergic neurons (demonstrated by immunocytochemical staining of rat and human brain and pancreatic islet cells in a pattern similar to anti-GAD staining from sheep anti-GAD antiserum), there were immunoreactive bands on Western blotting. A similar situation was reported by Gorin *et al.* (1990) in a patient with typical clinical features of the stiff-man syndrome. Anti-GABAergic antibodies were detected by immunocytochemistry and anti-GAD activity was evident by immunoprecipitation, but not immunoblotting. These authors concluded that there may be heterogeneity amongst GABAergic autoantigens and that more than one anti-GAD antibody may be associated with the stiff-man syndrome. Indeed, to date, anti-GAD activity in the stiff-man syndrome has been described against a 64 kd antigen (Baekkeskov *et al.*, 1990) and an 80 kd antigen (Darnell *et al.*, 1993). The use of the presence of an antibody against GAD as a diagnostic criterion must await further verification and, as suggested by Gorin *et al.* (1990), should not rely on a single immunological technique.

Oligoclonal IgG bands have been reported in several cases (Maida *et al.*, 1980; Meinck and Ricker, 1987; Solimena *et al.*, 1988, 1990; Harding *et al.*, 1989). Indeed, one of the original cases reported by Moersch had a positive Nonne curve. Not all cases have oligoclonal bands. In the series reported by Solimena *et al.* (1990b), oligoclonal IgG bands were detected in 3 of the 11 patients who were positive and 2 of the 7 who were negative for anti-GABAergic antibodies.

An association with the human leukocyte antigen B44 antigen was noted in 4 of the 5 patients reported by Williams *et al.* (1988). In 2 other patients (Harding *et al.*, 1989), DR3 and 4 antigens were demonstrated. Both B44 and D3,4 were present in the patient studied by Solimena *et al.* (1988). The D3 and 4 antigens are associated with diabetes mellitus (Todd *et al.*, 1988).

Imaging studies

Computed tomography of the brain has been normal in most cases, as has imaging of the spinal cord. Maida *et al.* (1980) described atrophic changes in a 60-year-old woman with stiff-man syndrome and elevated cerebrospinal fluid IgG. White matter lesions have been shown on magnetic resonance imaging in 2 patients (Meinck and Ricker, 1987; Gabellini *et al.*, 1991).

Pathology

Pathological examinations of the central nervous system in patients with the stiff-man syndrome have not shown any striking changes (Moersch and Woltman, 1956; Asher, 195; Trethowan *et al.*, 1960; Cohen, 1966; Martinelli *et al.*, 1978). Detailed histochemical studies of postmortem material have not been undertaken. In 2 cases the spinal cord was normal (Trethowan *et al.*, 1960; Martinelli *et al.*, 1978).

Treatment

Of the large number of therapies tried, benzodiazepines and baclofen have proven to be the most valuable. Howard (1963) was the first to report a dramatic improvement in the spasms of 2 patients with diazepam in doses of 60 mg/day. Clonazepam has also been reported to be beneficial in doses of 4–6 mg/day (Westblom, 1977). Several reports have also documented improvement with baclofen (Mertens and Ricker, 1968; Cobb, 1974; Mamoli *et al.*, 1977; Whelan, 1980; Miller and Korsvik, 1981). High doses (up to 100 mg/day) may be needed to realize maximum benefit. In practice most patients are helped by a combination of baclofen and diazepam, both in high dose but increased gradually over several weeks in order to minimize sedation. The spontaneous and stimulus-sensitive spasms respond best to treatment and may be completely abolished by treatment. However, the axial continuous motor unit activity and resultant abnormal posture and limitation of mobility do not respond as well and usually persist despite these high doses. Other drugs reported to be of benefit include sodium valproate (Spehlmann *et al.*, 1981) and tizanidine (Meinck and Conrad, 1986). Carbamazepine and phenytoin, in general, are not helpful, in contrast to their beneficial effects on continuous motor unit activity of peripheral nerve origin.

The effects of immunosuppression have been tried in a few cases on the grounds that evidence points towards an autoimmune basis for the stiff-man syndrome. Vicari *et al.* (1989) reported a dramatic improvement in a patient with anti-GAD antibodies following plasmapheresis and prednisolone. The rigidity disappeared after a course of plasmapheresis and the improvement was sustained at the end of 7 months' treatment with steroids. Brashear and Phillips (1991) reported clinical and electrophysiological improvement, the latter judged by a reduction in exteroceptive reflex activation of paraspinal muscles following median nerve stimulation, in a patient with stiff-man syndrome and anti-GAD immunoreactivity in serum (but not cerebrospinal fluid) following five plasma exchanges over a period of 12 days. Serum antibody titres began to fall after the first exchange and clinical and electrophysiological improvement was noted within 6 hours of the first exchange. This striking remission was not evident in the patients reported by Harding *et al.* (1989). Both patients had evidence of autoimmune disease but there was no change in rigidity or alteration in their diazepam and baclofen requirements after similar plasma exchanges and a period of immunosuppression with azathioprine and prednisolone. Since the autoimmune process is likely to be active within the central nervous system it is difficult to imagine how systemic immunotherapy could exert such a rapid effect. Prolonged treatment over many months may be required. Furthermore, it is not yet known what relationship the serological abnormalities have to the pathophysiology of the clinical manifestations of the stiff-man syndrome.

CASES OF THE STIFF-MAN SYNDROME WITH ATYPICAL FEATURES

Two further patients, described by Piccolo *et al.* (1988; Piccolo and Cosi, 1989) are of interest. Clinical diagnoses of the stiff-man syndrome were made. In one, rigidity was most pronounced in the legs, and in the other, in the arms with wasting and contracture of upper limb muscles. There was no evidence of immunoreactivity to GABAergic nerve terminals. The cerebrospinal fluid was abnormal in both cases. A slight lymphocytic pleocytosis was evident in one and oligoclonal IgG bands were detected in the other. Treatment with steroids led to an improvement in both. These patients were subsequently found to have systemic neoplasms (colon and breast). The patient with breast adenocarcinoma, arm and neck stiffness and oligoclonal IgG in cerebrospinal fluid was subsequently reported along with two other women with ductal breast carcinoma and the stiff-man syndrome (with leg involvement and oligoclonal IgG in one) (Folli *et al.*, 1993). In these case, autoantibodies to a 128-kd synaptic protein were identified but there were no anti-GAD autoantibodies, nor were there other organ-specific autoantibodies, suggesting the existence of a distinct form of 'paraneoplastic stiff-man' syndrome (Folli *et al.*, 1993). In another brief report, Piccolo and Cosi (1989) described the case of a middle-aged man who had a 6-year history of the stiff-man syndrome before a spontaneous remission occurred. This patient also failed to show evidence of immunoreactivity to GABAergic nerve terminals. He then developed myasthenia gravis, with an elevated acetylcholine receptor antibody titre, radiological evidence of a thymoma and chronic active hepatitis. The findings in this case are reminiscent of those in the patients reported by Halbach *et al.* (1987), in whom a peripheral cause for the muscular hyperactivity and rigidity was shown electrophysiologically (see below).

The 2 cases described in an abstract by Schwartzman *et al.* (1989) also exhibited additional clinical features that were atypical for the stiff-man syndrome. In one, 'extrapyramidal and brainstem ocular signs' were evident, and both died suddenly after developing autonomic instability. Both had anti-GAD antibodies. Pathological exmination revealed perivascular gliosis in the spinal cord in one and widespread lymphocytic perivascular infiltration in the other. A similar patient was described by Burn *et al.* (1991), in whom a clinical diagnosis of progressive encephalomyelitis with rigidity was made and antibodies to GABAergic neurons, thyroid, gastric parietal cells and acetylcholine receptors were detected.

These cases illustrate the potential difficulties in distinguishing between cases of the stiff-man syndrome and progressive encephalomyelitis with rigidity and paraneoplastic encephalomyelitis (see below). Atypical clinical features for the stiff-man syndrome include prominent limb rigidity with segmental signs and contracture, evidence of brainstem dysfunction, profound autonomic disturbances, cerebrospinal fluid pleocytosis and the pathological changes of an encephalomyelitis. The extent to which there may be overlap between the clinical expressions of these conditions is not clear, although the pathological changes are quite different, as will be discussed in the next section. These cases also stress the importance of defining clearly the clinical spectrum of the stiff-man syndrome.

PROGRESSIVE ENCEPHALOMYELITIS WITH RIGIDITY

This rare disease, also referred to as spinal interneuronitis, may present with similar clinical features to the stiff-man syndrome (Whiteley *et al.*, 1976; Howell *et al.*, 1979). It is likely that 'subacute myoclonic spinal neuronitis', described by Campbell and Garland (1956), is allied to progressive encephalomyelitis, differing largely in its more rapid course. These disorders are distinguished from the stiff-man syndrome by several features (Whiteley *et al.*, 1976; Howell *et al.*, 1979). These include a relentless and progressive course, the presence of cranial nerve signs, signs referable to spinal segmental and long tract involvement and pathological findings of encephalomyelitis. Few cases have been reported and the true incidence of this syndrome is not known. It may occur as an isolated illness or in the setting of neoplasia with an identical clinical picture and pathological changes of paraneoplastic encephalomyelitis.

Clinical features

The first symptoms of progressive encephalomyelitis with rigidity may be sensory with pain, dysaesthesiae and sensory loss in the limbs (Kasperek and Zebrowski, 1971), or motor with weakness, stiffness, clumsiness and rigidity (Lhermitte *et al.*, 1973; Whiteley *et al.*, 1976; Howell *et al.*, 1979; Rothwell *et al.*, 1986; McCombe *et al.*, 1989; Brown *et al.*, 1991b; case 7). The onset of symptoms is subacute, extending over weeks to months. Painful stimulus-sensitive spasms appear with dramatic and disabling extensor spasms of the trunk or generalized myoclonus. The spasms may be accompanied by profuse sweating. With progression the rigidity worsens. This type of rigidity has been referred to as plastic or alpha rigidity. The increase in muscle tone is uniform throughout the range of limb manipulation and is much more severe than that seen in basal ganglia disease. Voluntary movement of the limbs becomes impaired with incoordination, action tremor or myoclonus and varying degrees of paresis. Upper or lower limbs may be affected. The tendon reflexes often are absent with extensor plantar responses. There may be areas of sensory loss corresponding to spinal tract or root involvement. Cranial nerve involvement has been prominent in all cases described, with nystagmus, opsoclonus, ophthalmoplegia, deafness, dysarthria and dysphagia. In the cases reported to date the illness has progressed to death in about 3 years. Rigidity and spasms also have been described as the main manifestations of a more acute form of encephalomyelitis with progression to death over weeks to months.

Investigations

Continuous motor unit activity has been detected in all cases with particular involvement of trunk muscles. This disappears during sleep and after peripheral nerve, spinal nerve root or general anaesthesia, confirming a central origin. There also may be evidence of segmental denervation. Deailed neurophysiological studies of the generalized myoclonus in 2 cases (Rothwell *et al.*, 1986; Brown *et al.*, 1991b) suggested a brainstem origin. Stimulus sensitivity was most marked for taps to the mantle or touch around the perioral region. In one patient with a clinical diagnosis of progressive encephalomyelitis and rigidity, a variety of autoantibodies were found, including anti-GAD and acetylcholine receptor antibodies (Burn *et al.*, 1991). The cerebrospinal fluid usually is abnormal with a lymphocytic pleocytosis and elevated protein and immunoglobulin (gammaglobulin) levels and oligoclonal IgG bands. Imaging studies have revealed brainstem atrophy (Rothwell *et al.*, 1986), white matter lesions (Brown *et al.*, 1991b) and abnormal signal intensity throughout the length of the low brainstem and cervical spinal cord on magnetic resonance imaging (McCombe *et al.*, 1989).

Pathology

Postmortem examination has shown widespread encephalomyelitis with perivascular lymphocyte cuffing and infiltration and neuronal loss throughout the lower brainstem and spinal cord. The inflammatory response has been most marked in the region of the cervical spinal cord. The central grey zones of the spinal cord are the sites of maximal neuronal loss (Howell *et al.*, 1979). These areas contain spinal interneurons. This pattern of pathological involvement is thought to account for the profound rigidity seen in these patients by disconnecting the spinal alpha mononeurons from the influences of inhibitory interneuronal networks of the spinal cord. Anterior horn cell degeneration and loss in the ventral horn also are present to account for the segmental flaccid, areflexic paralysis. Degeneration of the long tracts in the cervical spinal cord gives rise to the upper motor neuron signs and sensory loss in the legs. The presence of these widespread pathological changes, in addition to the clinical features, distinguishes these cases from the stiff-man syndrome.

The importance of involvement of the central grey matter of the spinal cord in producing the rigidity and spasms seen in spinal cord disease is reinforced by the similar patterns of rigidity produced by experimental central spinal cord ischaemia in dogs (Gelfan and Tarlov, 1959). Indeed, central spinal cord lesions such as grey matter infarction may also have similar sequelae (see below).

Treatment

Symptomatic treatment of the jerks and spasms with large doses of diazepam and baclofen may be of help, but there is no treatment available for the underlying condition. McCombe *et al.* (1989) reported some improvement with methylprednisolone in 1 case with evidence of myelitis on spinal cord biopsy.

OTHER EXAMPLES OF PROGRESSIVE ENCEPHALOMYELITIS

Similar clinical and pathological features have been described in patients with paraneoplastic encephalomyelitis complicating Hodgkin's disease (Campbell and Garland, 1956) and oat cell carcinoma of the lung (Roobol *et al.*, 1987; Bateman *et al.*, 1990). The clinical features consisted of generalized or segmental muscle rigidity, painful stimulus-sensitive jerks and spasms, weakness and sensory loss. Continuous motor unit activity was present on electromyography. In the case reported by Roobol *et al.* (1987), the cerebrospinal fluid IgG index was elevated and the number of motor neurons in the spinal cord was reduced; no interneurons could be identified.

SPINAL CORD LESIONS AND RIGIDITY

The concept of spinal or alpha rigidity with continuous motor unit discharge as the result of isolation of the spinal alpha motor neurons from inhibitory interneuronal circuits arises from observations made in rare cases of structural spinal cord lesions. Trauma (Thorburn, 1887), syringomyelia (Babinski, 1913), tumour (Rushworth *et al.*, 1961; Lourie, 1968), hydromyelia (Tarlov, 1967) and myelitis (Martin *et al.*, 1990) have all been described as producing rigidity and continuous motor unit activity, presumably by such mechanisms. Most of these lesions involved the central cervical spinal cord and resulted in pain, stiffness, stimulus-induced spasms, rigidity and abnormal limb postures, often involving rigid adduction, extension and internal rotation (Penry *et al.*, 1960; Rushworth *et al.*, 1961). These postures are produced by continuous motor activity which is not influenced by voluntary effort or stimulation of reflex pathways, indicating functional isolation of the spinal motoneurons. Painful spasms may be produced by traction or passive manipulation of the limbs. Features that distinguish these spinal lesions with rigidity from the stiff-man syndrome include segmental muscle wasting and weakness, absent tendon reflexes in the arms and brisk tendon reflexes in the legs with extensor plantar responses, and segmental and tract sensory disturbances. As might be expected with such lesions, the clinical picture is more rapidly progressive than that of the stiff-man syndrome.

Experimental ischaemia of the central spinal cord in dogs also produces spinal rigidity with limb postures resembling decerebrate rigidity, but which are not influenced by posture. Pathologically these ischaemic lesions of the central spinal grey matter produce extensive destruction of interneurons in the central and posterior grey matter sparing anterior horn cells (Gelfan and Tarlov, 1959). These authors showed that the muscular rigidity was due to continuous spontaneous discharge of motoneurons and was not influenced by inhibitory or excitatory interneuronal activity. Watershed infarction of the central grey matter of the spinal cord may produce a similar clinical picture. Davis *et al.* (1981) reported an elderly patient who presented with leg and lower trunk rigidity and stimulus-sensitive spinal myoclonus in whom there was pathological evidence of interneuron loss due to spinal infarction. The importance of damage to spinal interneurons in producing this pattern of rigidity was illustrated in the case reported by Tarlov (1967). A 31-year-old woman had a 6-year history of a traumatic paraplegia with complete lower limb paralysis, severe rigidity and painful spontaneous flexor spasms. The rigidity persisted after section of the posterior roots and section of the spinal cord, but abated after section of the anterior roots. Pathological examination of the excised spinal cord below T12–L1 showed a large central hydromyelic cavity and a considerable reduction in the number of neurons in the L5 segment which was maximal for interneurons in the intermediate segment of the cord.

Segmental myoclonus, with spontaneous and stimulus-induced jerks, frequently accompanies rigidity and continuous motor unit activity in these lesions in humans. An example of myoclonus of the legs and trunk with involvement of the lumbar cord was reported by Lourie (1968). A 55-year-old man presented with a history of stiffness of the hips, pain and numbness of the lower back and was found to have a scoliosis, 'plastic' rigidity of the legs, slow leg movements and board-like rigidity of the abdomen and persistent contraction of the lumbar paraspinal muscles. A spinothalamic sensory loss with sacral sparing suggested an intramedullary lesion. There were spontaneous rhythmic contractions of the hip adductor muscles and independent contractions of the external oblique and paraspinal muscles. These persisted during sleep. Myelography and later surgery suggested a glioma of the low spinal cord. This example illustrates the combination of spontaneous activities that may arise from the spinal cord, including continuous motor unit activity.

MUSCLE ACTIVITY OF PERIPHERAL NERVE ORIGIN PRODUCING MUSCLE STIFFNESS AND CRAMPS

A variety of peripheral nerve disorders may produce continuous muscle activity and present with symptoms of muscle stiffness at rest and cramps with delay in muscle relaxation after voluntary contraction. Isaacs syndrome, Isaacs–Mertens syndrome, armadillo syndrome, quantal squander syndrome, neuromyotonia, neurotonia, pseudomyotonia, syndrome of continuous muscle fibre activity and syndrome of continuous motor unit activity are some of the names given to such syndromes. Some of the confusion surrounding the use of these terms is related to interchanging their intended use as electromyographic descriptions to refer to clinical phenomena.

Myokymia is defined clinically as a wave-like rippling of muscle and in an electromyographic sense as regular groups of motor unit discharges, especially doublets and triplets. Neuromyotonia refers to the clinical syndrome of myokymia with impaired muscle relaxation; it also is used to describe high-frequency muscle discharges ('complex repetitive discharges', 'bizarre high-frequency discharges') recorded by needle electromyography. Pseudomyotonia is another term used to describe the clinical phenomenon of abnormal delay in muscle relaxation after voluntary contraction in patients with peripheral nerve diseases or cervical cord lesions who do not have 'true myotonia' on electromyography or percussion myotonia as in myotonic myopathies. To complicate matters further, there is often no clear distinction between *motor unit* and *muscle fibre* activity in many reports of these syndromes. For example in the syndrome of 'continuous muscle fibre activity' (Isaacs, 1961), continuous motor unit activity also occurs, and may be more common. Spontaneous motor unit and muscle fibre activities may be distinguished by the stability of single fibre discharge. Trontelj and Stalberg (1983) have shown that myotonic and most bizarre high-frequency discharges consist of stereotyped sequences of muscle *fibre* activation. In contrast, single-fibre jitter in grouped discharges of myokymia was much greater, suggesting the impulses arose proximal to the terminal branchings of the motor axons and therefore recruited whole motor *units*.

In the following discussion, myokymia will be used to refer to the clinical sign of wave-like rippling of muscle; myokymic discharges will be used to refer to grouped discharges recorded on needle electromyography. Neuromyotonia will be used to describe the clinical syndrome of myokymia and delayed muscle relaxation which may be associated with a number of electromyographic patterns of activity including complex repetitive discharges and grouped discharges.

Most cases of muscle activity of peripheral nerve origin producing muscle stiffness and cramps conform to a stereotyped clinical picture which is distinguishable from the stiff-man syndrome. An important feature is the presence of abnormal muscle discharges that are not seen in any of the above conditions.

Clinical features

These syndromes may affect children or adults. The symptoms are of gradual onset. Muscle stiffness with continuous twitching or rippling of muscles is present at rest and becomes more pronounced during and after muscle contraction, giving rise to difficulties in moving and relaxing. Such symptoms are often described as cramps. The symptoms may improve with repeated movements. Pain is rarely a prominent complaint, although muscle aches are common (Greenhouse *et al.*, 1967). Distal, proximal and cranial muscles are involved, in contrast to the proximal emphasis of rigidity in the stiff-man syndrome. Profuse sweating may accompany the continuous motor unit activity. The symptoms persist during sleep, following peripheral nerve, spinal nerve root or general anaesthesia and are abolished by peripheral neuromuscular blockade with curare. Abnormal postures of the feet and hands are evident on examination with persistent flexion or extension of digits. The postures of the hands and feet can resemble the carpopedal spasm of tetany. The posture of the trunk is often abnormal and the gait may be stiff (Fig. 19.4). Inspection of muscles reveals continuous rippling (myokymia) and fasciculations. Muscle hypertrophy has been reported in some cases (Hughes and Matthews, 1969; Valenstein *et al.*, 1978; Zisfein *et al.*, 1983) and slight distal wasting and weakness may be present. The

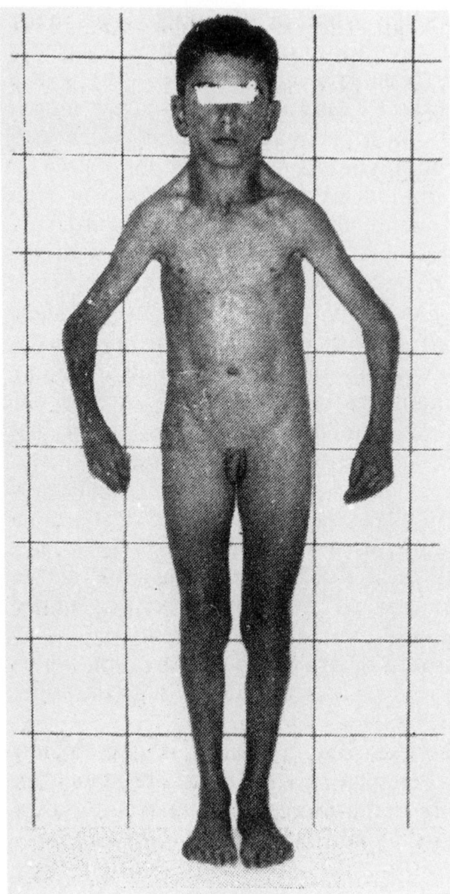

Figure 19.4 Abnormal posture in the original patient reported by Isaacs with the syndrome of continuous muscle fibre activity. Note the stiff posture and contraction of muscles with particular emphasis of the hand muscles. Contraction of the trapezius should not be mistaken for webbing. From Isaacs (1964) with permission.

tendon reflexes usually are absent. The latter is related to the phenomenon of occlusion (due to continuous muscle activity inhibiting spinal monosynaptic reflexes) since the tendon reflexes return after successful treatment in some cases (Isaacs and Heffron, 1974; Zisfein *et al.*, 1983; McGuire *et al.*, 1984). This response to treatment and the presence or absence of abnormal sensory signs depends on the nature of the underlying peripheral nerve disorder. Plantar responses are flexor. In the original cases described by Isaacs (1961), tachycardia and a raised basal metabolic rate were prominent features. Percussion myotonia occurs infrequently (Gamstrop and Wolfart, 1959; Valenstein *et al.*, 1978). Stimulus-sensitive myoclonus does not occur.

In many case reports of this syndrome there are few or only subtle signs of a peripheral neuropathy. In some the disorder has been inherited, without evidence of an associated neuropathy (Sheaff, 1952; Ashizawa *et al.*, 1983; Auger *et al.*, 1984). Similar sporadic cases also occur (Gardner-Medwin and Walton, 1969; Van den Burgh *et al.*, 1983). Other examples have evidence of an underlying peripheral neuropathy. These include hereditary motor and sensory neuropathy (Gamstrop and Wolfart, 1959; Lance *et al.*, 1979; Vasilescu *et al.*, 1984), chronic demyelinating neuropathy (Valenstein *et al.*, 1978), toxic neuropathies (Black *et al.*, 1962; Wallis *et al.*, 1970; Mitsumoto *et al.*, 1982), and neuropathies of unknown cause (Gamstrop and Wolfart, 1959; Greenhouse *et al.*, 1967; Negri *et al.*, 1977; Lublin *et al.*, 1979). Neuromyotonia also has been described as a paraneoplastic phenomenon in association with intrathoracic malignancy (Walsh, 1976) and oat cell carcinoma of the lung (Partanen *et al.*, 1980) without an overt peripheral neuropathy. In a review of 28 cases published between 1977 and 1985, Rowland (1985) noted that the great majority of cases had no evidence of a neuropathy.

Electrophysiology

The hallmark of this syndrome is the presence of continuous motor unit activity that persists during sleep and following peripheral nerve block. Activity may diminish after nerve block, implying that in some cases the abnormal activity is generated at many sites along the peripheral nerve, above and below the site of block (Irani *et al.*, 1977; Ashizawa *et al.*, 1983). Muscle activity disappears after local neuromuscular block with curare. Hyperventilation and ischaemia may increase the muscle activity. Fasciculations and the grouped discharges of myokymia are evident on electromyography (Fig. 19.5). Prolonged bursts of motor units of normal appearance and bizarre high-frequency discharges may be detected during attempts to relax after voluntary contraction (Lance *et al.*, 1979; Fig. 19.6). High-frequency discharges also occur spontaneously. These are of abrupt onset and offset, lacking the waxing and waning character of the myotonic discharges in myotonic dystrophies. Evidence of muscle denervation and reinnervation with large-amplitude, long-duration polyphasic motor unit potentials when present suggest an underlying peripheral neuropathy. Measurement of peripheral nerve conduction velocities will confirm this and indicate whether the neuropathy is axonal or demyelinating in type. Stimulation of peripheral nerves often reveals after-discharges following the direct compound muscle action potential (M-wave; Auger *et al.*, 1984; Fig. 19.7). Similar after-discharges are seen following voluntary activation of muscle. Gentle percussion of peripheral nerves also may elicit discharges, but percussion myotonia is not a feature. This after-discharge leads to the muscle stiffness, sustained postures and failure to relax after voluntary muscle contraction.

Pathology

Biopsy evidence of muscle denervation (Welch *et al.*, 1972; Ono *et al.*, 1989), and of nerve segmental demyelination (Welch *et al.*, 1972) and degeneration (Wallis *et al.*, 1970) is in keeping with the peripheral origin of this syndrome. In some hereditary

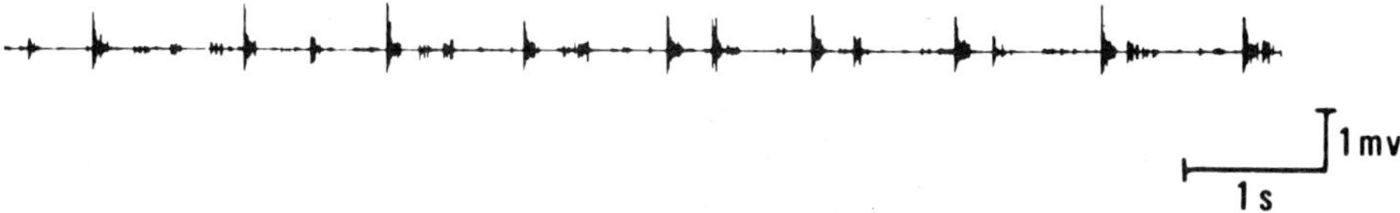

Figure 19.5 Spontaneous electromyographic activity in first dorsal interosseus muscle recorded with a concentric needle electrode in a patient with a hereditary form of continuous muscle activity of peripheral nerve origin, but without evidence of an underlying neuropathy. Regularly recurring bursts of motor unit potentials with a high intraburst firing frequency are evident (high-frequency myokymic discharges). From Auger *et al.* (1984) with permission.

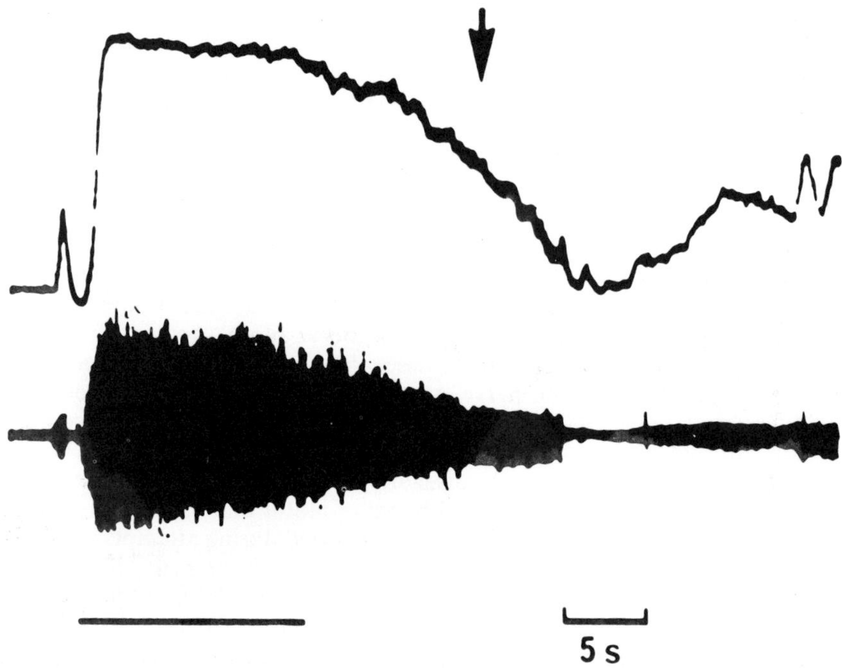

Figure 19.6 Electromyographic activity in flexor digitorum profundis recorded with surface electrodes during and following a strong voluntary contraction in a patient with a familial neuropathy resembling Charcot–Marie–Tooth disease. Horizontal bar indicates the duration of voluntary effort. Electromyogram (EMG) activity outlasts the effort by over 15 seconds. The remainder of the activity is 'spontaneous'. Lower trace depicts raw EMG activity; upper trace represents EMG activity 'integrated' by a low-pass filter with a time constant of 0.1 seconds. At rest there were fasciculations, fibrillations and repetitive discharges of simple motor units at high frequency. From Lance *et al.* (1979) with permission.

(Ashizawa *et al.*, 1983; Auger *et al.*, 1984) and sporadic (Greenhouse *et al.*, 1967; Nakanishini *et al.*, 1975) cases, nerve biopsies have been normal.

Abnormalities of terminal motor nerve fibre morphology (Isaacs, 1967; Lublin *et al.*, 1979) and the neuromuscular junction (Sroka *et al.*, 1975; Ono *et al.*, 1989) have been demonstrated. As discussed above, the results of nerve blocks in some patients indicate that the abnormal activity may arise more diffusely along the course of the peripheral nerves. In other cases the pathology is thought to lie in the proximal nerve trunks.

The origin of the abnormal muscle activity in these syndromes is debated. One theory is that ephaptic excitation in peripheral nerve trunks occurs after the passage of orthodromic impulses. Multiple discharges in different adjacent fibres of the nerve are then excited and can lead to local circuits of re-excitation. A disorder of membrane transport was postulated by Auger *et al.* (1984) to explain the nerve hyperexcitability in the absence of any evident pathological change within biopsied peripheral nerves. An autoimmune aetiology for neuromyotonia was suggested by Sinha *et al.* (1991). They reported the case of a 24-year-old man with a 7-year history of neuromyotonia in whom thyroid microsomal antibodies were detected. Treatment with plasma exchange alleviated his symptoms and reduced the electromyographic abnormalities

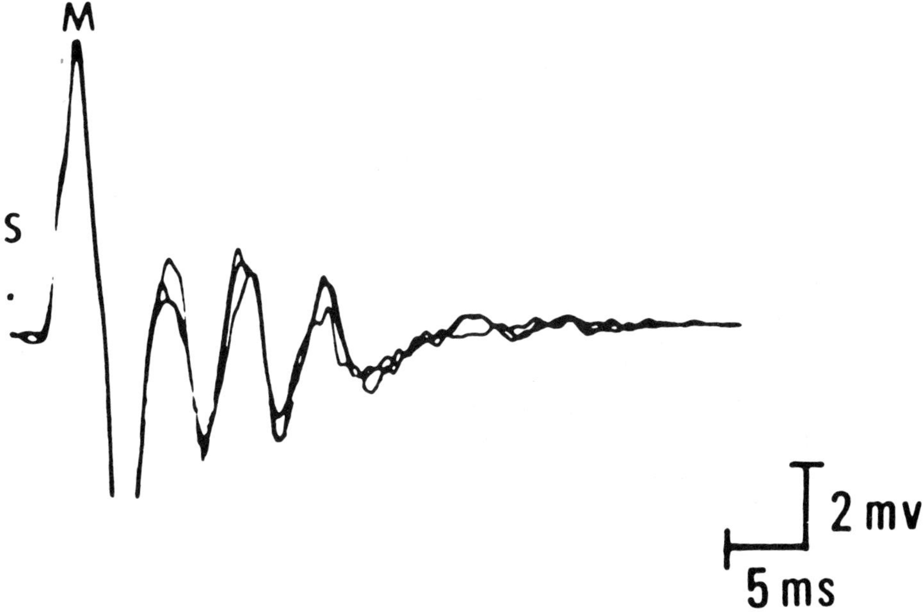

Figure 19.7 Three superimposed electromyographic responses recorded from abductor digiti minimi following stimulation of the ulnar nerve (S refers to stimulus arteface) in the same patient as shown in Figure 19.6. Repetitive after-discharges are seen following the initial M response. From Auger *et al.* (1984) with permission.

for 2–3 weeks. These authors have recently expanded this theme in a report of 5 patients with acquired neuromyotonia. Oligoclonal IgG was found in the spinal fluid of three patients and an improvement in symptoms followed plasma exchange in a further 2 (Newsom-Davis and Mills, 1993). The authors demonstrated the presence of pathogenic IgG antibodies and suggested that the condition might be an antibody-mediated ion channel disorder, perhaps to peripheral nerve potassium channels. A reduction in the number of functional potassium channels might lead to an increase in peripheral nerve excitability (Bostock and Baker, 1988).

Treatment

Carbamazepine and phenytoin are successful in abolishing most symptoms in these conditions. Muscle stiffness resolves and tendon reflexes may return to normal. Diazepam is not helpful.

Prognosis

A striking feature in cases without evidence of an underlying neuropathy (or other disease) has been the benign course. Isaacs treated his original 2 cases with phenytoin for several years but later reported that treatment was no longer necessary some 14 years after presentation (Isaacs and Heffron, 1974). Similar improvements over long periods of observation have been described in other cases (Hughes and Matthews, 1969; Irani *et al*., 1977; Wilton and Gardner-Medwin, 1990).

Related conditions

An autoimmune cause for continuous muscle activity, proven electrophysiologically to be peripheral in origin, was proposed in 2 cases reported by Halbach *et al*. (1987). Both were males and presented with symptoms of muscle stiffness and pain. Investigations revealed a thymoma and elevated acetylcholine receptor antibody titres, but no evidence of myasthenia gravis. Autonomic disturbances and psychosis were prominent, suggesting additional involvement of the central nervous system. These clinical features were said to correspond to previous descriptions of '*chorée fibrillaire de Morvan*' (DeBray *et al*., 1979; Halbach *et al*., 1987). The association of continuous motor unit activity with thymoma and peripheral neuropathy has also been reported in 2 further patients, one of whom had clinical myasthenia gravis with acetylcholine receptor antibodies (Garcia-Merino *et al*., 1991).

Continuous motor unit activity of peripheral nerve origin may be associated with other conditions such as *paroxysmal ataxia with myokymia* (Van Dyke *et al*., 1975; Hanson *et al*., 1977; Brunt and van Weerden, 1990).

Hereditary painful distal cramps comprise another group of syndromes attributed to motor unit hyperactivity of peripheral nerve origin, but which differ from Isaacs syndrome in several important respects. The disorder was inherited as an autosomal dominant trait affecting many family members from large pedigrees with spontaneous and exercise-induced cramps and painful spasms of predominantly distal muscles (Jusic *et al*., 1972; Lazaro *et al*., 1981; Ricker and Moxley, 1990). Tendon reflexes were normal or brisk. There was no evidence of continuous motor unit activity but subtle signs of a peripheral neuropathy, including fasciculations, were present in the cases of Lazaro *et al*. (1981) and Ricker and Moxley (1990). A peripheral origin for the cramps in the pedigree reported by Jusic *et al*. (1972) was supported by the persistence of cramps after peripheral nerve block and spinal anaesthesia. After-discharges also were present in 1 patient from this family. Muscle biopsies were normal in two families (Jusic *et al*., 1972; Lazaro *et al*., 1981) and showed changes of denervation in another (Ricker and Moxley, 1990). Treatment with carbamazepine was not helpful.

BENIGN (PHYSIOLOGICAL) CRAMPS

Painful nocturnal muscle cramps are very common in healthy people without apparent predisposing factors. Cramps may occur in association with a number of conditions such as dehydration, salt depletion and other electrolyte disturbances, pregnancy in association with autoimmune diseases and malabsorption (Sato *et al*., 1983).

Benign or physiological cramps are extremely painful. They often occur abruptly during or after exercise, with pain of sufficient severity to force the subject to stop activity. Cramps also may occur at rest or during sleep. The muscle contraction during a cramp forces the affected limb into an abnormal posture. A distinguishing feature of benign cramps is that the pain and muscle contraction may be overcome and terminated by stretching the affected muscle. It is generally thought that benign cramps originate from spontaneous activity in the terminal motor nerve fibres. Electromyography during cramp discloses variable recruitment of normal motor units (Norris *et al.*, 1957). This finding further distinguishes cramps from other syndromes of spontaneous muscle activity of peripheral nerve origin, and from myotonia or contracture of muscular origin.

THE SCHWARTZ-JAMPEL SYNDROME

This rare autosomal recessive condition is characterized by muscle stiffness due to continuous motor fibre activity associated with a variety of skeletal abnormalities, including spondyloepiphyseal dysplasia, often with short stature, and dysmorphic 'pinched' facies with blepharophimosis, puckered mouth and dimpled chin. The latter appearances are probable due to continuous contraction in facial muscles. Percussion myotonia may be present. Electromyography reveals continuous high-frequency complex repetitive muscle discharges of sudden onset and offset, often with abrupt changes in discharge frequency, giving rise to a 'gear-change' sound rather than the waxing and waning of myotonic discharges, although these also have been reported in this condition. After-discharges follow muscle activation by voluntary contraction or peripheral nerve stimulation (Fig. 19.8). The muscle stiffness and continuous muscle activity in this condition have been variously ascribed to neural and muscle origins. Muscle activity persists after peripheral nerve block and peripheral limb ischaemia; however, the effects of curarization have been variable (Taylor *et al.*, 1972; Spaans *et al.*, 1990). Persistence of activity after curare suggests a muscular origin (Spaans *et al.*, 1990), a finding supported by the demonstration of abnormal sodium channel opening in muscle fibres (Lehmann-Horn *et al.*, 1990). Procainamide, which blocks sodium channels in nerve, abolished both the spontaneous activity and after-discharges (Lehmann-Horn *et al.*, 1990). Phenytoin and carbamazepine are less helpful in relieving the muscle stiffness in this condition.

MUSCLE DISEASE AND SPASMS OR CRAMPS

Myotonic syndromes

Myotonia is defined as a delayed relaxation after muscle contraction which gives rise to symptoms of stiffness and limitation of movement. Myotonia may be the main symptom of a number of primary muscle diseases and is thought to be due to abnormalities of muscle fibres. Accordingly myotonia persists during sleep, after peripheral nerve or neuromuscular block, but is abolished by local infiltration of anaesthesia into muscle (Denny-Brown and Nevin, 1941; Landau 1952). Electromyography reveals typical waxing and waning myotonic discharges provoked by voluntary movement, percussion, cold, needle insertion and electrical stimulation of muscle. Myotonic discharges after muscle contraction result in a failure of the muscle to relax. The sustained posture after muscle contraction lasts for a minute or so. All skeletal muscle groups may be affected. In myotonia the twitch contraction time is normal but the relaxation phase is prolonged (in contrast to hypothyroidism).

Myotonic dystrophy is the commonest cause of myotonia and is associated with several other typical features, including an autosomal dominant pattern of inheritance, muscle wasting and extra neurological features which allow the diagnosis to be made.

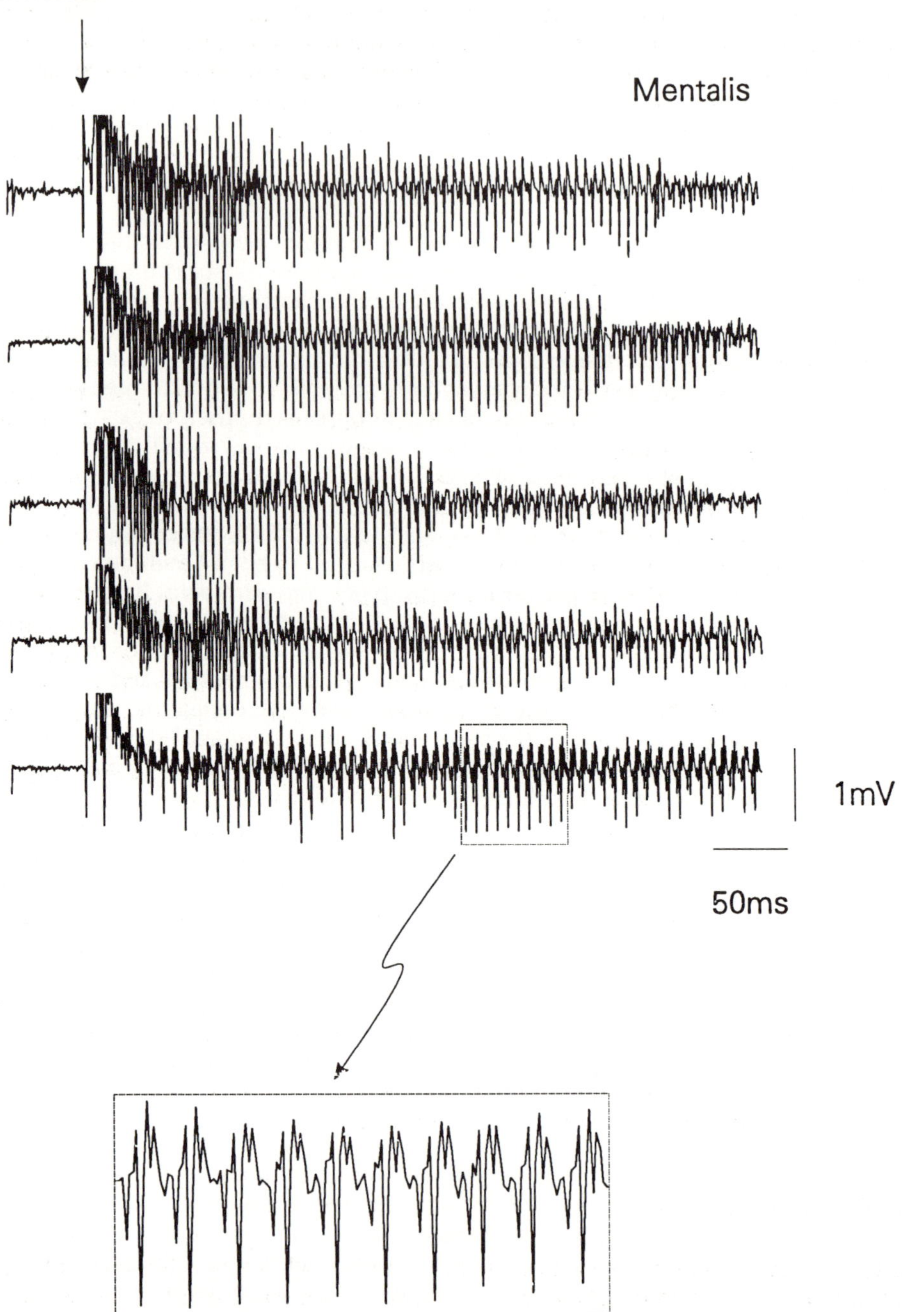

Figure 19.8 Concentric needle electromyogram recordings (five single traces) from mentalis muscle following stimulation of the facial nerve anterior to the mastoid process in a patient with the Schwartz–Jampel syndrome. After-discharges and complex repetitive high-frequency discharges follow the direct muscle response. The lower panel illustrates the morphology of the repetitive discharges.

Myotonia congenita, both the autosomal dominant (Thomsen's disease) and autosomal recessive (Becker) forms, are rarer conditions which produce similar myotonia but run relatively benign courses. Symptoms in these conditions often are related to the appearance of myotonia following sudden voluntary movement such as when standing to walk. Myotonia induced by cold and cold-induced electrically silent cramps or postmyotonic paresis are features of paramyotonia congenita (Eulenberg) which is thought to be related to an abnormality of the voltage-dependent sodium channel in adult skeletal muscle (Ebers *et al.*, 1991).

Metabolic myopathies

McArdle's disease and phosphofructokinase deficiency are well-recognized but rare disorders of muscle metabolism due to defects in the glycolytic pathways. Both conditions produce similar symptoms of fatigue, muscle aches and painful cramps after or during strenuous contraction. The painful cramps of McArdle's disease are due to muscle contracture, defined as shortening of muscle without the electrical activity of active muscle contraction (i.e. electrically silent muscle cramps). The cramps are thought to be due to failure of muscle relaxation after contraction due to a breakdown in the normal reuptake of liberated calcium. During this time the muscle is electrically silent. The cramps appear after variable levels of exertion and many patients limit their activities to avoid precipitating cramps. Attempts to straighten the muscle during cramp are accompanied by severe pain (in contrast to physiological cramps). Cramps may persist for hours. Some patients find that if they reduce the level of activity at the time when symptoms first appear, they can continue to exercise without symptoms. This is referred to as the 'second wind' phenomenon. Cramps are said to be less prominent in phosphofructokinase deficiency. Diagnosis is confirmed by an excessive rise in lactate during ischaemic muscle exercise and abnormal phosphorylase activity on muscle histochemistry.

Similar physiological mechanisms are thought to be responsible for the cramps and contractures following exertion in Brody's disease (Brody, 1969; Karpati *et al.*, 1986). These cramps also are electrically silent. They affect all muscle groups including the face and typically occur following brisk exercise. The stiffness produced at the onset of the cramp may force the patient to stop activity. Continued exercise exacerbates the cramp but, unlike McArdle's disease, the cramps are painless and of brief duration (Karpati *et al.*, 1986). The stiffness disappears after a few minutes rest. No localized swellings of muscle were evident in the patient reported by Brody and there was no percussion myotonia (Brody, 1969). A deficiency in the sarcoplasmic reticulum Ca^{2+} transport adenosine triphosphatase has been shown in 4 patients from two families with this condition (Karpati *et al.*, 1986).

Endocrine myopathies

Hypothyroidism commonly produces symptoms of muscle aches, stiffness and cramps. Prolongation of the contraction phase and a delay in the relaxation phase of muscle contraction are thought to be responsible for these symptoms. Muscle stiffness may be most marked during and after voluntary contraction. Percussion of muscle may produce a localized swelling of the muscle (myoedema). Muscle enlargement also may be seen.

Muscle contractures occur rarely in Addison's disease. These are poorly understood and have been attributed to various causes. Fibrosis of fascia (Adams *et al.*, 1962) and myopathic changes (Cambier *et al.*, 1970) have been described. Some are reported to be painful and associated with stimulus-sensitive spasms involving the axial musculature, suggesting a central rather than muscular origin. A further case has been described with signs suggesting neuromyotonia (Vilchez *et al.*, 1980).

Myopathies with contractures

Several other myopathies may cause permanent contractures with fibrosis and shortening of muscle. The shortened muscles are electrically silent and produce fixed abnormal limb postures. These include polymyositis, affecting elbows particularly, the rigid-spine syndrome, affecting muscles of the limbs and cervical and thoracic spine (Dubowitz, 1973), Bethlem muscular dystrophy, affecting the elbow, fingers and ankles (Morhire *et al.*, 1988) and Emery–Dreifuss muscular dystrophy, with contractures of spine, elbows and fingers (Rowland *et al.*, 1979). Diagnosis is made by the clinical features and demonstrating the presence of a dystrophy on muscle biopsy.

Other unclassified (presumed) muscle diseases

Muscle stiffness and cramps have been reported in a number of other poorly understood and unclassified disorders presumed due to muscle pathology. The patients described by Torbergson (1975), Alberca *et al.* (1980) and Ricker *et al.* (1989) presented similar clinical pictures with symptoms of difficulty relaxing after muscle contraction, slightly painful cramps and visible 'rolling' or 'rippling' muscle contractions. These contractions were electrically silent and were provoked by voluntary activity and percussion of the muscle. The latter produced a localized mounding of muscle lasting for several seconds. There was no clinical or electromyographic evidence of myotonia and the muscles were well-developed. In two of these reports the disorder was familial (Torbergson, 1975; Ricker *et al.*, 1989). No distinctive features were seen on detailed investigations to suggest a cause for these syndromes. Muscle biopsies were normal (Torbergson, 1975) or showed minor non-specific abnormalities (Alberca *et al.*, 1980; Ricker *et al.*, 1989). Dantrolene was helpful in relieving the symptoms in one family (Ricker *et al.*, 1989).

EXTRAPYRAMIDAL MUSCLE RIGIDITY AND SPASMS

Torsion dystonia affecting axial muscles typically produces abnormal postures of the thoracic and lumbar spine during walking. These postures subside during relaxation or when lying supine, thus distinguishing dystonia from the stiff-man syndrome. The age of onset also helps distinguish between dystonia and other causes of rigidity. Idiopathic torsion dystonia usually begins in childhood, unlike the stiff-man syndrome, which affects adults. A further clue to a dystonic cause of action-induced muscle spasms is the task specificity exhibited by many of the focal dystonias, the classical example of which is writer's cramp.

Axial rigidity in akinetic–rigid syndromes such as idiopathic Parkinson's disease, Steele–Richardson–Olszewski syndrome and drug-induced parkinsonism is accompanied by other clinical signs of basal ganglia and brainstem disease.

References

Adams RD, Denny-Brown D and Pearson CM (1962) Diseases of Muscle: A Study in Pathology, 2nd edn, New York, Harper & Row

Alberca R, Rafel E, Castilla JM, and Gil-Peralta A (1980) Increased mechanical muscle irritability syndrome. *Acta Neurol Scand*, **62**, 250–4

Alberca R, Romero M, and Chaparro J (1982) Jerking stiff-man syndrome. *J Neurol, Neurosurg Psychiatry*, **45**, 1159–60

Asher R (1958) A woman with the stiff-man syndrome. *Br Med J*, **i**, 265–6

Ashizawa T, Butler IJ, Harati Y, and Roongta SM (1983) A dominantly inherited syndrome with continuous motor neuron discharges. *Ann Neurol*, **13**, 285–90

Auger RD, Daube JR, Gomez MR, and Lambert EH (1984) Hereditary form of sustained muscle activity of peripheral nerve origin causing generalized myokymia and muscle stiffness. *Ann Neurol*, **15**, 13–21

Babinski J (1913) Contracture liée à une irritation des cornes antérieures de la moelle dans un cas de syringo myélie. *Rev Neurol*, **1**, 246–9

Baekkeskov S, Aanstoot H-J, Christgau S, Reetz A, Solimena M, Cascalho M *et al.* (1990) Identification of the 64K autoantigen in insulin dependent diabetes mellitus as the GABA-synthesizing enzyme glutamic acid decarboxylase. *Nature*, **347**, 151–6

Bateman DE, Weller RO, and Kennedy P (1990) Stiff-man syndrome. *J Neurol, Neurosurg Psychiatry*, **53**, 695–6

Black JT, Garcia-Mullin R, Good E, and Brown S (1962) Muscle rigidity in a newborn due to continuous peripheral nerve hyperactivity. *Arch Neurol*, **27**, 413–25

Blum P and Jankovic J (1991) Stiff-person syndrome: an autoimmune disease. *Movement Disorders*, **6**, 12–20

Boiardi A, Crenna P, Negri S, and Merati B (1980) Neurological and pharmacological evaluation of a case of stiff-man syndrome. *J Neurol*, **223**, 127–33

Bostock H and Baker M (1988) Evidence for two types of potassium channel in human motor axons in vivo. *Brain Res*, **462**, 354–8

Brashear HR and Phillips LH (1991) Autoantibodies to GABAergic neurones and response to plasmapharesis in stiff-man syndrome. *Neurology*, **41**, 1588–92

Brody I (1969) Muscle contracture induced by exercise. A syndrome attributable to decreased relaxing factor. *N Engl J Med*, **281**, 187–92

Brown P, Thompson PD, Rothwell JC, Day BL, and Marsden CD (1991a) A therapeutic trial of milacemide in myoclonus and the stiff person syndrome. *Movement Disorders*, **6**, 73–5

Brown P, Rothwell JC, Thompson PD, Britton TC, Day BL, and Marsden CD (1991b) The hyperekplexias and their relationship to the normal startle reflex. *Brain*, **114**, 1903–28

Brunt ERP and Weerden TW (1990) Familial paroxysmal kinesigenic ataxia and continuous myokymia. *Brain*, **113**, 1361–82

Burn DJ, Ball J, Lees AJ, Behan PO, and Morgan-Hughes JA (1991) A case of progressive encephalomyelitis with rigidity and positive antiglutamic acid dehydrogenase antibodies. *J Neurol, Neurosurg Psychiatry*, **54**, 449–51

Campbell AMG and Garland H (1956) Subacute myoclonic spinal neuronitis. *J Neurol, Neurosurg Psychiatry*, **19**, 268–74

Cambier J, Masson M, and Delaporte P (1970) Le syndrome de contracture abdomino-crurale au cours de la maladie d'Addison. *Presse Med (Paris)*, **78**, 2281–2

Cobb J (1974) Stiff-man syndrome: is the lesion at the spinal cord or brainstem level? *Proc R Soc Med*, **67**, 1065–6

Cohen L (1966) Stiff-man syndrome. *JAMA*, **195**, 222–4

Darnell RB, Victor J, Rubin M, Clouston P, and Plum F (1993) A novel antineuronal antibody in stiff-man syndrome. *Neurology*, **43**, 114–20

Davis SM, Murray NMF, Diengdoh JV, Galeo-Debono A, and Kocen RS (1981) Stimulus-sensitive spinal myoclonus. *J Neurol, Neurosurg Psychiatry*, **44**, 884–8

De Bray JM, Emile J, Basle M, Morer T, and Bastard J (1979) Choree fibrillaire de Morvan. *Rev Neurol*, **135**,. 827–33

Denny-Brown D and Nevin S (1941) The phenomenon of myotonia. *Brain*, **64**, 1–18

Dubowitz V (1973) Rigid spine syndrome: a muscle syndrome in search of a name. *Proc R Soc Med*, **66**, 219–20

Ebers GC, George AL, Barchi RL, Ting-Passador SS, Kallen RG, Lathrop GM *et al.* (1991) Paramyotonia congenita and hyperkalemic periodic paralysis are linked to the adult muscle sodium channel gene. *Ann Neurol*, **30**, 810–16

Folli F, Solimena M, Cofiell R, Austoni M, Tallini G, Fassetta G *et al.* (1993) Autoantibodies to a 128-kd synaptic protein in three women with the stiff-man syndrome and breast cancer. *NEJM*, **328**, 546–51

Gabellini A, Thompson PD, Stocchi F, Rothwell JC, Day BL, and Marsden CD (1991) Further observations on the stiff-man syndrome (in preparation)

Gamstrop I and Wolfart G (1959) A syndrome characterised by myokymia, myotonia, muscular wasting and increased perspiration. *Acta Psychiatr Scand*, **34**, 181–94

Garcia-Merino A, Cabello A, Mora JS, and Liano H (1991) Continuous muscle fibre activity, peripheral neuropathy and thymoma. *Ann Neurol*, **29**, 215–18

Gardner-Medwin D and Walton J (1969) Myokymia with impaired muscle relaxation. *Lancet*, **1**, 127–30

Gelfan S and Tarlov IM (1959) Interneurones and rigidity of spinal origin. *J Physiol*, **146**, 594–617

George TM, Burke JM, Sobotak PA, Greenberg HS, and Vinik AI (1984) Resolution of stiff-man syndrome with cortisol replacement in a patient with deficiencies of ACTH, growth hormone, and prolactin. *N Engl J Med*, **310**, 1511–13

Gordon EE, Januszko DM, and Kaufman L (1967) A critical survey of stiff-man syndrome. *Am J Med*, **42**, 582–99

Gorin F, Baldwin B, Tait R, Pathak R, Seyal M, and Mugnaini E (1990) Stiff-man syndrome: a disorder with autoantigenic heterogeneity. *Ann Neurol*, **28**, 711–14

Greenhouse AH, Bicknell JM, Pesch RN, and Seelinger DF (1967) Myotonia, myokymia, hyperhydrosis and wasting of muscle. *Arch Neurol*, **17**, 263–8

Guilleminault C, Sigwald J, and Castaigne P (1973) Sleep studies and therapeutic trial with L-Dopa in a case of stiff-man syndrome. *Eur Neurol*, **10**, 89–96

Halbach M, Homberg V, and Freund H-J (1987) Neuromuscular, automomic and central cholinergic hyperactivity associated with thymoma and acetylcholine receptor-binding antibody. *J Neurol*, **234**, 433–6

Hanson PA, Martinez LB, and Cassidy R (1977) Contractures, continuous muscle discharges and titubation. *Ann Neurol*, **1**, 120–4

Harding AE, Thompson PD, Kocen RS, Batchelor JR, Davey N, and Marsden CD (1989) Plasma exchange and immunosuppression in the stiff-man syndrome. *Lancet*, **ii**, 915

Howard FM (1963) A new and effective drug in the treatment of stiff-man syndrome: preliminary report. *Mayo Clin Proc*, **38**, 203–12

Howell DA, Lees AJ, and Toghill PJ (1979) Spinal internuncial neurones in progressive encephalomyelitis with rigidity. *J Neurol, Neurosurg Psychiatry*, **42**, 773–85

Hughes RC and Matthews WB (1969) Pseudomyotonia and myokymia. *J Neurol, Neurosurg Psychiatry*, **32**, 11–14

Irani PF, Purohit AV, and Wadia NH (1977) The syndrome of continuous muscle fibre activity. *Acta Neurol Scand*, **55**, 273–88

Isaacs H (1961) A syndrome of continuous muscle-fibre activity. *J Neurol, Neurosurg Psychiatry*, **24**, 319–25

Isaacs H (1967) Continuous muscle fibre activity in an Indian male with additional evidence of terminal motor fibre abnormality. *J Neurol, Neurosurg Psychiatry*, **30**, 126–33

Isaacs H (1979) Stiff-man syndrome in a black girl. *J Neurol, Neurosurg Psychiatry*, **42**, 988–94

Isaacs H and Heffron JJA (1974) The syndrome of 'continuous muscle fibre activity' cured: further studies. *J Neurol, Neurosurg Psychiatry*, **37**, 1231–5

Jusic A, Dogan S, and Stojanovic V (1972) Hereditary persistent distal cramps. *J Neurol, Neurosurg Psychiatry*, **35**, 379–84

Karpati G, Charuk J, Carpenter S, Jablecki C, and Holland P (1986) Myopathy caused by a deficiency of Ca^{++} adenosine triphosphatase in sarcoplasmic reticulum (Brody's disease). *Ann Neurol*, **30**, 38–49

Kasperek S and Zebrowski S (1971) Stiff-man syndrome and encephalomyelitis. *Arch Neurol*, **24**, 22–31

Klein R, Haddow JE, and DeLuca C (1972) Familial congenital disorder resembling the stiff-man syndrome. *Am J Dis Child*, **124**, 730–1

Kugelberg E, Eklund K, and Grimby L (1960) An electromyographic study of nociceptive reflexes of the lower limb. Mechanism of the plantar responses. *Brain*, **83**, 394–410

Kugelmass N (1961) Stiff-man syndrome in a child. *N Y State J Med*, **61**, 2483–7

Lance JW, Burke D, and Pollard J (1979) Hyperexcitability of motor and sensory neurons in neuromyotonia. *Ann Neurol*, **5**, 523–32

Landau WH (1952) The essential mechanisms in myotonia: an electromyographic study. *Neurology*, **2**, 369–88

Lazaro RP, Rollinson R, and Fenichel GM (1981) Familial cramps and muscle pain. *Arch Neurol*, **38**, 22–4

Lehman-Horn F, Iaizzo PA, Franke C, Hatt H, and Spaans F (1990) Schwartz–Jampel syndrome 2. Na^{+}

channel defect causes myotonia. *Muscle Nerve*, **13**, 528–35

Leigh PN, Rothwell JC, Traub M, and Marsden CD (1980) A patient with reflex myoclonus and muscle rigidity: 'jerking stiff-man syndrome'. *J Neurol, Neurosurg Psychiatry*, **43**, 1125–31

Lhermitte F, Chain F, Escourolle R, Chedru F, Guilleminault C, and Francoucal M (1973) Un noveau cas de contracture tétaniforme distinct du 'stiff-man syndrome'. *Rev Neurol*, **128**, 3–21

Lorish TR, Thorsteinsson G, and Howard FM (1989) Stiff-man syndrome updated. *Mayo Clin Proc*, **64**, 629–36

Lourie H (1968) Spontaneous activity of alpha motor neurones in intramedullary spinal cord tumour. *J Neurosurg*, **29**, 573–80

Lublin FD, Tsiaris P, Streletz LJ, Chambers RA, Riker WF, Van Poznack A *et al.* (1979) Myokymia and impaired muscular relaxation with continuous motor unit activity. *J Neurol, Neurosurg Psychiatry*, **42**, 557–62

Lutschg J, Jerusalem F, Ludin HP, Vasella F, and Mumenthaler M (1978) The syndrome of continuous muscle fibre activity. *Arch Neurol*, **35**, 198–205

McCombe PA, Chalk JB, Searle JW, Tannenberg AEG, Smith JJ, and Pender MP (1989) Progressive encephalomyelitis with rigidity: a case report with magnetic resonance imaging findings. *J Neurol, Neurosurg Psychiatry*, **52**, 1429–31

McGuire SA, Tomasovic JJ, and Ackerman NJR (1984) Hereditary continuous muscle fibre activity. *Arch Neurol*, **41**, 395–6

Maida E, Reisner T, Summer K, and Sandor-Eggerth H (1980) Stiff-man syndrome with abnormalities in CSF and computerized tomography findings. *Arch Neurol*, **37**, 182–3

Mamoli B, Heiss WD, Maida E, and Podreka I (1977) Electrophysiogical studies on the stiff-man syndrome. *J Neurol*, **217**, 111–21

Martin R, Meinck H-M, Schulte-Mattler W, Ricker K, and Mertens H-J (1990) *Borrelia burgdorferi* myelitis presenting as a partial stiff-man syndrome. *J Neurol*, **237**, 51–4

Martinelli P, Pazzaglia P, Montagna P, Coccagna G, Rizzuto N, Simonati S, and Lugaresi E (1978) Stiff-man syndrome associated with nocturnal myoclonus and epilepsy. *J Neurol, Neurosurg Psychiatry*, **41**, 458–62

Meinck HM and Conrad B (1986) Neuropharmacological investigations in the stiff-man syndrome. *J Neurol*, **233**, 340–7

Meinck HM and Ricker K (1987) Long-standing 'stiff-man' syndrome: a particular form of disseminated inflammatory CNS disease? *J Neurol, Neurosurg Psychiatry*, **50**, 1556–7

Meinck HM, Piesiur-Strhlow B, and Koehler W (1981) Some principles of flexor reflex generation in human leg muscles. *Electroencephalogr Clin Neurophysiol*, **52**, 140–50

Meinck HM, Ricker K, and Conrad B (1984) The stiff-man syndrome: new pathophysiological aspects from abnormal exteroceptive reflexes and the response to clomipramine, clonidine and tizanidine. *J Neurol, Neurosurg Psychiatry*, **47**, 280–7

Mertens HG and Ricker K (1968) Ubererregbarkeit der – Motoneurone beim 'stiff-man' syndrom. *Klin Wochenschr*, **46**, 33–42

Miller F and Korsvik H (1981) Baclofen in the treatment of stiff-man syndrome. *Ann Neurol*, **9**, 511–12

Mitsumoto H, Wilbourn AJ, and Subramony SH (1982) Generalised myokymia and gold therapy. *Arch Neurol*, **39**, 449–50

Moersch FP and Woltman HW (1956) Progressive fluctuating muscular rigidity and spasm ('stiff-man' syndrome): report of a case and some observations in 13 other cases. *Mayo Clin Proc*, **31**, 421–7

Mohire MD, Tandan R, Fries TJ, Little BW, Pendlebury WW, and Bradley WG (1988) Early onset benign autosomal dominant limb girdle myopathy with contractures (Bethlem myopathy). *Neurology*, **38**, 573–80

Nakanishi T, Sugira H, Shimada Y, and Toyokura Y (1975) Neuromyotonia. A mild case. *J Neurol Sci*, **26**, 599–604

Negri S, Caraceni T, and Boardi A (1977) Neuromyotonia. *Eur Neurol*, **16**, 35–41

Newsom-Davis J and Mills KR (1993) Immunological associations of acquired neuromyotonia (Isaac's syndrome). *Brain*, **116**, 453–69

Norris FH, Gasteiger EL, and Chatfield PO (1957) An electromyographic study of induced and spontaneous muscle cramps. *Electroencephalogr Clin Neurophysiol*, **9**, 139–47

Olafson RA, Mulder DW, and Howard FM (1964) Stiff-man syndrome: literature, report of three additional cases and discussion of pathology and therapy. *Proc Mayo Clin*, **39**, 131–44

Ono S, Munakata S, Kagao K, and Shimizu N (1989) The syndrome of continuous muscle fibre activity: light and electron microscopic studies in muscle and nerve biopsies. *J Neurol*, **236**, 377–81

Partanen VSJ, Soininen H, Saska M, and Riekkinen P (1980) Electromyographic and nerve conduction findings in a patient with neuromyotonia, normocalcaemic tetany and small-cell lung cancer. *Acta Neurol Scand*, **61**, 216–26

Penry JK, Hoefnagel D, Van der Noort S, and Denny-Brown D (1960) Muscle spasm and abnormal postures resulting from damage to interneurones in spinal cord. *Arch Neurol*, **34**, 500–12

Piccolo G and Cosi V (1989) Stiff-man syndrome, dysimmune disorder and cancer. *Ann Neurol*, **25**, 105

Piccolo G, Cosi V, Zandrini C, and Moglia A (1988) Steroid-responsive and dependent stiff-man syndrome: a clinical and electrophysiological study of two cases. *Ital J Neurol Sci*, **9**, 559–66

Ricker K and Moxley RT (1990) Autosomal dominant cramping disease. *Arch Neurol*, **47**, 810–12

Ricker K, Moxley FT, and Rohkamm R (1989) Rippling muscle disease. *Arch Neurol*, **46**, 405–8

Risk WS, Bosch EP, Kimura J, Cancilla PA, Fischbeck KH, and Layzer RB (1981) Chronic tetanus: clinical report and histochemistry of muscle. *Muscle Nerve*, **4**, 363–6

Roobol TH, Kazzaz BA, and Vecht CJ (1987) Segmental rigidity and spinal myoclonus as a paraneoplastic syndrome. *J Neurol, Neurosurg Psychiatry*, **50**, 628–31

Rossi B, Massetani R, Guidi M, Mondelli M, and Rossi A (1988) Electrophysiological findings in a case of stiff-man syndrome. *Electromyogr Clin Neurophysiol*, **28**, 137–40

Rothwell JC, Obeso JA, and Marsden CD (1986) Electrophysiology of somatosensory reflex myoclonus. *Adv Neurol*, **43**, 385–98

Rowland LP (1985) Cramps and stiffness. *Rev Neurol*, **141**, 261–73

Rowland LP, Fetell M, Olarte M, Hays A, Singh N, and Wanat FE (1979) Emery Dreifuss muscular dystrophy. *Ann Neurol*, **5**, 111–17

Rushworth G, Lishman WA, Trevor Hughes J, and Oppenheimer DR (1961) Intense rigidity of the arms due to isolation of motoneurones by a spinal tumor. *J Neurol, Neurosurg Psychiatry*, **24**, 132–42

Sander JE, Layzer RB, and Goldsobel AB (1979) Congenital stiff-man syndrome. *Ann Neurol*, **8**, 195–7

Sato A, Tsujihata M, Yoshimura T, Mori M, and Nagataki S (1983) Myasthenia gravis associated with Satoyoshi syndrome: muscle cramps, alopecia and diarrhoea. *Neurology*, **33**, 1209–11

Schmidt RT, Stahl SM, and Spehlmann R (1975) A pharmacologic study of the stiff-man syndrome. *Neurology*, **25**, 622–6

Schomburg EC (1990) Spinal sensorimotor systems and their supraspinal control. *Neurosci Res*, **7**, 265–340

Schwartzman MJ, Mitsumoto H, Chou SM, Estes ML, Raaf H, La Franchise EF *et al.* (1989) Sudden death in stiff-man syndrome with automatic instability. *Ann Neurol*, **26**, 166

Sheaff HM (1952) Hereditary myokymia. *Arch Neurol Psychiatry*, **68**, 236–47

Sinha S, Newsom-Davis J, Mills K, Bryne N, Lang B, and Vincent A (1991) Autoimmune aetiology for acquired neuromyotonia. *Lancet*, **338**, 75–7

Solimena M, Folli F, Denis-Donini S, Comi GC, Pozza G, De Camilli, and Vicari AM (1988) Autoantibodies to glutamic acid decarboxylase in a patient with stiff-man syndrome, epilepsy, and type 1 diabetes mellitus. *N Engl J Med*, **318**, 1012–20

Solimena M, Folli F, Morello F, Toso V, and De Camilli P (1990a) Autoantibodies directed against GABA-ergic synapses in a second case of stiff-man syndrome and epilepsy. In Berardelli A, Benecke R, Manfredi M, and Marsden CD, eds, *Motor Disturbances II*, London, Academic Press, 415–22

Solimena M, Folli F, Morello F, Bottazzo GP, Toso V, and De Camilli P (1990b) Autoantibodies to GABA-ergic neurones and pancreatic beta cells in stiff-man syndrome. *N Engl J Med*, **322**, 1555–60

Spaans F, Theunissen P, Reekers AD, Smit L, and Veldman H (1990) Schwartz–Jampel syndrome: 1 Clinical, electromyographic and histologic studies. *Muscle Nerve*, **13**, 516–27

Spehlmann R and Norcross K (1979) Stiff-man syndrome. In Klanvans HL, ed., *Clinical Neuropharmacology*, vol. 4, New York, Raven Press, 109–21

Spehlmann R, Norcross K, Rasmus SC, and Schlageter NL (1981) Improvement of stiff-man syndrome and sodium valproate. *Neurology*, **31**, 1162–3

Sroka H, Bornstein M, and Sandbank U (1975) Ultrastructure of the syndrome of continuous muscle fibre activity. *Acta Neuropathol*, **31**, 85–90

Struppler A, Struppler E, and Adams RD (1963) Local tetanus in man. *Arch Neurol*, **8**, 62–78

Tarlov IM (1967) Rigidity in man due to spinal interneuron loss. *Arch Neurol*, **16**, 536–43

Taylor KM and Laverty R (1969) The effect of chlordiazepoxide, diazepam and nitrazepam on catecholamine metabolism in regions of the rat brain. *Eur J Pharmacol*, **8**, 296–301

Taylor RG, Layzer RB, Davis HS, and Fowler WM (1972) Continuous muscle fibre activity in the Schwartz-Jampel syndrome. *Electroencephalogr Clin Neurophysiol*, **33**, 497–509

Thorburn W (1987) Cases of injury to the cervical region of the spinal cord. *Brain*, **9**, 510–43

Todd JA, Acha-Orebea H, Bell JI, Chao N, Fronek Z, Jacob CO *et al.* (1988) Molecular basis for MHC class II-associated autoimmunity. *Science*, **240**, 1003–9

Torbergson T (1975) A family with hereditary myotonia, muscular hypertrophy and increased muscular irritability distinct from myotonia congenita Thomsen. *Acta Neurol Scand*, **51**, 225–32

Trethowan WH, Allsop JL, and Turner B (1960) The stiff-man syndrome. *Arch Neurol*, **3**, 114–22

Trontelj J and Stalberg E (1983) Bizarre repetitive discharges recorded with single fibre EMG. *J Neurol, Neurosurg Psychiatry*, **46**, 310–16

Valenstein E, Watson RT, and Parker JL (1978) Myokymia, muscle hypertrophy and percussion 'myotonia' in chronic recurrent polyneuropathy. *Neurology*, **28**, 1130–4

Van Dyke DH, Griggs RL, Murphy MJ, and Goldstein MN (1975) Hereditary myokymia and periodic ataxia. *J Neurol Sci*, **25**, 109–18

Van den Bergh P, De Merisman J, Dom R, and Bulcke J (1983) Motor neuron rigidity. *J Neurol*, **230**, 183–92

Vasilescu C, Alexianu M, and Dan A (1984) Neuronal type of Charcot–Marie–Tooth disease with a syndrome of continuous motor unit activity. *J Neurol Sci*, **63**, 11–25

Vicari AM, Folli F, Pozza G, Comi CG, Comola M, Canal N *et al.* (1989) Plasmapheresis in the treatment of stiff-man syndrome. *N Engl J Med*, **320**, 1499

Vilchez JJ, Cabello A, Benedito J, and Villaroya T (1980) Hyperkalaemic paralysis, neuropathy and persistent motor neuron discharges at rest in Addison's disease. *J Neurol, Neurosurg Psychiatry*, **43**, 818–22

Wallis WE, van Poznack A, and Plum F (1970) Generalised muscular stiffness, fasciculations and myokymia of peripheral nerve origin. *Arch Neurol*, **22**, 430–9

Walsh JC (1976) Neuromyotonia: an unusual presentation of intrathoracic malignancy. *J Neurol, Neurosurg Psychiatry*, **39**, 1086–91

Warmolts JR and Mendell JR (1980) Neurotonia: impulse-induced discharges in peripheral neuropathy. *Ann Neurol*, **7**, 245–50

Welch LK, Appenzeller O, and Bicknell JM (1972) Peripheral neuropathy with myokymia, sustained muscular contraction and continuous motor unit activity. *Neurology*, **22**, 161–9

Werk EE, Sholiton LJ, and Marnell RT (1961) The 'stiff-man' syndrome and hyperthyroidism. *Am J Med*, **31**, 647–53

Westblom U (1977) Stiff-man syndrome and clonazepam. *JAMA*, **237**, 1930

Whelan JL (1980) Baclofen in treatment of the 'stiff-man' syndrome. *Arch Neurol*, **37**, 600–1

Whiteley AM, Swash M, and Urich H (1976) Progressive encephalomyelitis with rigidity. *Brain*, **99**, 27–42

Williams AC, Nutt JG, and Hare T (1988) Autoimmunity in stiff-man syndrome. *Lancet*, **ii**, 22

Wilton A and Gardner-Medwin D (1990) 21-year follow-up of myokymia with impaired muscle relaxation. *Lancet*, **ii**, 1138–9

Zisfein J, Sivak M, Aron A, and Bender AN (1983) Isaacs' syndrome with muscle hypertrophy reversed by phenytoin therapy. *Arch Neurol*, **40**, 241–2

20
Peripheral movement disorders

C. David Marsden

INTRODUCTION

Abnormal involuntary movements (dyskinesias) usually are caused by brain damage or dysfunction. Occasionally, however, lesions of the spinal cord, spinal roots, cervical or lumbar plexus, or even peripheral nerves may cause a variety of dyskinesias. A typical example is hemifacial spasm, where compression of the facial nerve by a cerebellopontine angle mass lesion, or by aberrent arteries in the posterior fossa, produces repetitive clonic and tonic contractions of one side of the face. Local pathology in the spinal cord may lead to focal spinal segmental myoclonus. Similar focal myoclonus is sometimes due to damage to spinal roots, the plexus or peripheral nerves. Such lesions also rarely cause other dyskinesias, such as dystonia and other forms of muscle spasms, sometimes associated with causalgia and reflex sympathetic dystrophy. Finally, a peripheral injury may act as the trigger to the appearance of dyskinesias thought to arise in the brain, as is the case in a significant proportion of patients with primary dystonia. In some way, the peripheral injury alters central nervous system activity to generate involuntary movements.

There is another category of pathological muscle contraction caused by peripheral nerve disease, namely the syndrome of neuromyotonia and continuous muscle fibre activity. This and other similar conditions is reviewed in this volume in Chapter 19.

SPINAL SEGMENTAL MYOCLONUS

The whole topic of spinal myoclonus is reviewed in this volume in Chapter 23. A brief summary is given below to highlight the concept that spinal cord disease can cause focal segmental myoclonus, as a prelude to later discussion of the mechanisms involved.

There is persuasive experimental evidence to show that local spinal cord disease can produce focal myoclonus. Newcastle disease virus injected into the lower spinal cord of the cat causes semirhythmic myoclonic jerks of the legs, which persist after high thoracic transection or deafferentation (Luttrell and Bang, 1958; Luttrell *et al.*, 1959). Likewise, local application of penicillin to the spinal cord can produce focal myoclonus which also persists after spinal transection (Kao and Crill, 1972).

A variety of spinal cord lesions have been recorded as producing focal segmental myoclonus in man (see Chapter 23). These include spinal cord tumours (Garcin *et al.*, 1968), ischaemia (Davis *et al.*, 1981), infection (such as herpes zoster and acquired immune deficiency syndrome; Dhaliwal and McGreal, 1974; Hoehn and Cherington, 1977; Berger *et al.*, 1986; Jankovic and Pardo, 1986), and trauma (Jankovic and Pardo, 1986), as well as demyelinating disease (Jankovic and Pardo, 1986), cervical spondylosis (Hoehn and Cherington, 1977; Jankovic and Pardo, 1986), and arteriovenous malformations (Levy *et al.*, 1983). Similar myoclonus also has been reported following spinal anaesthesia (Fox *et al.*, 1979).

Typically, spinal segmental myoclonus is rhythmic, at about 0.5–2 per second, and occurs spontaneously at rest, even persisting in sleep. Rarely it may appear on action or be stimulus-sensitive (Davis *et al.*, 1981). Those muscles innervated by the affected spinal segments are involved, hence the designation segmental myoclonus.

FOCAL MYOCLONUS DUE TO ROOT, PLEXUS OR PERIPHERAL NERVE LESIONS

Myoclonic jerking of the paraspinal muscles due to a malignant tumour involving the fifth thoracic root, without long tract signs of spinal cord involvement, has been described (Sotaniemi, 1985). Similar focal myoclonus of the legs has also occurred with lumbosacral radiculopathy, and after lumbar laminectomy for lumbar stenosis and root lesions (Jankovic and Pardo, 1986). Rhythmic myoclonus of the quadriceps muscle has been reported due to a Schwann-cell sarcoma of the femoral nerve (Said and Bathien, 1977).

Focal myoclonus of the right arm due to a brachial plexus lesion has been described following radiotherapy for carcinoma of the breast followed by abduction trauma of the right shoulder (Banks *et al.*, 1985). The latter case exhibited rhythmic muscle jerks at about 5 per second in the distribution of the axillary and radial nerves, but not in other muscles innervated by the lateral and medial cords of the brachial plexus. Electromyographic analysis of this case indicated that the myoclonus arose from a generator located in a segment of the posterior cord of the brachial plexus, between the departure of the axillary nerve and distal to the emergence of the suprascapular nerve. Another patient developed myoclonus of one arm after an electrical injury to the left brachial plexus (Jankovic and Pardo, 1986). Myoclonus of an arm has even occurred after a thoracic sympathectomy (Jankovic and Pardo, 1986).

THE MECHANISM OF SPINAL AND PERIPHERAL MYOCLONUS

The clinical characteristics of myoclonus due to spinal cord, root, plexus or peripheral nerve diseases are as follows:

1. It is focal, being confined to the muscles innervated by the affected spinal cord segments or peripheral lower motor neurons.
2. It is usually spontaneous and rhythmic, and it often persists in sleep.

These observations suggest that it is the result of repetitive, spontaneous discharge of groups of anterior horn cells.

Swanson *et al.* (1962) suggested two mechanisms which might be responsible for spinal segmental myoclonus: (1) enhanced neuronal excitability due to direct cellular exitation by inflammation or tumour; (2) enhanced neuronal excitability due to removal of inhibition. The former seems unlikely, for spinal segmental myoclonus can occur without evidence of damage to anterior horn cells. Loss of inhibition of anterior horn cell pools seems more probable.

Posterior rhizotomy or hemicordectomy leads to abnormal spontaneous discharge of some spinal neurons in the deafferented segments, which tend to fire in bursts at high frequency (Loeser and Ward, 1967). However, these bursting spinal neurons are found in the dorsal, not the ventral horns. Nevertheless, such spontaneous bursting of spinal interneurons following deafferentation might drive anterior horn cells to produce focal myoclonus.

Alternatively, loss of inhibitory spinal interneurons might liberate anterior horn cells to fire spontaneously in a rhythmic-burst fashion. In the case described by Davis *et al.* (1981), spinal myoclonus occurred following ischaemic damage to the cord, which at autopsy was found to have caused extensive loss of small and medium-sized interneurons, with relative preservation of large anterior horn cells. The loss of inhibitory spinal interneurons could well release anterior horn cells to discharge spontaneously, but what then determines their tendency to fire repetitively and rhythmically is less clear (Kiehn, 1991). Loss of spinal interneurons also is the pathological change held to be responsible for spinal rigidity (see Chapter 19).

In the case of focal myoclonus due to lesions of roots, the plexus, or peripheral nerves, the mechanism responsible is more difficult to perceive. However, the pathophysiology of hemifacial spasm, which has been studied extensively, provides a useful model.

HEMIFACIAL SPASM

The clinical characteristics of hemifacial spasm are well-known. It usually begins in middle life with clonic contractions of the muscles around one eye. These spread to involve those of the cheek and upper lip, and eventually the whole half of the face. The twitches occur in bursts, sometimes rhythmically, and may continue in sleep. The clonic spasms often are triggered by voluntary contraction of the facial muscles. In addition to the clonic spasms, prolonged tonic spasms of facial contraction also occur, closing the eye, lifting the forehead and retracting the angle of the mouth. With time, a mild degree of facial weakness becomes evident.

Rarely, hemifacial spasm is due to an obvious mass lesion in the cerebellopontine angle compressing the facial nerve. In the common idiopathic variety, exploration of the posterior fossa often reveals abnormal blood vessels compressing or pulsating on the facial nerve. If these are dissected away, the hemifacial spasm may be cured in a large majority of cases (Jannetta *et al.*, 1977). Rarely, injury to the peripheral branches of the seventh nerve in the face can provoke hemifacial spasm (Martinelli *et al.*, 1992).

One hypothesis to explain hemifacial spasm is that it is due to local irritation of the facial nerve causing ectopic excitation (spontaneous local initiation of action potentials) and ephaptic transmission (cross-talk during the passage of impulses in adjacent fibres via artificial synapses at the site of injury). Both have been claimed to have been demonstrated electrophysiologically in hemifacial spasm (Nielsen, 1984a,b), as has a local slowing of conduction in the compressed segment of the facial nerve due to focal segmental demyelination (Nielsen, 1984b). Ephaptic cross-talk was suggested by a delayed response in a distant muscle (orbicularis oculi or mentalis) on stimulating a distant branch of the facial nerve (mandibular or zygomatic). This was not due to stimulation of trigeminal sensory nerves, for the latency shortened when the stimulus was moved closer to the stylomastoid foramen but further from the exit of the trigeminal nerve. Nor was it due to an axon reflex in abberant regenerated nerve fibres, for the delayed distant response disappeared after decompression of the facial nerve (Nielsen and Jannetta, 1984). It was argued that it was not a distant F-wave due to antidromic excitation of the facial nucleus, for no such F-wave was seen in the directly activated muscle. Moller and Jannetta (1985), however, attributed these distant responses to activation of the facial nucleus (see below). Nielsen (1984a) also found after-discharges and late activity following peripheral facial nerve stimulation, suggestive of ectopic activity. This too disappeared after facial nerve decompression (Nielsen and Jannetta, 1984).

Nielsen (1984b) went on to suggest further evidence for both ephaptic transmission and ectopic activity in hemifacial spasm through indirect stimulation of the blink reflex. This also led to abnormal synkinetic contraction of mentalis and after-activity.

However, other evidence indicates that the facial nerve nucleus is hyperexcitable in this condition, and it has been argued that the widespread repetitive clonic movements and tonic spasms of the face cannot be generated by ectopic excitation and ephaptic transmission alone (Hjorth and Willison, 1973; Ferguson, 1978). The first component (R1) of the blink reflex is hyperactive on the affected side, and the second component (R2) shows less inhibition by a prior conditioning stimulus on the affected side (Esteban and Molina-Negro, 1986; Valls-Sole and Tolosa, 1989). The findings indicate a hyperactive facial nerve nucleus on the side of hemifacial spasm. Indeed, Moller and Jannetta (1986) found that under surgical anaesthesia, no R1 was evident on the unaffected side, but the R1 was obtained on the affected side; this pathological R1 component of the blink reflex disappeared when the facial nerve was decompressed.

One aftermath of injury to a motor nerve is loss of synapses on to the parent cell soma and dendrites, which is associated with changes in the excitability of the motoneuron. Thus, according to this hypothesis, hemifacial spasm is due to abnormal synchronous discharges of facial motoneurons within the facial nucleus itself.

The two theories can be combined by assuming that the partial lesion of the facial nerve, causing ectopic excitation and ephaptic transmission, results in both orthodromic and antidromic nerve activity combined with deafferentation (Ferguson, 1978), to produce a reorganization of the neuronal machinery within the facial nerve nucleus (Moller and Jannetta, 1986). This combined hypothesis introduces the principle that peripheral nerve injury can, on occasion, induce changes in the excitability of central motoneurons.

There are other situations in which such a mechanism appears to cause involuntary movements.

MUSCLE SPASMS ASSOCIATED WITH REFLEX SYMPATHETIC DYSTROPHY

In 1984, 5 patients were described who developed abnormal involuntary movements of a limb after injury (Marsden *et al.*, 1984). All subsequently developed reflex sympathetic dystrophy with Sudeck's atrophy, and then abnormal muscle spasms or jerks of the affected limb, lasting years. Two exhibited myoclonic jerks of the injured leg; 1 had both jerks and more prolonged muscle spasms of the injured foot; the remaining 2 patients developed more complex dystonic spasms of the injured arm. All had severe persistent causalgic pain in the damaged limb, as well as the vasomotor, sudomotor and trophic changes typical of reflex sympathetic dystrophy. Jankovic and Van der Linden (1988), Robberecht *et al.* (1988) and Schwartzman and Kerrigan (1990) also have drawn attention to a variety of involuntary movements associated with causalgia and reflex sympathetic dystrophy. These include fixed abnormal dystonic postures due to sustained muscle spasms, and tremor. Schwartzman and Kerrigan (1990) collected 43 patients with 'dystonia', spasms or tremor from 200 cases of reflex sympathetic dystrophy.

Recently, we (Bhatia *et al.*, 1993) have reviewed 18 patients with causalgia and dystonia, triggered by injury (usually trivial) in 15, and occurring spontaneously in 3 cases. Most were young women. All had the typical burning causalgic pain with hyperpathia and allodynia, along with the vasomotor, sudomotor and trophic changes in skin, subcutaneous tissue and bone, typical of reflex sympathetic dystrophy. All these patients developed deforming and often grotesque dystonic postures in the affected limb (the arm in 6, the leg in 12 cases), coincident with or after the causalgia. The dystonic spasms typically were sustained, producing a fixed dystonic posture, in contrast to the mobile spasms characteristic of idiopathic torsion dystonia. Both the dystonia and the causalgia spread to affect other limbs in 7 patients. All investigations were normal and all modes of conventional treatment failed to relieve either the pain or the dystonia, but 2 patients recovered spontaneously.

Thus, a relation between causalgia, reflex sympathetic dystrophy and a variety of involuntary movements, all precipitated by peripheral injury, seems established.

The classical clinical features of causalgia have been documented extensively (Mitchell, 1872; Schott, 1986a; Schwartzman and McLellan, 1987). The mechanisms responsible for causalgia and reflex sympathetic dystrophy have been the subject of much speculation, and appear relevant to the pathophysiology of the associated dyskinesias. At first sight, it would seem likely that some persisting peripheral abnormality must be responsible, but close analysis indicates that this is an inadquate explanation (Schott, 1986a; Schwartzman and McLellan, 1987). Most authors now also invoke altered central mechanisms, triggered by peripheral trauma, as the cause of reflex sympathetic dystrophy and causalgia.

Nathan (1947) proposed that the pain of reflex sympathetic dystrophy might arise from abnormal stimulation of somatic sensory axons in damaged nerves. Peripheral mechanisms (at sites of nerve damage, including neuromas) that have been invoked to explain causalgia and reflex sympathetic dystrophy (Janig, 1985; Schott, 1986a; Schwartzman and McLellan, 1987; Fields, 1990) include the following:

1. Activation of low-threshold mechanoreceptor afferents (pain and allodynia) by ephaptic sympathetic efferent activity.
2. Activation of nociceptor afferents by ephaptic sympathetic efferent activity.
3. Ectopic pacemaker discharges in damaged demyelinated axons, sensitive to circulating catecholamines or those released by sympathetic activity (Devor, 1983).

All these mechanisms might explain causalgic pain in the distribution of damaged peripheral nerves, but the trivial trauma provoking causalgia and dystonia often does not appear to cause detectable nerve damage. In these cases, it is assumed that the local trauma initiates changes in sensory input that have central consequences.

Schott (1986a) points out that causalgia is unlikely to arise solely from the peripheral nerve itself, for peripheral nerve section, rhizotomy, cordotomy and even sympathectomy are unlikely to relieve the pain (Sunderland, 1978; Noordenbos and Wall, 1981). He also reviews the numerous reports of causalgia provoked by disease of the central nervous system, such as strokes, multiple sclerosis and spinal cord trauma. The spread of pain (and dystonia) within the limb and to other limbs, sometimes bilaterally, points to a central process at spinal or supraspinal level. Persistent pain in a phantom limb also argues for a central origin.

So, trauma or damage to peripheral nerves is thought to give rise to abnormal impulse transmission in peripheral sensory and sympathetic nerves which, in turn, leads to reorganization of central processing of sensory (and motor) information to cause causalgia (and dystonia).

There is a close analogy between the postulated mechanisms responsible for hemifacial spasms and those causing reflex sympathetic dystrophy and causalgia. The idea is that both peripheral and central mechanisms interact to produce the motor, sensory and sympathetic phenomena.

JUMPY STUMPS AND BELLY DANCER'S DYSKINESIAS

Not only did Mitchell (1872) describe causalgia after gunshot wounds of peripheral nerves, he also recorded tremor, jerks and spasms of the remaining stump following amputation, sometimes associated with severe phantom pain (Mitchell, 1872). The 'painful, jumpy stump' has since been described by others (Ritchie, 1970; Steiner *et al.*, 1974; Marion *et al.*, 1989; Kulisevsky *et al.*, 1992), and even a phantom dyskinesia induced by metoclopramide has been recorded (Jankovic and Glass, 1985).

Jerking of the amputation stump (jactitation), coinciding with lancinating neuralgic stump pains, frequently occurs in the postoperative period but settles over weeks or months (Russell, 1970). The cases referred to above, however, experienced spasms and jerks of the stump for prolonged periods, for example, up to 40 years in 1 of the patients reported by Marion *et al.* (1989), who also reviewed many similar cases described in the earlier literature. Jerking of the stump frequently was preceded by severe pain in the stump, appearing weeks or months after the surgery. Upper or lower limb stumps could be affected. The stump jerks could be induced by voluntary movement or, sometimes, by cutaneous stimuli.

Steiner *et al.* (1974) considered involuntary stump movements to be a form of segmental myoclonus, caused by afferent impulses arising from the severed nerves. Marion *et al.* (1989) concluded that they were due either to 'the result of functional changes in spinal (or cortical) circuitry leading to redirection of afferent information through different spinal neurones, or structural reorganisation of local neuronal circuitry by axonal sprouting following nerve injury'.

Another bizarre condition sometimes related to abdominal trauma is 'belly dancer's dyskinesia' or the moving umbilicus syndrome. Iliceto *et al.* (1990) described 5 patients with odd abnormal movements of the abdomen. One had diaphragmatic flutter, but the remainder did not. The latter exhibited regular rhythmic contractions of the abdominal wall, which had a sinuous, writhing flowing character, often moving the umbilicus from side to side or in a circular rotatory fashion. Three of these 4 patients dated the onset of their abdominal dyskinesia to trauma (cholecystectomy and anal fistula, cystoscopic removal of a renal calculus and cystectomy) and 2 had severe pain.

PAINFUL LEGS (ARMS) AND MOVING TOES

There is another condition in which injury to peripheral nerves and roots may cause the combination of pain and abnormal involuntary movements. In 1971, Spillane *et al.* described 6 patients with severe pain in one or both feet accompanied by characteristic writhing movements of the toes and sometimes of the feet. Three of these patients had a history suggestive of lumbosacral root damage. Subsequently, further patients were described with local peripheral nerve damage, L5 herpes zoster, S1 root compression and caude equina lesions (Nathan, 1978), generalized peripheral neuropathy (Montagna *et al.*, 1983), as well as minor trauma to the legs (Schott, 1981). A similar condition has been recorded in the upper limb, with a painful arm and moving fingers, due to a brachial plexus lesion associated with a breast carcinoma and radiotherapy (Verhagen *et al.*, 1985).

Dressler *et al.* (1993) recently reviewed a further series of 18 patients with the syndrome of painful legs and moving toes. One case followed a bullet injury to the spinal cord and cauda equina; 4 cases were due to spinal nerve root injury (herpes zoster, 2 with lumbar disc prolapses, and an L5 haemangioma); 4 cases were due to peripheral leg trauma; 3 cases were associated with an axonal peripheral neuropathy; and in 6 cases no definite cause could be identified (although lumbosacral radiculopathies were suspected in at least 4 of these patients). Three other patients with identical toe movements but no pain also were described.

Pain usually was the first symptom, preceding the movements by days to years. The onset might be unilateral, with subsequent spread to the opposite limb, or bilateral. In many patients the pain and the movements appeared to be linked, with increasing pain associated with worsening movements. The pain typically was diffuse, not limited to a peripheral nerve or segmented dermatomal pattern, and was described as burning, crushing or throbbing. The characteristics of the pain and the common coexistence of hyperpathia and allodynia are typical of causalgia (Schott, 1986a).

The toe movements consist of complex sequences of flexion, extension, abduction and adduction, in various combinations at frequencies of 1–2 Hz. The electromyogram characteristics of such muscle contractions cannot be explained by a peripheral nerve mechanism alone, but point to an origin in the central nervous system.

The mechanism proposed to explain this condition again is that of peripheral injury to nerves, plexus or roots, causing an alteration in spinal and/or supraspinal sensory (the pain) and motor (the movements) machinery. However, the nature of the movements (slow, writhing and sustained, i.e. dystonic) is quite different to the type of movements seen in hemifacial spasm (myoclonic jerks) or, indeed, in spinal myoclonus. Whether the movements in this condition arise in the spinal cord, as suggested by Nathan (1978) and Schott (1981, 1986b), or supraspinally is unknown. Peripheral nerve injuries have been shown experimentally to alter the patterns of neuronal activity not only in the dorsal horn (Wall and Devor, 1982), but also in dorsal column nuclei (Wall and Devor, 1982), and in ventral thalamus and sensory cortex (Kass *et al.*, 1983). Alterations in basal ganglia neurotransmitters also occur following experimental peripheral injuries (De Ceballos *et al.*, 1986).

DYSTONIA INDUCED BY PERIPHERAL INJURY

There have been a few reports suggesting that peripheral nerve lesions apparently cause typical arm dystonia (Scherokman *et al.*, 1986), and action dystonia of the legs associated with severe lumbar canal stenosis has been described (Al-Kawi, 1987). However, caution must be exercised in attributing dystonia to a peripheral nerve injury, for nerve entrapment may be secondary to dystonia. Thus, for example, some 7% of patients with writer's cramp subsequently develop carpal tunnel compression of the median nerve as a consequence of their dystonia (Sheehy *et al.*, 1988), and secondary entrapment neuropathies are common in those with any form of dystonia.

More convincing is the association of trauma with the onset of dystonia. Sheehy and Marsden (1980) described 3 trauma-induced cases out of a series of 60 patients with torticollis and calculated that 9% of 414 cases of this focal dystonia had suffered preceding injuries. These authors (Sheehy and Marsden, 1982) also noted that writer's cramp could be precipitated by local hand injury, and subsequently identified 5 such cases amongst 91 patients (Sheehy *et al.*, 1988). Schott (1985) described 4 patients with axial or arm dystonia after local trauma, and later (1986b) described a further 10 patients with movement disorders which appeared to have been precipitated by peripheral trauma; 6 of these had developed dystonia, including writer's and pianist's cramps, cranial segmental dystonia, axial segmental dystonia and focal foot dystonia. The interval from injury to development of dystonia ranged from 24 hours to 3 years. In some patients, oromandibular dystonia has appeared after dental treatment (Thompson *et al.*, 1986; Koller *et al.*, 1989). Brin and colleagues (1986) briefly reported 23 patients in whom trauma precipitated dystonia in the injured region after an interval of between 1 day and 8 weeks. Jankovic and Van der Linden (1988) also described a number of patients with dystonia and tremor induced by peripheral trauma; of 28 cases, 13 had persistent dystonia (4 of a hand, 5 of a foot, 1 of an arm, 1 of a leg and 2 of craniocervical musculature) developing within 1 day to 12 months after a relevant injury. In blepharospasm, a history of preceding local ocular disease has been recorded in about 12% of cases (Grandas *et al.*, 1988).

Thus, there appears to be a significant association between local trauma and the onset of a variety of focal dystonias in a proportion of patients with this illness – perhaps some 5–10% overall.

Of course, the vast majority of those subjected to local injury do not develop dystonia, so trauma alone is unlikely to be the cause. Rather, it seems more probable that trauma acts as a trigger to the appearance of dystonia in those predisposed to develop this illness. Indeed, on occasion trauma may trigger a focal dystonia in patients who subsequently progress to develop generalized dystonia.

Primary idiopathic torsion dystonia is genetic in origin, so the trauma may be a significant trigger to onset of the illness in those carrying the abnormal gene. Fletcher *et al.* (1991a) recently examined the relationship between trauma and dystonia in 104 patients with idiopathic generalized, multifocal or segmental torsion dystonia. Genetic analysis of this population had indicated that the illness was caused by an autosomal dominant gene with reduced (40%) penetrance in about 85% of cases (Fletcher *et al.*, 1990). Seventeen (16.4%) of these 104 cases reported that their dystonia had been precipitated or exacerbated by local trauma. The dystonia appeared in the injured part of the body within days or up to 12 months after the trauma. Subsequently, the dystonia spread to other body regions. Some patients experienced a new dystonia in a different body part after a subsequent injury to that distant structure. Eight of these 17 patients had affected relatives, so were genetically at risk of developing dystonia before the injury. Brin *et al.* (1986) and Jankovic and Van der Linden (1988) also noted familial cases amongst patients with trauma-induced dystonia (i.e. 9 of 23, and 3 of 13 cases respectively). All this evidence is consistent with the hypothesis that peripheral injury might precipitate dystonia in those carrying the idiopathic torsion dystonia gene, although trauma amongst those with idiopathic torsion dystonia is no more frequent than in a matched control population (Fletcher *et al.*, 1991b).

The dystonia associated with trauma in these cases was similar in all respects to that occurring spontaneously. Inherited primary dystonia is thought to be due to basal ganglia dysfunction. If this is also the case in those who develop dystonia after injury, then it would seem that trauma may trigger abnormalities of the brain, as well as the spinal cord.

There are possible mechanisms whereby peripheral injury might alter basal ganglia function. A major projection of the spinothalamic tract is to the ventrobasal nucleus of the thalamus, which projects to the somatosensory cortex. This system probably subserves discriminative pain perception (Guillbaud *et al.*, 1984), while spinoreticular pathways may be involved in large-scale somatic and autonomic responses to pain (Willis, 1984). The main projection of the nociceptive component of the spinoreticular tract is to the nucleus gigantocellularis in which (in the rat) nearly all cells respond to noxious stimuli (Benjamin, 1970). Neurons in nucleus gigantocellularis project principally to the centrum medianum and parafascicular thalamic nuclei, which are a major source of projections to the striatum (Guillband *et al.*, 1984). Thus, nociceptive stimuli can gain access to the basal ganglia.

There also is direct experimental evidence that peripheral injury can alter basal ganglia chemistry. De Ceballos *et al.* (1986) found that a thermal injury to one hindlimb in the rat causes early (24 hours) bilateral reduction of leu-encephalin immunoreactivity in the globus pallidus, and later (1 week) bilateral (but most marked contralaterally) reduction of both met-encephalin and leu-encephalin immunoreactivity in globus pallidus, and of met-encephalin immunoreactivity in caudate and putamen. These late changes in basal ganglia encephalin content may reflect alterations in basal ganglia function that conceivably may be responsible for peripheral trauma precipitating dystonia in genetically susceptible individuals.

CONCLUSIONS

It seems established that lesions of peripheral nerves, plexi and spinal nerve roots, or peripheral injuries without overt nerve damage, can provoke a range of movement disorders. A number of mechanisms appear to be involved.

1. Peripheral nerve, plexus or spinal nerve root damage may result in local ectopic impulse generation and ephaptic cross-talk, but these mechanisms alone do not explain the resulting movement disorder.
2. Such abnormal peripheral nervous activity may lead to reorganization of spinal or brainstem motor machinery to cause myoclonus, as in the segmental myoclonus rarely seen in peripheral lesions and in hemifacial spasm.
3. Local lesions of the spinal cord may provoke similar spinal segmental myoclonus, perhaps by removal of interneuronal inhibition of anterior horn cell pools.
4. Peripheral nerve or spinal nerve root lesions also may cause more complex movement disorders, for example the curious athetoid digital movements often seen in the syndrome of painful legs and moving toes. Whether such complex movements again are generated by reorganization of spinal motor machinery or by changes in supraspinal sensorimotor integration is uncertain.

5. Likewise, amputation may provoke spasms of the stump, often associated with phantom pain, and abdominal dyskinesias also may appear to be precipitated by trauma often with pain.
6. The movement disorders precipitated by peripheral injury (with or without overt nerve damage) may or may not be associated with pain, often causalgic in nature, and sometimes with the full-blown syndrome of reflex sympathetic dystrophy. Many patients with reflex sympathetic dystrophy exhibit fixed dystonia, tremors and jerky muscle spasms.
7. The mechanisms responsible for the pain and the abnormal movements in reflex sympathetic dystrophy appear to involve reorganization of spinal, and perhaps supraspinal, sensory and motor mechanisms.
8. Peripheral trauma may provoke painless typical dystonia in those carrying the abnormal idiopathic torsion dystonia gene, perhaps by altering basal ganglia function.

Reorganization of spinal or supraspinal sensorimotor integration may account for a spectrum of disorders that develop after soft tissue or bone injury, or after damage to peripheral nerves, plexus or spinal nerve roots. Different degrees of interruption, or alteration in afferent input to the spinal cord or brain, and reorganization of its subsequent central processing may result in injury causing: (a) pain alone: causalgia; (2) pain and involuntary movements; painful legs and moving toes, painful arm and moving fingers, fixed dystonia or tremor and jerks associated with reflex sympathetic dystrophy and causalgia, painful jumpy amputation stumps, painful abdominal dyskinesias; and (3) involuntary movements alone: painless moving toes, painless jumpy amputation stumps or abdominal contractions, segmental myoclonus, hemifacial spasm, and even painless mobile dystonia in genetically susceptible individuals.

References

Al-Kawi MZ (1987) Focal dystonia in spinal stenosis. *Arch Neurol*, **44**, 692–3

Banks G, Nielsen VK, Short MP, and Kowal CD (1985) Brachial plexus myoclonus. *J Neurol, Neurosurg Psychiatry*, **48**, 582–4

Benjamin RM (1970) Single neurons in the rat medulla responsive to nocioceptive stimulation. *Brain Res*, **24**, 525–9

Berger JR, Bender A, Resnick L, and Perlmutter D (1986) Spinal myoclonus associated with HTLV III/LAV infection. *Arch Neurol*, **43**, 1203–4

Bhatia KP, Bhatt MH, and Marsden CD (1993) The causalgia–dystonia Syndrome. *Brain*, **116**, 843–51

Brin MF, Fahn S, Bressman SB, and Burke RE (1986) Dystonia precipitated by peripheral trauma. *Neurology*, **36** (suppl 1), 119

Davis SM, Murray, NMF, Diengdoh JV, Galea-Debono A, and Kocen RS (1981) Stimulus-sensitive spinal myoclonus. *J Neurol, Neurosurg Psychiatry*, **44**, 884–8

De Ceballos ML, Baker M, Rose J, Jenner P, and Marsden CD (1986) Do enkephalins in basal ganglia mediate a physiological motor rest mechanism? *Movement Disorders*, **1**, 223–33

Devor M (1983) Nerve pathophysiology and mechanisms of pain in causalgia. *J Auton Nerv Syst*, **7**, 371–84

Dhaliwal GS, and McGreal DA (1974) Spinal myoclonus in association with herpes zoster infection: two case reports. *Can J Neurol Sci*, **1**, 239–41

Dressler D, Thompson PD, Gledhill RF, and Marsden CD (1993) The syndrome of painful legs and moving toes: a review. *Movement Disorders*, in press

Esteban A and Molina-Negro P (1986) Primary hemifacial spasm: a neurophysiological study. *J Neurol, Neurosurg Psychiatry*, **49**, 58–63

Ferguson JH (1978) Hemifacial spasm and the facial nucleus. *Ann Neurol*, **4**, 97–103

Fields HL (ed) (1990) *Pain Syndromes in Neurology*, Oxford, Butterworth-Heinemann

Fletcher NA, Harding AE, and Marsden CD (1990) A genetic study of idiopathic torsion dystonia in the UK. *Brain*, **113**, 379–95

Fletcher NA, Harding AE, and Marsden CD (1991a) The relationship between trauma and idiopathic torsion dystonia. *J Neurol, Neurosurg Psychiatry*, **54**, 713–17

Fletcher NA, Harding, AE, and Marsden CD (1991b) A case-control study of idiopathic torsion dystonia. *Movement Disorders*, **6**, 304–9

Fox EJ, Villanueva R, and Schutta HS (1979) Myoclonus following spinal anaesthesia. *Neurology*, **29**, 379–80

Garcin R, Rondot P, and Guiot G (1968) Rhythmic myoclonus of the right arm as the presenting symptom of a cervical cord tumour. *Brain*, **91**, 75–84

Grandas F, Elston J, Quinn N, and Marsden CD (1988) Blepharospasm: a review of 264 patients. *J Neurol, Neurosurg Psychiatry*, **51**, 767–72

Guillbaud G, Peschanski M, and Besson J-M (1984) Experimental data related to nocioception and pain at the supraspinal level. In Wall PD and Melzack R, eds, *A Textbook of Pain*, Churchill Livingstone, London, 110–18

Hjorth RJ and Willison RG (1973) The electromyogram in facial myokimia and hemifacial spasm. *J Neurol Sci*, **20**, 117–26

Hoehn MM and Cherington M (1977) Spinal myoclonus. *Neurology*, **27**, 942–6

Iliceto G, Thompson PD, Day BL, Rothwell JC, Lees AJ, and Marsden CD (1990) Diaphragmatic flutter, the moving umbilicus syndrome and "belly dancer's" dyskinesia. *Movement Disorders*, **5**, 15–22

Janig W (1985) Causalgia and reflex sympathetic dystrophy: in which way is the sympathetic nervous system involved. *Trends Neurosci*, **8**, 471–7

Jankovic J and Glass JP (1985) Metoclopramide-induced phantom dyskinesia. *Neurology*, **35**, 432–5

Jankovic J and Pardo R (1986) Segmental myoclonus: clinical and pharmacological study. *Arch Neurol*, **43**, 1025–31

Jankovic J and Van der Linden C (1989) Dystonia and tremor induced by peripheral trauma: predisposing factors. *J Neurol, Neurosurg Psychiatry*, **51**, 1512–19

Jannetta PJ, Abbasy M, Maroon JC, Ramos FM, and Abir MS (1977) Aetiology and definitive microsurgical treatment of hemifacial spasms. *J Neurosurg*, **47**, 321–8

Kao LI and Crill WE (1972) Penicillin-induced segmental myoclonus. I. Motor responses and intracellular recording from motoneurons. *Arch Neurol*, **26**, 156–61

Kass JH, Merzenich MM, and Killackey HP (1983) The reorganization of sensory cortex following peripheral nerve damage in adult and developing mammals. *Ann Rev Neurosci*, **6**, 325–6

Kiehn O (1991) Plateau potentials and active integration in the 'final common pathway' for motor behaviour. *Trends Neurosci*, **14**, 68–73

Koller WC, Wong GF, and Lang A (1989) Post-traumatic movement disorders: a review. *Movement Disorders*, **4**, 20–36

Kulisevsky J, Marti-Fabregas J, and Grau JM (1992) Spasms of amputation stumps. *J Neurol, Neurosurg Psychiatry*, **55**, 626–7

Levy R, Plassche W, Riggs J, and Shoulson I (1983) Spinal myoclonus related to an arteriovenous malformation: response to clonazepam therapy. *Arch Neurol*, **40**, 254–5

Loeser D and Ward AA (1967) Some effects of deafferentation on neurons of the cat spinal cord. *Arch Neurol*, **17**, 629–36

Luttrell CN and Bang FB (1958) Newcastle disease encephalomyelitis in cats. I. Clinical and pathological features. *Arch Neurol*, **79**, 647–57

Luttrell CN, Bang FB, and Luxenberg K (1959) Newcastle disease encephalomyelitis in cats. II. Physiological studies on rhythmic myoclonus. *Arch Neurol*, **81**, 285–91

Marion MH, Gledhill RF, and Thompson PD (1989) Spasms of amputation stumps: a report of 2 cases. *Movement Disorders*, **4**, 1354–8

Marsden CD, Obeso JA, Traub MM, Rothwell JC, Kranz H, and LaCruz F (1984) Muscle spasms associated with Sudeck's atrophy after injury. *Br Med J*, **288**, 173–6

Martinelli P, Giuliani S, and Ippoloti M (1992) Hemifacial spasm due to peripheral injury of facial nerve: a nuclear syndrome? *Movement Disorders*, **7**, 181–4

Mitchell SW (1872) *Injuries of Nerves and their Consequences*, New York, JB Lippincott

Moller AR and Jannetta PJ (1985) Hemifacial spasm: results of electrophysiological recording during microvascular decompression operations. *Neurology*, **35**, 969–74

Moller AR and Jannetta PJ (1986) Blink reflex in patients with hemifacial spasm. Observations during microvascular decompression operations. *J Neurol Sci*, **72**, 171–82

Montagna P, Cirignotta F, Sacquegna T, Martinelli P, Ambrosetto G, and Lugaresi E (1983) 'Painful legs and moving toes' associated with polyneuropathy. *J Neurol, Neurosurg Psychiatry*, **46**, 399–403

Nathan PW (1947) On the pathogenesis of causalgia in peripheral nerve injuries. *Brain*, **70**, 145–70

Nathan PW (1978) Painful legs and moving toes: evidence on the site of the lesion. *J Neurol, Neurosurg Psychiatry*, **41**, 934–9

Nielsen VK (1984a) Pathophysiology of hemifacial spasm: I. Ephaptic transmission and ectopic excitation. *Neurology*, **34**, 418–26

Nielsen VK (1984b) Pathophysiology of hemifacial spasm: II. Lateral spread of the supraorbital nerve reflex. *Neurology*, **34**, 427–31

Nielsen VK and Jannetta PJ (1984) Pathophysiology of hemifacial spasm: III. Effects of facial nerve decompression. *Neurology*, **34**, 891–7

Noordenbos W and Wall PD (1981) Implications of the failure of nerve resection and graft to cure chronic pain produced by nerve lesions. *J Neurol, Neurosurg Psychiatry*, **44**, 1068–73

Ritchie RW (1970) Neurological sequela of amputation. *Br J Hosp Med*, **6**, 607–9

Robberecht W, Van Hess J, Adriansen H, and Carton H (1988) Painful muscle spasms complicating algodystrophy: central or peripheral disease? *J Neurol, Neurosurg Psychiatry*, **51**, 563–7

Russell WR (1970) Neurological sequelae of amputation. *Br J Hosp Med*, **6**, 607–9

Said G and Bathien N (1977) Myoclonies rhythmees du quadriceps en relation avec un envahissement sarcomateux du nerf crural. *Rev Neurol*, **133**, 191–8

Scherokman B, Gusain F, Cuetter A, Jabbari B, and Maniglia E (1986) Peripheral dystonia. *Arch Neurol*, **43**, 830–2

Schott GD (1981) 'Painful legs and moving toes': the role of trauma. *J Neurol, Neurosurg Psychiatry*, **44**, 344–6

Schott GD (1985) The relation of peripheral trauma and pain to dystonia. *J Neurol, Neurosurg Psychiatry*, **48**, 698–701

Schott GD (1986a) Mechanisms of causalgia and related clinical conditions. The role of the central nervous and of the sympathetic nervous systems. *Brain*, **109**, 717–38

Schott GD (1986b) Induction of involuntary movements by peripheral trauma: an analogy with causalgia. *Lancet*, **ii**, 712–15

Schwartzman RJ and Kerringan J (1990) The movement disorder of reflex sympathetic dystrophy. *Neurology*, **40**, 57–61

Schwartzman RJ and McLellan TL (1987) Reflex sympathetic dystrophy. *Arch Neurol*, **44**, 555–61

Sheehy MP and Marsden CD (1980) Trauma and pain in spasmodic torticollis. *Lancet*, **1**, 777–8

Sheehy MP and Marsden CD (1982) Writer's cramp – a focal dystonia. *Brain*, **105**, 461–80

Sheehy MP, Rothwell JC, and Marsden CD (1988) Writer's cramp. *Adv Neurol*, **50**, 467–72

Sotaniemi KA (1985) Paraspinal myoclonus due to spinal root lesions. *J Neurol, Neurosurg Psychiatry*, **48**, 722–3

Spillane JD, Nathan PW, Kelly RE, and Marsden CD (1971) Painful legs and moving toes. *Brain*, **94**, 541–56

Steiner JL, DeJesus PV, and Mancall EL (1974) Painful jumping amputation stumps: pathophysiology of a 'sore circuit'. *Trans Am Neurol Assoc*, **99**, 253–5

Sunderland S (1978) *Nerves and Nerve Injuries*, 2nd edn, Edinburgh, Churchill Livingstone, 377–420

Swanson PD, Luttrell CN, and Magladery JW (1962) Myoclonus – a report of 67 cases and review of the literature. *Medicine, Baltimore*, **41**, 339–56

Thompson PD, Obeso JA, DelGado G, Gallego G, and Marsden CD (1986) Focal dystonia of the jaw and differential diagnosis of unilateral jaw and masticatory spasm. *J Neurol, Neurosurg Psychiatry*, **49**, 651–6

Valls-Sole J and Tolosa ES (1989) Blink reflex excitability cycle in hemifacial spasm. *Neurology*, **39**, 1061–6

Verhagen WIM, Horstink MWIM, and Notermans SLH (1985) Painful arm and moving fingers. *J Neurol, Neurosurg Psychiatry*, **48**, 384–9

Wall PD and Devor M (1982) Consequences of peripheral nerve damage in the spinal cord and in neighbouring intact peripheral nerves. In Culp WJ and Ochoa J, eds, *Abnormal Nerves and Muscles and Impulse Generators*, Oxford, Oxford University Press, 588–603

Willis WD (1984) The original destination of pathways involved in pain transmission. In Wall PD, Melzack R, eds, *A Textbook of Pain*, London, Churchill Livingstone, 88–99

21
Startle syndromes

Joseph Matsumoto and Mark Hallett

The startle reflex is a rapid, generalized motor response to a sudden, surprise stimulus. It occurs throughout the mammalian world, but its adaptive significance is open to debate (Landis and Hunt, 1939). In normal humans, its persistence is most often a troublesome vestige, uncomfortable to experience, and amusing to behold. Over time, it has undergone considerable modulation by higher limbic and cortical influences, so that its intrusion into everyday life is usually minimal. The muscular jerk of startle is quick enough to satisfy the definition of myoclonus. Hence, the normal startle response is a form of physiological myoclonus. Some persons, however, appear to have an exaggeration of this response.

A startle disorder should be suspected when quick, involuntary movements are triggered by sudden stimuli in a manner deviant from the normal startle pattern. Differences may concern either the motor response or the eliciting stimulus. The motor response may seem too violent or consist of abnormally complex behaviours. A normal-appearing startle response may be deemed abnormal if it is triggered by a stimulus that is neither intense nor surprising enough to be effective in most people. Considerable confusion may result, however, if startle disorders are defined by these criteria alone. A case in point is the misnomer of an 'excessive startle reaction' in Creutzfeldt–Jakob disease, which has been demonstrated to be a cortically mediated myoclonic jerk (Shibasaki *et al.*, 1981). Similarly, the muscle jerks in Tay–Sachs disease or in certain stimulus-sensitive myoclonic disorders may be generated by neural circuits different from those that mediate normal human startle (Hallett *et al.*, 1977, 1979; Hallett, 1985). For a movement disorder to be correctly classified as a startle disorder, involvement of the primary startle circuit should be demonstrated through electrophysiological studies. Only recently has evidence begun to accrue in this regard for the best known of startle disorders, hyperekplexia (Brown *et al.*, 1990).

PRIMARY MAMMALIAN ACOUSTIC STARTLE CIRCUIT

A great deal has been learned about the neural mechanisms of mammalian startle through study of the whole-body jerk that occurs in response to intense acoustic stimuli in the rat. In elegant lesion and stimulation experiments, Davis *et al.* (1982a) showed that the earliest components of the acoustic startle response are generated

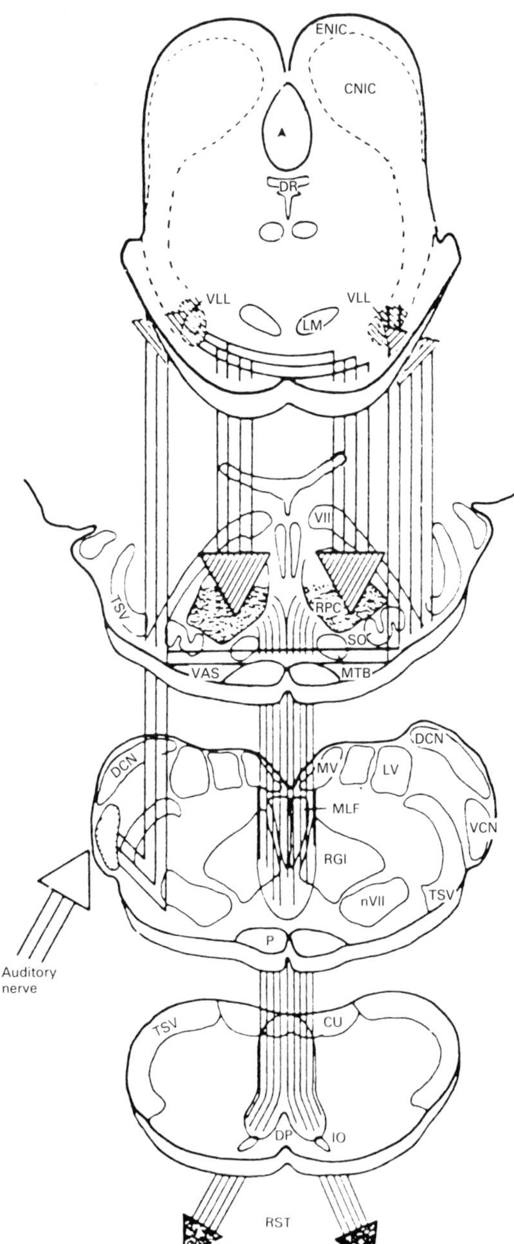

Figure 21.1 Schematic diagram of a primary acoustic startle circuit consisting of the ventral cochlear nucleus (VCN), ventral nucleus of the lateral lemniscus (VLL) and the nucleus reticularis pontis caudalis (RPC). A = Aqueduct; CNIC = central nucleus of the inferior colliculus; CU = cuneate nucleus; DCN = dorsal cochlear nucleus; DP = decussation of pyramids; DR = dorsal raphe nucleus; ENIC = external nucleus of the inferior colliculus; IO = inferior olive; LM = medial lemniscus; LV = lateral vestibular nucleus; MLF = medial longitudinal fasciculus; MTB = medial nucleus of the trapezoid body; MV = medial vestibular nucleus; nVII = nucleus of the seventh nerve; P = pyramids; RGI = nucleus reticularis gigantocellularis; RST = reticulospinal tract; SO = superior olive; TSV = spinal tract of the fifth nerve; VAS = ventral acoustic stria; VII = seventh nerve. From Davis *et al.* (1982a) with permission

by a pathway within the brainstem (Fig. 21.1). The auditory stimulus is received in the ventral cochlear nucleus and projects to auditory relay neurons within or near the ventral nucleus of the lateral lemniscus. This nucleus in turn projects to the pontomedullary reticular formation, which serves as the motor effector area for the startle response. More specifically, Davis *et al.* (1982a) found that bilateral lesions within the ventral portion of the nucleus reticularis pontis caudalis abolished acoustic startle. Reticulospinal spinal pathways involved in rat startle project from the nucleus reticularis pontis caudalis down the medial longitudinal fasciculus in the brainstem and in the ventral funiculus of the spinal cord before making monosynaptic connections with alpha motor neurons (Yeomans *et al.*, 1989). Single unit studies in the cat confirm that neurons in the pontomedullary reticular formation fire intensely during startle and project by fast conducting pathways down the spinal cord (Wu *et al.*, 1988).

In humans, startle can be observed in anencephalic infants, implicating a brainstem origin for the reflex (Landis and Hunt, 1939). However, direct evidence supporting the existence of a four-neuron reflex arc in humans is not available. The conservation of reticular nuclear structures across the animal kingdom (Neuman, 1985) and the similarity in behaviour between rat whole-body startle and the eyeblink component of human startle (Hoffman and Ison, 1980) provide some indirect evidence that a primary startle circuit similar to that described in the rat is active in humans.

NORMAL HUMAN STARTLE

The most extensively studied human startle response is that which occurs to loud noises. To elicit a startle response most effectively, acoustic stimuli must be about 100 dB and have a rapid rise time (less than 5 ms). The characteristics of the audiogenic startle response have been studied extensively (Landis and Hunt, 1939). Typically, the eyes close and the face tenses into a grimace. The head flexes forward and the arms take a defensive posture with abduction of the shoulders, flexion of the elbows, pronation of the forearms and clenching of the fists. Movements of the trunk and legs are less constant and, in general, consist of forward flexion of the torso and bending at the knees. Great individual variation exists, and in some persons, only the eyeblink may occur.

The signature of the normal startle response is equally distinctive on electromyogram (EMG) testing with surface electrodes (Wilkins *et al.*, 1986). The pattern is bilaterally symmetrical with an invariable blink; other craniocervical muscles almost always are activated, but recruitment in the limbs is variable. The onset latency of EMG activity is 30–40 ms in orbicularis oculi, 55–85 ms in masseter and sternocleidomastoid, 85–100 ms in biceps brachii, 100–125 ms in hamstrings and quadriceps, and 130–140 ms in tibialis anterior. There is synchronous activation of antagonist muscles with an EMG burst duration of 50–400 ms.

Whole-body startle responses to other stimulus modalities are less constantly observed. Landis and Hunt (1939), studying somasthetic and visual surprise stimuli, found that the typical startle pattern could be elicited by a non-auditory stimulus, such as a jet of ice water sprayed unexpectedly on the back. Visual startle to flash stimuli rarely consisted of more than an eyeblink. They concluded that startle is a general response in which auditory stimuli are the most efficacious, but not the sole trigger. Vestibular stimuli, such as a sudden free fall, can also elicit a startle response, and this reflex behaviour has been used in the assessment of otolith function (Halmagyi and Gresty, 1983).

Other physiological components of startle have been described. Autonomic reactions, as measured by galvanic skin response or heart rate acceleration, are common in startle and tend to habituate rapidly. A brief period of apnoea may also normally occur. Late components of startle are more varied and complex than the initial stereotyped motor discharge. Rhythmic EMG activity may occur 3–10 seconds after the initiating stimulus and has been called a B or orienting response (Davis, 1948; Gogan, 1970). Even more variable are the so-called secondary behaviours that convey emotions such as anger, disgust or amusement by means of body posture or facial expression after the reflex components of startle have passed (Landis and Hunt, 1939).

In infants, the Moro response can be distinguished from startle. Both are present at birth, startle presumably being recordable even *in utero* by ultrasonic imaging (Divon *et al.*, 1985). The Moro response is an extensor response, whereas the startle response is predominantly flexor. Early in life, the Moro response may conceal startle, but at 4 months of age it begins to disappear and startle becomes evident.

PLASTICITY OF THE STARTLE REFLEX

Several robust experimental phenomena have been described both in rat and in human startle that highlight the plastic changes occurring within the brainstem startle pathway. These paradigms provide a means of testing the complex modulatory influences acting on the mammalian startle reflex. Startle disorders could conceivably arise not only from dysfunction within the primary brainstem startle circuit, but also from altered behaviour of any of these modulatory pathways.

Habituation

Habituation refers to a decreasing magnitude of response with repetitive presentation of a triggering stimulus. Short-term habituation occurs with repeated stimulus presentation over seconds to minutes; long-term habituation happens with repeated trials over hours to days. In human audiogenic startle, short-term habituation generally occurs after four or five stimuli (Wilkins *et al.*, 1986). With habituation, the EMG bursts shorten and onset latencies prolong until activity disappears. The orbicularis oculi activity persists, but it too undergoes short- and long-term habituation of amplitude (Geyer and Braff, 1982; Ornitz and Guthrie, 1989). Habituation appears to involve structures on the sensory side of the startle reflex arc (Davis *et al.*, 1982b). Short-term habituation may occur within the ventral cochlear nucleus. Autoradiographic studies indicate that long-term habituation is correlated with increased activity within the superior olivary nucleus, nucleus of the lateral lemniscus, inferior colliculus and cerebellum, and suppression of activity is correlated with activity in the midbrain reticular formation (Gonzalez-Lima *et al.*, 1989).

Sensitization

Sensitization results in increased amplitude or decreased latency of startle responses with repeated stimuli. It is often masked by the larger simultaneous effects of habituation. The locus for sensitization is on the motor half of the reflex arc, most likely within the nucleus reticularis pontis caudalis (Davis *et al.*, 1982b).

Prepulse inhibition

Prepulse inhibition occurs when a brief, non-startling sensory stimulus in any modality precedes a startle auditory stimulus by 30–200 ms. Under these conditions, the amplitude of the startle response will be reduced compared with that obtained without a prepulse stimulus. This phenomenon has been amply demonstrated for rat and human eyeblink startle (Graham, 1975), but not for the body component of the human startle response. Pathways from the inferior colliculus to the nucleus reticularis pontis caudalis are likely to be responsible for this effect (Leitner and Cohen, 1985).

Fear-conditioned potentiation

Fear-conditioned potentiation of startle may be a probe into the effect of emotion on the startle reflex. In this paradigm, rats receive light and shock stimuli simultaneously until the animal is conditioned to experience fear at the presentation of the light alone. If the light is then presented before a loud auditory stimulus, the magnitude of the startle response is greatly enhanced (Brown *et al.*, 1951). The central representation of conditioned fear may arise in the central amygdaloid nucleus and project to the nucleus reticularis pontis caudalis through the ventral amygdalofugal tract (Davis, 1989). Similarly, in humans, pleasant and unpleasant visual experiences have inhibitory and excitatory effects on the eyeblink component of startle, providing a measure of limbic projections to this brainstem reflex pathway (Vrana *et al.*, 1988).

PHARMACOLOGY OF THE STARTLE RESPONSE

The primary startle circuit neurons in the brainstem appear to use an excitatory amino acid transmitter such as glutamate or aspartate. Miserendino and Davis (1988) found that non-NMDA (*N*-methyl-D-aspartate) receptor antagonists infused into the ventral cochlear nucleus completely abolished startle. Similar effects occur with both NMDA and non-NMDA receptor blockade in the ventral nucleus of the lateral lemniscus and spinal cord (Spiera and Davis, 1988). The neurotransmitter mediating startle in the reticular formation has not been identified.

In addition, a wide variety of neurotransmitters modulate the amplitude of the startle response in a manner reflecting the complex regulation of this reflex (Davis, 1979). Serotonin (5-HT) has a net inhibitory effect on startle, but its actions at different levels are conflicting. In the brainstem, the action is inhibitory through 5-HT_{1B} receptors, and in the spinal cord 5-HT_{1A} receptors are stimulated to augment the startle response. Similarly, alpha$_2$-adrenergic receptors are inhibitory in the brainstem, and alpha$_1$-adrenergic receptors are excitatory in the spinal cord. Gamma-aminobutyric acid acts at multiple sites that have not been clearly unravelled, but its net effect is strongly inhibitory. It appears to play a specific role in fear-potentiated startle, as benzodiazepines can attenuate this effect without affecting the baseline level of startle (Davis, 1986). Dopamine is also conflicting in its effects on startle. D_1 agonists are excitatory and D_2 agonists inhibitory, with a net excitatory effect for dopamine itself. This transmitter may modulate startle through pathways that are responsible for prepulse inhibition (Mansbach *et al.*, 1988).

STARTLE SYNDROMES

Major difficulties confront any attempts to classify the startle syndromes. The primary one, alluded to earlier, is the lack of physiological or anatomical evidence for involvement of startle pathways in many disorders that traditionally have come to be known as syndromes of excessive startle (Wilkins *et al.*, 1986). In addition, controversy about use of the term hyperekplexia must be resolved.

Hyperekplexia is often used synonymously with any presumed startle disorder. Suhren *et al.* (1966) originally used the term hyperexplexia (to jump excessively) to describe an autosomal dominant disease in a large Dutch kindred with exaggerated startle reflexes and many other associated abnormalities. Gastaut and Villeneuve (1967) then reported 12 patients with a sporadic form of exaggerated startle, which they called hyperekplexia. A psychiatric aetiology was suspected in many of these sporadic cases, and it seems likely that a separate disease entity with a different name was being proposed. Andermann *et al.* (1980) noted a markedly variable penetrance in the hereditary disease described by Suhren *et al.* (1966), with many mildly affected family members being symptomatic only with illness or stress. They felt that a positive family history could easily be missed in mildly affected kindreds and that a common genetic abnormality caused both the hereditary and so-called sporadic forms of the disease. The term hyperekplexia, which was a more faithful representation of the Greek, was adopted as a unifying term for a major form of the disease in which associated abnormalities occurred and a minor form in which exaggerated startle was the sole abnormality. Others have objected to such a unification and propose the continued use of hyperexplexia for hereditary disease and hyperekplexia for sporadic disease (Morley *et al.*, 1982).

We believe that the continued use of two terms so similar in spelling and meaning will lead to increasing confusion. No classification scheme can reconcile the previous literature, but we would propose the use of the proper Greek term hyperekplexia to denote any movement disorder in which there is a physiological demonstration of exaggerated startle reflexes (Table 21.1). Hereditary hyperekplexia is only clearly diagnosed in the presence of a definite family history and can be strongly suspected when symptoms begin in the neonatal period. Symptomatic hyperekplexia refers to all other disorders resulting in exaggerated startle reflexes, regardless of their severity. Use of this term will encourage the clinician to consider a wide range of pathological

Table 21.1 Startle syndromes

Hyperekplexia
Hereditary
Symptomatic
Brainstem lesions (encephalitis, haemorrhage, Chiari malformation)
Perinatal hypoxic–ischaemic encephalopthy
Thalamic lesions (inflammatory, vascular, traumatic)
Posttraumatic stress syndrome
Tourette's syndrome
Drugs (amphetamines, cocaine)
Idiopathic
Startle epilepsy
Latah syndrome

processes that might impinge on the primary startle circuit or its modulation. In the future, genetic markers or physiological analysis may aid in the further classification of hyperekplexia.

Two presumed startle disorders should be separated from hyperekplexia on the basis of clinical phenomenology. In startle epilepsy, an apparent exaggerated startle response evolves into a seizure disorder. The latah syndrome typifies a group of startle disorders recognized by complex and prolonged behavioural responses to startling stimuli.

Hereditary hyperekplexia

Hereditary hyperekplexia is an autosomal dominant disorder characterized by exaggerated startle and other characteristic motor phenomena. The syndrome was described in detail by Suhren *et al.* (1966), and the literature has been reviewed by Andermann and Andermann (1988).

CLINICAL MANIFESTATIONS

The clinical manifestations of hereditary hyperekplexia are hypertonia in infancy, exaggerated startle reflexes, nocturnal and diurnal leg jerks, gait disorder, exaggerated head retraction reflexes, and somatic abnormalities.

At birth, the infants are continuously stiff in a flexor posture, often with tightly clenched fists. Suhren *et al.* (1966) reported leg stiffness so severe that mothers put their heads between their babies' legs in order to change nappies. The stiffness disappears during sleep. The stiffness may resemble spastic quadriparesis, but it slowly disappears over the first few months of life (Andermann and Andermann, 1988). Apnoea and cardiorespiratory arrest occur with disturbing frequency in affected infants and may result from stiffness of the chest wall (Kurczynski, 1983; Vigevano *et al.*, 1989). A congenital stiff-baby syndrome has been described and likely represents a form of hyperekplexia (Lingam *et al.*, 1981). There is also a familial form of stiff-man syndrome that also shares many features with hereditary hyperekplexia, but differs in that continuous normal EMG activity is present at rest (Klein *et al.*, 1972).

Immediately after birth, severely affected children startle excessively to sudden stimuli, such as movement of their cribs or loud noises. Mothers in large kindreds recognize affected children, because their arms flex in a startle response rather than extend in the Moro response. The startle responses become more of a handicap when the children begin to walk. A sudden sound or touch will cause them to stiffen and fall. The muscular contractions prevent protective arm movements, and falls often result in head lacerations and concussions. There is no loss of consciousness unless severe head injury complicates a fall. Mild urinary incontinence may occur as the result of contraction of the abdominal muscles. Some affected children quickly learn the hazards of erect posture and regress to crawling, walking on their knees or squatting in anticipation of a loud sound.

In severely affected patients, startle attacks and falls occur throughout life. In school, children are teased and provoked to have attacks (Suhren *et al.*, 1966). There is often worsening of the illness in adolescence (Dooley and Andermann, 1989) and variable improvement with ageing. Mildly affected family members may have isolated exaggerated startle responses, which may be manifest only during periods of emotional stress or physical illness (Andermann and Andermann, 1988).

Patients frequently have violent bilateral flexor jerks of the legs during the night.

These often arise during the descent into slow-wave sleep. DeGroen and Kamphuisen (1978) found that the jerks were associated with electroencephalogram (EEG) evidence of arousal and that their frequency correlated with the respiratory rhythm. Rarely, similar jerks may occur during the daytime.

Severely affected patients walk with a slow, wide-based gait, the arms held motionless in flexion at the elbows and slightly abducted at the shoulders. One hypothesis holds that the patients walk in such a manner out of fear of falling (Andermann and Andermann, 1988). Patients feel much more secure when touching a wall or squeezing an object (Suhren *et al.*, 1966). Muscular stiffness may also contribute to the gait disorder. Many patients complain of continual muscular stiffness, which is exacerbated by cold weather. Brisk reflexes, clonus and spasticity often are found in the legs of such patients (Andermann *et al.*, 1980). Slow movements of the limbs accompany this sense of stiffness.

Suhren *et al.* (1966) noted brisk stiffening of the neck and retraction of the head with taps to the bridge of the nose in patients with hereditary hyperekplexia. Several other kindreds displayed myoclonic head jerks when tapped about the head, but the effective location of the tap varied (Andermann *et al.*, 1980; Kurczynski, 1983). In one family, the tip of the nose was the only field which stimulated the reflex, and in another the glabella was effective.

Inguinal and abdominal hernias occurred with a high frequency in two families of patients with hyperekplexia (Suhren *et al.*, 1966; Kurczynski, 1983). Congenital hip dislocations may also be more frequent in these patients (Morley *et al.*, 1982). Continuous muscle contractions in early life or *in utero* may explain these associated abnormalities.

PATHOPHYSIOLOGY

The physiological observations in patients with hyperekplexia are controversial. Although hyperekplexia has been intuitively known as startle disease, clear evidence relating the muscle jerks of hyperekplexia to normal startle has been lacking until recently.

Suhren *et al.* (1966) first implicated brainstem pathways in noting shortening of the latencies of EMG bursts in the orbicularis oculi and trapezius muscles to pistolshot stimuli in patients with hyperekplexia. They theorized that there was loss of inhibition from the 'rhombomesencephalic' reticular formation, resulting in an abnormal release of startle pathways. Wilkins *et al.* (1986) reviewed the available evidence and concluded that the shortened EMG onset latencies argued against the involvement of normal startle pathways in hyperekplexia. Recently, Brown *et al.* (1990) presented preliminary evidence that the EMG pattern in hyperekplexic jerks is very similar to that of normal startle. In both responses, initial activation occurs in the orbicularis oculi followed by early and intense activity in the sternocleidomastoid. Conduction down the spinal cord both in patients with hyperekplexia and in subjects with normal startle reflex appeared to use a slowly conducting pathway of approximately 15–20 m/s. Testing of patients with hyperekplexia in our laboratory (Matsumoto *et al.*, 1992) has confirmed the normal startle pattern noted by Brown *et al.* (1990; Fig. 21.2). It is now clear that the audiogenic jumps in hyperekplexia are generated through the primary startle circuit. Given the patterned jumps to both acoustic and trigeminal stimuli in these patients, it seems justified to assume that the hyperexcitibility exists on the motor side of the reflex arc, in the pontomedullary reticular formation.

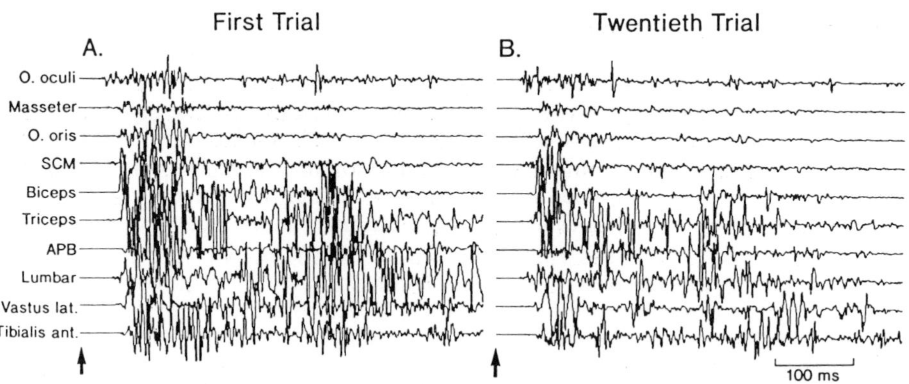

Figure 21.2 Multichannel surface electromyogram (EMG) recordings of startle responses in a 13-year-old girl with hereditary hyperekplexia. (A) An initial 103 dB acoustic stimulus given at the time indicated by the arrow is followed by a generalized EMG startle response. Note the early activation of the orbicularis oculi followed by the sternocleidomastoid (SCM). (B) The 20th startle response after repetitive acoustic stimuli given at 1-minute intervals shows little habituation. (Matsumoto *et al.*, 1992)

Several lines of evidence also implicate cerebral hyperexcitability in hyperekplexia. EEG spikes in the frontocentral regions have been associated with exaggerated startle (Gastaut and Villeneuve, 1967; Andermann *et al.*, 1980). In certain cases, however, detailed analysis of such potentials indicates that they are an artefact of eye movement and scalp muscle activity (Morley *et al.*, 1982). Other non-specific EEG abnormalities, such as intermittent generalized slow waves, activation of generalized spike-and-wave discharges and focal epileptiform abnormalities, are reported in all kindreds. In addition, seizures and mental deficiency occur with increased frequency in hyperekplexia, providing clinical evidence for cortical dysfunction (Andermann and Andermann, 1988). Enlarged somatosensory evoked potentials and 'long-loop' reflexes have been observed in hyperekplexia and are thought to support the presence of cortical excitability in this disorder (Markand *et al.*, 1984).

Hereditary hyperekplexia is best conceived of as a syndrome of widespread neural hyperexcitability in normal pathways, the most important of which is the startle circuit. The gene causing hyperekplexia has been located to chromosome 5q (Ryan *et al.*, 1992). The underlying cause at the neuronal level is unknown, but it is attractive to hypothesize an inborn dysfunction of a neurotransmitter system to explain the diffuse alterations in function. Andermann *et al.* (1990) speculated that a deficiency of serotonin is at fault, given the marked response of patients to clonazepam.

THERAPY

Clonazepam is the therapy of choice in hyperekplexia. When it is effective, the severity of startle reactions and frequency of falls are markedly decreased. Patients may report improvement in muscle stiffness and the ability to move faster. Even with a good response, the brisk head retraction reflexes persist (Andermann and Andermann, 1988). Other benzodiazepines, such as diazepam and chlordiazepoxide, have been used with similar results. Valproic acid is also effective, often in patients who have failed to respond to clonazepam. 5-Hydroxytryptophan and piracetam also have been used successfully in a few cases (Sáenz-Lope *et al.*, 1984b).

Symptomatic hyperekplexia

Only rudimentary knowledge is currently available concerning the types of disease processes that can affect the startle reflex. Brainstem lesions conceivably could result in reduced or absent startle, but it is unlikely that such a state would be clinically significant. Of greater importance is the accumulation of case reports suggesting that exaggerated startle can occur with acquired structural disease of the brain and perhaps even with prolonged fear. Almost all of these reports lack the physiological precision to prove involvement of the startle reflex, but it is expected that future reports will include such data and permit sharper clinicopathological correlation.

BRAINSTEM LESIONS

Inflammatory brainstem diseases are associated with exaggerated startle reflexes similar in severity to those seen in hereditary hyperekplexia. Duensing (1952) reported 3 patients with poorly defined inflammatory processes with brainstem signs who jerked to auditory and tactile stimuli. The clinical description of the muscle jerks, with maximal involvement of the orbicularis oculi and paraspinal muscles, as well as the EMG onset latencies, recorded in 1 patient supports the conclusion that these patients suffered from exaggerated and poorly habituating startle reflexes. The first patient in this series, who may have had paraneoplastic brainstem encephalitis, exhibited startle and head retraction reflexes similar in severity to those occurring in hereditary hyperekplexia.

Fenzi *et al.* (1988) provided pathological correlation in a patient with 'massive myoclonias' presumed to be startle associated with subacute encephalomyelitis with lymphocytic infiltration of the pons and medulla. Brainstem haemorrhages have released exaggerated startle in 2 patients (Duensing, 1952; Shibasaki *et al.*, 1988). A child with neonatal onset of apparent exaggerated startle reflexes was found to have a Chiari malformation, and the presumed hyperekplexia improved after surgical decompression (Winston, 1983).

CEREBRAL OR DIENCEPHALIC LESIONS

Exaggerated startle has been reported in several patients with perinatal hypoxic–ischaemic encephalopathy (Duensing, 1952; Baier, 1980; Sáenz-Lope *et al.*, 1984b). It may be difficult to discern the precise role of perinatal anoxia, because hyperekplexia itself predisposes to cardiorespiratory arrest. Duensing (1952) studied several patients who had vague inflammatory, traumatic or vascular thalamic lesions and postulated that lesions of the diencephalon or midbrain were the basis for exaggerated startle. More precise information was given by Fariello *et al.* (1983), who described exacerbation of hyperekplexia by occlusion of the posterior thalamic arteries. The patient had exaggerated startle at the age of 35 years which disappeared several years later. At age 65, he suffered a left thalamic infarction with angiographic evidence of left thalamoperforate artery occlusion and recurrence of the exaggerated startle response. Although the implication of these cases is that interruption of descending cortical inhibitory influences can release exaggerated startle reflexes, much more work is necessary before such a hypothesis can be accepted.

PSYCHIATRIC DISEASE

Posttraumatic stress disorder may follow periods of intense fear and is associated with clinical evidence of hyperarousal, including insomnia, hyperalertness and exaggerated startle. Children with this disorder were tested by Ornitz and Pynoos (1989) for the eyeblink component of startle. Baseline responses were reduced in amplitude, but prepulse inhibition was diminished. This pattern may reflect stress-induced regression in the normal maturational control of startle. When interpreted in light of the experimental paradigm of fear-conditioned startle, these findings suggest that intense or prolonged fear can disinhibit startle pathways in humans through limbic modulation.

Landis and Hunt (1939) observed increased startle reactions in patients with catatonic schizophrenia, and in one of Duensing's (1952) patients, exaggerated startle developed after postpartum psychosis. Braff *et al.* (1978) reported decreased prepulse inhibition in patients with schizophrenia and hypothesized that this represented an abnormality of sensorimotor gating. None of the patients, however, appeared to display significant exaggerated startle responses. Therefore, while these observations may be useful in the study of schizophrenia, it does not appear that hyperekplexia is a common movement disorder in this disease.

TOURETTE'S SYNDROME

Exaggerated startle responses complicate Tourette's syndrome in approximately 5% of cases (Lees *et al.*, 1984). The distinction between startle and stimulus-sensitive tics is seldom made, and physiological data are lacking. However, the startle reactions may respond to clonazepam even when tics and vocalizations persist, suggesting that the phenomena are distinct.

DRUG INTOXICATION

Maternal cocaine exposure can lead to convulsions and increased startle in newborns (Kramer *et al.*, 1990). A quantitative increase was demonstrated in the eyeblink component of startle in cocaine-exposed infants (Anday *et al.*, 1989). Both cocaine (Davis, 1985) and amphetamines (Davis *et al.*, 1975) increase the amplitude of acoustic startle in rats. It is, therefore, likely that exaggerated startle would be a common sign in acute and chronic human abuse syndromes with both of these drugs.

IDIOPATHIC CASES

Many cases of exaggerated startle occur late in life in patients without a family history of hyperekplexia and have no identifiable cause. Indeed, such cases constitute most cases of acquired hyperekplexia. Gastaut and Villeneuve's (1967) 12 cases of 'essential startle disease' fall into the category of idiopathic hyperekplexia. Physiological analysis was lacking in these cases and many had emotional precipitants, raising the possibility that psychiatric disease may have been a contributing factor. Andermann *et al.* (1980) believe such cases represent a minor form of hereditary hyperekplexia, but clearly a genetic or biochemical marker is necessary before this issue can be unequivocally resolved.

A recent report (Colebatch *et al.*, 1990) clearly implicated the startle response in a case of sporadic late-onset exaggerated startle. The patient was a 76-year-old woman with a 5-year history of exaggerated startle without any other, apparently related, neurological problem. She would startle 30–40 times a day to unexpected noise or touch. The element of surprise was clearly important, since repeated stimuli were generally ineffective. Many various medications were tried, but were ineffective. Physiological studies showed that the timing of the involuntary movement was consistent with startle. We have studied a 41-year-old woman with a 12-year history of exaggerated startle to sound, touch, or sudden changes in illumination (B. Geller and M. Hallett, 1988, unpublished observations). No medications were useful. Physiological studies showed onset latencies and burst durations typical of exaggerated startle on many occasions, but on other occasions, the latencies ranged from 200 to 300 ms. She sometimes exhibited apparently hysterical behaviour. We concluded that she had a mixture of true exaggerated startle and hysterical movements.

Startle epilepsy

Startle epilepsy is principally characterized by epileptic seizures triggered by sudden, unexpected stimuli and initiated by a startle. Startling stimuli can be in any modality, but sound is typically most effective. Startle epilepsy has been described in the setting of severe brain damage, most commonly perinatal encephalopathy from anoxia (Gastaut and Tassinari, 1966). Other conditions include hexosaminidase A deficiency (Tay–Sachs disease; Gastaut and Tassinari, 1966), Down's syndrome (Giménez-Roldán and Martin, 1980), and Sturge–Weber syndrome (Nakamura *et al.*, 1975). In the series of Sáenz-Lope *et al.* (1984a), 12 patients had perinatal anoxic encephalopathy, 1 had encephalitis and 1 had Down's syndrome; 2 patients also had Lennox–Gastaut syndrome. Of the 16 patients of Aguglia *et al.* (1984), 5 had perinatal anoxia, 3 had encephalitis, and 4 had West's syndrome; 6 patients also had Lennox–Gastaut syndrome.

Sáenz-Lope *et al.* (1984a) divided their patients into two groups. One group had predominantly hemispheric lesions with hemiparesis, IQ of 50–95, and normal EEG background. The other group had more severe, diffuse brain damage, with marked intellectual impairment, generalized seizures not related to startle, and background EEG abnormalities.

Startle epilepsy often begins early in life, but may begin any time in the first two decades. In very young patients, audiogenic violent starts, compatible with startle responses, are characterized by limb and trunk flexion in association with desynchronization of ongoing EEG activity. Subsequently, the starts blend into more prolonged (1–30 seconds) tonic spasms emphasizing extensor mechanisms in those body areas displaying the greatest paresis. In hemiparetic patients, for example, the spasms involve the paretic hemibody (Sáenz-Lope *et al.*, 1984a). While the tonic spasm is itself accompanied by EEG desynchronization, occasionally epileptiform discharges, bilaterally symmetrical or even focal, with or without associated clonic jerks, may evolve within seconds. A generalized seizure may follow. The events appear to be a non-habituating startle reflex followed by tonic extensor spasms which, on occasion, degenerate further into an epileptic seizure (Wilkins *et al.*, 1986). In some patients, an atonic seizure may follow the startle (Aguglia *et al.*, 1984).

Brain imaging often shows abnormalities. In 6 of 10 patients, computed tomography showed atrophy of the mesial surface of one or both hemispheres ('mesial hypodensity'; Aguglia *et al.*, 1984).

Treatment of startle epilepsy is difficult. Sáenz-Lope *et al.* (1984a) found carbamazepine useful in all 6 of their patients with the hemiparetic form. In the generalized form, 4 patients improved with valproic acid, 2 with carbamazepine, and the 2 with Lennox–Gastaut syndrome improved with clonazepam. Clobazam can be useful. It effected good control (91.5% reduction of reflex seizures) in 8 of 13 patients who were previously on an ineffective regimen (Tinuper *et al.*, 1986).

Jumping, latah, myriachit

The essential features of 'jumping' (jumping Frenchmen of Maine), latah and myriachit are considered by some to represent a single entity (Andermann *et al.*, 1980). There is much debate over this group of conditions. Some consider them to be conditioned behavioural responses rather than startle phenomena. Characteristic is an initial violent start in response to sudden, unexpected sensory stimulation (most commonly sound), which is often immediately followed by automatic speech or behaviour (e.g. echolalia or echopraxia), coprolalia, striking out or the assumption of a defensive posture.

Latah has been known for centuries in primitive societies in the East and in Africa, but is best known in Malaysia. The disease is most common in women. The jumping Frenchmen of Maine were first described to the American Neurological Association in 1878 by George Beard, who drew an analogy to latah. He emphasized their quick, involuntary and uninhibitable execution of sudden commands (automatic obedience) such as 'jump', 'strike' or 'throw'. The disorder was endemic in the Moosehead Lake region, was familial, occurred largely in men, began in childhood, and lasted throughout life. Kunkle (1967) noted that aggressive gestures or actual blows directed to the nearest bystander were common. Men with this propensity are sometimes known as 'killer jumpers'. William Hammond in 1884 described myriachit as being a similar disorder found in Siberia.

In three jumpers studied by Stevens (1965), the EEGs were normal, even during the jumping. The results of neurological examinations were normal in 15 patients seen by Kunkle (1967).

Each of these disorders occurs in a different geographical area and has some culture-bound features (Simons, 1980). For example, latah is seen virtually entirely in women of low social class. Similar disorders in other societies include yaun in Burma, bah-tsche in Thailand, mali-mali in the Philippines, Lapp panic in Lapland, imu in Japan, goosey in the southern USA, and ragin' Cajuns in Louisiana. There are enough similarities in the different disorders, however, to make it likely they represent culturally modified variations of the same phenomenon. As Simons (1980) and Andermann *et al.* (1980) pointed out, one essential similarity is the increased startle, which is the initial event. Recent clinical observations by Tanner and Chamberland (1989) support the idea that the initial event is an exaggerated startle. They noted the prominence of the eyeblink and the lack of habituation in patients with latah. This initial event, however, requires electrophysiological analysis before its definitive identification as a startle reflex.

The echolalia, echopraxia and other automatic behaviours are somewhat more varied than the initial jump and appear to reflect cultural differences, but the similarities from culture to culture are more remarkable than the differences. The nature of these events is not at all understood, although they may well represent in part either late startle components (Davis, 1948; Gogan, 1970) or secondary behaviours.

Acknowledgement

The skilful editing of B. J. Hessie is gratefully acknowledged.

References

Aguglia U, Tinuper P, and Gastaut H (1984) Startle-induced epileptic seizures. *Epilepsia*, **25**, 712–20

Anday EK, Cohen ME, Kelley NE, and Leitner DS (1989) Effect of *in utero* cocaine exposure on startle and its modification. *Dev Pharmacol Ther*, **12**, 137–45

Andermann F and Andermann E (1988) Startle disorders of man: hyperekplexia, jumping and startle epilepsy. *Brain Dev*, **10**, 214–22

Andermann F, Keene DL, Andermann E, and Quesney LF (1980) Startle disease or hyperekplexia: further delineation of a syndrome. *Brain*, **103**, 985–97

Baier WK (1980) The 'startle disease' in brain-damaged patients: report of a case. *Neuropaediatrie*, **11**, 72–5

Beard GM (1878) Remarks on 'Jumpers or Jumping Frenchmen'. *J Nerve Ment Dis*, **5**, 526

Braff D, Stone C, Callaway E, Geyer M, Glick I, and Bali L (1978) Prestimulus effects on human startle reflex in normals and schizophrenics. *Psychophysiology*, **15**, 339–43

Brown JS, Kalish HI, and Farber IE (1951) Conditioned fear as revealed by magnitude of startle response to an auditory stimulus. *J Exp Psychol*, **41**, 317–28

Brown P, Rothwell RC, Thompson PD, Britton TC, Day BL, and Marsden CD (1990) Reticular reflex myoclonus and its relationship to the normal startle reflex in humans. *Neurology*, **40** (suppl 1), 386

Colebatch JG, Barrett G, and Lees AJ (1990) Exaggerated startle reflexes in an elderly woman. *Movement Disorders*, **5**, 167–9

Davis M (1979) Neurochemical modulation of sensory-motor reactivity: acoustic and tactile startle reflexes. *Neurosci Behav Rev*, **4**, 241–63

Davis M (1985) Cocaine: excitatory effects on sensorimotor reactivity measured with acoustic startle. *Psychopharmacology*, **86**, 31–6

Davis M (1986) Pharmacologic and anatomical analysis of fear conditioning using the fear-potentiated startle paradigm. *Behav Neurosci*, **100**, 814–24

Davis M (1989) Neural systems involved in fear-potentiated startle. *Ann NY Acad Sci*, **563**, 165–83

Davis M, Svensson TH, and Aghajanian GK (1975) Effects of *d-l*-amphetamine on habituation and sensitization of the acoustic startle response in rats. *Psychopharmacologia (Berlin)*, **43**, 1–11

Davis M, Gendelman DS, Tischler MD, and Gendelman PM (1982a) A primary acoustic startle circuit: lesion and stimulation studies. *J Neurosci*, **2**, 791–805

Davis M, Parisi T, Gendelman DS, Tischler M, and Kehne JH (1982b) Habituation and sensitization of startle reflexes elicited electrically from the brainstem. *Science*, **218**, 688–90

Davis RC (1948) Motor effects of strong auditory stimuli. *J Exp Psychol*, **38**, 257–75

DeGroen JHM and Kamphuisen HAC (1978) Periodic nocturnal myoclonus in a patient with hyperekplexia (startle disease). *J Neurol Sci*, **38**, 207–13

Divon MY, Platt LD, Cantrell CJ, Smith CV, Yeh S, and Paul RH (1985) Evoked fetal startle response: a possible intrauterine neurological exam. *Am J Obstet Gynecol*, **153**, 454–6

Dooley JM and Andermann F (1989) Startle disease or hyperekplexia: adolescent onset and response to valproate. *Pediatr Neurol*, **5**, 126–7

Duensing F (1952) Schreckreflex und Schreckreaktion als hirnorganische Zeichen. *Arch Psychiatr Z Neurol*, **188**, 162–92

Fariello RG, Schwartznab RJ, and Beall SS (1983) Hyperekplexia exacerbated by occlusion of the posterior thalamic arteries. *Arch Neurol*, **40**, 244–6

Fenzi F, Bongiovanni G, Fincati E, Pampanin M, Tomelleri G, and Rizzuto N (1988) Anatomical and clinical study of a case of subacute encephalomyelitis with hyperekplexia syndrome. *Ital J Neurol Sci*, **9**, 505–8

Gastaut H and Tassinari CA (1966) Triggering mechanisms in epilepsy: the electroclinical point of view. *Epilepsia*, **7**, 85–138

Gastaut H and Villeneuve A (1967) The startle disease or hyperekplexia: pathological suprise reaction. *J Neurol Sci*, **5**, 523–42

Geyer MA and Braff DL (1982) Habituation of the blink reflex in normals and schizophrenic patients. *Psychophysiology*, **19**, 1–6

Giménez-Roldán S and Martin M (1980) Startle epilepsy complicating Down syndrome during adulthood. *Ann Neurol*, **7**, 78–80

Gogan P (1970) The startle and orienting reactions in man. A study of their characteristics and habituation. *Brain Res* **18**, 117–35

Gonzalez-Lima F, Finkenstadt T and Ewert JP (1989) Neural substrates for long-term habituation of the acoustic startle reflex in rats: a 2-deoxyglucose study. *Neurosci Lett*, **96**, 151–6

Graham FK (1975) The more or less startling effects of weak pre-stimulation. *Psychophysiology*, **12**, 238–48

Hallett M (1985) Myoclonus: relation to epilepsy. *Epilepsia*, **26** (suppl 1), S67–77

Hallett M, Chadwick D, Adam I, and Marsden CD (1977) Reticular reflex myoclonus. *J Neurol, Neurosurg Psychiatry*, **40**, 253–64
Hallett M, Chadwick D, and Marsden CD (1979) Cortical reflex myoclonus. *Neurology*, **29**, 1107–25
Halmagyi GM and Gresty MA (1983) Eye blink reflexes to sudden free falls: a clinical test of otolith function. *J Neurol, Neurosurg Psychiatry*, **46**, 844–7
Hammond WA (1884) Myriachit: newly described disease of nervous system and its analogues. *NY Med J*, **39**, 191–2
Hoffman HS and Ison JR (1980) Reflex modification in the domain of startle. I. Some empirical findings and their implications for how the nervous system processes sensory input. *Psychol Rev*, **87**, 175–89
Klein R, Haddow JE, and DeLuca C (1972) Familial congenital disorder resembling stiff-man syndrome. *Am J Dis Child*, **124**, 730–1
Kramer LD, Locke GE, Ogunyemi A, and Nelson L (1990) Neonatal cocaine-related seizures. *J Child Neurol*, **5**, 60–4
Kunkle EC (1967) The 'jumpers' of Maine: a reappraisal. *Arch Intern Med*, **119**, 355–8
Kurczynski TW (1983) Hyperekplexia. *Arch Neurol*, **40**, 246–8
Landis C and Hunt WA (1939) *The Startle Pattern*, New York, Farrar and Rinehart
Lees AJ, Robertson M, Trimble MR, and Murray NMF (1984) A clinical study of Gilles de la Tourette syndrome in the United Kingdom. *J Neurol, Neurosurg Psychiatry*, **47**, 1–8
Leitner DS and Cohen ME (1985) Role of the inferior colliculus in the inhibition of acoustic startle in the rat. *Physiol Behav*, **34**, 65–70
Lingam S, Wilson J, and Hart EW (1981) Hereditary stiff-baby syndrome. *Am J Dis Child*, **135**, 909–11
Mansbach RS, Geyer MA, and Braff DL (1988) Dopaminergic stimulation disrupts sensorimotor gating in the rat. *Psychopharmacology*, **94**, 507–14
Markand OM, Garg BP, and Weaver DD (1984) Familial startle disease (hyperekplexia): electrophysiologic studies. *Arch Neurol*, **41**, 71–4
Matsumoto J, Fuhr P, Nigro M, and Hallett M (1992) Physiological abnormalities in hereditary hyperekplexia. *Ann Neurol*, **32**, 41–50
Miserendino MJD and Davis M (1988) Blockade of the acoustic startle reflex by local infusion of excitatory amino acid antagonists into the ventral cochlear nucleus. *Soc Neurosci Abstr*, **14**, 1263
Morley DJ, Weaver DD, Garg BP, and Markand O (1982) Hyperexplexia: an inherited disorder of the startle response. *Clin Genet*, **21**, 388–96
Nakamura M, Kanai H, Miyamoto Y *et al.* (1975) A case of Sturge–Weber syndrome with startle epilepsy. *No To Shinkei*, **27**, 325–31
Neuman DB (1985) Distinguishing rat brainstem reticulospinal nuclei by their neuronal morphology. II. Pontine and mesencephalic nuclei. *J Hirnforsch*, **26**, 385–448
Ornitz EM and Guthrie D (1989) Long-term habituation and sensitization of the acoustic startle response in the normal adult human. *Psychophysiology*, **26**, 166–73
Ornitz EM and Pynoos RS (1989) Startle modulation in children with posttraumatic stress disorder. *Am J Psychiatry*, **146**, 866–70
Ryan SG, Dixon MJ, Nigro MA, Kelts KA, Markand ON, Terry JC, Shiang R, Wasmuth JJ, and O'Connel P (1992) Genetic and radiation hybrid mapping of the hyperekplexia region on chromosome 5q. *Am J Human Genet*, **51**, 1334–43
Sáenz-Lope E, Herranz FJ, and Masdeu JC (1984a) Startle epilepsy: a clinical study. *Ann Neurol*, **16**, 78–81
Sáenz-Lope E, Herranz-Tanarro FJ, Masdeu JC, and Chacon-Pena JR (1984b) Hyperekplexia: a syndrome of pathological startle responses. *Ann Neurol*, **15**, 36–41
Shibasaki H, Motomura S, Yamashita Y, Shii H, and Kuroiwa Y (1981) Periodic synchronous discharge and myoclonus in Creutzfeldt–Jacob disease: diagnostic application of jerk-locked averaging method. *Ann Neurol*, **9**, 150–6
Shibasaki H, Kagigi R, Oda KI, and Masukawa SI (1988) Somatosensory and acoustic brain stem reflex myoclonus. *J Neurol, Neurosurg Psychiatry*, **51**, 572–5
Simons RC (1980) The resolution of the latah paradox. *J Nerv Ment Dis*, **168**, 195–206
Spiera RF and Davis M (1988) Excitatory amino acid antagonists depress acoustic startle after infusion into the ventral nucleus of the lateral lemniscus or paralemniscal zone. *Brain Res*, **445**, 130–6
Stevens H (1965) Jumping Frenchmen of Maine. *Arch Neurol*, **12**, 311–14
Suhren O, Bruyn GW, and Tuynman JA (1966) Hyperexplexia: a hereditary startle syndrome. *J Neurol Sci*, **3**, 577–605
Tanner CM and Chamberland GF (1989) Latah in Indonesians. *Neurology*, **39** (suppl 1), 140
Tinuper P, Aguglia U, and Gastaut H (1986) Use of clobazam in certain forms of status epilepticus and in startle-induced epileptic seizures. *Epilepsia*, **27** (suppl 1), S18–26
Vigevano F, Dicapua M, and Bernardina BD (1989) Startle disease: an avoidable cause of sudden infant death. *Lancet*, **1**, 216

Vrana SR, Spence EL, and Lang PJ (1988) The startle probe response: a new measure of emotion? *J Abnorm Psychol*, **97**, 487–91

Wilkins DE, Hallett M, and Wess MM (1986) Audiogenic startle reflex of man and its relationship to startle syndromes. *Brain*, **109**, 561–73

Winston K (1983) Hyperekplexia relieved by surgical decompression of the cervicomedullary junction. *Neurosurgery*, **13**, 708–10

Wu M, Suzuki SS, and Siegel JM (1988) Anatomical distribution and response patterns of reticular neurons active in relation to acoustic startle. *Brain Res*, **457**, 399–406

Yeomans JS, Rosen JB, Barbeau J, and Davis M (1989) Double-pulse stimulation of startle-like responses in rats: refractory periods and temporal summation. *Brain Res*, **486**, 147–58

22
Odd tremors

Lynn Cleeves, Leslie J. Findley and C. David Marsden

The most frequently encountered tremor disorders such as Parkinson's disease (PD), essential tremor (ET) and cerebellar tremor have been dealt with in many articles including those in volumes 1 and 2 of the present series. This chapter is concerned with 'odd' tremors which, owing to their relative rarity or unusual clinical characteristics, may present problems in classification and diagnosis.

ACTION TREMOR IN PARKINSON'S DISEASE

One of the cardinal signs of PD is rest tremor (tremor present when the limb is fully supported against gravity). It is now known that action tremor (present on maintenance of posture and on movement) is also common in PD (De Jong, 1926; Lance *et al.*, 1963; Findley *et al.*, 1981). This may occur in addition to, or in the absence of, a separate rest tremor.

The action tremor of PD has received relatively little attention in the clinical and experimental literature. For example, it remains to be established how much of the disability arising from tremor in PD is due to the action tremor (which by definition is present during motor activity) rather than the rest tremor which often diminishes during movement. In addition the majority of clinical trials have not separated rest and postural tremors in evaluating drug effects.

The action tremor of PD is clinically indistinguishable from ET (Fig. 22.1). In their classical forms PD and ET may be readily distinguished by the clinical characteristics of the tremors and the absence of extrapyramidal or other neurological signs in ET. However, misdiagnosis is surprisingly common (Rautakorpi, 1978; Dupont, 1980; Findley, 1988a).

The study of the action tremor of PD is difficult because in some cases the typical 4–5 Hz rest tremor does not attenuate with movement, or it may become re-established, unchanged in frequency and waveform characteristics, during the maintenance of posture. Thus, clinically, it may be difficult to differentiate a rest tremor which persists in posture from a 'true' postural tremor.

In an elegant neurophysiological study, Lance *et al.* (1963) clearly separated the lower-frequency rest tremor from a higher-frequency action tremor which they considered to be an exaggeration of physiological tremor.

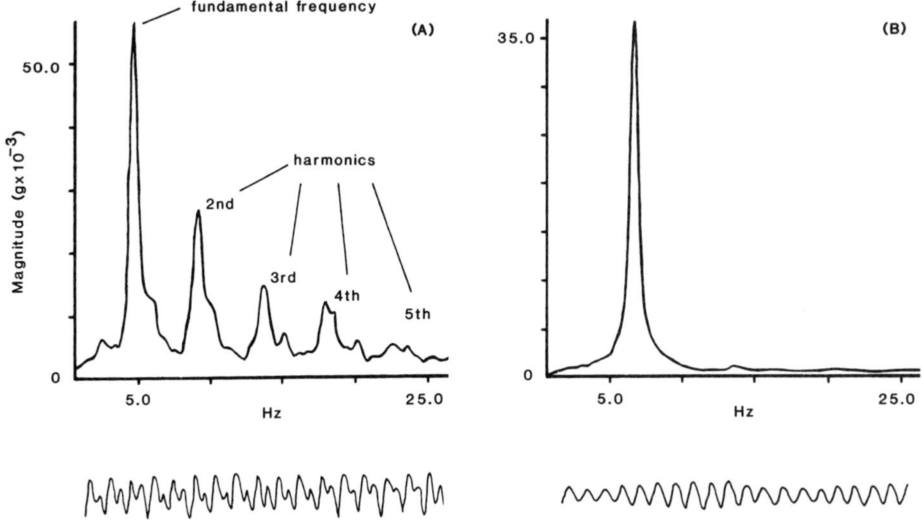

Figure 22.1 (Top) Raw records and (bottom) derived spectra from patients with (A) rest tremor of Parkinson's disease and (B) essential tremor.

Using techniques of spectral analysis Findley *et al.* (1981) showed that an action tremor on maintenance of posture (modal frequency 6 Hz) could be identified in many patients with PD. In some patients the 6 Hz postural tremor could be separated from a higher-frequency (8–11 Hz) tremor of posture and movement which was considered to be an enhanced physiological tremor. Action tremor was as common as the classical rest tremor, and in many patients the two types of tremor (4–5 and 6 Hz) could be identified concurrently in the tremor spectrum. The authors considered this latter finding to be pathognomonic of PD.

The relationship of action tremor in Parkinson's disease to essential tremor

The clinical similarity of the action tremor of PD to ET is one factor contributing to the long-standing (and continuing) debate as to whether ET, which is more prevalent in the population (Dupont, 1980), predisposes to, or is genetically linked to PD.

Using available prevalence data one would expect PD to occur, by chance, in around 1–2% of ET patients (Dupont, 1980). Geraghty *et al.* (1985) showed a surprisingly high prevalence of PD (24 times the expected rate) in patients with ET. However, the majority of epidemiological and retrospective clinical studies have failed to show any significant association between these two disorders (Larsson and Sjogren, 1960; Marttila *et al.*, 1984; Rajput *et al.*, 1984; Cleeves *et al.*, 1988b; Marttila and Rinne, 1988).

Due to clinical similarity between parkinsonian action tremor and ET, it is futile to attempt to estimate the prevalence of ET in patients with established PD. Cleeves *et al.* (1988b) found no evidence of an increased prevalence of monosymptomatic action tremor *preceding* the onset of classical tremulous PD. However, until parkinsonian action tremor can be shown to be a nosologically distinct entity (arising from the primary pathology of PD), the possibility that it represents an associated ET cannot be excluded.

No increase in the prevalence of PD in families of patients with ET has been found. However, a slight increase in the prevalence of ET in families of patients with PD compared with controls has been found (Lang *et al.*, 1986; Cleeves *et al.*, 1988b). This is consistent with the finding of Barbeau and Pourcher (1982) of a high prevalence of ET in the families of patients with young-onset (under age 40), predominantly tremulous PD.

In summary, the available evidence suggests that there may be a genetic link between ET and young-onset, tremulous PD. However, in general, there are no grounds for supposing that a given individual with ET is more predisposed to developing classical PD than the general population (For a recent review of this topic, see Pahwah and Koller, 1993).

The pharmacology of parkinsonian action tremor

One area where it may be possible to differentiate the action tremor of PD from ET is pharmacological responsiveness. In contrast to ET, little is known of the pharmacology of parkinsonian action tremor. Some studies found propranolol to be of benefit in parkinsonian tremor (Owen and Marsden, 1965; Abramsky *et al.*, 1971; Schwab and Young, 1971; Kissel *et al.*, 1974), but others reported no effect (Strang, 1965; Vas, 1966). These conflicting findings may be due to the fact that action tremor was not specifically differentiated from rest tremor in these studies.

In a selected group of 5 PD patients with action tremor as the predominant symptom, Rajput *et al.* (1975) reported improvement in all patients on propranolol.

Foster *et al.* (1984) noted improvement in resting, postural and intention tremor in PD patients after nadolol treatment. Koller and Herbster (1987) reported improvement in resting and postural tremor but not movement tremor after propranolol. In both of these studies, however, it was reported that tremor frequency did not differ between rest and action, so it is still unclear as to whether these patients had a separate, 'true' action tremor of the type which resembles ET.

Action tremor in PD has been reported to be less responsive to alcohol than ET (Rajput *et al.*, 1975) and to be unresponsive both to primidone (which is as effective as propranol in ET) and to clonazepam (Koller and Herbster, 1987).

Thus, although there is some evidence for a role of beta-blockers in the management of parkinsonian tremor generally, particularly when used in combination with dopaminergic drugs, the issue of whether *specific* action tremor in PD responds, pharmacologically, in a similar way to ET remains unresolved.

Benign tremulous Parkinsonism

Most research criteria for the diagnosis of PD require clear evidence of at least two of the cardinal signs of the disorder (tremor, rigidity, bradykinesia). Occasionally, however, patients may present with isolated rest tremor (with or without postural tremor) affecting an arm, or more rarely a leg. Other cardinal signs of PD are absent or minimal. Some reduction in arm-swing on the affected side may be detected when the patient walks, the shoulder may exhibit a delayed shrug and some cogwheel rigidity may be present on passive movement of the wrist. The face may be somewhat lacking in expression.

Such patients present a diagnostic problem; a firm diagnosis of PD is not fully justified and yet the presence of 'classical' parkinsonian rest tremor (in the absence of central nervous system trauma) would seem to preclude alternative diagnoses. On follow-up there may be little or no progression over many years. Hence this entity has been termed benign tremulous parkinsonism.

The recognition of a benign, tremulous form of PD adds to the debate about the relationship between ET and PD, particularly since Barbeau and Pourcher (1982) reported an increased incidence of tremor in family members of patients with young-onset predominantly tremulous PD.

Benign tremulous PD may or may not respond to levodopa, anticholinergics or propranolol. As yet no such patient's brain has been reported to show Lewy body degeneration of the substantia nigra. ^{18}Fluorodopa positron emission tomography (PET) scanning of such individuals shows dopamine depletion in the majority of such cases, suggestive of PD (Brooks *et al.*, 1992).

TRAUMA AND TREMOR

Central nervous system trauma and tremor

Any of the diagnostic categories of tremor can result from trauma to the brain.

Critchley (1957) identified parkinsonian rest tremor as a common feature of the 'punch-drunk' state (progressive traumatic encephalopathy of boxers). Parkinsonism may also result from other forms of severe trauma to the head (see review by Factor *et al.*, 1988).

Acute trauma to the brain with midbrain damage may result in a tremor which is often loosely termed 'rubral tremor' (see below) as it has many features in common with tremor arising from lesions involving the red nucleus and/or superior cerebellar peduncle (Kremer *et al.*, 1947; Samie *et al.*, 1990). Such tremors are often complex, involving both proximal and distal muscles and present when the limb is at rest, in posture and frequently exacerbated with movement. Invariably such patients have widespread damage to the brainstem and its connections, hence the tremor is often complicated by weakness, dysmetria, and other signs of ataxia. In its severest form there is complete decomposition of movement and the appearance is indistinguishable from the gross tremor seen in multiple sclerosis with multiple brainstem lesions.

Action tremor indistinguishable from ET and responsive to propranolol has been reported in children following severe head injury (Ellison, 1978; Obeso and Narbona, 1983). Action tremor as a late complication of severe closed head injury has also been described in adults (Andrew *et al.*, 1982).

An interesting feature of these patients is that there is almost always a delay, sometimes up to 18 months, in the development of tremor following trauma (Andrew *et al.*, 1982), a finding which may have medicolegal significance. The mechanisms underlying the late development of tremor are not understood. It has been suggested that late-onset, posttraumatic dyskinesias could be related to receptor sensitivity changes, axonal sprouting or transsynaptic neuronal degeneration (Mitchell, 1974; Burke *et al.*, 1980) but these hypotheses are, at present, only speculative.

Most tremors due to midbrain damage persist once they appear, but on occasions they may gradually remit. Recovery may take as long as 2 years; this should be borne in mind when stereotactic surgery is contemplated.

CASE 1

A 19-year-old girl suffered severe head injury in a motor-cycle accident. She sustained a basal skull fracture and a linear fracture of the left temperoparietal area. She was unconscious for 4 weeks. She made a slow recovery over 12 months. At this stage she was emotionally labile and dysarthric. She had a pseudobulbar palsy and left hemiplegia (mild spastic weakness of pyramidal distribution, MRC grade 4). In addition, she had moderate dysmetria of the left upper limb. Over a 2-month period (14 months post accident) she developed a severe 3 Hz tremor involving distal and proximal muscles of the left upper limb which was present at rest and in posture and was exacerbated on movement. The tremor, which became the patient's main disability, was unresponsive to primidone, levodopa, bromocriptine and clonazepam. She refused further trials of medication or to be considered for stereotaxis. Her family found difficulty in accepting that the tremor was due to the brain trauma because of the delay in onset. The tremor has remained unchanged for 18 months.

CASE 2

A 51-year-old right-handed man suffered a subarachnoid haemorrhage associated with loss of consciousness at the age of 28. Angiography revealed an arteriovenous malformation arising near the tip of the basilar artery in the interpeduncular fossa with a large anomalous vein to the right of the midline, passing through the midbrain. He had a mild left-sided spastic hemiparesis. Six weeks after the acute episode he developed involuntary movements of the left hand, which became worse over 6 months to affect the whole arm and the left leg. The arm tremor was a large-amplitude, mainly distal tremor at rest which persisted and was exaggerated by voluntary movement and maintenance of posture. The tremor of the leg was intermittent and less severe and did not significantly impair gait. The tremor remained unchanged over a period of 20 years. Various drugs, including tetrabenazine, diazepam, clonazepam and orphenadrine, were ineffective. Levodopa in the form of Sinemet 220 mg three times daily produced marked attenuation of the tremor and he has maintained this response over 5 years.

'Rubral' or midbrain tremor

Damage to the midbrain tegmentum in the region of the red nucleus or its connections may give rise to tremor. However, the term rubral or midbrain tremor is sometimes used as a descriptive term for tremors with similar clinical characteristics, even when no nervous system lesion can be identified.

The classical description of midbrain tremor is that of Holmes (1904) who described a series of 9 patients exhibiting an unusual type of tremor which could occur in any part of a limb, was of low frequency (3–5 Hz) and large amplitude and arose from alternating contractions of agonist and antagonist muscle groups. A similarity with the rest tremor of PD was noted. However the tremor occurred at rest, in posture and during movement and was often exacerbated on approaching a goal. Patients were unable to exert volitional control over the tremor for more than a short time; indeed, attempts to inhibit the tremor often resulted in enhancement.

From the clinical findings and, in 2 cases, postmortem examination, it was concluded that a lesion occupied or involved the midbrain tegmentum. Tremor was attributed to damage to the red nucleus and/or adjacent superior cerebrellar peduncles. However, as these tremors were posttraumatic, damage beyond the environs of the red nucleus and superior cerebellar peduncles would almost certainly have been present.

Masucci *et al.* (1984) described the clinical findings in 24 patients with 'extremity myorhythmia', a term first used by Herz (1931). Masucci *et al.* (1984) described a low-frequency tremor occurring invariably in the limbs and frequently involving other body parts such as face, palate, head, jaw, tongue, eyes and trunk. The behavioural features have many similarities with Holmes's (1904) description of rubral tremor, being described as a course alternating tremor, present at rest and during movement with a frequency range of 2–3 Hz. As with rubral tremor, the other features of PD were not seen.

Six patients were followed to autopsy and the most common aetiologies were brainstem vascular disease and cerebellar degeneration secondary to chronic alcoholism and nutritional deficiency. Clinicopathological correlation indicated that this tremor could arise from ipsilateral lesions of the dentate nucleus or superior cerebellar peduncle or from contralateral inferior olive involvement.

The appearance of these tremors may be indistinguishable from the grosser tremors of multiple sclerosis, midbrain posttraumatic tremors and the tremors in the severest forms of ET, including those associated with peripheral neuropathy.

Tremor with the behavioural characteristics of midbrain tremor or 'extremity myorhythmia' need not be associated with structural brain damage. We have seen a number of patients who developed monosymptomatic unilateral tremor of the upper limbs in the absence of other extrapyramidal signs. Intensive investigations failed to reveal any underlying cause. Perhaps this entity should be categorized as 'idiopathic tremor of midbrain type'.

It may be difficult to distinguish such tremors from atypical benign tremulous PD (Barbeau and Roy, 1984). Features that may indicate idiopathic tremor of midbrain type include a long history, the absence of other extrapyramidal signs and the lack of response to dopaminergic medication.

Assessment of striatal dopamine transmission in these patients by ^{18}F PET studies may provide further means of separating them from patients with PD.

This section has emphasized that 'rubral' or midbrain tremor may arise in the absence of obvious traumatic damage to the nervous system. However, it should be borne in mind that such tremors may result from other pathologies, for example demyelinating disease or small (cryptic) arteriovenous malformations.

CASE 3

A 72-year-old right-handed man noted the onset of tremor of the right hand at the age of 18 during war service. The tremor slowly progressed in severity over 54 years. He related the onset to the shock of seeing a friend shot by the enemy. The tremor did not interfere with his capacity to work as a labourer. There was no family history of tremor. On examination he had a large-amplitude tremor of the right hand and arm present at rest, in posture and throughout action. There were no other relevant signs in the upper limbs; in particular, there was no rigidity or bradykinesia. There was slight loss of associative movement in the right arm. There was a small-amplitude rest tremor of the right leg. There was no tremor on the left. Investigations, including full metabolic screen and magnetic resonance imaging (MRI) scan of the brain and brainstem were normal. The tremor was not affected by alcohol (30 g), primidone (250 mg four times daily) or levodopa (Sinemet 275 mg four times daily).

Minimal trauma and tremor

In the case of posttraumatic tremor described above, tremor was associated with clinical evidence of neurological injury. However, it is now recognized that postural and kinetic tremor may result from minimal or indirect head trauma, not necessarily associated with loss of consciousness and without evidence of neurological damage.

Biary *et al.* (1989) described 7 patients who developed postural tremor of the hands or head within 1–4 weeks of a mild head injury with no (or very brief) loss of consciousness. There were no other neurological signs, with the exception of myoclonic jerking which occurred in 5 (71%) patients. Neuroimaging studies were normal. Features suggestive of a psychogenic origin (see below), such as inconsistent symptomatology, disappearance of tremor with distraction of attention, were not present. Litigation was pending in only 1 patient.

Although this minimal trauma tremor was clinically indistinguishable from ET, it may be different in terms of pharmacological responsiveness. Propranolol, effective in a majority of patients with classical ET, was generally ineffective in minimal trauma tremor; only 1 patient showed improvement on a relatively high dose (400 mg/day). Primidone, which is as effective as propranolol in ET (Findley *et al.*, 1985) was ineffective in the 5 patients with minimal trauma tremor who received it. Three patients showed mild to moderate improvement on clonazepam (1.5–2 mg/day).

There are two important differences between posttraumatic tremor and minimal trauma tremor. Firstly, in minimal trauma tremor neuroimaging fails to reveal underlying structural lesions. This indicates that the responsible lesions are very small or that the tremor arises from functional changes in neuronal networks.

Secondly, the onset of minimal trauma tremor appears to follow a relatively close temporal relationship to the traumatic event. Once established, minimal trauma tremor does not remit, though clearly, in the initial stages following any traumatic or emotional shock, it must be distinguished from enhanced physiological tremor.

CASE 4

A 64-year-old man presented with tremor of the hands, present since 1945, when he had been forced to bail out of an aeroplane over the North Atlantic. He remembers being conscious at the time of rescue and there was no evidence of direct trauma to the head or nervous system. He noticed mild tremor of the hands immediately after the event, and this persisted unchanged until the age of 63 when there was a marked deterioration so that activities such as writing and drinking from a cup were impaired. General and neurological examination was unremarkable, apart from a large-amplitude 5.5 Hz postural tremor of both hands persisting throughout movement and exacerbated with intention pointing. There was no tremor at rest. There was no relevant family history. Tremor responded well to propranolol-LA 400 mg daily.

CASE 5

A 55-year-old science teacher slipped backwards, striking her head on the floor. She was not unconscious but felt anxious and shocked. Approximately 1 month later she developed a tremor of both upper limbs which interfered with her ability to carry out classroom experiments. There was no family history of tremor. On examination a rapid (7.5 Hz) distal, postural and action tremor was observed in both hands. There was no tremor at rest. General and neurological examination was otherwise unremarkable. Tremor responded only minimally to propranolol-LA 320 mg daily. The tremor remains unchanged after 2 years.

Peripheral trauma and tremor

When trauma (albeit relatively mild) involves the head, a proposed aetiological link between the traumatic event and tremor is valid even if unconfirmed. More contentious is the possibility that tremor may be a sequela of any kind of physical or, indeed, psychological trauma.

Pelnar (1913) recognized tremor as a sequel to various kinds of trauma other than head injury. He noted 4 cases of tremor onset after severe chills due to immersion in water, 1 case after 'very strenuous exertion', and 2 cases associated with the climacteric, though one of the latter ladies had also been 'frightened by a gamekeeper' which 'may have contributed and produced the trembling'.

A number of more recent reports have described the onset of movement disorders, including tremor, subsequent to acute peripheral trauma (Marsden *et al.*, 1984; Brin *et al.*, 1986; Schott, 1986; Jankovic and Van der Linden, 1988; Cole *et al.*, 1989; see Chapter 20).

Jankovic and Van der Linden (1988) described 23 cases of dystonia and/or tremor apparently resulting from peripheral injury (fractures, sprains, lacerations etc.). Tremor (6 cases) commenced between 1 day and 9 months after injury.

In a survey of our own ET patients (Findley, 1988b) we found 16 of 185 (8.6%) patients who related the onset of their tremor to a non-neurological emotionally traumatic event. These events were bereavement (7); following surgical operations (4); road traffic accident not involving head injury (3); childbirth (1); shock of learning a relative had been badly injured (1). In these cases the tremor appeared to have commenced suddenly and within a day or two of the emotional trauma. Furthermore, the tremor was persistent and not associated with clinical signs or subjective reports of chronic anxiety.

It has been suggested that emotional or peripheral physical trauma may unmask a pre-existing mild or subclinical ET. This may, indeeed, be the case in some patients. Pelnar (1913) described a patient who 'suffered for three months from trembling of the left extremities; he was then run over by a carriage which dislocated one hand and crushed one foot and the chest. When he recovered consciousness, the extremities of the right side also trembled'.

More recently, Cole *et al.* (1989) described a patient with a pre-existing mild tremor of the outstretched fingers who developed a marked postural tremor of the right hand after falling downstairs and fracturing his right wrist.

There was no family history of tremor in the patients with tremor subsequent to minimal head trauma described by Biary *et al.* (1989) or tremor subsequent to peripheral trauma described by Jankovic and Van der Linden (1988). Interestingly, however, 2 patients in the latter study who developed dystonia subsequent to peripheral trauma had a pre-existing tremor and 3 had a family history of ET.

Clearly, an aetiological link between peripheral trauma and tremor cannot be proven and the mechanisms by which peripheral injury might produce central effects are not known. Parallels have been drawn between movement disorders induced by peripheral trauma and similarly induced sensory phenomena such as causalgia and reflex sympathetic dystrophies (Schott, 1986; Jankovic and Van der Linden, 1989).

Trauma-induced tremor does appear to be relatively uncommon but its prevalence may have been underestimated due to a tendency on the part of clinicians to regard the two events as purely coincidental.

TASK-SPECIFIC TREMOR

Occasionally patients are encountered who complain of tremor only during the performance of specific activities. Tremor during writing is the most commonly encountered form of task-specific tremor. This entity has been termed primary writing tremor but there is no reason to suppose that it is fundamentally different from other forms of task-specific tremor such as tremor when using a golf club or other sporting equipment or whilst playing a musical instrument. The relationship of task-specific tremors to ET and dystonia is, however, a subject of debate.

Primary writing tremor

Difficulty with writing is common in all tremor disorders. Many patients with ET complain only of tremor on writing but, on examination, a clearly developed bilateral postural hand tremor may be seen. It is not uncommon for patients with early PD to present with writing difficulties. However, thorough neurological examination usually reveals other, characteristic signs. In classical ET and PD other manual tasks in addition to writing are generally also affected.

Differentiating primary writing tremor from writer's cramp, which is now recognized as a form of focal dystonia (Sheehy and Marsden, 1982), may be difficult. Patients with focal dystonia often have an associated tremor and some patients with writing tremor attempt to suppress the tremor by isometric contraction of forearm and hand muscles, producing a clinical picture which is difficult to distinguish from true focal dystonia. However, isolated writing tremor is now recognized as a clinical entity, though its aetiological relationship to dystonia is unclear (see below).

Rothwell *et al.* (1979) described a patient who, at age 13, developed shaking and jerking movements of the right hand when holding a pen. The disorder progressed in severity over a 7-year period but did not spread to involve the other limbs. On investigation, it was found that any motor act involving pronation of the right forearm, for example, lifting a cup or using a screwdriver, also elicited a short burst of tremor activity. There was no tremor with the arms held outstretched in static posture or on movement, provided the movement did not involve forearm pronation or supination. There was no evidence of focal dystonia. Despite the jerky appearance, electromyogram (EMG) studies showed the jerks to be the initial part of a tremor burst. Thus, the disorder was considered to be consistent with true tremor rather than segmental myoclonus, in which jerking occurs spontaneously and may persist for many minutes or hours irrespective of the manual task.

Kachi *et al.* (1985) summarized the clinical features of a group of 9 patients with a diagnosis of primary writing tremor. By definition, tremor was present during writing in all patients but in 3 patients tremor was present during certain other specific tasks. In all cases tremor resulted from a rhythmic 5–6 Hz pronation-supination of the forearm.

A family history of tremor appears to be rare in patients with primary writing tremor, in contrast to ET where a family history is reported in around 50% of cases. In five reports involving a total of 31 patients with primary writing tremor, only 4 subjects had a family history of bilateral hand tremor (Klawans *et al.*, 1982; Ohye *et al.*, 1982; Kachi *et al.*, 1985; Ravits *et al.*, 1985; Koller and Martyn, 1986). However, Cohen *et al.* (1987) studied 6 members of a single family, 2 of whom had typical ET, 2 (twins) writer's cramp, 1 ET with writer's cramp and 1 primary writing tremor. This study suggests that ET, writing tremor, writer's cramp and perhaps other focal dystonias may represent a spectrum of movement disorders which are genetically linked. Others have considered some cases of primary writing tremor to be a manifestation of focal dystonia (Rosenbaum and Jankovic, 1988; Elble *et al.*, 1990).

Katchi *et al.* (1985) reported that primary writing tremor responded to drugs effective in classical ET. Three patients reported that alcohol improved their tremor. Tremor was attenuated in 4 patients given intravenous propranolol (1.7–2.0 mg) and in 6 patients given oral propranolol (120–240 mg/day).

In contrast, Klawans *et al.* (1982) found propranolol (minimum dose 120 mg/day) to be ineffective in all 5 patients with primary writing tremor who received it. Sinemet was also ineffective. A therapeutic effect was, however, observed after anticholinergics. One patient improved after intramuscular scopolamine. Another showed improvement after intravenous benztropine (1 mg), with reversal of the therapeutic effect after intravenous administration of the anticholinesterase physostigmine (1 mg). The only medication which proved useful on chronic therapy was benztropine, with all patients showing improvement described as moderate to marked. Ravits *et al.* (1985) noted some degree of improvement in 2 patients with writing tremor who were treated with trihexyphenidyl though, in both, the drug had to be discontinued due to side-effects.

The reasons for these contradictory findings regarding the efficacy of propranolol is not clear. There is no indication that the patients of Klawans *et al.* (1982) differed clinically from those of Kachi *et al.* (1985). In both studies, however, the number of patients tested was relatively small and even in classical ET it is known that interpatient response to drugs is variable. The possibility that primary writing tremor, unlike classical ET, may respond to anticholinergics deserves further investigation.

Thalamotomy (ventralis intermedius nucleus) has been reported to abolish primary writing tremor (Ohye *et al.*, 1982).

Physiological studies of primary writing tremor have yielded conflicting results. Rothwell *et al.* (1979) found that tendon taps delivered to pronator teres provoked a burst of tremor. Partial motor point anaesthesia (with no reduction in voluntary power) of pronator teres abolished tremor elicited by tendon taps and tremor occurring during writing. The authors therefore concluded that the tremor was generated by proprioceptive input from pronator teres, though the level within the nervous system at which this was occurring could not be determined.

Ravits *et al.* (1985) found that long-latency responses to stretch of pronator teres were absent in the 4 patients studied, in contrast to the single patient of Rothwell *et al.* (1979) in whom long-latency responses were present.

EMG studies have little diagnostic value as it has been shown that writing tremor, like ET, may involve alternating (Ravits *et al.*, 1979) or synchronous (Rothwell *et al.*, 1979) activity in antagonist muscles or rhythmic activity in a single muscle, namely pronator teres (see case 6).

CASE 6

A 69-year-old man complained of a 9-year history of tremor of the right hand. Initially this was confined solely to the act of writing. However, recently, tremor had been present during other specific tasks such as using cutlery or a screwdriver. His mother had a yes-yes tremor of the head in the last 7 years of her life. On examination, he had a small-amplitude 6 Hz pronation-supination tremor of the right forearm which was most prominent during writing. There was no evidence of dystonia. General and neurological examination was otherwise normal. EMG studies revealed tremor bursts in the right pronator teres which were responsible for the movements. Passive supination of the right forearm increased tremor amplitude. Surface EMG recordings from other muscles showed no segmentation of the record. Reciprocal inhibition from the right forearm extensor muscles on to the right forearm flexor muscles was normal in both early and late stages.

The patient did not wish to take regular medication.

Other task-specific tremors

Task-specific tremors may occur in situations other than writing. For example Kachi *et al.* (1985) described a patient with tremor occurring only during the backswing in golf. In their study of focal dystonia of golfers (the 'yips'), McDaniel *et al.* (1989) noted tremor in some subjects occurring only during specific actions, most commonly putting. We have encountered patients with tremors specific to aiming darts, cueing in snooker, playing the violin and a wide variety of other musical instruments.

CASE 7

A 57-year-old professional violinist complained of a 10-year history of tremor of the right hand which occurred when the right arm was held with the shoulder abducted and elbow flexed during bowing. Sustaining a single note was impossible. Tremor did not occur during other aspects of playing and was not a manifestation of performance anxiety or stage fright. Tremor did not occur during other activities. The tremor was suppressed by alcohol. However, tolerance developed over a number of years so that eventually the amount of alcohol required to suppress the tremor also produced intoxication, incapacity and liver impairment. There was no relevant family history. There were no other clinical abnormalities, in particular no evidence of dystonia. The patient was successfully treated with a combination of propranolol and primidone, plus a small quantity of alcohol prior to public performance. Liver function returned to normal.

Clearly, these tremors are provoked by specific patterns of activity in specific muscles groups, although the level in the nervous system at which tremor is generated is not known. We have, however, studied a patient who exhibited a 5.6 Hz tremor in the right hand when writing with that hand. There was no tremor when the right hand was simply held in static posture. Interestingly, writing with the left hand did not produce tremor in the left hand but provoked a clear 5.6 Hz postural tremor in the *right* hand. This finding suggests that, in this individual at least, the expression of tremor is closely linked with execution of the motor program for writing.

DYSTONIA AND TREMOR

A connection between tremor and dystonic syndromes has long been recognized. A high incidence of postural hand tremor having the characteristics of ET has been reported in patients with generalized dystonia (Larsson and Sjogren, 1966; Eldridge, 1970; Yanagisawa *et al.*, 1971; Marsden and Harrison, 1974), torticollis (Patterson and Little, 1943; Couch, 1976) and writer's cramp (Sheehy and Marsden, 1982).

A high incidence of tremor has also been noted in family members of patients with dystonia (Larsson and Sjogren, 1966; Yanagisawa *et al.*, 1971; Couch, 1976). Cohen *et al.* (1987) found cases of ET, writer's cramp, ET with writer's cramp, and primary writing tremor in members of one family. These findings have lead to the suggestion that tremor and dystonia may be aetiologically (possibly genetically) linked. Some authors have regarded tremor as an integral part of the dystonic syndrome and tremor in family members as a *forme fruste* of dystonia (see Couch, 1976).

Whether the tremor associated with dystonia is identical to ET remains to be established. Clinically, however, one can encounter a spectrum of disorders ranging from a pure tremor (classical ET) to a pure dystonic syndrome with, in between, diverse combinations of tremor in association with dystonia. Both disorders may be generalized (whole-body involvement), segmental (both arms, both legs, trunk, neck) or focal (e.g. writer's cramp, primary writing tremor).

At the clinical level the association of tremor with dystonia could be categorized in two ways: firstly, the occurrence of the two disorders in separate body parts, for example torticollis with bilateral postural hand tremor. This may be termed tremor associated with dystonia; and secondly, the occurrence of tremor and dystonia in the same body part, which may be termed dystonic tremor (see below). Included in this latter group would be patients who exhibit dystonia clinically and also patients in whom dystonia may only be recognized on electrophysiological assessment, i.e. impaired reciprocal inhibition or prolonged (greater than 200 ms) synchronous bursts in antagonist muscles.

CASE 8

A 52-year-old right-handed housewife developed pain in the right hand and wrist on writing at the age of 22. After 1 year this remitted but reappeared after a further 2 years. At the age of 30, she developed tremor of the right hand on writing which worsened over 5 years so that she changed over to using her left hand for writing. At 35 she noticed a postural tremor in the right hand and a tremor in the left hand on writing. Propanolol had a modest effect on the tremor. Clonazepam and alcohol were ineffective. Her mother (aged 79) developed tremor of the right arm at age 50. On examination, she demonstrated dystonic posturing in the right arm and a cramp in the right hand when writing. She had a distal postural tremor in the right arm and writing tremor in both hands. Surface EMG records revealed alternating (5 Hz) agonist/antagonist EMG bursts in the wrist flexors and extensors of the right arm in posture and synchronous EMG activity at the same frequency in biceps and deltoid muscles. At times synchronous bursts of EMG activity lasting 200 ms were visible in the biceps and deltoid muscles. Reciprocal inhibition in the right forearm was normal.

SITE-SPECIFIC TREMORS

Classical ET is a tremor of the hands, although in a significant proportion of patients tremor is present in other body parts as well. However, isolated tremors of different body parts may occur without involvement of the hands.

These site-specific tremors present diagnostic problems. Traditionally such tremors, in the absence of other neurological signs, have been considered as focal manifestations of ET (essential head tremor, essential leg tremor, etc.).

The fact that many patients with focal dystonia (e.g. writer's cramp, spasmodic torticollis) exhibit a tremor of the affected part (see above) raises the possibility that focal tremor and focal dystonia share a common pathology. In this case, focal tremor could be viewed as a manifestation of a covert dystonia.

A third possibility is that there are true primary focal tremors different from both ET and dystonia.

These nosological considerations are not merely academic since each has different implications for management. A number of approaches may help to resolve the issue: (1) extensive observations of families with essential tremor or dystonia may establish whether site-specific or task-specific tremors can be the sole manifestation of the abnormal gene(s) in these conditions; (2) long-term follow-up of patients with isolated tremor to see if they subsequently develop essential tremor elsewhere, or obvious dystonia; (3) careful neurophysiological investigations to establish whether evidence of subclinical dystonia (see above) exists in all cases of site-specific tremors.

In a recent study of 20 families with classical ET in which family members were examined personally, no examples of task-specific or site specific tremors were found (Bain *et al.*, unpublished observations). In contrast patients with task-specific or site specific tremors may develop dystonia (Marsden, personal observations). So most, if not all such tremors may be manifestations of dystonia rather than ET.

Head and trunk tremor

Head tremor may occur in a number of clinical conditions. However, as originally emphasized by Charcot (1989), head tremor does not occur as a feature of PD.

Midline cerebellar lesions may give rise to slow (3–4 Hz), predominantly anteroposterior oscillations of the head and trunk (titubation). However, in such cases other cerebellar signs such as truncal ataxia and hypotonia are present.

Head tremor in association with hand tremor is relatively common in ET. The tremor may manifest as a no-no oscillation (yaw), a yes-yes oscillation (pitch), or a complex combination of both types of movement. There may be a family history of head tremor, hand tremor or torticollis.

Isolated tremor of the trunk has also been described. Tremor is absent when the patient is lying down, but oscillations about the pelvis occur on sitting, standing or walking.

Rivest and Marsden (1990) studied a series of patients with head and trunk tremor in a variety of manifestations. Interestingly, several patients had a history of head tremor preceding the development of torticollis and 1 patient had a history of arm, head and voice tremor with subsequent development of dystonia of the arm and torticollis. Some patients found their head or trunk tremors could be ameliorated by changes in posture, a feature which is characteristic of dystonia.

On the basis of their findings, Rivest and Marsden (1990) suggested that some patients with isolated tremors of the head and trunk may have primary or idiopathic dystonia rather than ET. On clinical observation patients with isolated complex head tremors often have subtle dystonic features. As yet there are insufficient neurophysiological data on this group of patients.

Head and trunk tremors do not generally respond to the drugs used in the treatment of ET. In a clinical trial of primidone in patients diagnosed as having ET of the hands and head, Findley *et al.* (1985) found primidone to be effective in hand tremor but generally ineffective in head tremor in the same patients. Koller (1984) did find propranolol to be effective in attenuating head tremor. However, none of the head or trunk tremors described by Rivest and Marsden (1990) were responsive to propranolol or primidone, though 1 patient with isolated trunk tremor did show considerable improvement on an anticholinergic (trihexyphenidyl).

It is apparent, therefore, that head and trunk tremors respond less predictably to drugs than hand tremor. However, patients presenting with head and trunk tremors should be given therapeutic trials of propranolol, primidone and anticholinergics.

Tremors of the face, chin, lips and tongue

Rarely, patients with tremor confined to the facial muscles, jaw, lips or tongue (or combinations of these) may be encountered. Tremor of these structures, particularly the chin, may be seen in PD but those patients have no other neurological signs.

A number of cases of hereditary chin tremor have been reported. Chin tremor may commence in childhood (Grossman, 1957; Lawrence *et al.*, 1968). Koller *et al.* (1987) described 2 cases of isolated chin tremor commencing in later life. In 1 case the patient's mother had also developed isolated chin tremor late in life. Levodopa was ineffective in both patients. One patient was successfully treated with propranolol (120 mg/day) and the other responded well to primidone (250 mg/day) but not propranolol.

Rosenberg and Clark (1987) documented a family with 8 cases of isolated chin tremor over four generations. EMG studies in 2 patients revealed rhythmical discharges (8–10 Hz) in the affected muscles. Abnormal motor unit discharges were recorded in all muscles of the face, even though clinical tremor was only evident in the chin.

Episodic repetitive (2–3 Hz) tongue movements have been reported in children with epilepsy (Jabbari and Coker, 1981). Episodic desynchronization of the EEG coincided with the tongue movements which the authors attributed to subcortical seizures. Rhythmical tongue movements have also been reported in adults after head trauma (Troupin and Kamm, 1974; Keane, 1984). In these cases there were no synchronous surface EEG discharges. Both patients described by Keane (1984) had evidence of pontine injury. The abnormal tongue movements were not permanent but disappeared within a few days or weeks of the trauma.

Tongue tremor may occur in ET. Biary and Koller (1987) described 20 patients with 'essential' tongue tremor. Hand tremor was present in 17 patients but in 2 patients tongue tremor was the only finding. One patient had isolated tongue tremor and spasmodic torticollis. A family history of hand tremor was present in 2 patients with isolated tongue tremor. In individual patients, the frequency of tremor recorded in the tongue (4–8 Hz) was similar to the frequency of hand tremor. Tongue tremor was reduced in 9 of 9 patients after alcohol; in 6 of 12 patients after propranolol; in 4 of 6 patients after clonazepam and in 1 of 2 patients after primidone.

Isolated leg tremor

Isolated rest tremor of the legs is most likely to be due to PD. ^{18}Fluorodopa positron emission tomography (PET) scanning of such patients frequently shows dopamine depletion (Brooks *et al.*, 1992). Tremor of the legs on standing occurs in a wide variety of conditions, including spasticity, cerebellar disease, action myoclonus and dystonia. Strictly speaking, these tremors could all be classified as orthostatic. However, the presence of other neurological signs clearly indicates their origin. We would suggest that these be classified as secondary orthostatic tremor, as distinct from primary orthostatic tremor, as described by Heilman (1984).

ORTHOSTATIC TREMOR

In 1984, Heilman described 3 patients with an unusual tremulous condition which had not previously been recorded in the clinical literature. This was characterized by a rapid, irregular tremor of the legs and sometimes also of the trunk, on standing but not on walking, sitting or when leaning against a support. Tremor commenced several seconds after standing and increased in amplitude over time until, after a minute or so, the patients felt as if they were about to fall and required support to prevent them from doing so. Heilman termed this condition orthostatic tremor (OT) and considered it to be a distinct neurological entity related to dysfunction in the maintenance of static body posture.

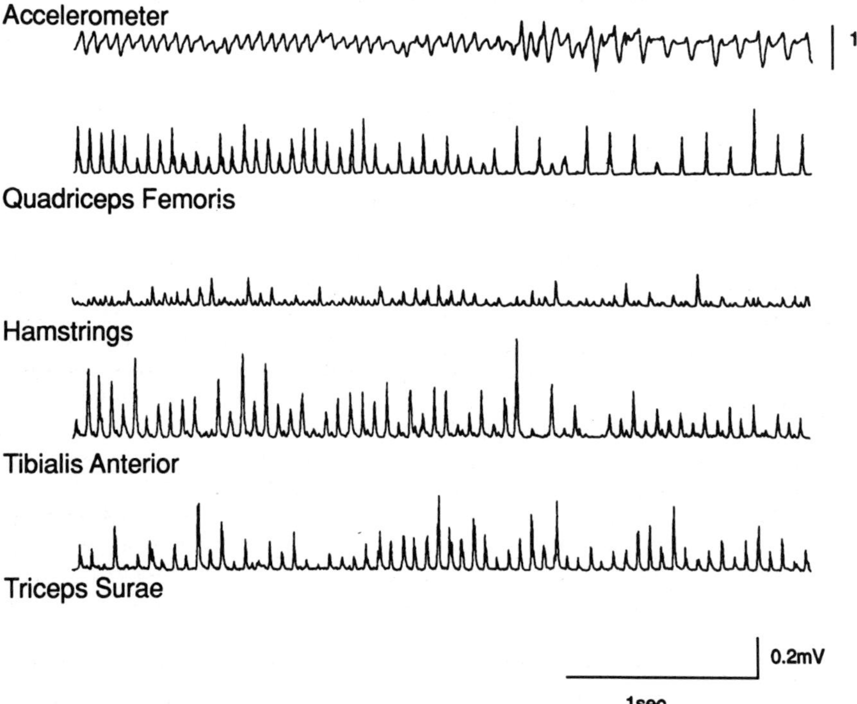

Figure 22.2 Accelerometer (placed over right quadriceps near the patellar tendon) and rectified and filtered electromyogram recordings from the muscles of right leg while a patient with orthostatic tremor was standing. Note the change in tremor frequency in quadriceps from 16 to 8 Hz. Tremor frequency remained constant at 16 Hz in other muscles. From Thompson *et al.* (1986) with permission.

Involvement of the legs is not uncommon in classical ET. In our own survey of 185 consecutive ET patients (Findley, 1988b), leg tremor was found to be present in 29 (15.7%). However, isolated leg tremor in the absence of concurrent hand tremor was less common and occurred in only 4 patients (2.2%).

Despite certain features which distinguish primary OT from classical ET, there is some overlap in the phenomenology of the two disorders. This raises the issue of whether primary OT should be classified as a separate diagnostic entity or as a variant of ET (Britton *et al.*, 1992).

Like ET, primary OT has an insidious onset and may slowly progress, in terms of severity, over many years. However, the oscillation frequency of primary OT has been reported to be between 14 and 18 Hz (Thompson *et al.*, 1986; Deuschl *et al.*, 1987; Kelly and Sharbrough, 1987; Papa and Gershanik, 1988; Gabellini *et al.*, 1990; Britton *et al.*, 1992; Fig. 22.2). This is far higher than the frequency range of classical ET which rarely exceeds 10 Hz (Gresty and Findley, 1984).

ET of the legs is generally present during any voluntary muscle activity but may be exacerbated on standing. In a single case study, Thompson *et al.* (1986) noted that high-frequency (16 Hz) primary OT was not present during all types of voluntary muscle activity. Tremor was present when the patient was standing or pressing the feet against the floor as if preparing to stand but was absent when the patient was seated and extending the leg horizontally against gravity. Thompson *et al*. suggested, therefore, that primary OT arises from an abnormality in the organization of the motor program for standing.

Deuschl *et al*. (1987), however, described a patient with a similar 16 Hz leg tremor which was present during all kinds of muscle activation in sitting, lying or standing positions. They postulated that a central oscillator was involved in tremor production and that mechanisms involved in stance regulation had a 'predominant access' to this oscillator.

Electrophysiological studies of primary OT have invariably shown synchronous tremor activity in the corresponding muscles of the two legs at a frequency (14–18 Hz) higher than is found in any other type of tremor (Thompson *et al*., 1986; Deuschl *et al*., 1987; Veilleux *et al*., 1987; Britton *et al*., 1992). This is pathognomonic of the disorder. This synchronicity, together with the finding that the frequency of primary OT could not be reset by peripheral nerve stimulation (Thompson *et al*., 1986), suggests that primary OT has a central, rather than a peripheral, origin. ET, too, is considered to arise from a central generator, although the tremor may be modified to varying degrees by peripheral factors (Marsden, 1984).

No other significant neurophysiological abnormalities have been found in the higher-frequency primary OT. Sensory evoked potentials from stimulation of the tibial nerve at the ankle and central motor conduction to the leg muscles using transcranial motor cortex stimulation are normal. Short- and long-latency stretch reflexes are also within the normal range (Rothwell, 1989).

Thompson *et al*. (1986) observed that, at certain times, the frequency of tremor in quadriceps suddenly slowed to 8 Hz whilst the frequency in the other muscles recorded (hamstrings, tibialis anterior and triceps surae) remained at 16 Hz (Fig. 22.2). The EMG discharges in the quadriceps then occurred at every other beat of the tremor cycle. Deuschl *et al*. (1987) recorded an 8 Hz peak at the patella, caused by alternating large and small bursts in the ongoing 16 Hz EMG activity. In both these studies it was noted that the slower, 8 Hz tremor was more associated with subjective and objective unsteadiness in the patients' stance than the 16 Hz tremor. Veilleux *et al*. (1987) also noted that the frequency of leg tremor recorded with an accelerometer was often a subharmonic of the basic firing frequency of the motor units.

Thus, there is evidence that the very-high-frequency EMG activity seen in primary OT may produce mechanical oscillations of the legs at a lower frequency, although the high-frequency EMG bursts invariably produce a clinically visible quivering of the muscles.

This small-amplitude tremor produces a disproportionate degree of disability and distress. All patients with high-frequency primary OT complain of feelings of unsteadiness associated with the upright posture and can experience actual falls. The factor or factors producing postural instability in primary OT are not clear. It could be postulated that the high-frequency discharges are approaching a partial tetanic fusion of muscle and therefore the normal voluntary and involuntary postural adjustments are impaired. It may be that the sudden changes of frequency of tremor may add to the instability and that subjective feelings of imminent falling are more likely to occur at these times.

There is some evidence that ET and primary OT may be differentially responsiveness to drugs. The marked attenuation of tremor by alcohol which has often been reported in ET has not been observed in primary OT. Propranolol, the drug of choice in ET, has also been found to be ineffective in primary OT (Heilman, 1984; Wee *et al.*, 1986). Phenobarbitone may be effective in OT and ET (Papa and Gershanik, 1988; Gabellini *et al.*, 1990). It should, however, be borne in mind that relatively few patients with primary OT have been investigated and ET, itself, shows a variable response to drug treatment.

The benzodiazepine derivative clonazepam has been reported to be beneficial in primary OT (Heilman, 1984; Wee *et al.*, 1986; Kelly and Sharbrough, 1987), whereas its efficacy in essential (hand) tremor is highly inconsistent (Fung, 1981; Thompson *et al.*, 1984).

However, ET of the legs may also be attenuated by clonazepam. Cleeves *et al.* (1988a) described a patient with familial ET involving the hands and legs. Tremor frequency was 6.4 Hz. EMG studies were not carried out but there was no clinical evidence of the high-frequency quivering of the leg muscles characteristic of primary OT. On incremental doses of clonazepam, objective measures showed no effect on hand tremor, but a dose-related decrease (up to 80% reduction on 4 mg/day) in the amplitude of leg tremor. Thus, response to clonazepam is not specific to the high-frequency primary orthostatic leg tremor, but can be effective in leg tremor (though not hand tremor) which is clinically consistent with classical ET. Interestingly, clonazepam has also been found effective in controlling myoclonic-like repetitive movements of the legs occurring during sleep (Ohanna *et al.*, 1985).

A finding of some interest is the occurrence of upper limb tremor consistent with ET in some primary OT patients or in members of their families (Heilman, 1984; Wee *et al.*, 1986). Wee *et al.* (1986) described a single family in which some members had a 7–8 Hz tremor of the hands which was responsive to propranolol, and others had a 6–7 Hz tremor of the legs on standing which was responsive to clonazepam but not to beta-blockers.

In a small survey of 15 patients with monosymptomatic tremor involving the legs, Papa and Gershanik (1988) distinguished three groups on the basis of clinical and EMG characteristics.

Five patients were classified as having classical ET of upper and lower limbs. Tremor frequency in these patients ranged from 5 to 8 Hz. In individual patients the frequency was similar in all four limbs. Frequency and amplitude did not change significantly upon standing and there was no subjective feeling of instability.

Seven patients had a 6–8 Hz postural tremor of the upper and lower limbs. However, on standing both amplitude and frequency of leg tremor increased, producing a marked 10–13 Hz oscillation. Despite reported feelings of unsteadiness these patients did not fall.

The last group of 3 patients was considered to meet the criteria for primary OT. They had a 6–8 Hz postural tremor of the hands and legs. However, a 16 Hz tremor of the legs (tibialis anterior and gastrocnemius) appeared on standing, causing severe instability and falling if no support was given. This high-frequency tremor was also seen in the supine position when pressing the feet against a hard surface. Interestingly, a similar high-frequency tremor was recorded from the hands when pressing the palms against a hard surface.

The patients described by Papa and Gershanik differ from the earlier reports of Heilman (1984) and Thompson *et al.* (1986) in that they all, clearly, had ET of the hands and in many cases a family history of hand tremor also. The finding of interest is that, in addition to a postural tremor of the legs within the frequency range of ET, some patients showed a higher-frequency OT. Papa and Gershanik (1988) suggested that primary OT may represent part of the spectrum of ET. The two disorders share the common feature of being initiated by the adoption of certain patterns of muscular activity. In primary OT the initiating factors arise from the muscle activity required to stand though, as several studies have shown, primary OT is not invariably associated with upright posture (Deuschl *et al.*, 1987; Papa and Gershanik, 1988).

CASE 9

A 45-year-old schoolteacher had a history of chronic asthma and had used a Ventolin inhaler intermittently for 20 years. She noticed postural and action tremor of the upper limbs for 25 years (i.e. before Ventolin use). Five years prior to consultation she noticed shaking in the legs associated with a feeling of unsteadiness occurring immediately on standing. On two occasions she fell. She was unable to stand without support for more than 2 minutes. There was no family history of tremor. Alcohol had no effect on tremor. On examination she had a fine postural tremor of the hands, and a rapid tremor in the muscles of both legs occurring immediately upon standing which was barely visible but could be felt as a fine vibration. Gait was normal.

On standing, an 18 Hz, alternating EMG pattern was recorded from hamstrings, quadriceps, soleus, tibialis anterior and abductor hallucis brevis on both sides. The tremor was absent when sitting, even when the muscles of the leg were voluntarily activated. There was no tremor in the outstretched arms when sitting. However, 18 Hz rhythmic EMG activity occurred in the arms when the patient was standing and bracing her arms against a vertical wall or supporting herself on all fours. Auditory startle when the patient was standing increased the amount of EMG activity but did not alter the phase of tremor. Near motor threshold stimulation of the median nerve at the wrist produced normal M and H responses and a late response with a latency of 38.5 ms and with an amplitude greater than the preceding H response (abnormal early type 1 long-latency reflex). Cross-correlation studies on single motor units in tibialis anterior showed that when sitting and voluntarily activating tibialis anterior, the cross-correlogram between single motor units in the two muscles was flat, implying units firing independently of each other. When standing, cross-correlograms revealed multiple peaks, 30 ms wide at the base and 60 ms apart over a time period of 0.5 seconds, implying that firing of the motor unit in one tibialis anterior was closely linked to the firing of the motor unit in the other and that there was little frequency modulation in either unit.

Owing to a tendency to bronchospasm, beta-blocking drugs were not tried. Phenobarbitone 30 mg twice daily produced improvement so she could stand comfortably. Clonazepam 1 mg three times daily produced an improvement. However, the side-effects of sedation precluded continuation of therapy.

TREMOR IN PERIPHERAL NEUROPATHY

Tremor may occur in association with any type of peripheral neuropathy. The clinical characteristics of neuropathic tremor are not, however, uniform and it can mimic any of the common pathological tremors. In some patients the tremor may resemble ET; in others the tremor may be indistinguishable from the rest tremor seen of PD or the intention tremor of cerebellar disease.

A number of reports have described tremor in chronic relapsing polyneuropathy. Usually the tremor takes the form of an irregular postural and movement tremor of the hands (Shahani and Young, 1978; Dalakas and Engel, 1981). However Thomas *et al.* (1969) described a coarse intention tremor of the arms occurring in a case of chronic relapsing Guillain–Barré polyneuritis. Matthews *et al.* (1970) described a patient with relapsing polyneuritis who had a regular 6 Hz postural tremor and, in addition, a 'pill-rolling' rest tremor indistinguishable from that of PD.

In all these cases tremor commenced some time after the onset of the neuropathy, usually during relapse. Dalakas and Engel (1981) reported that tremor was not related to the severity or distribution of muscle weakness, to sensory loss (which was absent or minimal) or to corticosteroid therapy. Such tremor does not respond to propranolol (Shahani and Young, 1978; Dalakas and Engel, 1981).

Tremor may occur in hereditary motor and sensory neuropathies (HMSN) and is more common in type I than in type II (Dyck, 1975; Harding and Thomas, 1980). HMSN in which tremor is dominant is often classified as the Roussy–Lévy syndrome. The tremor is usually postural, regular and indistinguishable from ET. It may respond to propranolol.

Smith *et al.* (1983) described tremor in 10 of 12 patients with chronic demyelinating neuropathy associated with benign immunoglobulin M paraproteinaemia. All showed an irregular tremor of the outstretched arms and in 3 patients a rest tremor was also present. These authors noted that the tremor involved different antagonistic muscle groups at different times, giving it a variable and complex character. Tremor was not related to muscle weakness or deficits in proprioception. The tremor was not responsive to propranolol or antiparkinsonian drugs.

Said *et al.* (1982) summarized the findings in 14 patients with tremor in association with acquired peripheral neuropathies of different origin (including diabetic, uraemic and alcoholic neuropathy). Tremor was present in posture and limited to the limbs (upper or lower) affected by the neuropathy.

Given the variation in its presenting characteristics, it seems likely that different mechanisms are involved in the development of tremor in peripheral neuropathies. However, these mechanisms are not yet known.

One possibility is that tremor results from increased conduction time in peripheral motor servoloops. However, not all patients with reduced nerve conduction velocities have tremor. Conversely, some patients with normal conduction velocities do have tremor (Adams *et al.*, 1972; Thomas, 1975; Dalakas and Engel, 1981). Smith *et al.* (1984) observed a positive correlation between nerve conduction velocity and tremor frequency in a small group of patients with paraproteinaemic neuropathy. However, no such correlation was found by Said *et al.* (1982) in a heterogeneous group of neuropathies.

Dyck (in Adams *et al.*, 1972) suggested a central origin of tremor in neuropathy, particularly paraproteinaemic neuropathy in which central abnormalities are common. According to this view the tremor mechanism is separate from the neuropathy *per se*. This would explain why only some patients with neuropathy have tremor, why the tremor may manifest in a variety of clinical forms, and why in some patients the appearance and progression of tremor does not mirror the neuropathic process. However, the nature of the proposed central abnormality in neuropathic tremor remains obscure.

As yet, the relationship between peripheral neuropathy and tremor is not understood. However, the possibility of neuropathy must be considered in any patient presenting with isolated tremor and the electrophysiological examination of periopheral nerves is important in the investigation of these patients.

HYSTERICAL TREMOR

By its nature hysteria, or its modern designation of conversion disorder (American Psychiatric Association, 1980), does not lend itself to precise definition. The term covers diverse symptomatology and the very concept of hysteria has been the subject of much controversy (Slater, 1965; Lewis, 1975). However, as Marsden (1986) has commented, neurologists 'would be hard put to it if they could no longer make a diagnosis of hysteria'. The frequency of diagnosis of hysteria in two major neurological centres has been estimated to be around 1% (Trimble, 1981; Marsden, 1986). Trimble (1981) found no significant change in the frequency of diagnosis of hysteria over a time period spanning three decades.

The critical features of hysterical psychogenic tremor are that the clinical characteristics do not meet the diagnostic criteria for other, recognized tremor disorders and, after full investigations the tremor is considered not to be due to physical disease. Clearly, however, these features, in themselves, are not definitive. It is important to attempt to formulate a broader set of criteria for the diagnosis of hysterical tremor in order to avoid the error of consigning all 'odd' tremors to this category simply because they do not fit any other.

Charcot (1889) believed hysteria to be 'governed in the same way as other morbid conditions, by rules and laws which attentive and sufficiently numerous observations always permit us to establish'. Unfortunately, observations of hysterical tremor have not been very numerous and usually take the form of anecdotal descriptions.

Koller *et al.* (1989) have summarized the findings in 24 patients with a diagnosis of hysterical tremor. Tremor usually had an abrupt onset (bilaterally), often with a non-progressive course and fluctuating severity. In some cases there was abrupt resolution of tremor.

It has long been postulated that variability in tremor frequency is indicative of hysterical tremor. Gowers (1893) noted that hysterical tremor was 'rarely constant' and varied in 'degree and time'. Inconsistencies such as changing tremor frequency and abrupt changes in direction from flexion-extension to pronation-supination were noted by Koller *et al.* (1989). The frequency of other pathological tremors such as ET or the tremors of PD is generally remarkably constant but in some patients variations of up to 1 Hz may occur from day to day or with changes in limb position. However, sudden marked changes in frequency within a single period of observation are not seen (Cleeves *et al.*, 1986; Cleeves and Findley, 1987).

It has been suggested that hysterical tremor is more influenced by conscious attention than other tremors (Campbell, 1979). Gowers noted that hysterical tremors were 'always increased, and sometimes distinctly induced, by attention and when the mind is diverted the tremor may cease'.

There is, however, a danger of tautology in using suppression-with-distraction as a defining feature of hysterical tremor. It needs to be established that patients diagnosed as hysterical on *other* grounds invariably show suppression. Furthermore, the effect of distraction upon other tremor disorders has not been systematically investigated. There is some evidence that diverting attention to some other activity increases parkinsonian tremor (Cleeves *et al.*, 1986). Provisional findings from a study we are currently conducting suggest that some patients with ET may show marked suppression of tremor when attention is diverted to the performance of cognitive tasks. Diverting attention may also markedly suppress the tremor of Wilson's disease.

Koller and Biary (1989) studied voluntary suppression in a number of movement disorders. A majority of patients with parkinsonian tremor or neuroleptic-induced tremor were able to suppress their tremor by voluntary effort for brief periods of time, but only 2% of ET patients were able to do this and, indeed, the attempt to suppress made the tremor worse in 24% of patients. No patients with hysterical tremor were studied.

La belle indifférence has been regarded as indicative of hysterical symptoms. However, in our experience this is not common in patients with hysterical tremor. Furthermore we have encountered patients with quite marked organic tremors who are surprisingly indifferent to their symptoms.

Fahn (1984) stated that to be certain that the tremor is due to a conversion reaction, remission must occur 'either spontaneously, with psychotherapy, or with placebo'. Gowers (1893) regarded hysterical tremors as extremely 'obstinate', requiring 'great patience and perseverance' in their treatment, a view with which we would concur. Ljungberg (1957) found hysterical tremor to have a less favourable prognosis than other conversion symptoms such as astasia-abasia or fits. Of 38 patients with a diagnosis of hysterical tremor, 62% still had symptoms after 1 year and 50% still had symptoms after 5 years.

Contrary to popular belief, obvious motives for secondary gain are not typical in hysterical tremor. Only 5 of 24 patients studied by Koller *et al.* (1989) had litigation or compensation claims pending. Ljunberg (1957) stated that only a small number of hysterical patients were rendered unfit for work as a result of their symptoms. Adopting symptoms for personal gain is more indicative of malingering which, by definition, involves conscious deception. Great caution should, however, be exercised in attributing significance to a medicolegal context since this may be present in cases of organic tremor (see the section on trauma and tremor, above).

A number of studies have indicated that the majority of patients with a diagnosis of hysteria seen in neurological clinics do not conform to the histrionic personality type (Ljunberg, 1957; Chodoff and Lyons, 1958; Merksey and Trimble, 1979). This has recently been reiterated in a study of patients with hysterical tremor (Ranawaya *et al.*, 1990).

In summary, a number of features may be indicative of hysterical tremor though, with the exception of marked changes in frequency, no single feature can be considered diagnostic. Caution must be exercised in making the diagnosis since follow-up studies have shown that a high proportion of 'hysterical' patients subsequently develop an organic illness (Tissenbaum *et al.*, 1951; Slater and Glithero, 1965). Furthermore, a diagnosis of hysterical tremor does not rule out the possibility of concurrent organic tremor, which may be subconsciously exaggerated or masked by a hysterical overlay (Ranawaya *et al.*, 1990).

CASE 10

A 15-year-old schoolgirl was referred with a 12-month history of abrupt-onset, large-amplitude tremor of hands, head and legs. Tremor was intermittent but present for some part of every day. On examination, low-frequency intermittent tremor was seen. The behavioural characteristics, frequency and body part affected changed from moment to moment. Distraction completely abolished the tremor. If a tremulous body part was restrained, tremor would immediately appear in another part of the body. General and neurological examination was otherwise normal.

The patient's elder brother had been adopted and for many years had exhibited violent behaviour towards her parents, completely disrupting family life. During counselling she admitted that her tremor resulted from her 'bottled-up' feelings towards her brother, but she felt she had no control over it. Group therapy and, finally, removal of the brother into care resulted in remission of tremor.

CASE 11

A 35-year-old refuse collector gave a 6-month history of action tremor of the upper limbs since falling from his lorry during the course of his work. He described generalized bruising but there was no evidence of direct trauma to the nervous system. He was seen in an emergency department, reassured and discharged. He had not worked since the accident because of the tremor. A compensation claim was pending. There was no significant previous personal or family history. On examination he showed a distal action tremor of the upper limbs. The tremor varied in frequency from moment to moment and was completely abolished with simple distraction tasks. General and neurological examination was otherwise normal. He exhibited a *belle indifférence* and talked enthusiastically about his abilities as a guitarist. Outside the neurological department the patient was observed reading a newspaper with no sign of tremor. Referral to a psychologist was suggested. He refused and did not attend for follow-up. No medical report was requested.

References

Abramsky O, Carmon A, and Lavy S (1971) Combined treatment of parkinsonian tremor with propranolol and levodopa. *J Neurol Sci*, **14**, 491–4

Adams RD, Shahani BT, and Young RR (1972) Tremor in association with polyneuropathy. *Trans Am Neurol Assoc*, **97**, 44–8

American Psychiatric Association (1980) *Diagnostic and Statistical Manual of Mental Disorders*, 3rd edn, Washington DC, American Psychiatric Association

Andrew J, Fowler CJ, and Harrison MJ (1982) Tremor after head injury and its treatment by stereotaxic surgery. *J Neurol, Neurosurg Psychiatry*, **45**, 815–19

Barbeau A and Pourcher E (1982) New data on the genetics of Parkinson's disease. *Can J Neurol Sci*, **9**, 53–60

Barbeau A and Roy M (1984) Familial subsets in idiopathic Parkinson's disease. *Can J Neurol Sci*, **11**, 144–50

Biary N and Koller WC (1987) Essential tongue tremor. *Movement Disorders*, **2**, 25–9

Biary N, Cleeves L, Findley LJ, and Koller W (1989) Post-traumatic tremor. *Neurology*, **39**, 103–6

Brin MF, Fahn S, Bressman SB, and Burke RE (1986) Dystonia precipitated by trauma. *Neurology*, **36** (suppl 1), 119

Britton TC, Thompson PD, Van der Kamp W, Rothwell JC, Day BL, and Marsden CD (1992) Primary orthostatic tremor: further observations in six cases. *J Neurol*, **239**, 209–17

Brooks DJ, Playford ED, Ibantz V, Sawle GV, Thompson PD, Findley LJ, and Marsden CD (1992) Isolated tremor and disruption of the nigrostriatal dopaminergic system. An F^{18}-dopa PET study. *Neurology*, **42**, 1554–60

Burke RE, Fahn S, and Gold AP (1980) Delayed onset dystonia in patients with 'static' encephalopathy. *J Neurol, Neurosurg Psychiatry*, **48**, 650–2

Campbell J (1979) The shortest paper. *Neurology*, **29**, 1633

Charcot JM (1889) *Clinical Lectures on Diseases of the Nervous System*, vol 3, London, The New Sydenham Society

Chodoff P and Lyons H (1958) Hysteria, the hysterical personality and hysterical conversion. *Am J Psychiatry*, **114**, 734–40

Cleeves L and Findley LJ (1987) Variability in amplitude of untreated essential tremor. *J Neurol, Neurosurg Psychiatry*, **50**, 704–8

Cleeves L, Findley LJ, and Gresty MA (1986) Assessment of rest tremor in Parkinson's disease. In Yahr MD and Bergmann KJ, eds, *Parkinson's Disease, Advances in Neurology*, vol 45, New York, Raven, 349–52

Cleeves L, Cowan J, and Findley LJ (1988a) Orthostatic tremor: diagnostic entity or variant of essential tremor? *J Neurol, Neurosurg Psychiatry*, **52**, 130–1

Cleeves L, Findley LJ, and Koller WC (1988b) Lack of association between essential tremor and Parkinson's disease. *Ann Neurol*, **24**, 23–6

Cohen LG, Hallett M, and Sudarsky L (1987) A single family with writer's cramp, essential tremor, and primary writing tremor. *Movement Disorders*, **2**, 109–16

Cole JD, Illis LS, and Sedgwick EM (1989) Unilateral essential tremor after wrist immobilisation: a case report. *J Neurol, Neurosurg Psychiatry*, **52**, 286

Critchley M (1957) Medical aspects of boxing, particularly from a neurological standpoint. *Br Med J*, **1**, 357–62

Couch JR (1976) Dystonia and tremor in spasmodic torticollis. In Eldridge R and Fahn S, eds, *Dystonia, Advances in Neurology*, vol 14, New York, Raven, 245–58

Dalakas MC, Teravainen, and Engel WK (1984) Tremor as a feature of chronic relapsing and dysgammaglobaemic polyneuropathies. *Arch Neurol*, **41**, 711–14

De Jong H (1926) Action tremor. *J Nerv Ment Dis*, **64**, 1–11

Deuschl G, Lucking CH, and Quintern J (1987) Orthostatischer tremor: klinik, pathophysiologie und therapie. *Z EEG-EMG*, **18**, 13–19

Dupont E (1980) Parkinson's disease and essential tremor: differential diagnosis and epidemiological aspects. In Rinne UK, Klingler M, and Stamm G, eds, *Parkinson's Disease – Current Progress, Problems and Management*, Elsevier, North Holland Biomedical Press, 165–79

Dyck PJ (1975) Inherited neuronal degeneration and atrophy affecting peripheral motor, sensory and autonomic neurons. In Dyck PJ, Thomas PK, and Lambert EH, eds, *Peripheral Neuropathy*, Philadelphia, W.B. Saunders, 825–67

Elbe RJ, Moody C, and Higgins C (1990) Primary writing tremor: a form of focal dystonia? *Movement Disorders*, **5**, 118–26

Eldridge R (1970) The torsion dystonias: literature review and genetic and clinical studies. *Neurology*, **20**, 1–78

Ellison PH (1978) Propranolol for severe post-head injury action tremor. *Neurology*, **28**, 197–9

Factor SA, Sanchez-Ramos J, and Weiner WJ (1988) Trauma as an etiology of parkinsonism: a historical review of the concept. *Movement Disorders*, **3**, 30–6

Fahn S (1984) Atypical tremors, rare tremors and unclassified tremors. In Findley LJ and Capildeo R, eds, *Movement Disorders: Tremor*, 431–43

Findley LJ (1988a) Tremors: differential diagnosis and pharmacology. In Jankovic J and Tolosa E, eds, *Parkinson's Disease and Movement Disorders*, Blatimore, Urban and Schwarzenberg, 243–61

Findley LJ (1988b) Essential tremor: a clinical and pharmacological study. MD Thesis, University of Sheffield, UK

Findley LJ, Gresty MA, and Halmagyi M (1981) Tremor, the cogwheel phenomenon and clonus in Parkinson's disease. *J Neurol, Neurosurg Psychiatry*, **44**, 534–46

Findley LL, Cleeves L, and Calzetti S (1985) Primidone in essential tremor of the hands and head: a double blind controlled clinical study. *J Neurol, Neurosurg Psychiatry*, **48**, 911–15

Foster NL, Newman RP, LeWitt P *et al.* (1984) Peripheral beta-adrenergic blockage treatment of parkinsonian tremor. *Ann Neurol*, **16**, 505–8

Fung D (1981) Clonazepam in the treatment of essential tremor. *Proc World Congress Neurol*,

Gabellini AS, Martinelli P, Gulli MR, Ambrosetto G, Ciucci G, and Lugaresi E (1990) Orthostatic tremor: essential and symptomatic cases. *Acta Neurol Scand*, **81**, 113–17

Geraghty JJ, Jankovic J, and Zetusky WJ (1985) Association between essential tremor and Parkinson's disease. *Ann Neurol*, **17**, 329–33

Gresty MA and Findley LJ (1984) Definition, analysis and genesis of tremor. In Findley LJ and Capildeo R, eds, *Movement Disorders: Tremor*, London, Macmillan, 15–26

Grossman BJ (1957) Trembling of the chin – an inheritable dominant character. *Pediatrics*, **19**, 453–5

Gowers WR (1893) *A Manual of Disease of the Nervous System*, vol 2, London, J & A Churchill, 1001

Harding AE and Thomas PK (1980) Autosomal recessive forms of hereditary motor and sensory neuropathy. *J Neurol, Neurosurg Psychiatry*, **43**, 669–78

Heilman K (1984) Orthostatic tremor. *Arch Neurol*, **41**, 880–1

Herz E (1931) Die amyostatischen Unruheerscheinungen. Klinisch kinemategraphische Analyse ihrer Kennzeichen und Beleiterscheinungen. *J Psychol Neurol*, **43**, 146–63

Holmes G (1904) On certain tremors in organic cerebral lesions. *Brain*, **27**, 327–75

Jabbari B and Coker SB (1981) Paroxysmal rhythmic lingual movements and chronic epilepsy. *Neurology*, **31**, 1364–7

Jankovic J and Van der Linden C (1988) Dystonia and tremor induced by peripheral trauma: predisposing factors. *J Neurol, Neurosurg Psychiatry*, **51**, 1512–19

Kachi T, Rothwell JC, Cowan JM, and Marsden CD (1985) Writing tremor: its relationship to benign essential tremor. *J Neurol, Neurosurg Psychiatry*, **48**, 545–50

Keane JR (1984) Galloping tongue: post-taumatic, episodic, rhythmic movements. *Neurology*, **34**, 251–2

Kelly JJ and Sharbrough FW (1987) EMG in orthostatic tremor. *Neurology*, **37**, 1434

Kissel P, Tridon P, and Andre JR (1974) Levodopa-propranolol therapy in parkinsonian tremor. *Lancet*, **1**, 403–4

Klawans HL, Glantz R, Tanner CM, and Goetz CG (1982) Primary writing tremor: a selective action tremor. *Neurology*, **32**, 203–6

Koller WC (1984) Propranolol therapy for essential tremor of the head. *Neurology*, **34**, 1077–9

Koller WC and Biary NM (1989) Volitional control of involuntary movements. *Movement Disorders*, **4**, 153–6

Koller WC and Martyn B (1986) Writing tremor: its relationship to essential tremor. *J Neurol, Neurosurg Psychiatry*, **49**, 220

Koller WC and Herbster G (1987) Adjuvant therapy of parkinsonian tremor. *Arch Neurol*, **44**, 921–3
Koller WC, Glatt S, Biary N, and Rubino F (1987) Essential tremor variants: effect of treatment. *Clin Neuropharmacol*, **10**, 342–50
Koller WC, Lang A, Vetere-Overfield B, Findley L, Cleeves L, Factor S *et al.* (1989) Psychogenic tremors. *Neurology*, **39**, 1094–9
Kremer M, Russell WR, and Smyth GE (1947) A mid-brain syndrome following head injury. *J Neurol, Neurosurg Psychiatry*, **10**, 49–60
Lance JW, Schwab RS, and Peterson EA (1963) Action tremor and the cogwheel phenomenon in Parkinson's disease. *Brain*, **86**, 95–110
Lang AE, Kierans C, and Blair RD (1986) Family history of tremor in Parkinson's disease compared to controls and patients with idiopathic dystonia. In Yahr MD and Bergmann KJ, eds, *Parkinson's Disease, Advances in Neurology*, vol 45, New York, Raven, 313–16
Larsson T and Sjogren T (1960) Essential tremor. A clinical and genetic population study. *Acta Psychiatr Neurol Scand*, **36**, 1–176
Larsson T and Sjogren T (1966) Dystonia musculorum deformans. *Acta Neurol Scand*, **42** (suppl 17), 1–232
Lawrence BM, Matthews W, and Diggle JA (1968) Hereditary quivering of the chin. *Arch Dis Child*, **43**, 249–54
Lewis A (1975) The survival of hysteria. *Psychol Med*, **5**, 9–12
Ljungberg L (1957) Hysteria: a clinical, prognostic and genetic study. *Acta Psychiatr Neurol Scand*, **32** (suppl 112), 1–162
McDaniel KD, Cummings JL, and Shain S (1989) The 'yips': a focal dystonia of golfers. *Neurology*, **39**, 192–5
Marsden CD (1984) Origins of normal and pathological tremor. In Findley LJ and Capildeo R, eds, *Movement Disorders: Tremor*, London, Macmillan, 37–84
Marsden CD (1986) Hysteria – a neurologist's view. *Psychol Med*, **16**, 277–88
Marsden CD and Harrison MJG (1974) Idiopathic torsion dystonia (dystonia musculorum deformans). *Brain*, **97**, 793–810
Marsden CD, Obeso JA, Traub MM *et al.* (1984) Muscle spasms associated with Sudeck's atrophy after injury. *Br Med J*, **288**, 173–6
Marttila RJ and Rinne UK (1988) Parkinson's disease and essential tremor in families of patients with early onset Parkinson's disease. *J Neurol, Neurosurg Psychiatry*, **51**, 429–31
Marttila RJ, Rautakorpi I, and Rinne UK (1984) The relation of essential tremor to Parkinson's disease. *J Neurol, Neurosurg Psychiatry*, **47**, 734–5
Masucci EF, Kurtzke JF, and Saini N (1984) Myorhythmia: a widespread movement disorder. Clinicopathological correlations. *Brain* **107**, 53–79
Matthews WB, Howell DA, and Hughes RC (1970) Relapsing corticosteroid-dependent polyneuritis. *J Neurol, Neurosurg Psychiatry*, **33**, 330–7
Merksey H and Trimble MR (1979) Personality, sexual adjustment and brain lesions in patients with conversion symptoms. *Am J Psychiatry*, **136**, 179–82
Mitchell SW (1974) Post-paralytic chorea. *Br H Med Sci*, **68**, 342–52
Obeso JA and Narbona J (1983) Post-traumatic tremor and myoclonic jerking. *J Neurol, Neurosurg Psychiatry*, **46**, 788
Ohanna N, Peled R, Rubin AE, Zomer J, and Lavie P (1985) Periodic leg movements in sleep: effect of clonazepam treatment. *Neurology*, **35**, 408–11
Ohye C, Miyazaki M, Hirai T, Shibazaki T, Nakajima H, and Nagaseki Y (1982) Primary writing tremor treated by stereotactic surgery. *J Neurol, Neurosurg Psychiatry*, **45**, 988–97
Owen DA and Marsden CD (1965) Effect of adrenergic beta-blockage on parkinsonian tremor. *Lancet*, **2**, 1259–62
Pahwa R and Koller WC (1993) Is there a relationship between Parkinson's disease and essential tremor? *Clinical Neuropharmacol*, **16**, 30–35
Papa SM and Gershanik OS (1988) Orthostatic tremor: an essential tremor variant? *Movement Disorders*, **3**, 97–108
Patterson RM and Little SC (1943) Spasmodic torticollis. *J Nerv Ment Dis*, **98**, 571–99
Pelnar J (1913) *Das Zittern*, Berlin, Springer
Rajput AH, Jamieson H, Hirsh S, and Quraishi A (1975) Relative efficacy of alcohol and propranolol in action tremor. *Can J Neurol Sci*, **2**, 31–5
Rajput AH, Offord KP, Beard CM, and Kurland LT (1984) Essential tremor in Rochester, Minnesota: a 45-year study. *J Neurol, Neurosurg Psychiatry*, **47**, 466–70
Ranawaya R, Riley D, and Lang A (1990) Psychogenic dyskinesias in patients with organic movement disorders. *Movement Disorders*, **5**, 127–33
Rautokorpi I (1978) *Essential Tremor: an Epidemiological, Clinical and Genetic Study*. Research report

no. 12, Department of Neurology, University of Turku, Finland

Ravits J, Hallett M, Baker M, and Wilkins D (1985) Primary writing tremor and myoclonic writer's cramp. *Neurology*, **35**, 1387–91

Rivest J and Marsden CD (1990) Trunk and head tremor as isolated manifestations of dystonia. *Movement Disorders*, **5**, 60–5

Rosenberg ML and Clark JB (1987) Familial trembling of the chin. *Neurology*, **37** (suppl 1), 190

Rosenbaum R and Jankovic J (1988) Focal task-specific tremor and dystonia: categorization of occupational movement disorders. *Neurology*, **38**, 522–7

Rothwell JC (1989) Orthostatic tremor. In Quinn NP and Jenner PG, eds, *Disorders of Movement*, London, Academic Press, 521–8

Rothwell JC, Traub MM, and Marsden CD (1979) Primary writing tremor. *J Neurol, Neurosurg Psychiatry*, **42**, 1106–14

Said G, Bathien N, and Cesaro P (1982) Peripheral neuropathies and tremor. *Neurology*, **32**, 480–5

Samie MR, Selhorst JB, and Koller WC (1990) Post-traumatic midbrain tremors. *Neurology*, **40**, 62–6

Schott GD (1986) Induction of involuntary movements by peripheral trauma: an analogy with causalgia. *Lancet*, **2**, 712–16

Schwab RS and Young RR (1971) Non-resting tremor in Parkinson's disease. *Trans Am Neurol Assoc*, **96**, 305–7

Shahani BR and Young RR (1978) Action tremors: a clinical neurophysiological review. In Desmedt JE, eds, *Progress in Clinical Neurophysiology*, vol 5, Basel, Karger, 129–37

Sheehy MP and Marsden CD (1982) Writer's cramp – a focal dystonia. *Brain*, **105**, 461–80

Slater E (1965) Diagnosis of hysteria. *Br Med J*, **1**, 1395–9

Slater E and Glithero E (1965) A follow-up of patients diagnosed as suffering from hysteria. *J Psychosom Res*, **9**, 9–13

Smith IS, Kahn SN, Lacey BW, King RH, Eames RA, Whybrew DJ *et al.* (1983) Chronic demyelinating neuropathy associated with benign IgM paraproteinaemia. *Brain*, **106**, 169–95

Smith IS, Furness P, and Thomas PK (1984) Tremor in peripheral neuropathy. In Findley LJ and Capildeo R, eds, *Movement Disorders: Tremor*, London, Macmillan, 399–406

Strang RR (1965) Clinical trial with a beta-receptor antagonist (propranolol) in parkinsonism. *J Neurol, Neurosurg Psychiatry*, **28**, 404–6

Thomas PK (1975) Clinical features and differential diagnosis. In Dyck PJ, Thomas PK, and Lambert EH, eds, *Peripheral Neuropathy*, Philadelphia, W.B. Saunders, 495–512

Thomas PK, Lascelles RG, Hallpike JF, and Hewer RL (1969) Recurrent and chronic relapsing Guillain–Barre polyneuritis. *Brain*, **92**, 589–606

Thompson C, Lang A, Parkes JD, and Marsden CD (1984) A double-blind trial of clonazepam in benign essential tremor. *Clin Neuropharmacol*, **7**, 83–8

Thompson PD, Rothwell JC, Day BL, Berardelli A, Dick JP, Kachi T *et al.* (1986) The physiology of orthostatic tremor. *Arch Neurol*, **43**, 584–7

Tissenbaum MJ, Harter HM, and Friedman AP (1951) Organic neurological syndromes diagnosed as functional disorders. *JAMA*, **147**, 1519–21

Trimble MR (1981) *Neuropsychiatry*, Chichester, John Wiley

Troupin AS and Kamm RF (1974) Lingual myoclonus: a case report and review. *Dis Nerv System*, **35**, 378–80

Vas CJ (1966) Propranolol in parkinsonian tremor. *Lancet*, **1**, 182–3

Veilleux M, Sharborough SN, Kelly JJ, and Westmoreland BF (1987) Shaky-leg Syndrome. *J Clin Neurophysiol*, **4**, 304–305

Wee AS, Subramony SH, and Currier RD (1986) Orthostatic tremor in familial essential tremor. *Neurology*, **36**, 1241–5

Yanagisawa N, Goto A, and Narabayashi H (1971) Familial dystonia musculorum deformans and tremor. *J Neurol Sci*, **16**, 125–36

23
Spinal myoclonus

Peter Brown

Friedreich in 1881 first suggested that myoclonus could originate in the spinal cord, and Turtschaninow in 1894 provided the first important experimental evidence to support Friedreich's contention. Turtschaninow gave intravenous injections of 4–5% phenol solution to dogs and produced asymmetrical myoclonus which persisted after brainstem and higher spinal cord transection, and was therefore of spinal origin. Lhermitte, in 1919, established myoclonus of spinal origin as a clinical entity when he reported a case of traumatic transection of the spinal cord complicated by myoclonus below the level of the transection. The latter was later confirmed at postmortem.

Several reports of spinal myoclonus followed Lhermitte's description (Patrikios, 1938; Penfield and Jasper, 1954; Campbell and Garland, 1956; Sikes, 1959; Norris, 1965). Halliday (1967, 1975) summarized this experience of spinal myoclonus in his description of segmental myoclonus. He defined the latter as rhythmic myoclonus confined to muscles innervated by a few spinal segments and often persisting in sleep. Local spinal pathology is believed to cause enhanced cellular excitability, either due to direct cellular inflammation, or due to removal of inhibition by interneurons (Swanson *et al.*, 1962).

The spinal cord, however, possesses not only local segmental organization, but also long propriospinal pathways linking activity in many segments (Lloyd, 1942). Recently a form of more extensive myoclonus of spinal origin has been described, in which many spinal segments are involved, linked by activity in long propriospinal pathways (Brown *et al.*, 1991a).

SEGMENTAL SPINAL MYOCLONUS

Despite Halliday's careful description of segmental myoclonus (Halliday, 1967, 1975), confusion still exists over the characteristics of segmental spinal myoclonus. Thus segmental spinal myoclonus has since been described as rhythmic (Shivapour and Teasdall, 1980; Berger *et al.*, 1986; Roobol *et al.*, 1987), semirhythmic (Daniel and Webster, 1984), and even arrhythmic (Fox *et al.*, 1979; Levy *et al.*, 1983). Other authors have considered segmental spinal myoclonus as persisting in sleep (Gupta and Tandon, 1973; Levy *et al.*, 1983), or disappearing in sleep (Hoehn and Cherington,

1977; Shivapour and Teasdall, 1980). Some of this confusion has been due to the failure to establish a definite spinal aetiology in some cases of reported spinal segmental myoclonus. Indeed spinal myoclonus has been considered as myoclonus involving a few spinal segments (Swanson *et al.*, 1962), although this clearly does not exclude focal myoclonus of supraspinal origin, such as epilepsia partialis continua, or peripheral origin, as seen with lesions of the spinal roots (Sotaniemi, 1985), cervical or lumbosacral plexi (Banks *et al.*, 1985), or peripheral nerves (Said and Bathien, 1977). As such, cases of 'spinal' myoclonus have been reported where the known pathology is supraspinal (Jankovic and Pardo, 1986).

Implicit in any description of segmental spinal myoclonus must be a spinal aetiology for the jerks. Table 23.1 reviews those cases of reported segmental spinal myoclonus in whom a spinal aetiology has been reasonably established on clinical, radiological or electrophysiological grounds.

Pathophysiology

Experimental evidence indicates that all the necessary components for segmental myoclonus exist at the spinal level (Turtschaninow, 1894; Luttrell *et al.*, 1959; Kao and Crill, 1972; Lothman and Somjen, 1976). In particular, Luttrell *et al.* (1959) have shown that the rhythmic myoclonus of the hindquarters in cats, produced by inoculation of the lumbar spinal cord with Newcastle disease virus, persists after thoracic transection and intradural deafferentation of both hindlimbs. The segmental myoclonus which follows the topical application of penicillin to the spinal cord also persists after spinal transection (Kao and Crill, 1972; Lothman and Somjen, 1976).

Swanson *et al.*, in their authoritative review of myoclonus in 1962, distinguished two possible mechanisms of segmental myoclonus: enhanced neuronal excitability due to direct cellular inflammation, and enhanced neuronal excitability due to removal of inhibition. Subsequent studies have tended to support the latter hypothesis. Direct involvement of anterior horn cells has been thought unlikely, as weakness and denervation potentials are usually absent (Hopkins and Michael, 1974; Shivapour and Teasdall, 1980). Histologically, destruction of small and medium-sized neurons in the spinal cord grey matter dominates (Figs 23.1 and 23.2), and large anterior horn cells are often remarkably spared (Campbell and Garland, 1956; Howell *et al.*, 1979; Davis *et al.*, 1981). The majority of the small and medium-sized neurons in the grey matter are spinal interneurons, and it is the loss of these cells which is thought to lead to increased excitability of anterior horn cells and myoclonus. Loss of such interneurons could cause myoclonus either by removal of interneuronal inhibitory effects, as occurs in the myoclonus that follows the parenteral administration of strychnine in the spinal animal (Alvord and Fuortes, 1954), or by denervation hypersensitivity, as proposed to be responsible for palatal myoclonus (Matsuo and Ajax, 1979).

There is good evidence that the selective loss of spinal interneurons may, through increased anterior horn cell excitability, also lead to rigidity in the experimental animal (Gelfan and Tarlov, 1959, 1963) and in humans (Penry *et al.*, 1960; Rushworth *et al.*, 1961; Tarlov, 1967). However, rigidity has been reported in only a minority of cases of segmental myoclonus (Patrikios, 1938; Lourie, 1968; Whiteley *et al.*, 1976; Howell *et al.*, 1979; Roobol *et al.*, 1987). An increased anterior horn cell excitability through the selective loss of spinal interneurons also fails to explain the rhythmicity seen in the majority of cases of segmental spinal myoclonus.

Table 23.1 Characteristics of those cases of segmental myoclonus in whom clinical, electrophysiological or pathological evidence indicates a spinal origin for the myoclonus

Authors	*Aetiology*	*Distribution*	*Frequency*	*Stimulus sensitivity*	*Effect of mental stress/action*	*Effect of sleep*
Lhermitte (1919)	Traumatic transection of cord at T6–7 level (confirmed at autopsy)	Lower abdominal wall	Rhythmic 32/minute	No	N/A	N/A
Patrikios (1938)	Bullet wound to cord at C4	Right trapezius, levator scapulae, rhomboids and serratus anterior	Rhythmic 10–12/minute	No	N/A	N/A
Penfield and Jasper (1954)	Infiltrating glioma of grey matter of thoracic cord	Abdominal wall	Rhythmic 1–2/minute	N/A	N/A	N/A
Campbell and Garland (1956)	Viral spinal neuronitis (confirmed at autopsy in 2 out of 3 cases)	Initially abdominal wall and both legs. Later in course of illness more rostral muscles involved	20/minute	Yes	N/A	N/A
Sikes (1959)	Intradural extrinsic tumour at T8–9 level with compression degeneration of cord at this level (confirmed at autopsy)	Both legs	N/A	Yes	N/A	N/A
Garcin *et al.* (1968)	Cervical astrocytoma at C3–5 (confirmed at operation)	Right deltoid, biceps, supinator, triceps and diaphragm	Preoperatively: rhythmic 43/minute Postoperatively: irregular, less frequent	Yes	Amplitude increased by action and mental arithmetic	Present in sleep
Lourie (1968)	Intramedullary tumour at T10–11	Right paraspinal muscles, lower intercostal muscles, abdominal wall muscles, abductor muscles of hip and gluteus maximus	Irregular 29/minute	No	N/A	Present in sleep

Table 23.1 (continued)

Authors	*Aetiology*	*Distribution*	*Frequency*	*Stimulus sensitivity*	*Effect of mental stress/action*	*Effect of sleep*
Castaigne *et al.* (1969)	Myoclonus followed drainage of an intramedullary cyst of the cervical cord	Right biceps and triceps	Semirhythmic 10/minute	No	Amplitude increased by mental arithmetic but not by action	N/A
Robertson (1969)	Ependymoma of cervical cord	Left shoulder	Rhythmic Frequency N/A	N/A	N/A	N/A
Snyder and Appenzeller (1971)	Lower thoracic meningomyelocele	Right and left glutei and legs	Rhythmic Frequency N/A	N/A	N/A	N/A
Gupta and Tandon (1973)	Intramedullary tumour at T8–12 (confirmed at operation)	Both lower limbs and trunk below subcostal margin	Rhythmic 22–24/minute	No	N/A	Present in sleep
Hopkins and Michael (1974)	Possible viral neuronitis (suggested by CSF changes), spinal origin confirmed by latency of reflex response	Both legs	Rhythmic 100–150/minute	Yes (latency of reflex response in both gastrocnemii was about 40 ms following electrical stimulation of medial popliteal nerve)	Action had no effect	Present in sleep
Aminoff (1976)	Cervical arteriovenous malformation (confirmed at operation)	Left thumb	N/A	N/A	N/A	N/A
Whiteley *et al.* (1976) (case 2)	Progressive encephalomyelitis with rigidity (confirmed at autopsy)	Trunk and limbs	N/A	Yes	N/A	N/A
Frenken *et al.* (1976) (case 2)	Recurrent extramedullary cyst (confirmed at operation)	Right pectoral muscles, elbow and hand	Rhythmic 40–60/minute	N/A	Increased in amplitude by emotion and action	Present in sleep

Nori *et al.* (1978)	Intramedullary astrocytoma at C3–8 (confirmed at operation)	Neck left shoulder and both forearms	Rhythmic 60–100/minute	N/A	Increased in frequency by emotion and action	Absent during deeper sleep
Fox *et al.* (1979)	Spinal anaesthesia	Both legs	Irregular	N/A	N/A	N/A
Howell *et al.* (1979)	Progressive encephalomyelitis with rigidity (confirmed at autopsy)	Left arm and leg	N/A	Yes	Increased in frequency by emotion	N/A
Shivapour and Teasdall (1980)	Extradural metastasis leading to compression of cord at T3–8 (confirmed at autopsy)	Abdomen and both legs	Rhythmic 20–40/minute	No	N/A	Absent in sleep
Davis *et al.* (1981) (case 2)	Ischaemic myelopathy (confirmed at autopsy) spinal origin supported by latency of reflex response	Both legs	Semirhythmic 10–30/minute	Yes (latency of reflex response in both gastrocnemii was 42–45 ms following electrical stimulation of each posterior tibial nerve in popliteal fossa	Increased in frequency and amplitude by mental stress	Absent during deeper sleep
Levy *et al.* (1983)	Thoracic arteriovenous malformation	Thorax and upper abdomen	Paroxysmal and irregular	No	Increased by mental stress	Present in sleep
Jankovic and Pardo (1986) Case 27	Spinal extradural block	Both legs	N/A	N/A	N/A	N/A
Case 29	Cervical laminectomy for syringomyelia	Right arm	Rhythmic 240/minute	N/A	N/A	N/A
Roobol *et al.* (1987)	Paraneoplastic syndrome	Left lower leg	Rhythmic	No	N/A	N/A

CSF = Cerebrospinal fluid; N/A = not available.

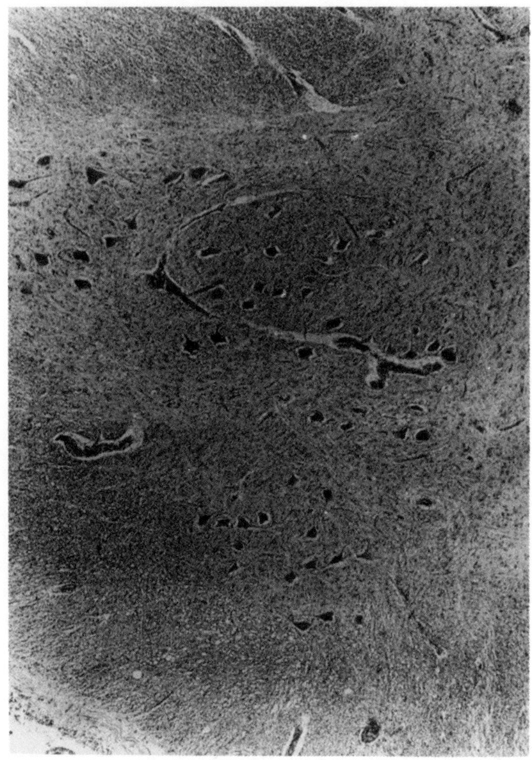

Figure 23.1 The loss of small and intermediate-sized neurons in the anterior horn of a patient with progressive encephalomyelitis with rigidity and myoclonus. The anterior horn of the fifth cervical segment was stained by Nissl's method; original magnification ×52. From Howell *et al.* (1979) with permission.

The second mechanism for segmental spinal myoclonus proposed by Swanson *et al.* (1962) involved an increase in neuronal excitability due to direct cellular injury. Dempsher *et al.* (1955) recorded spontaneous periodic burst discharges in isolated rat sympathetic ganglia infected with pseudorabies virus. The importance of this observation was twofold. Firstly, it showed that rhythmical burst discharges may be generated in the absence of neuronal loops. Secondly, the synchronous firing of neurons implied an abnormal lateral spread of activity within the ganglion. Direct injury of alpha motoneurons might also lead to rhythmic myoclonus. Histological evidence of such injury has been reported in two cases of segmental spinal myoclonus (Shivapour and Teasdall, 1980; Roobol *et al.*, 1987).

Aetiology

Spinal myoclonus may have many aetiologies. Rarely, it has been due to developmental neural tube defects (Snyder and Appenzeller, 1971), and arteriovenous malformations may present with segmental myoclonus in later life (Aminoff, 1976; Levy *et al.*, 1983). Most commonly, however, the cause is acquired. Reports of

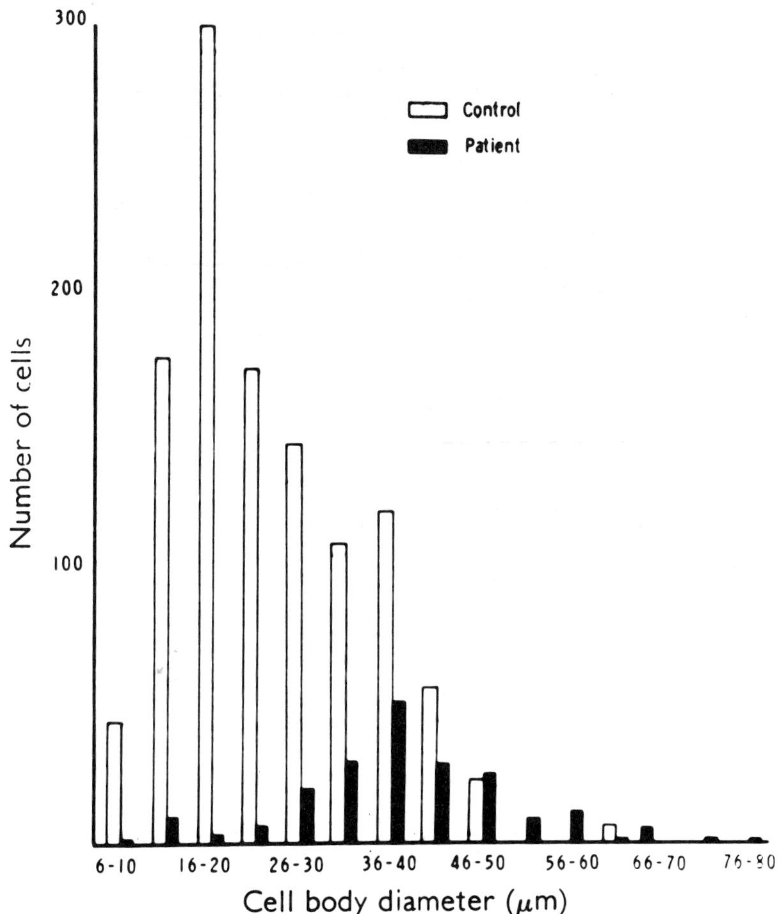

Figure 23.2 Histogram showing the numbers of neuronal perikarya of different diameters in the ventral horns in equal lengths of the eighth thoracic segment of a patient with progressive encephalomyelitis with rigidity and myoclonus, and a control patient of the same age and sex. The selective reduction in the numbers of small and medium-sized neurons, most of which are spinal internuncial neurons, may release alpha motor neurons from their normal control, and cause the myoclonus. From Howell *et al.* (1979) with permission.

intradural spinal malignancies presenting with segmental myoclonus (Penfield and Jasper, 1954; Sikes, 1959; Garcin *et al.*, 1968; Lourie, 1968; Robertson, 1969; Gupta and Tandon, 1973; Nohl *et al.*, 1978) provide clear evidence that myoclonus may be spinal in origin. In addition, compression of the spinal cord by extradural malignancies (Shivapour and Teasdall, 1980) or even paraneoplasic subacute motor neuronopathy (Roobol *et al.*, 1987) may lead to segmental myoclonus.

Extramedullary cysts may also cause spinal myoclonus. Frenken *et al.* (1976) described a case who developed spinal segmental myoclonus with recurrence of an extramedullary cyst. The myoclonus ceased following surgery to seal the communication between the cyst and the arachnoid space. Marinesco (1897) and

Norris (1965) reported spinal myoclonus as a complication of syringomyelia, although pathological proof of syringomyelia was lacking in these 2 cases. Spinal segmental myoclonus has been frequently reported as a complication of cervical spondylosis (Hoehn and Cherington, 1977; Daniel and Webster, 1984; Jankovic and Pardo, 1986), although often in the absence of significant cord compression (Daniel and Webster, 1984). Some of these cases may represent the existence of coincidental spondylosis, while others might represent the effects of spinal root compression, which itself may lead to a segmental myoclonus (Sotaniemi, 1985).

Spinal segmental myoclonus is rarely seen in vascular disease, although Davis *et al.* (1981) reported a case in whom jerking of the lower limbs developed acutely, and subsequent pathology confirmed an ischaemic myelopathy. The latter was also the proposed aetiology in a case described by Frenken *et al.* (1976), but pathological proof was lacking and there was clinical evidence of additional, suprasinal deficits.

Spinal myoclonus has also been reported in amyotrophic lateral sclerosis (Patrikios, 1951) and spinal muscular atrophy (Frenken *et al.*, 1974). Norris (1965) provided electrophysiological support for a central origin for such myoclonus in amyotrophic lateral sclerosis, by showing that synchronous spontaneous activity may occur in different muscles supplied from the same spinal segment by different peripheral nerves.

Viral infections have frequently been associated with segmental myoclonus. Walshe (1920) argued that the myoclonus seen in encephalitis lethargica originated at an anterior horn cell or peripheral nerve level in view of its association with neuralgic pains of a segmental distribution, fibrillations and weakness of a lower motor neuron type. Histological evidence that viral spinal neuronitis may cause segmental myoclonus came with the reports of subacute myoclonic spinal neuronitis by Campbell and Garland (1956), and of progressive encephalomyelitis with rigidity by Whiteley *et al.* (1976), and Howell *et al.* (1979). The virus responsible remained a mystery in these and other cases (Hopkins and Michael, 1974; Davis *et al.*, 1981). However, more recently, circumstantial evidence has accrued to implicate herpes zoster (Castaigne *et al.*, 1969; Dhaliwal and McGreal, 1974; Hoehn and Cherington, 1977; Jankovic and Pardo, 1986) and human T-lymphotrophic virus III (HTLV III) myelitis (Berger *et al.*, 1986) in some cases of segmental myoclonus.

Trauma to the spinal cord may be complicated by segmental myoclonus (Lhermitte, 1919; Patrikios, 1938). Reports of myoclonus developing after spinal surgery in patients with syringomyelia (Castaigne *et al.*, 1969; Jankovic and Pardo, 1986) and acquired immunodeficiency syndrome-related myelopathy (Jankovic and Pardo, 1986) are therefore difficult to interpret. Segmental myoclonus rarely may develop after spinal irradiation (Askenasy *et al.*, 1988). Short-lived segmental myoclonus has also been described following spinal anaesthesia (Fox *et al.*, 1979).

Clinical and electrophysiological features

Hitherto, there has been some confusion over the clinical and electrophysiological features of spinal segmental myoclonus. The following account will be based on a review of only those cases of segmental myoclonus in which there is good clinical, electrophysiological or pathological support for a spinal origin for the jerks (Table 23.1). In most cases of segmental myoclonus jerking is, as described by Halliday (1975), limited to muscles innervated by one or a few contiguous spinal segments. When these spinal segments include the fourth and fifth cervical segments, then the diaphragm is also involved (Garcin *et al.*, 1968; Sagisaka *et al.*, 1989). Occasionally the spinal pathology is extensive and many contiguous spinal segments are involved, as seen with some spinal arteriovenous malformations (Levy *et al.*, 1983) and in some cases of viral neuronitis (Campbell and Garland, 1956; Hopkins and Michael, 1974). The myoclonus may be unilateral or bilateral (Table 23.1), and may follow months after the occurrence of the causative lesion (Lhermitte, 1919; Patrikios, 1938).

Classical spinal segmental myoclonus is rhythmic (Halliday, 1967, 1975). However, cases have been reported in which the jerks are semirhythmic (Lourie, 1968; Castaigne *et al.*, 1969; Davis *et al.*, 1981) irregular (Fox *et al.*, 1979) or even paroxysmal (Levy *et al.*, 1983). The case of segmental myoclonus due to an astrocytoma of the cervical cord reported by Garcin *et al.* (1968) is particularly interesting as the jerks in the right arm were initially rhythmic (Fig. 23.3), but became irregular following surgical biopsy. In the case described by Patrikios (1938) myoclonus was rhythmic in those muscles supplied by the third to sixth cervical segments, but irregular in the hand.

In those cases in which spinal myoclonus is rhythmic, the frequency of the jerks may vary from 1–2 per minute (Penfield and Jasper, 1954) to 240 per minute (Jankovic and Pardo, 1986). Segmental myoclonus is usually synchronous bilaterally (Gupta and Tandon, 1973; Hopkins and Michael, 1974; Shivapour and Teasdall, 1980), as stated by Halliday (1975), but may be asynchronous in the contralateral limb (Davis *et al.*, 1981), or even within segments of the same limb (Nohl *et al.*, 1978). The duration of electromyogram (EMG) activity in each jerk may vary from 20 ms (Shivapour and Teasdall, 1980) to 1000 ms (Davis *et al.*, 1981).

Spinal segmental myoclonus has been considered relatively unaffected by supraspinal influences (Halliday, 1975), but several authors have reported an increase in amplitude or frequency of the jerks with action or mental stress (Garcin *et al.*, 1968; Castaigne *et al.*, 1969; Frenken *et al.*, 1976; Nohl *et al.*, 1978; Davis *et al.*, 1981; Levy *et al.*, 1983), or even sound (Sikes, 1959; Davis *et al.*, 1981). The myoclonus tends to persist in sleep, but this is not the rule, and Nohl *et al.* (1978), Shivapour and Teasdall (1980) and Davis *et al.* (1981) have reported cases in whom the myoclonus disappeared in sleep.

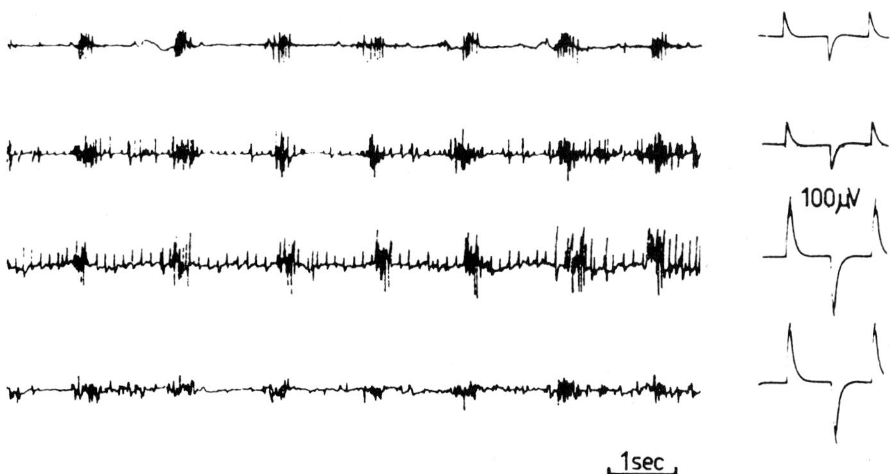

Figure 23.3 Rhythmic spinal segmental myoclonus in a patient with an astrocytoma of the cervical cord. From Garcin *et al.* (1968) with permission.

Spinal segmental myoclonus has also been considered relatively unaffected by peripheral afferent information (Halliday, 1967; Hoehn and Cherington, 1977; Daniel and Webster, 1984), but both Hopkins and Michael (1974), and Davis *et al.* (1981) have provided evidence for stimulus sensitivity, with reflex responses of short latency in some cases (Fig. 23.4). Stimulus sensitivity was also a feature of the jerks reported in subacute myoclonic spinal neuronitis (Campbell and Garland, 1956), and in progressive encephalomyelitis with rigidity (Whiteley *et al.*, 1976; Howell *et al.*, 1979), although this was not studied electrophysiologically. Sikes (1959) reported dramatic stimulus sensitivity in a case of spinal myoclonus due to an intradural tumour. Sagisaka *et al.* (1989) have suggested that stimulus sensitivity in segmental spinal myoclonus may be masked when the duration of the refractory period is close to the interval between spontaneous jerks. They reported a case in whom stimulus sensitivity was only apparent once the frequency of the segmental myoclonus was reduced with medication.

Treatment

The treatment of segmental spinal myoclonus is that of the underlying cause, where this is possible. This may abolish the jerks (Frenken *et al.*, 1976; Daniel and Webster, 1984; Roobol *et al.*, 1987). When definitive treatment is not possible, or the aetiology elusive despite investigation, then symptomatic treatment is moderately effective.

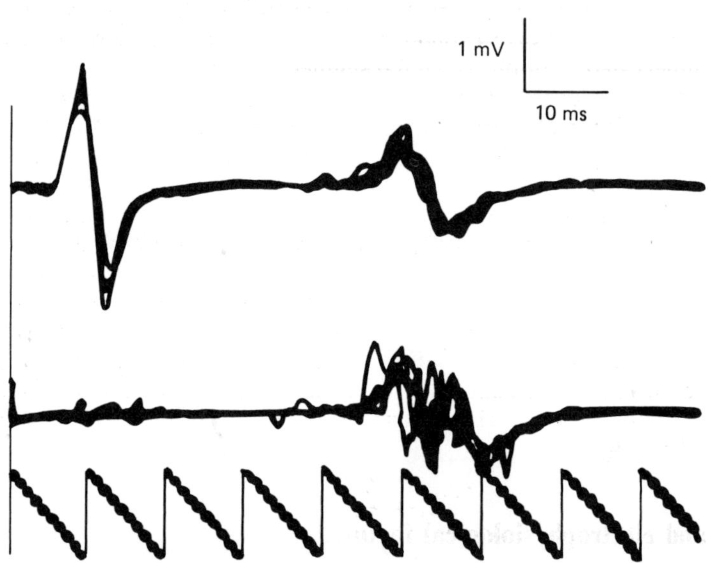

Figure 23.4 Stimulus-sensitive myoclonus in a patient with ischaemic myelopathy. Following electrical stimulation of the right posterior tibial nerve in the popliteal fossa an early ipsilateral direct (M) response and a later bilateral reflex response were recorded in the gastrocnemeii. At the same time widespread myoclonic jerking occurred in both legs. The short latency of this reflex myoclonic response (44 ms) indicates conduction through a pathway confined to the spinal cord. From Davis *et al.* (1981) with permission.

Clonazepam is the drug of first choice and, in dosages up to 6 mg daily, may diminish or completely abolish the myoclonus (Hoehn and Cherington, 1977; Shivapour and Teasdall, 1980; Davis *et al.*, 1981; Levy *et al.*, 1983; Jankovic and Pardo, 1986). Diazepam, in dosages up to 30 mg daily (Hopkins and Michael, 1974), carbamazepine in dosages up to 1000 mg daily (Askenasy *et al.*, 1988) and tetrabenazine, in dosages up to 200 mg daily (Hoehn and Cherington, 1977; Jankovic and Pardo, 1986), may also be effective.

SUMMARY

A review of those cases with clinical, electrophysiological or pathological evidence indicating a spinal origin for repetitive myoclonic jerking in muscles innervated by a single or several contiguous spinal segments, suggests that not all cases of segmental spinal myoclonus conform to Halliday's original description (1967). In particular, irregularity in rhythm, response to supraspinal influences and stimulus sensitivity do not mitigate against a spinal origin.

PROPRIOSPINAL MYOCLONUS

A second type of spinal myoclonus has recently been described, which is not segmental in distribution, but involves activity over extensive lengths of the spinal cord (Bussel *et al.*, 1988; Brown *et al.*, 1991a,b). Myoclonic activity is thought to spread up and down the length of the spinal cord via long propriospinal pathways intrinsic to the cord (Brown *et al.*, 1991a). A spinal generator at one level is therefore able to recruit muscles innervated by multiple spinal segments.

Experimental evidence that activity in propriospinal pathways could underlie an extensive form of spinal myoclonus has been provided by Luttrell *et al.* (1959). They showed that the intraspinal inoculation of Newcastle disease virus in cats led, initially, to segmental myoclonus at the level of the injection, followed later by the development of generalized rhythmical myoclonus. Spinospinal pathways, rather than viral spread, were thought to mediate the development of this generalized rhythmical myoclonus, since the myoclonus in segments rostral to a lower thoracic inoculation site, or caudal to a cervical inoculation site, was abolished by thoracic spinal cord transection. The myoclonus in this animal model persisted after high cervical cord transection, confirming a spinal origin for the jerks. Interestingly, in some animals the generalized rhythmic myoclonic movements took the form of quasi-locomotory movements, with flexor movements in the forelimbs being succeeded immediately by extensor thrust of the hindlimbs.

Clinical and electrophysiological features

The first report of an extensive form of spinal myoclonus in humans was that of Bussel *et al.* in 1988. They described a patient in whom rhythmic extension movements of the trunk and lower limbs supervened 15 months after a spinal cord injury. At times the involuntary jerks were rigorous enough to propel the patient from his bed or wheelchair. The myoclonus was spontaneous, and sensitive to stimuli applied to the trunk or legs. It was absent during sleep. Clinical evidence and magnetic resonance imaging indicated complete spinal cord transection at the level of the lower cervical cord. EMG recordings showed that the myoclonus had a frequency of 0.3–0.6 Hz, and was bilaterally symmetrical. The relative onset latencies of the bursts of EMG activity in different muscles were not measured, but the phase shift between the activity in different muscles remained fixed, implying that the myoclonus was due to the rhythmic discharge of a single spinal generator. Mechanical or electrical stimulation of flexor reflex afferents could induce, slow or interrupt the rhythmic activity. Interestingly, when stimulation of flexor reflex afferents induced a flexion reflex, it occurred between extensor EMG bursts, and induced alternating flexion-extension activity, which could last for several cycles. The myoclonus was completely controlled by treatment with carbamazepine and sodium valporate. A spontaneous and sustained remission occurred several months later.

The report by Bussel *et al.* (1988) provided clear evidence that the isolated spinal cord in humans is capable of generating myoclonic movements of a more extensive distribution and complex nature than simple segmental myoclonus. We have since studied 5 cases of axial myoclonus of spinal origin in intact humans (Table 23.2). These differed from the case reported by Bussel *et al.* (1988) in that the myoclonus was non-rhythmic, and led to axial flexion, rather than extension. In one of these 5 cases, axial myoclonus developed following excision of a cervical haemangioblastoma, and worsened during subsequent distortion of the cervical cord by dural adhesions. The latter were confirmed during surgical exploration, and division of the dural adhesions led to a marked improvement in the spinal myoclonus. The aetiology of the axial myoclonus was unknown in the remaining 4 cases, although in 1 patient (case 5, Table 23.2) the myoclonus developed 3 weeks after a blow to the neck. In all 5 of the cases myoclonic jerks were repetitive and caused symmetrical, often violent, axial flexion. This involved flexion of the neck, trunk, hips and knees in cases 1, 2, 3 and 4 (Table 23.2), and of the neck and trunk in case 5. The jerks were spontaneous, and often occurred in sleep. They were more pronounced when supine in 3 of the patients. The axial jerks could also be elicited by taps to the trunk and limbs in 4 of the cases. The myoclonus partially improved on treatment with clonazepam or carbamazepine, but spontaneous remissions were not seen.

Electrophysiologically, the jerks were very similar between patients (Brown *et al.*, 1991a). They consisted of irregular bursts of EMG activity in the axial musculature, occurring up to twice per second, with a duration varying between 40 ms and 4 seconds. Homologous muscles were activated synchronously bilaterally and co-contraction was evident in agonist and antagonist muscle pairs. Four of the 5 patients were stimulus-sensitive. The latency of the most marked reflex response was long, with EMG activity being recorded about 100 ms after taps to the limbs or trunk in cases 2, 3 and 5, and even later in case 4. Long reflex latencies do not exclude a spinal origin for the jerks, and spinal reflex latencies up to 450 ms have been reported in patients with cord transections (Shahani and Young, 1971; Roby-Brami and Bussel, 1987). Two of the cases also exhibited a reflex response of short latency in the abdominal recti (Fig. 23.5). EMG activity was recorded in the abdominal recti about 35 ms after a tap to the left abdomen or neck in cases 3 and 5 respectively. In case 5 sustained passive or active flexion or lateral rotation of the neck led to an increase in frequency and amplitude of spontaneous myoclonus. Nohl *et al.* (1978) reported a similar effect of neck flexion on spontaneous spinal segmental myoclonus in a patient with a cervical astrocytoma.

The most striking feature of the myoclonus was the pattern of muscle recruitment in both spontaneous and stimulus-sensitive jerks. In 4 of the 5 cases the order of

Table 23.2 Propriospinal myoclonus

Source	*Aetiology*	*Clinical features*	*Stimulus sensitivity*	*Effect of posture*	*Order of recruitment of muscles in the jerk*
Bussel *et al.* (1988)	Trauma leading to cervical cord transection	Rhythmic extension jerks below level of cord transection	Yes	N/A	N/A
Brown *et al.* (1991a) Case 1	Unknown	Arrhythmic axial flexion jerks	None	Increased in frequency and amplitude when supine	Muscles recruited up and down cord from myoclonic generator in the lower half of thoracic cord
Case 2	Distortion of cervical cord by dural adhesions following excision of a cervical haemangioblastoma	Arrhythmic axial flexion jerks	Yes	None	Muscles recruited up and down cord from a myoclonic generator near the cervicothoracic junction
Case 3	Unknown	Arrhythmic axial flexion jerks	Yes	Increased in frequency and amplitude when supine	Muscles recruited up and down cord from a myoclonic generator in the lower half of thoracic cord
Brown *et al.* (1991b) Case 4	Cervical myeloradiculopathy of unknown cause	Paroxysmal axial flexion jerks giving the clinical appearance of spasms of jerky truncal flexion	Yes	None	N/A
Previously unreported (Case 5)	Unknown	Arrhythmic axial flexion jerks with prominent diaphragmatic involvement	Yes	Increased in frequency and amplitude when supine or with flexion of the neck	Muscles recruited up and down cord from a high thoracic myoclonic generator

N/A = Not available.

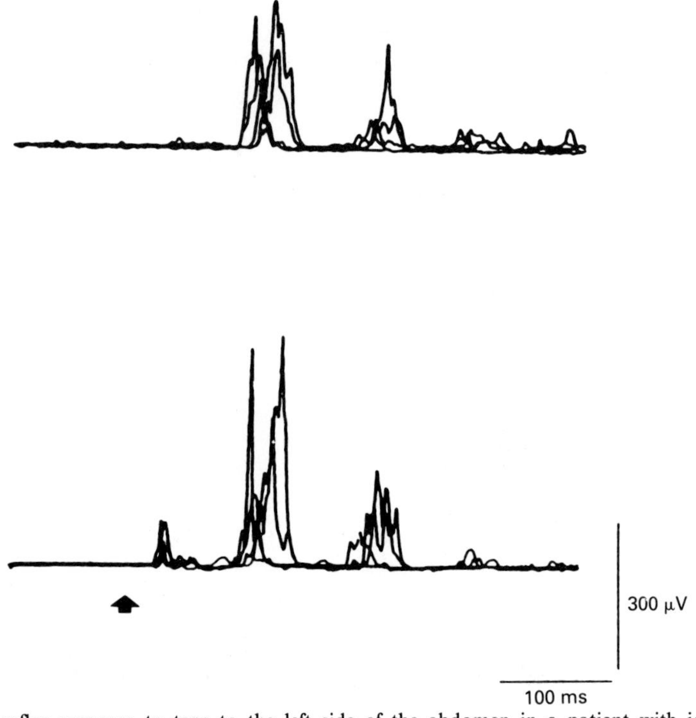

Figure 23.5 The reflex response to taps to the left side of the abdomen in a patient with idiopathic propriospinal myoclonus. Taps to this site evoked a response at about 33 ms in the left rectus abdominis, evident as the first electromyogram (EMG) burst in the lower trace. Taps to the abdomen also elicited a later response in both recti at about 100 ms, followed by smaller and less consistent repetitive discharges. The superimposed rectified EMG records of the responses to five taps (given at 100 ms at arrow) to the left abdomen are illustrated. From Brown *et al.* (1991a) with permission.

recruitment of muscles during the jerks suggested that the myoclonic discharge spread up and down the spinal cord from a spinal generator (Fig. 23.6). In cases 1 and 3 (Table 23.2), EMG activity was first recorded in the abdominal recti during each jerk, indicating that the myoclonic discharge arose in the lower half of the thoracic spinal cord. Muscles with more rostral and caudal segmental innervations were then recruited later in an orderly fashion. In cases 2 and 5, the pattern of muscle recruitment in the reflex jerks indicated that the myoclonic discharge arose near the cervicothoracic junction. In each case the difference in relative latencies of muscles innervated by different spinal segments indicated that the conduction velocity in the spinal efferent pathways subserving the axial myoclonus was slow.

Pathophysiology

Thus axial myoclonus, involving multiple segments of the spinal cord, may have a spinal origin in humans. We have previously suggested that such myoclonus is subserved by long propriospinal systems intrinsic to the cord (Brown *et al.*, 1991a). Histological (Giok, 1958; Nathan *et al.*, 1990) and electrophysiological (Kearney and

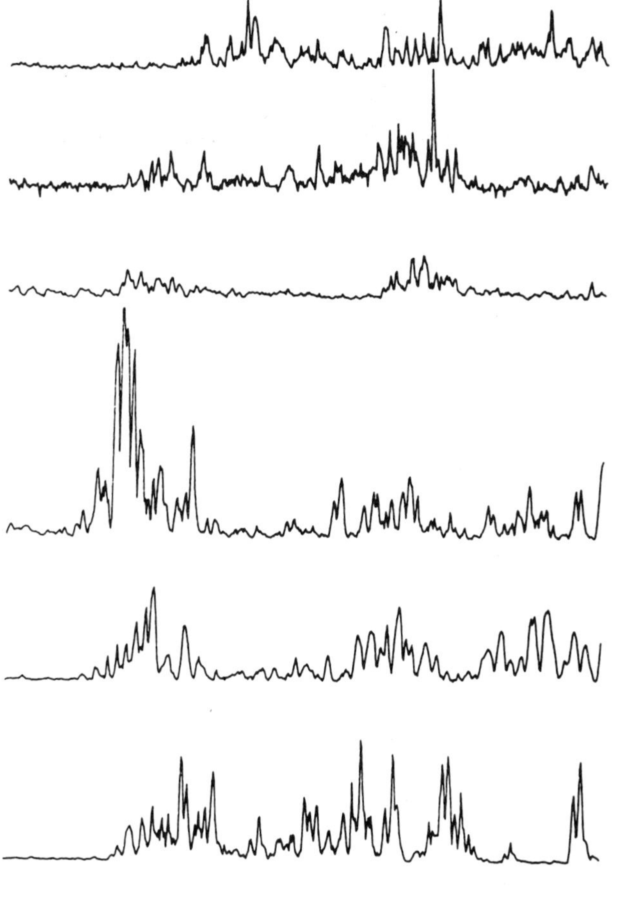

Figure 23.6 The rectified electromyogram of a single spontaneous jerk in a patient with idiopathic propriospinal myoclonus. Myoclonic activity is recorded first in the rostral aspect of rectus abdominis, and then spreads slowly to muscles innervated by more rostral and caudal spinal segments. This pattern of muscle recruitment indicates a spinal origin for the myoclonus in this patient. The vertical calibration line represents 200 μV and 100 μV for the bottom and top three channels respectively. The horizontal calibration line represents 50 ms. From Brown *et al.* (1991a) with permission.

Chan, 1979; Meinck and Piesiur-Strehlow, 1981) evidence suggests that such propriospinal pathways may exist in humans, although these pathways have been most extensively investigated in the cat. In the latter, long propriospinal pathways originate in the cervical (Lloyd, 1942; Jankowska *et al.*, 1974; Vasilenko, 1975) or mid thoracic (Baldissera *et al.*, 1972) segments and project to lumbar segments, or originate in lumbar segments and project rostrally (Gernandt and Megirian, 1961; Barilari and Kuypers, 1969; Miller *et al.*, 1973). These long propriospinal pathways are similar in character to those subserving axial spinal myoclonus in humans. They are relatively slowly conducting (Lloyd, 1942), and recruit mainly trunk (Baldissera *et al.*, 1972) and proximal limb (Vasilenko, 1975) motoneurons bilaterally (Barilari and Kuypers, 1969), without a reciprocal action upon antagonists (Lloyd, 1942; Vasilenko, 1975). In addition, long cervical propriospinal neurons receive very large vestibular and proprioceptive inputs in the cat (Alstermark *et al.*, 1987a,b). Axial spinal myoclonus is often sensitive to postural influences.

Long propriospinal pathways are particularly suited to a role in the spinal organization of locomotion, as the pattern of the response generated by propriospinal projections varies systematically with limb position (Grillner and Rossignol, 1978) in static situations, and with the phase of the step cycle during locomotion (Forssberg *et al.*, 1977; Miller *et al.*, 1977). The isolated spinal cord itself can generate rhythmic locomotory movements in animals (Grillner, 1975; Miller and Van der Meche, 1976), and Bussel *et al.* (1988) speculated that the rhythmic axial myoclonus seen in their patient was due to the partial release of a central rhythmic stepping generator.

CONCLUSION

Halliday (1967, 1975) defined spinal segmental myoclonus as rhythmic myoclonus confined to muscles innervated by a few spinal segments and often persisting in sleep. He believed such spinal myoclonus to be unresponsive to supraspinal influences or peripheral stimulation. However, a review of those cases in whom clinical, electrophysiological or pathological evidence indicates a spinal origin for repetitive myoclonic jerking of segmental distribution suggests that the concept of spinal segmental myoclonus should be expanded. Focal myoclonus of spinal origin may be rhythmic or arrhythmic, may persist or disappear in sleep, and may or may not respond to supraspinal influences and peripheral stimulation.

In addition, Brown *et al.* (1991a) have recently proposed a second type of spinal myoclonus. This propriospinal myoclonus consists of predominantly axial and often arrhythmic flexor or extensor jerks involving many spinal segments linked by long propriospinal pathways. The expansion of the concept of spinal myoclonus means that a spinal origin should be considered in any segmental or axial myoclonus. Recognition of the varied forms of spinal myoclonus, however, also means that diagnosis is seldom possible on the basis of clinical features alone, and comprehensive electrophysiological investigation and imaging studies are always necessary.

References

Alstermark B, Lundberg A, Pinter M, and Sasaki S (1987a) Vestibular effects in long C3–C5 propriospinal neurones. *Brain Res, Amsterdam*, **404**, 388–94

Alstermark B, Lundberg A, Pinter M, and Sasaki S (1987b) Long C3–C5 propriospinal neurones in the cat. *Brain Res, Amsterdam*, **404**, 382–8

Alvord EC and Fuortes MGF (1954) A comparison of generalised reflex myoclonic reactions elicitable in cats under chloralose anaesthesia and under strychnine. *Am J Physiol*, **176**, 253–61

Aminoff MJ (1976) *Spinal Angiomas*, Oxford, Blackwell Scientific Publications

Askenasy JJM, Brunet P, Leger JM, Bouche P, Lafont F, Cathala HP *et al.* (1988) Postradiation segmental myoclonus selectively inhibited by REM sleep (sleep-wake myoclonus). *Eur Neurol*, **28**, 317–20

Baldissera F, Lundberg A, and Udo M (1972) Activity evoked from the mesencephalic tegmentum in descending pathways other than the rubrospinal tract. *Exp Brain Res*, **15**, 133–50

Banks G, Nielsen VK, Short MP, and Kowal CD (1985) Brachial plexus myoclonus. *J Neurol, Neurosurg Psychiatry*, **48**, 582–4

Barilari MG and Kuypers HGJM (1969) Propriospinal fibres interconnecting the spinal enlargements in the cat. *Brain Res, Amsterdam*, **14**, 321–30

Berger JR, Bender A, Resnick L, and Perlmutter D (1986) Spinal myoclonus associated with HTLV III/LAV infection. *Arch Neurol*, **43**, 1203–4
Brown P, Thompson PD, Rothwell JC, Day BL, and Marsden CD (1991a) Axial myoclonus of propriospinal origin. *Brain* **114**, 197–214
Brown P, Thompson PD, Rothwell JC, Day BL, and Marsden CD (1991b) Paroxysmal axial spasms of spinal origin. *Movement Disorders*, **VI**, 43–8
Bussel B, Roby-Brami A, Azouvi PH, Biraben A, Yakovleff A, and Held JP (1988) Myoclonus in a patient with spinal cord transection. *Brain*, **111**, 1235–45
Campbell AMG and Garland H (1956) Subacute myoclonic spinal neuronitis. *J Neurol, Neurosurg Psychiatry*, **19**, 268–74
Castaigne P, Cambier J, Laplane D, Cathala HP, Brunet P, and Pierrot-Deselligny E (1969) Myoclonies rhythmees segmentaires d'origine medullaire: a propos de deux observations. *Rev Oto-Neuro-Ophthal*, **41**, 241–50
Daniel GD and Webster DL (1984) Spinal segmental myoclonus: successful treatment with cervical spinal decompression. *Arch Neurol*, **41**, 898–9
Davis SM, Murray NMF, Diengdoh JV, Galea-Debono A, and Kocen RS (1981) Stimulus-sensitive spinal myoclonus. *J Neurol, Neurosurg Psychiatry*, **44**, 884–8
Dempsher J, Larrabee MG, Bang FB, and Bodian D (1955) Physiological changes in sympathetic ganglia infected with pseudorabies virus. *Am J Physiol*, **182**, 203–16
Dhaliwal GS and McGreal DA (1974) Spinal myoclonus in association with herpes zoster infection: two case reports. *Can J Neurol Sci*, **1**, 239–40
Fox EJ, Villaneuva R, and Schutta HS (1979) Myoclonus following spinal anaesthesia. *Neurology*, **29**, 379–80
Forssberg H, Grillner S, and Rossignol S (1977) Phasic gain control of reflexes from the dorsum of the paw during spinal locomotion. *Brain Res, Amsterdam*, **132**, 121–39
Frenken CWGM, Korten JJ, Gabreels FJM, and Joosten EMG (1974) Spinal myoclonus. *Clin Neurol Neurosurg*, **77**, 44–53
Frenken CWGM, Notermans SLH, Korten JJ, and Horstink MWIM (1976) Myoclonic disorders of spinal origin. *Clin Neurol Neurosurg*, **79**, 107–18
Friedreich N (1881) Neuropathologische beobachtungen. I. Paramyoklonus multiplex. *Virch Archiv Pathol Anat Physiol Klin*, **86**, 4211–30
Garcin R, Rondot P, and Guiot G (1968) Rhythnic myoclonus of the right arm as the presenting symptom of a cervical cord tumour. *Brain*, **91**, 75–84
Gelfan S and Tarlov IM (1959) Interneurones and rigidity of spinal origin. *J Physiol, Lond*, **146**, 594–617
Gelfan S and Tarlov IM (1963) Altered neuron population in L7 segment of dogs with experimental hind-limb rigitity. *Am J Physiol*, **205**, 606–16
Gernandt BE and Megirian D (1961) Ascending propriospinal mechanisms. *J Neurophysiol*, **24**, 364–76
Giok SP (1958) The fasciculus intermediolateralis of Loewenthal in man. *Brain*, **81**, 577–87
Grillner S (1975) Locomotion in vertebrates: central mechanisms and reflex interaction. *Physiol Rev*, **55**, 247–304
Grillner S and Rossignol S (1978) Contralateral reflex reversal controlled by limb position in the acute spinal cat injected with clonidine i.v. *Brain Res, Amsterdam*, **144**, 411–14
Gupta PC and Tandon PN (1973) Rhythmic myoclonus of spinal origin. *Ind J Med Sci*, **27**, 31–5
Halliday AM (1967) The electrophysiological study of myoclonus in man. *Brain*, **90**, 241–84
Halliday AM (1975) The neurophysiology of myoclonic jerking – a reappraisal. In Charlton HH, ed, *Myoclonic Seizures*, Excerpta Medica International Congress Series, vol 307, Amsterdam, Excerpta Medica, 1–29
Hoehn MM and Cherington M (1977) Spinal myoclonus. *Neurology*, **27**, 942–6
Hopkins AP and Michael WF (1974) Spinal myoclonus. *J Neurol, Neurosurg Psychiatry*, **37**, 1112–15
Howell DA, Lees AJ, and Toghill PJ (1979) Spinal internuncial neurones in progressive encephalomyelitis with rigidity. *J Neurol, Neurosurg Psychiatry*, **42**, 773–85
Jankovic J and Pardo R (1986) Segmental myoclonus. *Arch Neurol*. **43**, 1025–31
Jankowska E, Lundberg A, Roberts WJ, and Stuart D (1974) A long propriospinal system with direct effect on motoneurones and on interneurones in the cat lumbosacral cord. *Exp Brain Res*, **21**, 169–94
Kao LI and Crill WE (1972) Penicillin-induced segmental myoclonus: I. Motor responses and intracellular recording from motoneurons. *Arch Neurol*, **26**, 156–61
Kearney RE and Chan CWY (1979) Reflex response of human arm muscles to cutaneous stimulation of the foot. *Brain Res, Amsterdam*, **170**, 214–17
Levy R, Plassche W, Riggs J, and Shoulson I (1983) Spinal myoclonus related to an arteriovenous malformation: response to clonazepam therapy. *Arch Neurol*, **40**, 254–5
Lhermitte J (1919) *La section totale de la moelle dorsale*, Bourges, Tardy Pigelet

Lloyd DPC (1942) Mediation of descending long spinal reflex activity. *J Neurophysiol*, **5**, 435–58
Lothman EW and Somjen GG (1976) Motor and electrical signs of epileptiform activity induced by penicillin in the spinal cords of decapitate cats. *Electroencephalogr Clin Neurophysiol*, **41**, 237–52
Lourie H (1968) Spontaneous activity of alpha motor neurons in intramedullary spinal cord tumour. *J Neurosurg*, **29**, 573–80
Luttrell CN, Bang FB, and Luxenberg K (1959) Newcastle disease encephalomyelitis in cats. II. Physiological studies on rhythmic myoclonus. *Arch Neurol Psychiatry, Chicago*, **81**, 285–91
Marinesco G (1897) On the existence of clonic movements during the cause of syringomyelia. *Sem Med*, **17**, 324
Matsuo F and Ajax ET (1979) Palatal myoclonus and denervation supersensitivity in the cental nervous system. *Ann Neurol*, **5**, 72–8
Miller S and Van der Meche FGA (1976) Coordinated stepping of all four limbs in the high spinal cat. *Brain Res, Amsterdam*, **109**, 395–8
Miller S, Reitsma DJ, and Van der Meche FGA (1973) Functional organisation of long ascending propriospinal pathways linking lumbosacral and cervical segments in the cat. *Brain Res, Amsterdam*, **62**, 169–88
Miller S, Ruit JB, and Van der Meche FGA (1977) Reversal of sign of long spinal reflexes dependent on the phase of the step cycle in the high decerebrate cat. *Brain Res, Amsterdam*, **128**, 447–59
Nathan PW, Smith MC, and Deacon P (1990) The corticospinal tracts in man: course and location of fibres at different segmental levels. *Brain*, **113**, 303–24
Nohl M, Doose H, Gross-Selbeck G, and Jensen H (1978) Spinal myoclonus. *Eur Neurol*, **17**, 129–35
Norris FH (1965) Synchronous fasciculation in motor neuron disease. *Arch Neurol*, **13**, 405–500
Patrikios MJ (1938) Sur un cas d'automatisme moteur particulier des membres superieurs apres traumatisme de la moelle cervicale. *Rev Neurol*, **69**, 179–88
Patrikios MJ (1951) Sclerose laterale amyotrophiques avec mouvement involuntaire des doights et du poignet gauches de caractere extrapyramidal. *Rev Neurol*, **85**, 60–2
Penfield W and Jasper H (1954) *Epilepsy and the Functional Anatomy of the Human Brain*, Boston: Little, Brown
Penry JK, Hoefnagel D, Van den Noort S, and Denny-Brown D (1960) Muscle spasm and abnormal postures resulting from damage to interneurones in spinal cord. *Arch Neurol*, **34**, 500–12
Robertson (1969) *Proc Aust Assoc Neurol*, **6**, 69
Roby-Brami A and Bussel B (1987) Long latency spinal reflex in man after flexor reflex afferent stimulation. *Brain*, **110**, 707–25
Roobol TH, Kazzaz BA, and Vecht ChJ (1987) Segmental rigidity and spinal myoclonus as a paraneoplastic syndrome. *J Neurol, Neurosurg Psychiatry*, **50**, 628–31
Rushworth G, Lishman WA, Hughes JT, and Oppenheimer DR (1961) Intense rigidity of the arms due to isolation of motoneurones by a spinal tumour. *J Neurol, Neurosurg Psychiatry*, **24**, 132–42
Sagisaka H, Kakigi R, Shibasaki H, Oda K, and Kuroda Y (1989) A case of stimulus-sensitive segmental spinal myoclonus. *Clin Neurol, Jpn*, **29**, 310–14
Said G and Bathien N (1977) Myoclonies rhythmees du quadriceps en relation avec un envasalessment sarcomateux du nerf crural. *Rev Neurol, Paris*, **133**, 191–8
Shahani BT and Young RR (1971) Human flexor reflexes. *J Neurol, Neurosurg Psychiatry*, **34**, 616–27
Shivapour E and Teasdall RD (1980) Spinal myoclonus with vacuolar degeneration of anterior horn cells. *Arch Neurol*, **37**, 451–3
Sikes ZS (1959) Stiff-man syndrome. *Dis Nerv System*, **20**, 254–8
Snyder RD and Appenzeller O (1971) Segmental myoclonus in meningomyelocele. *Trans Am Neurol Assoc*, **96**, 97–8
Sotaniemi KA (1985) Paraspinal myoclonus due to spin root lesion. *J Neurol, Neurosurg Psychiatry*, **48**, 723–4
Swanson PD, Luttrell CN, and Magladery JW (1962) Myoclonus – a report of 67 cases and review of the literature. *Medicine, Baltimore*, **41**, 339–56
Tarlov IM (1967) Rigidity in man due to spinal interneuron loss. *Arch Neurol*, **16**, 536–43
Turtschaninow P (1894) Experimentelle studien uber den ursprungsort einiger klinisch wichtiger toxischer krampfformen. *Arch Exp Pathol Pharmalol* (*Leipzig*), **34**, 208–46
Vasilenko DA (1975) Propriospinal pathways in the ventral funicles of the cat spinal cord: their effects on lumbosacral motoneurones. *Brain Res, Amsterdam*, **93**, 502–6
Walshe FMR (1920) On the symptom-complexes of lethargic encephalitis with special reference to involuntary muscular contractions. *Brain*, **43**, 197–219
Whiteley AM, Swash M, and Urich H (1976) Progressive encephalomyelitis with rigidity: its relationship to 'subacute myoclonic spinal neuronitis' and to the 'stiff-man syndrome'. *Brain*, **99**, 27–42

24
Botulinum toxin therapy*

P. Greene, S. Fahn, M. F. Brin and A. Blitzer

INTRODUCTION

Botulinum toxin type A (BTX-A) has provided a dramatically effective therapy for many focal dystonias. Although it was first used for the treatment of childhood strabismus (Scott, 1980), it is most commonly used today in the treatment of focal dystonia. It has also been used to treat other hyperkinetic movement disorders such as hemifacial spasm (see below), synkineses developing after Bell's palsy (Biglan *et al.*, 1988), myokymia (Ruusuvaara and Setala, 1990), muscle spasm in multiple sclerosis and stroke (see below), tremor (Jankovic and Schwartz, 1991a), and other involuntary facial movements (e.g. benign lid fasciculations; Kraft and Lang, 1988). In addition to treating movement disorders and strabismus, the use of botulinum toxin injections has been reported in the treatment of endocrine orbital myopathy (Scott, 1984), lateral rectus palsy (Scott and Kraft, 1985), entropion (Carruthers and Stubbs, 1987), to induce 'protective ptosis' in corneal ulceration (Adams *et al.*, 1987), detrusor-sphincter dyssynergia (Dykstra and Sidi, 1990), anismus in intractable constipation (Hallan *et al.*, 1988) and nystagmus (Helveston and Pogrebniak, 1988). Botox injections have also been used to treat 'apraxia of eyelid opening' in parkinsonism which, although not strictly speaking a hyperkinetic disorder, seems to respond to injections in a manner similar to that of blepharospasm (see below).

Several investigators had suggested treating strabismus by chemically weakening extraocular muscles, but Scott and colleagues were the first to test this approach in an animal model (Scott *et al.*, 1973). Using rhesus monkeys as a model, they located the extraocular muscles using electromyogram (EMG) under ketamine anaesthesia and injected varying doses of alcohol, di-isopropyl-fluorophosphate, alpha-bungarotoxin and BTX. Only BTX produced weakness of the muscles without severe local or systemic toxicity. Scott *et al.* speculated that the technique might prove valuable in treating strabismus, endocrine exophthalmos, blepharospasm and skeletal muscle hyperactivity (Scott *et al.*, 1973). Medical use of botulinum toxin was first reported by Scott (1980), who used injections of BTX-A to correct strabismus in children.

* BTX refers to generic botulinum toxins. BTX-A refers to type A botulinum toxin. BOTOX® refers to type A BTX produced by Allergen, Inc USA. DYSPORT® refers to type A BTX produced by Porton Downs, UK. Trade names are used when specific dosages are reported. See also p. 478

BIOCHEMISTRY AND PHARMACOLOGY

There are seven antigenically distinct neurotoxins produced by strains of *Clostridium botulinum*. All types of the neurotoxin act on the presynaptic cholinergic nerve terminal to inhibit the release of acetylcholine. Type A toxin is the most potent: it has been estimated that no more than several hundred molecules of type A toxin are necessary to block neuromuscular transmission at a synapse (Hanig and Lamanna, 1979). If this is the case, neuromuscular blockade results from about one molecule of botulinum toxin at each presynaptic release site (Hanig and Lamanna, 1979). The duration of action of the toxins is also extremely long, from 3 to 6 months for type A. The action of the toxin at the neuromuscular junction has been intensively studied, but the exact mechanism of action is still not clearly understood. Calcium-mediated quantal release of acetylcholine is dramatically reduced by botulinum toxin, but calcium entry into the terminal is probably not affected (Kao *et al.*, 1976). The toxin seems to desensitize the release process to the presence of intracellular calcium (Simpson, 1986). Toxin injected into muscle is also transported centrally into the spinal cord and can bind to brain synaptosomes (Habermann, 1974), although the functional significance of this is not known (Simpson, 1986).

The structure of botulinum toxins is known in detail for type A, and the other types appear to have similar structure. Type A toxin consists of a 150 kDa neurotoxin moiety, a 150 kDa non-toxic protein and a 200–400 kDa haemagglutinin (Hambleton *et al.*, 1987). The non-toxic associated proteins are necessary to stabilize the neurotoxin. The neurotoxin requires proteolytic cleavage into a 100 kDa (heavy) and a 50 kDa (light) subunit for full activity. The two subunits must remain linked by at least one disulphide bond for activity. It is believed that the heavy subunit is necessary for binding to the presynaptic nerve terminal, and that the light subunit is responsible for blockade of transmitter release (Hambleton *et al.*, 1987).

Botox is usually measured in units of biological activity, with 1 unit being the mouse LD_{50} by intraperitoneal administration. Unfortunately, the toxin is also sometimes measured by weight, either as nanograms of neurotoxin or of toxin–haemagglutinin complex. To make matters worse (Brin and Blitzer, 1993), the potency in mouse units of 1 ng of toxin produced in the USA (BOTOX®) is different from that produced in the UK (DYSPORT®: 1 UK ng of toxin–haemagglutinin complex is 40 units while 1 US ng is 2.5 units (Quinn and Hallett, 1989). It has been suggested that doses of toxin should be expressed in biological units and by weight of toxin–haemagglutinin complex (Quinn and Hallett, 1989). Doses in this review will refer to biological units of toxin as produced in the USA unless otherwise noted.

Botulinum toxin is freeze-dried and shipped under vacuum. It is diluted with normal saline (without preservative to reduce local irritation). It is recommended that alcohol should not be used on the stopper, but we use alcohol swabs and have not had difficulty. Once saline is added to the desired concentration, BTX-A is drawn up in 1 ml tuberculin syringes; we change the needle before injection to reduce pain, since the rubber stopper on the vial blunts the needle. About 1–3 days after injection, injected muscles atrophy and become weak; maximal weakness usually takes about 1 week to appear. Similarly, the adverse effects of BTX-A described below usually appear 1–3 days after injection. Occasionally, benefit (or adverse effects), may not appear for about 2 weeks after injection.

There are no absolute contraindications to the use of BTX-A. Pregnancy is a relative contraindication since the effect of BTX-A on the fetus is unknown. Botulism during pregnancy may not produce clinical botulism in the infant (St Clair *et al.*, 1985), but there has not been sufficient experience to be reassuring. At least 9 women have been injected for strabismus or blepharospasm while pregnant without obvious adverse effects on the fetus (A. Scott, 1989, personal communication). Four pregnant women with torticollis have been injected with BOTOX during the first trimester and delivered normal full-term infants: 2 in Vancouver (J. Tsui, 1990, personal communication), and 2 at our institution. Likewise, injection of toxin during lactation is discouraged, although a single case has been reported in which an infant was unaffected after breast-feeding while her mother developed botulism (Middaugh, 1978).

Patients with known disorders of synaptic transmission such as myasthenia gravis or Eaton–Lambert syndrome could theoretically experience worsening of their symptoms. The amount of toxin entering the systemic circulation after injection is minute, however, and this theoretical concern should be balanced against the severity of the hyperkinetic symptoms. A patient with motor neuron disease has been injected with BOTOX for blepharospasm by Dr A. Scott and evaluated at our institution without any increase in systemic weakness (S. Fahn, 1991, personal communication).

Although BTX-A has been used therapeutically in human beings since 1980 without evidence of direct effect of botulinum toxin on uninjected muscles, the long-term consequences of chronic injections are unknown. Weakness or routine EMG changes in muscles distal to the site of injection have not been reported. However, there are detectable abnormalities on single-fibre EMG (Sanders *et al.*, 1986; Lange *et al.*, 1987, 1991; Olney *et al.*, 1988). It is not known how long these abnormalities persist, or whether they have any clinical significance. For this reason, children should receive chronic injections only when alternative therapies have failed, and when the severity of symptoms justifies this risk.

No case of anaphylaxis to BTX has been reported. There have been reports of rash or hives developing after BTX injections, but patients receiving placebo in double-blind studies have also developed skin reactions. Even if injections of BTX can trigger an allergic reaction, other components of the BTX mixture besides botulinum toxin itself may provide the allergen. It is believed that survivors of botulism do not have detectable antibodies to the toxin (Paton *et al.*, 1982), but some patients injected chronically for torticollis may develop immunity to BTX-A (see below). Scott and Suzuki (1988) have estimated that in the monkey *Macaca fascicularis* the LD_{50} of BOTOX by intramuscular injection is about 39 u/kg. The threshold for any systemic effect was quite close to this – about 33 u/kg. If humans have the same threshold as monkeys in u/kg, then the LD_{50} for a 60 kg person would be about $39 \times 60 = 2340$ units.

Use of BTX-A will be described separately for each of the most commonly injected focal dystonias. Patients with segmental dystonia or other combinations of focal dystonias can be treated with combinations of the appropriate protocols.

BLEPHAROSPASM

Indications

Blepharospasm was the first focal dystonia to be treated with BTX-A (Scott *et al.*, 1985). Since then, Scott has collected data on over 2000 patients injected with botox (A. Scott, 1990, personal communication). Publications on BTX-A treatment of blepharospasm, including two double-blind studies, have reported a success rate ranging from 69 to 100% (Table 24.1). BTX-A is an effective treatment for idiopathic blepharospasm, blepharospasm arising after birth injury or after neuroleptic exposure

Table 24.1 Published studies on blepharospasm

Report	*Number improved*	*Mean dose*	*Duration of benefit*	*Rating scale*
Double-blind studies				
Fahn *et al.* (1985)	5/5	10 u (1 eye)	?	Video and EMG
Jankovic and Orman (1987)	12/12	25 u	12.5 weeks	Subjective and video
Open studies				
Arthurs *et al.* (1987)	26/27	24–48 u	7–11.2 weeks	8.6/12 (before)→ 2.8/12 (after)
Berlin *et al.* (1987)	10/10	25–100 u	8.6–12.9 weeks	Improved by 2–4/4
Biglan *et al.* (1988)	58/61	31–325 u	4.5 months	
Borodic and Cozzolino (1989)	56/61	25.5–61.9 u	2.7–3.4 months	
Brin *et al.* (1987)	29/42	47.3 u	12.9 weeks	Improved by 2–3/3
Carruthers and Stubbs (1987)	47/47	25–50 u	14.5–16.9 weeks	
Cohen *et al.* (1986)	58/75	25–50 u	10.7–12.6 weeks	3.1/4 (before)→ 0.6/4 (after)
Defazio *et al.* (1990)	12/13	30–60 u	14.5 weeks	3.2/4 (before)→ 1.6/2.4 (after)
Dutton and Buckley (1988)	167/172	25–150 u	13.1 weeks	3.2/4 (before)→ 0.5–0.7/4 (after)
Elston (1992)	199/234	0.4–2.2 ng*	12–15 weeks	184/234 'almost normal'
Engstrom *et al.* (1987)	76/76	about 100 u	14.4–22.9 weeks	
Frueh and Musch (1986)	39/42	25–100 u	11–17 weeks	
Jankovic and Schwartz (1991b)	66/70	32 u	12 weeks	3.6/4
Kalra and Magoon (1990)	65/69	?	?	
Lingua (1985)	10/10	?	?	
Mauriello *et al.* (1987)	77/79	25–115 u	13 weeks	90% were 75% better patient/ physician rating
Maurri *et al.* (1988)	16/16	20–85 u	13 weeks	3.06/4 (before)→ 0.86/4 (after)

Table 24.1 (continued)

Report	*Number improved*	*Mean dose*	*Duration of benefit*	*Rating scale*
Osako and Keltner (1991)	49/53	35–140 u	17.6 weeks	
Perman *et al.* (1986)	28/28	25–130 u	2.5–3 months	
Ruusuvaara and Setala (1990)	29/36	About 60 u	3.4 months	
Scott *et al.* (1985)	39/39	10–100 u	9.9 weeks	Decreased force of eyelid closure
Shore *et al.* (1986)	25/26	?	8.5 weeks	
Shorr *et al.* (1985)	17/17	25 u	6–8 weeks	3.27/4 (before)→ 2.67/4 (after)
Taylor *et al.* (1991)	231/235	30–120 u	14.4 weeks	
Tsoy *et al.* (1985)	37/38	25–50 u	9.3–25.7 weeks	2.82/4 1.94/4
Waller *et al.* (1985)	19/20	25 u		

*Dosage in nanograms of toxin–haemagglutinin complex, UK preparation.
The most recent study is cited in most cases where several studies appeared from the same group.
EMG = Electromyogram.

(tardive blepharospasm), blepharospasm as a dystonic tic, and blepharospasm occurring as a peak-dose dystonia during levodopa treatment in patients with parkinsonism. BTX-A treatment has largely supplanted medication trials and surgical procedures in the treatment of blepharospasm. We treat blepharospasm with medications when patients refuse BTX-A injections or are BTX-A failures. If blepharospasm is part of widespread dystonia requiring medication trials, BTX-A injections can provide immediate relief of the blepharospasm.

Methods

Investigators have differed somewhat in the concentration of BTX-A, exact location and number of injection sites, and volume of injection per site for the treatment of blepharospasm. Most investigators have reported using 12.5–70 u of BOTOX per eye in 5–7 sites around each eye, with a concentration of 2.5–5 u/0.1 ml (0.1–0.2 ml per site). For an initial injection series, we inject 5 u in each of 5–6 sites in the orbicularis oculi of each eye: 1–2 intramuscular sites above the brow, 1 subcutaneous site each at the lateral canthus and in the lower lid, and 2 subcutaneous sites in the upper lid for a total of 25–30 u per eye (Fig. 24.1). Some patients who continue to have spasms at these doses will improve at double or triple this dose. We usually use 30-gauge

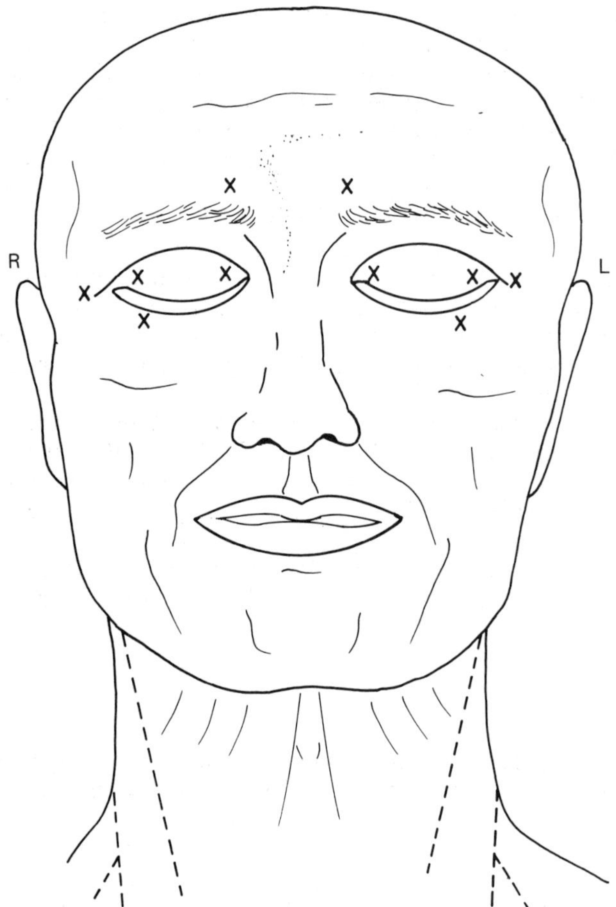

Figure 24.1 Injections for blepharospasm. × =0.2 ml; 2.5 u/0.1 ml.

needles for facial injections. Several patients consistently developed diplopia with 30-gauge needles, but not with 26-gauge needles. We suspect that the higher pressure necessary to express toxin from the 30-gauge needle may have increased spread of toxin from the injection site, resulting in weakening of the lateral rectus.

Benefit after injections seems to be similar for all techniques. Larger total doses probably result in longer duration of benefit, although the increase in duration is not dramatic (Frueh and Musch, 1986). The spectrum of adverse effects does depend on the technique of injection (see below).

The levator palpebrae inserts into the tarsal plate in the mid-portion of the upper lid. Subcutaneous spread of toxin from sites over the upper lid to the levator palpebrae causes blepharoptosis (ptosis). Most investigators minimize the risk of spread to the levator by injecting the upper lid as far from the midline as possible and pointing the tip of the needle away from the midline. In addition, some investigators inject subcutaneously over the pretarsal component of the orbicularis oculi just above the eyelashes (Fig. 24.1). These sites are far from the insertion of the levator palpebrae and minimize ptosis. These pretarsal injection sites are over the globe; the needle can be inserted safely by first retracting the upper lid, so that the needle tip is actually superior to the globe while the needle is inserted. The lid is then released, and BTX is injected while the tip of the needle is angled slightly up, away from the globe. In patients who cannot remain still (e.g. patients with marked torticollis or head tremor), the globe can be protected with lid shields inserted under the upper lid after the cornea is anaesthetized. On rare occasions, patients with severe jerky dystonia of the face or neck cannot be injected safely without sedation. When reassurance fails, sedation may also be necessary with the extremely anxious patient.

Most patients tolerate the injections well even at ages over 80. It is prudent, however, intially to reduce the dose in patients over about 70 years of age. It is also prudent to reduce the initial dose in patients with reason to have some degree of denervation (e.g. history of Guillain–Barré syndrome, prior myectomy for blepharospasm), as they may be more sensitive to BTX-A.

Occasionally, paranasal contractions over the levator labii superioris alaeque nasi will be troublesome to the patient. Injections of 2.5–5 u subcutaneously over each levator labii are usually effective. Rarely, frontalis, corrugator supercilii or procerus contractions are severe and troublesome and, if so, one can inject 2.5 or 5 u into 2–4 sites subcutaneously over these muscles with good results.

Patients usually request repeat injections approximately 3 months after the injections. At this time, some weakness of lid closure is still apparent, even though spasms have returned.

Adverse effects

Ptosis is the most troublesome common side-effect, occurring in approximately 10% of injections in our centre. Ptosis generally lasts up to 2 weeks, while benefit from injections lasts about 3 months. All patients may occasionally experience troublesome unilateral or bilateral ptosis, although some patients seem prone to developing repeated ptosis. In addition to the techniques described above for minimizing ptosis, the concentration of BTX-A can be increased and the volume of injection decreased. This may decrease the extent of subcutaneous spread of toxin and seems to reduce the incidence of ptosis.

Ecchymoses occasionally occur. Mild dermatochalasis (baggy skin) is common; patients who complain of this beneath the eyes may do well without any lower lid injections (Frueh *et al.*, 1988). Excess tearing for 1–2 weeks after the injection is common – presumably from a weakened contribution of the orbicularis oculi to the 'lacrimal pump' (Patrinely *et al.*, 1988). Avoiding injections in the medial lower lid may minimize excess tearing. Some patients will complain of dry eyes after the injection, possibly from decreased blink rate. Occasionally, patients develop diplopia after injections (from spread of BTX-A to the extraocular muscles). In addition, there have been reports of brow ptosis, entropion, ectropion and exposure keratopathy from lagophthalmos. There has been one report of herpes simplex keratitis appearing after injection for strabismus (Lingua, 1985).

Results

There are two published double-blind, placebo-controlled studies demonstrating significant benefit from BTX-A injections for blepharospasm. In the study by Jankovic and Orman (1987), all 11 patients injected with BTX-A showed improvement of about 40–70% on three blepharospasm rating scales, while 4 placebo-injected patients showed no improvement. In a study of our patients comparing BTX-A injections around one eye with placebo injections around the other, there was a shorter duration of eyelid closure, less forceful spasm and decreased EMG amplitude after BTX-A injection in one eye compared to the saline-injected contralateral eye of 5 patients (Fahn *et al.*, 1985).

Results in published, open label trials vary from about 70 to 100% response rate (see Table 24.1). In a survey of 54 patients with idiopathic blepharospasm from our institution, only 6/54(11%) of patients received no benefit. Some 35/54(64%) received substantial benefit, returning to almost normal functioning. The remaining 13/54(24%) received benefit from BTX-A injections but continued to have some troublesome symptoms (P. Greene, 1991, personal communication).

Failure to respond

The most common reason for failure to improve is inadequate dose. Many patients with residual spasm after injection will improve after repeat injections with a larger dose. Some patients have been reported to develop an enhanced Bell's phenomenon after injection, which obscured vision (Elston, 1987). In a survey of our patients, reasons for inadequate response included persistent blinking (even though forceful spasms disappeared) and short duration of response despite increased dose. Some of our poor responders had eyelid closure without obvious forceful contractions (similar to apraxia of eyelid opening, although none of these patients had signs of parkinsonism). Some patients with persistent blinking after injection, or with short duration of benefit, may benefit from the use of ptosis crutches.

APRAXIA OF EYELID OPENING (LEVATOR INHIBITION)

Indications and methods

Apraxia of eyelid opening describes an inability to open the eyelids in the absence of blepharospasm, dysfunction of the third cranial nerve or of the orbicularis oculi muscle. The condition is most commonly seen in progressive supranuclear palsy (PSP), but also has been described in other Parkinson-plus syndromes and, rarely, in idiopathic Parkinson's disease, Huntington's disease and several other conditions (Lepore, 1988). Some patients with PSP and apraxia of eyelid opening will improve with BTX-A injections. The technique of injection is identical to that used for blepharospasm. Our patients with apraxia have required larger doses of BTX-A than patients with blepharospasm, but there is not enough published experience to define the optimal doses.

Results

There have been no controlled studies of the use of BTX-A for apraxia of eyelid opening. There is a case report of a single patient with apraxia of eyelid opening who improved with botox (Katz and Rosenberg, 1987) and several studies of BTX-A treatment of blepharospasm have included patients with apraxia (Brin *et al.*, 1987; Mauriello *et al.*, 1987). Of 6 patients we have injected, 3 had sustained benefit, 1 had brief benefit after each injection series, and 2 had no benefit.

LOWER FACIAL DYSTONIA

Indications

In some patients with dystonia involving the lower facial muscles, the quality of life may be improved if symptoms are relieved in a few muscles. BTX may be used in these patients to achieve rapid relief of symptoms. When there is extensive involvement of lower facial muscles, medication trials are necessary because it is difficult to localize and inject all the involved muscles.

Methods

The toxin is used in a concentration of 2.5–5 u/01 ml. Some muscles, such as the depressor anguli oris and orbicularis oris, can easily be injected without EMG control. In patients with lip-puckering dystonia, the orbicularis oris can be injected. These injections are painful, and should be performed only if the patient is determined to have the puckering stop. Excess weakness of the orbicularis oris can cause food to pool between the lips and teeth.

Other lower facial muscles such as the zygomaticus, risorius, platysma, etc. can be injected without EMG guidance, but the effects may vary from session to session even when the dose is kept constant. Injecting through a hollow-core EMG needle under EMG control produces reproducible results. For example, 3–4 injections of 0.1 ml (2.5 u) spaced 2.5–5 cm apart subcutaneously over the platysma on one side will often eliminate dystonic contractions, and excess platysma weakness has not so far produced symptoms. The zygomaticus major can be injected with 1.25–7.5 u at its insertion in the mandibular arch.

Adverse effects

Excess weakness and its consequences (facial paresis, eating difficulties) are the only adverse effects of these injections, in general.

Results

There have been no controlled studies of BTX-A injections for lower facial muscles in dystonia. Many series of patients with blepharospasm and hemifacial spasm reported some injections of involved lower facial muscles, usually with success. However, a minority of patients develop unacceptable weakness of the injected muscle before involuntary movements disappear.

HEMIFACIAL SPASM

Indications

Several of the earliest reports of the use of botox injections in the treatment of blepharospasm included patients with hemifacial spasm (HFS; Frueh and Musch, 1986). Patients with HFS respond at least as well to BTX-A as patients with blepharospasm. We no longer require drug trials for HFS before recommending BTX-A injections (Fahn and Greene, 1990). No one has compared the results of BTX-A injections with seventh nerve surgical decompression.

Methods and adverse effects

The methods and adverse effects of BTX-A injections for HFS are similar to those outlined for upper and lower facial dystonia above, applied to half the face. Patients with HFS are more sensitive to BTX-A than patients with dystonia – possibly as a result of underlying nerve damage. The duration of benefit tends to be longer in HFS (3–6 months in our patients, with an average of almost 4 months). Unfortunately, the incidence and severity of ptosis seem to be increased. Initial injections should use reduced dose over the upper lid. Injecting over the pretarsal component of the orbicularis will also help reduce the risk of ptosis.

Injecting lower facial muscles requires use of a hollow-core EMG needle to ensure reproducible results and avoid facial droop. Small differences in needle tip placement result in dramatic differences in muscle weakness after injection. In addition, patients with HFS vary considerably in response to the same dose of BTX-A: some patients will require 5–10 units in the zygomaticus before twitching stops, while others will have severe facial droop at these doses. When first injecting a patient in the lower face, it is necessary to start with tiny doses (2.5 units or less) and use the response to titrate the dose gradually at future injections.

Response and failure to respond

There has been one single-blind, placebo-controlled study of BTX-A injections for HFS published as an abstract (Yoshimura *et al.*, 1990). Most published studies have reported close to a 100% success rate, although many patients had only the periorbital muscles injected. For review, see Tolosa *et al.* (1988). Over 100 patients have been injected at our institution. All obtained dramatic relief of periorbital spasms from the injections, although a few developed severe ptosis and were unwilling to have further injections. Several patients have developed marked lower facial weakness lasting up to 2 months after lower facial injections. Several patients continue to feel twitching even when no contractions can be seen or palpated (generally in the lower face, occasionally in the upper face as well). Several patients are bothered by the contrast between the briskly blinking uninjected eye and the sluggishly blinking injected eye, although none has been willing to have injections in the unaffected side. Similarly, small degrees of ptosis which would be insignificant in blepharospasm may be an annoyance in HFS because of contrast with the uninjected eye.

OROMANDIBULAR DYSTONIA

Indications

According to the American Academy of Neurology Technology Assessment report, BTX-A injections for oromandibular dystonia are considered accepted (American Academy of Neurology, 1990); although drug therapy is often attempted initially. In patients who are losing weight because of oromandibular dystonia, BTX-A may allow resumption of a relatively normal diet and should be attempted promptly. Lingual injections entail a significant risk of severe dysphagia and aspiration and should be attempted only for severe disease.

Methods

The muscle of the masseter and temporalis can be easily injected for jaw-closing dystonia. Initial doses of 25–40 u divided into 3–4 sites for each masseter and about 25 u divided into 2 sites for each temporalis will minimize excess weakness, although may not be sufficient for severe cases. If necessary, repeat injections can be performed with EMG guidance to ensure proper placement. In some cases, the internal pterygoid may also require injection for jaw-closing dystonia.

For jaw-opening and jaw-deviating dystonia, the external pterygoids (and sometimes the anterior belly of the digastrics) can be injected. The external pterygoids can be approached intraorally with an initial dose of about 6–15 u per muscle. As with all BTX injections, these injections need to be performed by someone familiar with the anatomy, with EGM guidance. For tongue-protruding dystonia, the hyoglossus and genioglossus can be injected, but only if the risk of severe dysphagia is justified.

Adverse effects

Excess weakness of jaw closure may result from masseter and temporalis injections. This may make chewing difficult, but is transient and patients can usually get adequate nutrition with a soft diet until strength returns. More serious dysphagia and aspiration may result from injection of other jaw, tongue and pharyngeal muscles.

Results

One double-blind study included patients with oromandibular dystonia (Jankovic and Orman, 1987), but the results of the oromandibular injections were not analysed separately. In a review of BTX-A injections in a series of 20 patients with oromandibular dystonia at our institution, 12/20 (60%) improved, and 9/20 (45%) were rated by the treating physician as markedly improved (Blitzer *et al.*, 1989). In our recent series 96 patients, function was improved by 40% or better in most cases (Brin *et al.*, 1993)

LARYNGEAL DYSTONIA (SPASMODIC DYSPHONIA, DYSTONIC DYSPHONIA)

Background and classification

Idiopathic spasmodic dysphonia and laryngeal dystonia (LD) are clinical terms used to describe an action-induced laryngeal movement disorder (for review, see Brin *et al.*, 1991a). Two distinct types of LD have been distinguished (Darley *et al.*, 1975): *adductor*, due to irregular hyperadduction of the vocal folds; and *abductor*, due to intermittent abduction of the vocal folds. Some patients appear to have a combination of the two. Patients with adductor LD exhibit a choked, strained or strangled voice quality with abrupt initiation and termination of voicing resulting in short breaks in phonation. Patients with abductor LD exhibit a breathy, effortful voice quality with abrupt termination of voicing resulting in aphonic whispered segments of speech. Because many patients with LD present with a tremulous voice, the differential diagnosis between LD with essential tremor versus dystonic tremor can be difficult (Blitzer, 1988).

Indications

Long-term treatment of LD was unrewarding until the advent of local injections of BTX-A. Systemic pharmacotherapy provides little relief of symptoms. Dedo (1976) described dramatic relief of symptoms by sectioning the recurrent laryngeal nerve. The initial favourable reports were temporized by Aronson's review of 33 patients (Aronson, 1983) treated with surgery. By 3 years, only 36% of patients had some persistent improvement and only 1 of 33 achieved a persistent normal voice. Adverse effects included breathiness, hoarseness, diplophonia and falsetto. Although Dedo recently reported an outstanding follow-up among his cohort (Dedo and Behlau, 1991), a double-blind assessment of these patients has not been performed.

In 1984, using EMG guidance, we began injecting BTX-A into the vocalis muscles for the treatment of adductor LD (Brin *et al.*, 1987). At that time, no one had ever injected toxin into the vocalis muscle complex.

Compared to alternative methods of therapy, treatment with BTX-A is preferred by most patients with LD, and is currently offered as primary therapy for adductor LD. For all forms of LD, we recommend that injections into the vocalis muscle be performed by a physician trained in the anatomy and physiology of the larynx. Because reflex laryngeal stridor occasionally occurs during laryngeal EMG, it is recommended that the injections be administered in an environment equipped to treat laryngeal stridor (American Academy of Neurology, 1990; American Academy of Otolaryngology – Head and Neck Surgery, 1990).

Methods

We use BTX-A reconstituted to a final concentration of 1.25–2.5 u/0.1 ml injected through a monopolar hollow Teflon-coated EMG needle connected to an EMG recorder via an alligator clip attached to the hub of the needle. A physician with experience in performing laryngeal EMGs performs the injections. The needle is placed into the thyroarytenoid vocalis complex by impaling the muscle through the cricothyroid cartilage, using a previously described technique (Blitzer *et al.*, 1985). Once the muscle is identified, the toxin is slowly injected.

The calculation of the dose to be injected evolved as we gained experience with injecting this small muscle. Our initial experience with bilateral, low-dose, vocalis muscle complex injections was encouraging. Aiming to minimize the total dose of injected toxin, our group developed a programme of injecting both cords with small doses (0.625–2.5 u) of toxin in an effort to decrease the degree of adduction by causing mild bilateral weakness (Brin *et al.*, 1989, 1991a; Blitzer and Brin, 1991). The Baylor and National Institutes of Health Centers have injected higher doses (15–30 u botox) into one vocalis complex in order to effect a unilateral paralysis (Miller *et al.*, 1987; Ludlow *et al.*, 1988, 1990; Jankovic *et al.*, 1990), and have reported comparable results.

Adverse effects

Adverse experiences using the unilateral and bilateral approaches include transient breathy hypophonia, hoarseness and usually clinically insignificant aspiration of fluids. In over 600 cases treated in this country, there have been no cases of documented pneumonia.

Results

All centres agree that, regardless of technique, there is a dramatic improvement in symptoms (Gacek, 1987; Ludlow *et al.*, 1988, 1990; Jankovic *et al.*, 1990; Brin *et al.*, 1991a; Troung *et al.*, 1991; Zwirner *et al.*, 1991) in non-surgical and surgical patients with an 80–100% improvement in speech function during therapy. Patients with adductor LD, who have already undergone recurrent laryngeal nerve section, have a marked improvement from BTX-A therapy, but the degree of benefit is somewhat less than in the non-surgical patient. Although all centres report benefit from treatment, we hope our current double-blind protocol will help elucidate the relative benefits of unilateral versus bilateral injections.

Treatment of abductor laryngeal dystonia

We have recently reported out technique in treating abductor LD with BTX-A (Brin *et al.*, 1990, 1991a; Blitzer *et al.*, 1992). Percutaneous injections are guided by EMG control with the Teflon-coated hollow EMG recording needle placed posterior to the thyroid lamina, directly impalling the posterior cricoarytenoid (PCA) muscle overlying the cricoid cartilage. We first weaken one PCA muscle with 2.5–3.75 u BOTOX. If bringing this muscle closer to the midline does not provide adequate relief of symptoms, then conservative serial small doses (1.25–2.5 u) of BOTOX are injected to weaken one or both PCA muscles. Marked improvement was seen in 7 of the initial 10 patients treated; benefit persisted for up to 19 weeks. Because the technique requires chemically bringing the vocal folds towards the midline, there is a significant risk of stridor requiring tracheostomy. In our series of 32 patients, 2 patients have developed transient, non-disabling exercise-induced stridor. This form of therapy is effective in many cases and recommended when available at treatment centres.

When BTX-A treatment does not provide an adequate response, patients are considered for a type I thyroplasty to assist in maintaining one vocal cord near the midline.

TORTICOLLIS (CERVICAL DYSTONIA)

Indications

There are no generally accepted guidelines for initial therapy of torticollis. Therapy with anticholinergics and other medications is effective in a minority of patients, and these drugs have been in use for a sufficient time to assure patients about long-term safety (Fahn, 1983). Although anticholinergics will benefit the largest percentage of patients, substantial benefit will occasionally result from a number of agents, including baclofen, carbamazepine, clonazepam and other benzodiazepines (Greene *et al.*, 1988), tetrabenazine (possibly in combination with lithium; Jankovic and Orman, 1988) and dopamine receptor blockers (Marsden *et al.*, 1984). Successful medical treatment often requires trials with multiple agents over substantial time. BTX injections produce more benefit for a higher percentage of patients in a shorter time than medications. It is particularly important that pain is often dramatically improved, even when head control is not dramatically affected. Because of the risks involved in surgery for torticollis (e.g. rhizotomy, neurectomy, myectomy or ramicectomy), it seems reasonable to try BTX injections before surgery. For the moment, timing of therapy with BTX or medications must be decided on a case-by-case basis.

Cervical dystonia can involve many neck muscles in different combinations (Chan *et al.*, 1991), and so considerable experience is required to decide what muscles to inject and the dose per muscle. Complicating this decision is the fact that patients may have compensatory contraction of non-dystonic muscles. Common patterns of cervical dystonia are rotation, tilt, extension, flexion and shift of the head. It is best to consider these patterns separately when discussing methods and results of injections. Unfortunately, reports to date have not analysed each of these separately.

We have injected a small number of patients with prior surgery (myectomy, denervation, thalamotomy or combinations), tardive torticollis and torticollis secondary to a variety of other conditions. It appears that all these groups may improve after BTX-A injections.

Methods

There is considerable variation in technique in published reports of the treatment of torticollis with BTX-A. Several groups have injected 2–3 of the most active muscles (Tsui *et al.*, 1986; Stell *et al.*, 1988). Others (Jankovic and Orman, 1988; Gelb *et al.*, 1989; Greene *et al.*, 1990) inject multiple muscles depending on the combination of tilt, turn, retrocollis and pain. The number of sites per muscle has varied from 2 sites per muscle (Tsui *et al.*, 1986; Stell *et al.*, 1988) to multiple sites per muscle (up to 10 or more sites in our group). The reported concentration of toxin has varied from 2.5 u/0.1 ml to greater than 10 u/0.1 ml. A few published reports have included the use of EMG to select target muscles and guide injections after muscles have been selected (Dubinsky *et al.*, 1991; Poewe *et al.*, 1992). Comella *et al.* found greater magnitude of response after EMG selection of muscles and EMG-guided injections, compared to injection without the use of EMG (Comella *et al.*, 1992). There have been double-blind, placebo-controlled studies documenting the efficacy of several of these techniques (Table 24.2), but there have been few studies comparing differing techniques. The optimal technique for use of BTX-A remains to be defined.

At our centre, toxin at a concentration of 5–10 u/0.1 ml is injected in from 2 to about 8 sites per muscle depending on the size of the muscle. We vary the initial

Table 24.2 Published studies on torticollis

Report	*Number improved*	*Number with pain improved*	*Mean dose*	*Duration of benefit*
Double-blind studies				
Tsui *et al.* (1986)	10–12/21	14/16	100 u	?
Jankovic and Orman (1987)	3/8	?	114 u	11.7 weeks
Gelb *et al.* (1989)	16/20	?	100–280 u	Most 1–3 months
Greene *et al.* (1990)	17/28	7/11	145 u	?
Blackie and Lees (1990)	14/19	12/16	960 u*	12 weeks
Koller *et al.* (1990)	1/29	?	150 u	?
Lorentz *et al.* (1991)	14–20/23	12/19	150 u	12.5 weeks
Moore and Blumhardt (1991)	12/20	?	25 ng†	8–10 weeks
Open studies				
Borodic *et al.* (1991)	28/35	26/32	100–250 u	5.1 months
Comella *et al.* (1992)	45/52	?	150–560 u	?
D'Costa and Abbott (1991)	11/12	6/?	10–15 ng†	3 months
Defazio *et al.* (1990)	1/4	?	60–160 u	4 weeks
Dubinsky *et al.* (1991)	70/84	?	180–300 u	15.3 weeks
Jankovic and Schwartz (1990)	145/205	68/89	183–237.5 u	9.6–11.7 weeks
Kostic *et al.* (1990)	13/15	6/9	25–40 ng†	8–15 weeks
Lees *et al.* (1992)	75/89	85% of visits	4–32 ng†	3–28 weeks
Poewe *et al.* (1992)	35/37	26/31	160–1000 u*	13.6 weeks
Stell *et al.* (1988)	7–9/10	5/5	30 ng†	10.8 weeks

*Dosage in mouse units, UK preparation.
†Dosage in nanograms of toxin–haemagglutinin complex, UK preparation.
?Cannot determine from study.
The most recent study is cited in most cases where several studies appeared from the same group.

injection pattern and dose per muscle depending on the nature of the torticollis and the size of the muscles (Figs 24.2–24.4). Patients with simple rotation initially receive injections in the sternocleidomastoid contralateral to direction of turning and the trapezius and splenius capitus ipsilateral to direction of turning (Fig. 24.2). Patients with significant retrocollis initially receive injections in both trapezeii and splenii (Fig. 24.3). Patients with tilt usually receive injections into the ipsilateral sternocleidomastoid, muscles in the posterior triangle (the ipsilateral levator scapulae

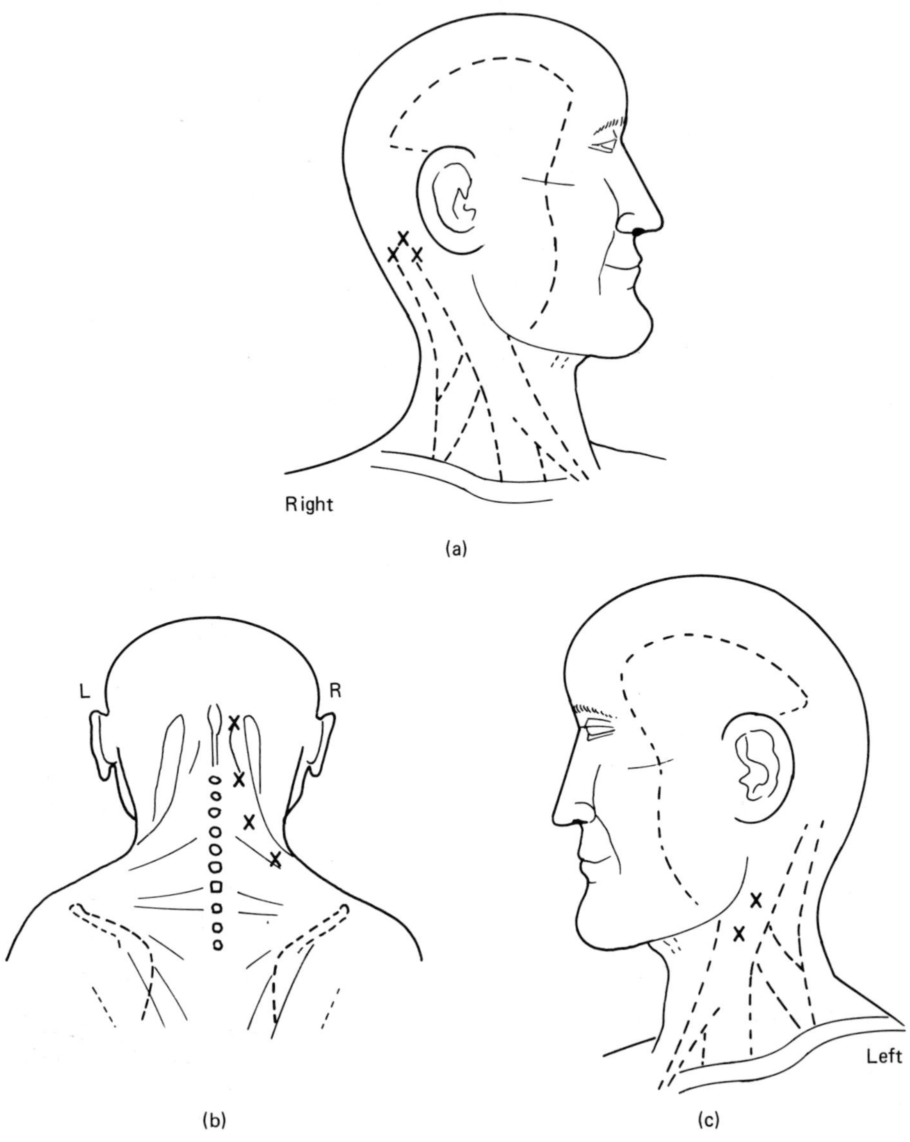

Figure 24.2 Injections for torticollis consisting of right rotation. (a) Splenius capitus: × =0.5 ml; 5 u/0.1 ml; (b) trapezius: × =0.5 ml; 5 u/0.1 ml; (c) sternocleidomastoid: × =0.4 ml; 5 u/0.1 ml.

or scalenus medius) and the ipsilateral trapezius and splenius capitus (Fig. 24.4). All these muscles are superficial and, when actively contracting, are easily palpated. We find palpation to be adequate to identify muscles that require injection, and superior to EMG recording of muscle activity in that muscles can easily be palpated during walking or other activities that activate torticollis. Occasionally, patients with rotation will have pain in the trapezius contralateral to the direction of turning, which we then inject.

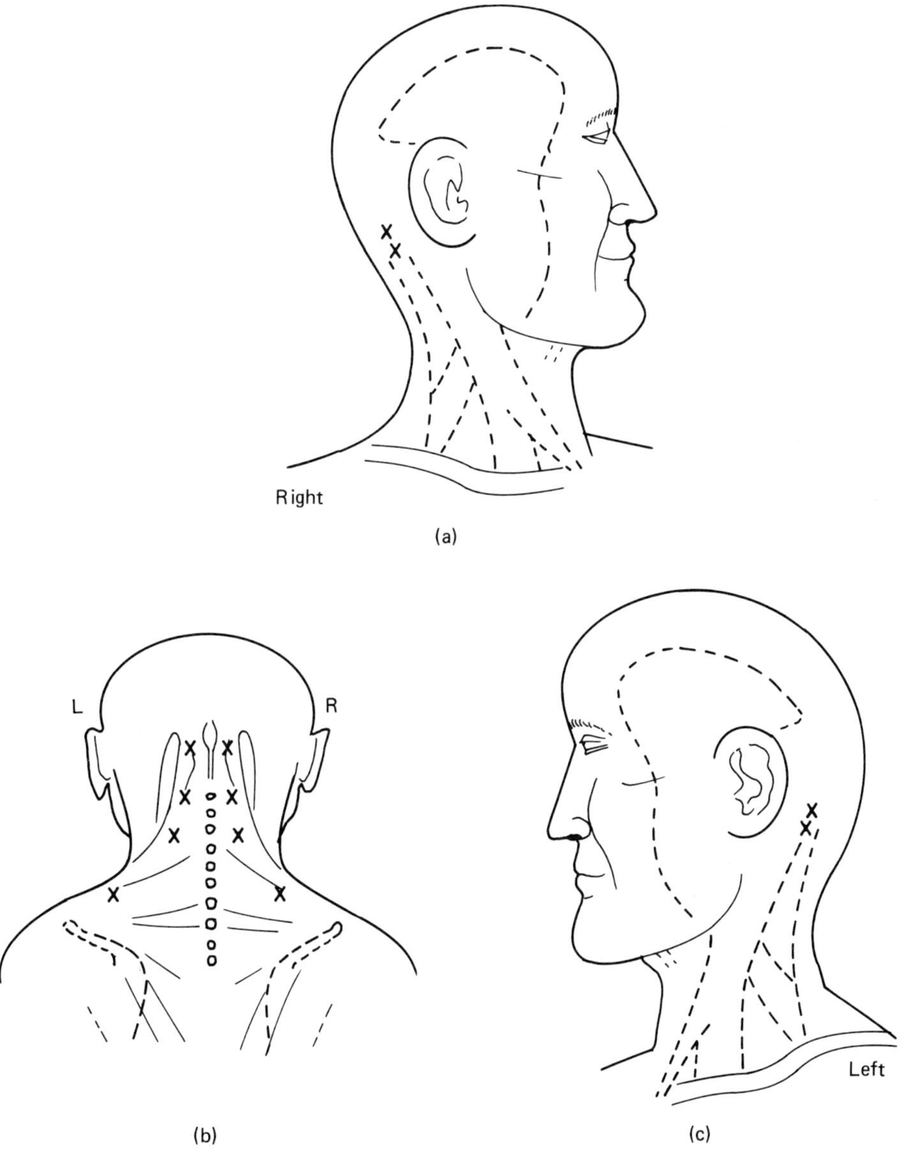

Figure 24.3 Injections for torticollis consisting of retrocollis. (a) Splenius capitus; (b) right and left trapezius; (c) splenius capitus. All × =0.5 ml; 5 u/0.1 ml.

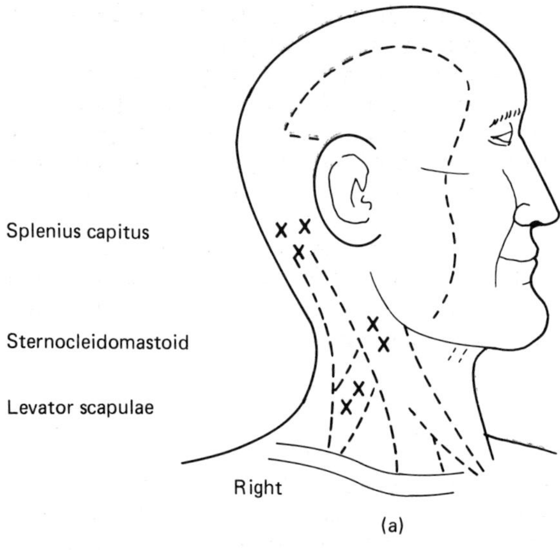

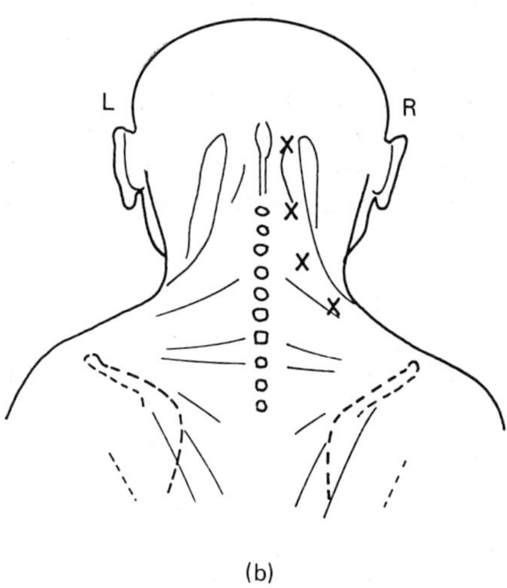

Figure 24.4 Injections for torticollis consisting of right laterocollis. All × =0.5 ml; 5 u/0.1 ml.

We have been unable accurately to estimate the optimal dose per muscle on the first visit. There is significant variation in individual sensitivity to BTX-A, and the average treatment dose of BTX-A at our centre is sufficient to produce symptomatic neck weakness in a small percentage of patients. In addition, we believe that the risk of developing immunity to BTX-A increases as the dose of BTX-A goes up. We, therefore, initially inject a modest dose of toxin, and have patients return in 4 weeks for supplemental injections if necessary. Reasonable doses for an initial set of injections are 40–50 u into the sternocleidomastoid, 75–100 u into the trapezius, and 25–75 u each into the splenius capitus and levator scapulae.

Typical doses for a second session might range from 50 to 150 u divided into actively contracting muscles. Because of the risk of developing antibodies to BTX-A (see below), we prefer to inject patients as infrequently as possible, in the lowest possible doses, and avoid booster injections whenever possible. We explain the rationale for this to patients, and most agree to determine the optimal dose gradually.

These doses usually produce detectable but mild weakness of head turning and extension. Most patients request repeat injections about 3 months after the injection series. At this time, some atrophy of muscles is still apparent, although weakness of head turning is not usually detectable.

Adverse effects

The most serious reported side-effect of BTX-A injections for torticollis has been swallowing difficulty, usually mild. This may last several weeks when severe. At our centre, several patients have required a soft food diet for about a week, but aspiration has not occurred. We suspect that this results from direct spread of toxin to underlying pharyngeal muscles.

Other complaints include excess local weakness (usually a feeling of head heaviness or lack of head control), persistent or shifting pain for several days to 2 weeks after the injections, headache, nausea, fatigue, generalized aching and malaise.

Some of our patients who ultimately improved felt that their torticollis was temporarily worse before benefit was experienced. Several patients have had a change in the quality of their torticollis after injections (e.g. development of tilt after injection for rotation). A few patients complaining of a 'floppy head' did not have excess weakness, but had the head pulled forward by the development of anterocollis transiently after injections. These changes may represent unmasking of previously present contractions, or development of contractions in new muscles. Most of these changes have resolved as the BTX-A effect diminished.

Patients have now been reported with antibodies to botulinum toxin after therapeutic BTX-A injections (Brin *et al.*, 1987; Tsui *et al.*, 1988; Jankovic and Schwartz, 1991b; Hambleton *et al.*, 1992). Patients at our centre have had antibotulinum toxin antibodies confirmed by mouse neutralization assay in the laboratory of Dr Charles Hatheway at the Centers for Disease Control in Atlanta, Georgia, or in the laboratory of Dr Alan Scott at the Smith-Kettlewell Eye Institute in San Francisco, California. These patients did not develop muscle atrophy after injection, and lost all benefit from BTX-A. We estimate the prevalence of antibodies at 7–10% of our population of patients with torticollis, although this probably is an underestimate (P. Greene, 1992, personal communication). With the technique we use, the risk of developing antibodies seems to increase with increasing frequency of injection treatments, and with increasing dose per treatment. Clarification of the risk factors for developing antibodies awaits further research, including a more sensitive assay for antibodies.

Patients with antibodies may be treatable with injections of other botulinum toxin serotypes. The first use of botulinum toxin type F in patients with antibodies to BTX-A was reported in 2 patients with torticillis, 1 patient with ornomandibular dystonia, and 1 patient with stuttering (Ludlow *et al.*, 1992). We have also used botulinum toxin type F to treat successfully 10/15 patients with torticollis who had serological evidence of antibodies to botulinum toxin type A (P. Greene, 1992, personal communication).

Results

There have been eight double-blind, placebo-controlled studies published evaluating BTX-A injections for torticollis (Table 24.2). Tsui *et al.* (1986) reported objective improvement in 63%, subjective improvement in 53%, and improvement of pain in 88% of patients injected (compared to 35%, 15% and 24%, respectively, in placebo-treated patients). Jankovic and Orman (1987) found that only 3 of 8 patients with cervical or oromandibular dystonia improved after BTX-A, but they did not analyse patients with torticollis alone. Gelb *et al.* (1989) found subjective benefit in 80% of patients injected, but no significant objective benefit compared to placebo. They concluded that their objective rating system was not sensitive enough to detect improvement. Blackie and Lees (1990), using the same rating scale as Tsui *et al.* and Gelb *et al.*, reported subjective improvement in 74% of patients, objective improvement in 84% of patients, and improvement in pain in 75% of patients with pain. Lorentz *et al.* (1991) also used the rating scale of Tsui *et al.* and found subjective benefit in 78% of patients, objective improvement in 61%, and improvement in pain in 63% of patients – all significantly better than the placebo group. Moore and Blumhardt (1991) reported objective improvement in 60% of patients, subjective improvement in 80%, and improvement in tremor – all significantly superior to placebo response. Koller *et al.* (1990) is the only reported controlled study that did not detect superiority of BTX-A over placebo, possibly because of insufficient dose, or because the same three muscles (sternocleidomastoid and both trapezii) were injected in all patients. In our double-blind study (Greene *et al.*, 1990), we found subjective improvement in 58% of patients treated with botox, compared to 4% with placebo. Botox-treated patients had a mean 15° improvement in head turning at rest and walking, compared to 2–5° with placebo. Pain improved a mean 41% in BTX-A-treated patients compared to 0% with placebo. In our study, a second, open trial phase found the subjective response rate to be 75% at a higher total dose than that given in the double-blind phase. In addition to double-blind studies, several open trials have been published (Table 24.2). These studies also found dramatic improvement of pain and significant improvement in head control.

Failure to respond

All investigators have found the success rate in torticollis lower than that in blepharospasm. The reasons for this are not known. Most injections have been limited to superficial muscles, and it is likely that the participation of deeper, uninjected muscles accounts for many failures. Although Gelb *et al.* (1989) were unable to detect a clear relationship between dose and response, patients in our study did significantly better after injection with 240 u than with 145 u, so that inadequate dose may also account for some failures. A minority of patients appear to develop dystonic contractions in new muscles after botox injection, and this may also account for failure in some patients. A number of patients at our centre who do not improve after injections at a reasonable dose will be found to have residual contracting muscles when examined 2–3 weeks after injection. In some of these, atrophy of superficial muscles may make deeper contracting muscles apparent. Injection of these muscles may then produce significant benefit. About 20% of patients at our centre do not get significant benefit from botox (primary response failure).

Some patients with initial benefit from BTX-A appear to lose benefit after 6 months to about 2 years of regular injection series (secondary failure). Most of these have developed antibodies to BTX-A, as indicated by failure of the sternocleidomastoid to atrophy after injection of 60–80 u of BTX-A. Several of these patients were reinjected after about 1 year and failed to develop atrophy.

LIMB DYSTONIA

Indications

Some patients with brachial dystonia may benefit from BTX-A injections into a small number of muscles, even in the presence of more widespread involvement of upper extremity muscles. Similarly, patients with dystonic equinovarus posturing of the lower extremities may have improved gait after injection into the posterior tibial and gastronemius muscles. In these patients, benefit is achieved without producing weakness that is disabling. Other patients with severe idiopathic or symptomatic limb dystonia may also benefit from BTX-A injections. In these severe patients, spasm, pain or extreme postures resulting in skin abrasion can be relieved by injecting multiple muscles, although it may be difficult to avoid weakness in some of these muscles. There have been relatively few publications on limb dystonia, and this use of BTX-A has to be considered investigational until doses and criteria for selection of patients are better defined.

There have been preliminary, encouraging reports of successful use of BTX-A injections for spasticity from multiple sclerosis (Snow *et al.*, 1990), stroke (Das and Park, 1989), and upper extremity tremor (Jankovic and Schwartz, 1991a).

Methods

There have been five reports describing the use of BTX-A for brachial dystonia. Yoshimura *et al.* (1992) performed a single-blind, placebo-controlled study of BTX-A injections in 13 patients with idiopathic brachial dystonia and 4 patients with secondary dystonia. Dystonic muscles were identified by wire electrode during tasks, and by clinical evaluation, and in all but 1 patient all muscles judged abnormal were injected with one of three dose schedules. Patients had from 3 to 5 muscles injected to about 30, 60 and 120 u for the limb. Fourteen of 17 had subjective improvement, with 10 of 17 reporting substantial subjective improvement. Review of video tapes by blinded observers was not able to confirm objective improvement compared to placebo. Excess local weakness was the major side-effect, but several patients also developed muscle twitching, paraesthesias or nausea after BTX-A injection. Cohen *et al.* (1989) used EMG recording and clinical examination to identify dystonic muscles for injections. Patients were injected every 2 weeks increasing doses for up to four sessions. Doses were increased gradually until the target dystonic movements improved, or excess weakness supervened. Change in the pattern of contraction at follow-up sessions sometimes required injections in new muscles. They found no advantage in injecting at the motor point. Rivest, Lees and co-workers (Rivest *et al.*, 1991; Lees *et al.*, 1992) used clinical criteria to choose muscles for injection, and then used EMG recording to identify those muscles for injection: 11 of 12 patients received some benefit, and 7 of 12 reported significant benefit. Poungvarin (1991) reported improvement in writing in 14 of 21 patients with brachial dystonia, and 12 of 12 had improvement in pain.

We have used a similar strategy. We have found that it is difficult to distinguish dystonic movements from patients' attempts to compensate for their dystonia (e.g. a patient with dystonic extension of the thumb and forefinger will grip the pen tightly). The underlying dystonia may emerge if the patient grips the pen in a novel manner (e.g. with the first, or between the knuckles of the third and fourth digits). Once the dystonic movements are identified, we attempt to find the optimal dose in small increments, as described above. In patients with severe spasms and pain, the most active muscles are injected. In severe patients, the relief of pain or severe postures is the most important goal, and significant weakness of some muscles may be acceptable.

We and others have injected small numbers of patients with multiple sclerosis and lower extremity adductor spasms and post-stroke spasticity. There is insufficient information so far to define a reliable technique.

Adverse effects

Ecchymoses and excess weakness in injected or nearby muscles have been the only adverse effects. Despite maximal care, patients may have spread of toxin to uninjected muscles, especially in attempting to inject individual finger fascicles in muscles such as the extensor digitorum communis.

Results

Cohen *et al.* (1989) found benefit in 16 of 19 patients and 'major' improvement in 13 of 19 lasting 1–6 months. Rivest *et al.* (1991) found benefit in 11 of 12, with 7 of 12 patients judging the improvment 'significant'. Injection of patients with dystonic involvement of the lower extremity has been described in abstract form (Dubinsky and Gray, 1990), and mentioned in several studies (Jankovic *et al.*, 1990; Yoshimura *et al.*, 1992). At our institution, we have injected about 45 patients with limb dystonia, including 11 patients with severe dystonia, 7 musicians and 1 surgeon (S. Pullman, unpublished data). Of 14 patients with dystonia involving a small number of muscles, 12 (86%) improved, with 5 (36%) having dramatic improvement in writing or typing. Of 11 severe patients, often with pain, 5 (45%) improved. Two of the musicians improved sufficiently to play their instruments, and 2 others experienced improvement in writing, but not in playing. Overall, 22 of 45 (49%) of our patients had definite, functional improvement.

In a preliminary report, 8 patients with post-stroke spasticity of the upper extremities had marked reduction in spasticity, increase in range of movement and some improvement in functional ability after BTX-A injections (Das and Park, 1989). A double-blind study (Snow *et al.*, 1990) found decreased adductor spasticity in the lower extremities in 7 of 9 patients with multiple sclerosis, resulting in greater ease of patient care. Although there were no adverse effects, patients were injected with 400 units of BOTOX, considerably higher than most doses used to treat torticollis, raising concern about possible development of antibodies to botox. Jankovic and Schwartz (1991a) reported that Botox injections resulted in functional improvement in upper-extremity tremor due to Parkinson's disease, essential tremor and possibly other causes, but no details were given.

Acknowledgement

The authors wish to acknowledge support from PR-00645, FD-000195, DC-01139 and the Dystonia Medical Research Foundation.

References

Adams GGW, Kirkness DM, and Lee JP (1987) Botulinum toxin A induced protective ptosis. *Eye*, **1**, 603–8

AAO-HNS: American Academy of Otolaryngology – Head and Neck Surgery Policy Statement (1990) Botox for spasmodic dysphonia. *AAO-HNS Bulletin*, **9**, 8

American Academy of Neurology (1990) Assessment: the clinical usefulness of botulinum toxin-A in treating neurologic disorders. Report of the Therapeutics and Technology Assessment subcommittee of the American Academy of Neurology. *Neurology*, **40**, 1332–6

Aronson AE (1983) Adductor spastic dysphonia: three years after recurrent laryngeal nerve resection. *Laryngoscope*, **93**, 1–8

Arthurs B, Flanders M, Codere F, Gauthier S, Dresner S, and Stone L (1987) Treatment of blepharospasm with medication, surgery and type A botulinum toxin. *Can J Ophthalmol*, **22**, 24–8

Berlin AJ, Cassen JH, DeNelsky G, Hanson MR, and Sweeney PJ (1987) Benign essential blepharospasm treated with botulinum toxin. *Cleveland Clin J Med*, **54**, 421–6

Biglan AW, May M, and Bowers RA (1988) Management of facial spasm with *Clostridium botulinum* toxin, type A (Oculinum). *Arch Otolaryngol – Head Neck Surg*, **114**, 1407–12

Blackie JD and Lees AJ (1990) Botulinum toxin treatment in spasmodic torticollis. *J Neurol, Neurosurg Psychiatry*, **53**, 640–3

Blitzer A and Brin M (1991) Laryngeal dystonia: a series treated with botulinum toxin therapy. *Ann Otol, Rhinol Laryngol*, **100**, 85–9

Blitzer A, Lovelace RE, Brin MF, Fahn S and Fink ME (1985) Electromyographic findings in focal laryngeal dystonia (spastic dysphonia). *Ann Otol Rhinol Laryngol*, **94**, 591–4

Blitzer A, Brin MF, Greene PE, and Fahn S (1989) Botulinum toxin injection for the treatment of oromandibular dystonia. *Ann Otol, Rhinol, Laryngol*, **98**, 93–7

Blitzer A, Brin MF, Fahn S, Lovelace RE (1988) Clinical and Laboratory Characteristics of Focal Laryngeal Dystonia: Study of 110 Cases. *Laryngoscope*, **98**, 636–640

Blitzer A, Brin M, Fahn S, Lovelace RE (1988) The Use of Botulinum Toxin in the Treatment of Focal Laryngeal Dystonia (Spastic Dystonia). *Laryngoscope*, **98**, 193–97

Blitzer A, Brin MF, Stewart C, Aviv JE, and Fahn S (1992) Abductor laryngeal dystonia: a series treated with botulinum toxin. *Laryngoscope*, **102**, 163–67

Borodic GE and Cozzolino D (1989) Blepharospasm and its treatment with emphasis on the use of botulinum toxin. *Plast Reconstr Surg*, **83**, 546–54

Borodic GE, Mills L, and Joseph M (1991) Botulinum A toxin for the treatment of adult-onset spasmodic torticollis. *Plast Reconstr Surg*, **87**, 285–9

Brin MF and Blitzer A (1993) Botulinum Toxin – Dangerous Terminology Errors. *J R Soc Med*, **86**, 494

Brin MF, Fahn S, Moskowitz C, Friedman A, Shale HM, Greene PE *et al.* (1987) Localized injections of butolinum toxin for the treatment of focal dystonia and hemifacial spasm. *Movement Disorders*, **2**, 237–54

Brin MF, Blitzer A, Fahn S, Gould W, and Lovelace RE (1989) Adductor laryngeal dystonia (spastic dysphonia): treatment with local injections of botulinum toxin (Botox). *Movement Disorders*, **4**, 287–96

Brin MF, Blitzer A, Stewart C, and Fahn S (1990) Botulinum toxin: now for abductor laryngeal dystonia. *Neurology*, **40** (suppl 1), 381

Brin MF, Blitzer A, Stewart C, and Fahn S (1991a) Treatment of spasmodic dysphonia (laryngeal dystonia) with local injections of botulinum toxin: review and technical aspects. In Blitzer A, Brin MF, Sasaki CT, Fahn S, and Harris KS, eds, *Neurological Disorders of the Larynx*, New York, Theime, 214–28

Brin MF, Fahn S, Blitzer A, Ramig LO, and Stewart C (1991b) Laryngeal motion disorders. In Blitzer A, Brin MF, Sasaki CT, Fahn S, and Harris KS, eds, *Neurological Disorders of the Larynx*, New York, Theime, 248–78

Brin MF, Blitzer A, Herman S, and Stewart C (1993) Oromandibular dystonia: treatment of 96 patients with botulinum toxin A. In: Jankovic J, Hallett M (eds) *Therapy with botulinum toxin*, Marcel Dekker, New York

Carruthers J and Stubbs HA (1987) Botulinum toxin for benign essential blepharospasm, hemifacial spasm and age-related lower eyelid entropion. *Can J Neurol Sci*, **14**, 42–5

Chan J, Brin MB, and Fahn S (1991) Idiopathic cervical dystonia: clinical characteristics. *Movement Disorders*, **6**, 119–26

Cohen DA, Savino PJ, Stern MB, and Hurtig HI (1986) Botulinum injection therapy for blepharospasm: a review and report of 75 patients. *Clin Neuropharmacol*, **9**, 415–29

Cohen LG, Hallett M, Geller BD, and Hochberg F (1989) Treatment of focal dystonias of the hand with botulinum toxin injections. *J Neurol, Neurosurg Psychiatry*, **52**, 355–63

Comella CL, Buchman AS, Tanner CM, Brown-Toms NC, and Goetz CG (1992) Botulinum toxin injection for spasmodic torticollis. *Neurology*, **42**, 878–82

Darley FL, Aronson AE, and Brown JR (1975) *Motor Speech Disorders*, Philadelphia, WB Saunders

Das TK and Park DM (1989) Botulinum toxin in treating spasticity. *Br J Clin Pract*, **43**, 401–3

D'Costa DF and Abbott RJ (1991) Low dose botulinum toxin in spasmodic torticollis. *J R Soc Med*, **84**, 650–1

Dedo HH (1976) Recurrent laryngeal nerve section for spastic dysphonia. *Ann Otol, Rhinol and Laryngol*, **85**, 451–9

Dedo HH and Behlau MS (1991) Recurrent laryngeal nerve section for spastic dysphonia: 5- to 14-year preliminary results in the first 300 patients. *Ann Otol, Rhinol Laryngol*, **100**, 274–9

Defazio G, Lepore V, Lamberti P, Livrea P, and Ferrari E (1990) Botulinum A toxin treatment for eyelid spasm, spasmodic torticollis and apraxia of eyelid opening. *Ital J Neurol Sci*, **11**, 275–80

Dubinsky RM and Gray CS (1990) Botulinum toxin for dystonic foot inversion. *Movement Disorders*, **5** (suppl 1), 75

Dubinsky RM, Gray CS, Vetere-Overfield B, and Koller WC (1991) Electromyographic guidance of botulinum toxin treatment in cervical dystonia. *Clin Neuropharmacol*, **14**, 262–7

Dutton JJ and Buckley EG (1988) Long-term results and complications of botulinum A toxin in the treatment of blepharospasm. *Ophthalmology*, **95**, 1529–34

Dykstra DD and Sidi AA (1990) Treatment of detrusor-sphincter dyssynergia with botulinum A toxin: a double-blind study. *Arch Phys Med Rehab*, **71**, 24–6

Elston JS (1987) Long-term results of treatment of idiopathic blepharospasm with botulinum toxin injections. *Br J Ophthalmol*, **71**, 664–8

Elston JS (1992) The management of blepharospasm and hemifacial spasm. *J Neurol*, **239**, 5–8

Engstrom PF, Arnoult JB, Mazow ML, Prager TC, Wilkins RB, Byrd WA *et al.* (1987) Effectiveness of botulinum toxin therapy for essential blepharospasm. *Ophthalmology*, **94**, 971–5

Fahn S (1983) High dosage anticholinergic therapy in dystonia. *Neurology*, **339**, 1255–61

Fahn S and Greene P (1990) Hemifacial Spasm. In Johnson RT, ed, *Therapy in Neurologic Diseases*, vol 3, Philadelphia, BC Decker, 274–5

Fahn S, List T, Moskowitz C, Brin MF, Bressman S, Burke R *et al.* (1985) Double-blind controlled study of botulinum toxin for blepharospasm. *Neurology*, **35** (suppl 1), 271

Frueh BR and Musch DC (1986) Treatment of facial spasm with botulinum toxin: an interim report. *Ophthalmology*, **93**, 917–23

Frueh BR, Nelson CC, Kapustiak JF, and Musch DC (1988) The effect of omitting botulinum toxin from the lower eyelid in blepharospasm treatment. *Am J Ophthalmol*, **106**, 45–7

Gacek RR (1987) Botulinum toxin for relief of spasmodic dysphonia. *Arch Otolaryngol Neck Surg*, **113**, 1240

Gelb DJ, Lowenstein DH, and Aminoff MJ (1989) Controlled trial of botulinum toxin injections in the treatment of spasmodic torticollis. *Neurology*, **39**, 80–4

Greene P, Shale S, and Fahn S (1988) Analysis of open-label trials in torsion dystonia using high dosages of anticholinergics and other drugs. *Movement Disorders*, **3**, 46–60

Greene P, Kang U, Fahn S, Brin M, Moskowitz C, and Flaster E (1990) Double-blind, placebo-controlled trial of botulinum toxin injections for the treatment of spasmodic torticollis. *Neurology*, **40**, 1213–18

Habermann E (1974) ^{125}I-labeled neurotoxin from *Clostridium botulinum* A: preparation, binding to synaptosomes and ascent to the spinal cord. *Naunyn-Schmiedebergs Arch Pharmacol*, **281**, 47–56

Hallan RI, Melling J, Womack NR, Williams NS, Waldron DJ, and Morrison JFB (1988) Treatment of anismus in intractable constipation with botulinum A toxin. *Lancet*, **2**, 714–16

Hambleton P, Shone CC, and Melling J (1987) Botulinum toxin – structure, action and clinical uses. In Jenner P, ed, *Neurotoxins and Their Pharmacological Implications*, pp. 233–60. New York, Raven Press

Hambleton P, Cohen HE, Palmer BJ, and Melling J (1992) Antitoxins and botulinum toxin treatment. *Br Med J*, **304**, 959–60

Hanig JP and Lamanna C (1979) Toxicity of botulinum toxin: a stochiometric model for the locus of its extraordinary potency and persistence at the neuromuscular junction. *J Theor Biol*, **77**, 107–13

Helveston EM and Pogrebniak AE (1988) Treatment of acquired nystagmus with botulinum A toxin. *Am J Ophthalmol*, **106**, 584–6

Jankovic J and Orman J (1987) Botulinum A toxin for cranial-cervical dystonia: a double-blind, placebo-controlled study. *Neurology*, **37**, 616–23

Jankovic J and Orman J (1988) Tetrabenazine therapy of dystonia, chorea, tics and other dyskinesias. *Neurology*, **38**, 391–4

Jankovic J and Schwartz K (1990) Botulinum toxin injections for cervical dystonia. *Neurology*, **40**, 277–80

Jankovic J and Schwartz K (1991a) Botulinum toxin treatment of tremors. *Neurology*, **41**, 1185–8

Jankovic J and Schwartz KS (1991b) Clinical correlates of response to botulinum toxin injections. *Arch Neurol*, **48**, 1253–6

Jankovic J, Schwartz K, and Donovan DT (1990) Botulinum toxin treatment of cranial-cervical dystonia, spasmodic dysphonia, other focal dystonias and hemifacial spasm. *J Neurol Neurosurg Psychiatry*, **53**, 633–9

Kalra HK and Magoon EH (1990) Side effects of the use of botulinum toxin for treatment of benign essential blepharospasm and hemifacial spasm. *Ophthalm Surg*, **21**, 335–8

Kao I, Drachman DB, and Price DL (1976) Botulinum toxin: mechanism of presynaptic blockade. *Science*, **193**, 1256–8

Katz B and Rosenberg JH (1987) Botulinum therapy for apraxia of eyelid opening. *Am J Ophthalmol*, **103**, 718–19

Koller W, Vetere-Overfield B, Gray C, and Dubinsky R (1990) Failure of fixed-dose, fixed muscle injection of botulinum toxin in torticollis. *Clin Neuropharmacol*, **13**, 355–8

Kostic V, Covickovic-Sternic N, and Filipovic S (1990) Local treatment of spasmodic torticollis with botulinum toxin. *Neurologiija*, **39**, 29–33

Kraft SP and Lang AE (1988) Botulinum toxin injections in the treatment of blepharospasm, hemifacial spasm and eyelic fasciculations. *Can J Neurol Sci*, **15**, 276–80

Lange DJ, Brin MF, Warner CL, Fahn S, and Lovelace RD (1987) Distant effects of local injection of botulinum toxin. *Muscle Nerve*, **10**, 552–5

Lange DJ, Rubin M, Greene PE, Kang UJ, Moskowitz CB, Brin MF *et al.* (1991) Distant effects of local injected botulinum toxin: a double-blind study of single fiber EMG changes. *Muscle Nerve*, **14**, 672–5

Lees AJ, Trujanski N, Rivest J, Lorch M, and Brookes G (1992) Treatment of cervical dystonia, hand spasms and laryngeal dystonia with botulinum toxin. *J Neurol*, **239**, 1–4

Lepore FE (1988) So-called apraxias of lid movement. *Adv Neurol*, **49**, 85–90

Lingua RW (1985) Sequelae of botulinum toxin injections. *Am J Ophthalomol*, **100**, 305–7

Lorentz IT, Subramaniam SS, and Yiannikas C (1991) Treatment of idiopathic spasmodic torticollis with botulinum toxin A: a double-blind study on twenty-three patients. *Movement Disorders*, **6**, 145–50

Ludlow CL, Naunton RF, Sedory SE, Schulz GM, and Hallett M (1988) Effects of botulinum toxin injections on speech in adductor spasmodic dysphonia. *Neurology*, **38**, 1220–5

Ludlow CL, Naunton RF, Fujita M, and Sedory SE (1990) Spasmodic dysphonia: botulinum toxin injection after recurrent nerve surgery. *Otolaryngol Head Neck Surg*, **102**, 122–31

Ludlow CL, Hallett M, Rhew K, Cole R, Shimizu T, Sakaguchi E *et al.* (1992) Therapeutic use of type F botulinum toxin. *N Engl J Med*, **326**, 349–50

Marsden CD, Marion MH, and Quinn N (1984) The treatment of severe dystonia in children and adults. *J Neurol Neurosurg Psychiatry*, **47**, 1166–73

Mauriello JA, Coniaris H, and Haupt EJ (1987) Use of botulinum toxin in the treatment of one hundred patients with facial dyskinesias. *Ophthalmology*, **94**, 976–9

Maurri S, Brogelli S, Alfieri G, and Barontini F (1988) Beneficial effect of botulinum A toxin in blepharospasm: 16 months experience with 16 cases. *Ital J Neurol Sci*, **9**, 337–44

Middaugh J (1978) Botulism and breast milk. *N Engl J Med*, **298**, 343

Miller RH, Woodson GE, and Jankovic J (1987) Botulinum toxin injection of the vocal fold for spasmodic dysphonia. A preliminary report. *Arch Otolaryngol Head Neck Surg*, **113**, 603–5

Moore AP and Blumhardt LD (1991) A double-blind trial of botulinum toxin-A in torticollis, with one year follow up. *J Neurol Neurosurg Psychiatry*, **54**, 813–16

Olney RK, Aminoff MJ, Gelb DJ, and Lowenstein DH (1988) Neuromuscular effects distant from the site of botulinum neurotoxin injection. *Neurology*, **38**, 1780–3

Osako M and Keltner JL (1991) Botulinum A toxin (Oculinum) in ophthalmology. *Surv Ophthalmol*, **36**, 28–46

Paton JD, Lawrence AJ, and Manson JI (1982) Quantitation of *Clostridium botulinum* organisms and toxin in the feces of an infant with botulism. *J Clin Microbiol*, **15**, 1–4

Patrinely JR, Whiting AS, and Anderson RL (1988) Local side effects of botulinum toxin injections. *Adv Neurol*, **49**, 493–500

Perman KI, Baylis HI, Rosenbaum AL, and Kirschen DG (1986) The use of botulinum toxin in the medical management of benign essential blepharospasm. *Ophthalmology*, **93**, 1–3

Poewe W, Schelosky L, Kleedorfer B, Heinen F, Wagner M, and Deuschl G (1992) Treatment of spasmodic torticollis with local injections of botulinum toxin. *J Neurol*, **239**, 21–5

Poungvarin N (1991) Writer's cramp: the experience with botulinum toxin injections in 25 patients. *J Med Assoc Thailand*, **74**, 239–46

Quinn N and Hallett M (1989) Dose standardisation of botulinum toxin. *Lancet*, **1**, 964

Rivest J, Lees AJ, and Marsden CD (1991) Writer's cramp: treatment with botulinum toxin injections. *Movement Disorders*, **6**, 55–9

Ruusuvaara P and Setala K (1990) Long-term treatment of involuntary facial spasms using botulinum toxin. *Acta Ophthalmol*, **68**, 331–8

St Clair EH, DiLiberti JH, and O'Brien ML (1985) Observations of an infant born to a mother with botulism. *J Pediatr*, **87**, 658

Sanders DB, Massey EW, and Buckley EG (1986) Botulinum toxin for blepharospasm: single-fiber EMG studies. *Neurology*, **36**, 545–7

Scott AB (1980) Botulinum toxin injection into extraocular muscles as an alternative to strabismus surgery. *Ophthalmology*, **87**, 1044–9

Scott AB (1984) Injection treatment of endocrine orbital myopathy. *Doc Ophthalmol*, **58**, 141–5

Scott (1989) Clostridial toxins as therapeutic agents. In: Simpson LL (ed) *Botulinum neurotoxin and tetanus toxin*, Academic Press, New York, 399–412

Scott AB and Kraft SP (1985) Botulinum toxin injection in the management of lateral rectus paresis. *Ophthalmology*, **92**, 676–83

Scott AB and Suzuki D (1988) Systemic toxicity of botulinum toxin by intramuscular injection in the monkey. *Movement Disorders*, **3**, 333–5

Scott AB, Rosenbaum A, and Collins CC (1973) Pharmacologic weakening of extraocular muscles. *Invest Ophthalmol*, **12**, 924–7

Scott AB, Kennedy RA, and Stubbs HA (1985) Botulinum A toxin injection as a treatment for blepharospasm. *Arch Ophthalmol*, **103**, 347–50

Shore JW, Leone CR, O'Connor PS, Neuhaus RW, and Arnold AC (1986) Botulinum toxin for the treatment of essential blepharospasm. *Ophthalm Surg*, **17**, 747–53

Shorr N, Seiff SR, and Kopelman J (1985) The use of botulinum toxin in blepharospasm. *Am J Ophthalmol*, **99**, 542–6

Simpson LL (1986) Molecular pharmacology of botulinum toxin and tetanus toxin. *Ann Rev Pharmacol Toxicol*, **26**, 427–53

Snow BJ, Tsui JKC, Bhatt MH, Varelas M, Hashimoto SA, and Calne DB (1990) Treatment of spasticity with botulinum toxin: a double-blind study. *Ann Neurol*, **28**, 512–15

Stell R, Thompson PD, and Marsden CD (1988) Botulinum toxin in spasmodic torticollis. *J Neurol Neurosurg Psychiatry*, **51**, 920–3

Taylor JDN, Kraft SP, Kazdan MS, Flanders M, Cadera W, and Orton RB (1991) Treatment of blepharospasm and hemifacial spasm with botulinum A toxin: a Canadian multicentre study. *Can J Ophthalmol*, **26**, 133–8

Tolosa E, Marti MJ, and Kulisevsky J (1988) Botulinum toxin injection therapy for hemifacial spasm. *Adv Neurol*, **49**, 479–91

Truong DD, Rontal M, Rolnick M, Aronson AE, and Mistura K (1991) Double-blind controlled study of botulinum toxin in adductor spasmodic dysphonia. *Laryngoscope*, **101**, 630–4

Tsoy EA, Buckley EG, and Dutton JJ (1985) Treatment of blepharospasm with botulinum toxin. *Am J Ophthalmol*, **99**, 176–9

Tsui JKC, Eisen A, Stoessl AJ, Calne S, and Calne DB (1986) Double-blind study of botulinum toxin in spasmodic torticollis. *Lancet*, **2**, 245–7

Tsui JK, Wong NLM, Wong E, and Calne DB (1988) Production of circulating antibodies to botulinum-A toxin in patients receiving repeated injections for dystonia. *Ann Neurol*, **23**, 181

Waller RR, Kennedy RH, Henderson JW, and Kesty KR (1985) Management of blepharospasm. *Trans Am Ophthalmol Soc*, **83**, 367–86

Yoshimura DM, Aminoff MJ, and Tami TA (1990) Botulinum toxin therapy for hemifacial spasm. *Neurology*, **40** (suppl 1), 381

Yoshimura DM, Aminoff MJ, and Olney RK (1992) Botulinum toxin therapy for limb dystonias. *Neurology*, **42**, 627–30

Zwirner P, Murry T, Swenson M, and Woodson G (1991) Acoustic changes in spasmodic dysphonia after botulinum toxin injection. *J Voice*, **5**, 78–84

25
Stereotypies

Joseph Jankovic

Introduction

The term stereotypy is often used to describe patterned and repetitive movements, but no clear definition of this movement disorder has been formulated. For the purposes of this review, stereotypy is defined as an involuntary or unvoluntary, coordinated, patterned, repetitive, rhythmic, purposeless, but seemingly purposeful or ritualistic, movement, posture or utterance. In the context of this definition it is important to first clarify the terms voluntary, involuntary, unvoluntary, and automatic movements (Jankovic, 1992). *Voluntary* movements are either intentional (planned, willed, self-initiated) or responsive (occurring in response to an external auditory, visual or tactile stimulus). Studies showing a delay in the execution of voluntary movements by electrical or magnetic brain stimulation suggest that the motor programs for the initial sequence of agonist–antagonist activity required for voluntary movement are stored outside the motor cortex, but that coded instructions are released to the motor cortex immediately prior to the execution of the movement (Day *et al*., 1989; Papa *et al*., 1991). *Involuntary* movements can be subdivided into non-suppressible (e.g. reflexes, seizures, myoclonus and some hyperkinetic movement disorders) and suppressible (e.g. most hyperkinetic movement disorders, particularly tics, and some tremors, dystonias, choreas and stereotypies). Besides willpower, abnormal movements can be suppressed by other techniques or manoeuvres, such as sensory tricks (e.g. self-induced sensory feedback by *geste antagonistique* in patients with torticollis), self-hypnosis and sleep (Koller and Biary, 1989; Silvestri *et al*., 1990). *Unvoluntary* movements occur in response to or are driven by either somatic sensations (local feeling of discomfort, pain, tension or tightness) or unwanted psychic phenomenon (an inner feeling of urge, anxiety and compulsion). *Automatic* movements are those that occur unconsciously (e.g. respiratory, cardiac, intestinal and other smooth muscle contractions) or they are learned and do not require conscious effort (e.g. gait, oromandibular movements in the act of speaking, chewing, crying or smiling). Stereotypies can be both involuntary and unvoluntary; when not accompanied by severe cognitive deficit, they can be temporarily suppressed.

Stereotypical behaviour is common in animals in lower species up to and including the primates. Some studies have suggested that stereotypies are more common in farm and zoo animals housed in restraining environments with low stimulation

(Dantzer, 1986). With the development of stereotypies, there is a reduction in the broad behavioural repertoire normally displayed by unrestrained animals. Therefore, stereotypy has been viewed as either a self-generating sensory stimulus or a motor expression of underlying tension and anxiety. The repetitive and ritualistic behaviour displayed by some animals has been used as an experimental model of obsessive-compulsive disorders (Pitman, 1989). Indeed, studies of animal and human stereotypies have provided important insights into relationships between motor function and behaviour. It is well-known that stereotypies often accompany a variety of behavioural disorders such as anxiety, obsessive-compulsive disorders, Tourette's syndrome, schizophrenia, akathisia, autism and mental retardation. Thus, stereotypy is a motor–behavioural disorder found most frequently in patients who are in the borderland between neurology and psychiatry.

PATHOPHYSIOLOGY OF STEREOTYPIES

Most studies of stereotypical behaviour in experimental animals have focused on the role of dopaminergic systems in the basal ganglia and limbic structures (Cooper and Dourism, 1990). Intrastriatal injection of dopamine and systemic administration of both presynaptically active dopaminergic drugs, such as amphetamine, and postsynaptically active dopamine agonists, such as apomorphine, in rats produce dose-related repetitive sniffing, gnawing, licking, biting, rearing, head bobbing, grooming and other stereotyped learned activities (Costall *et al.*, 1977; Chipkin *et al.*, 1987; Koller and Herbster, 1988; Tschanz and Rebec, 1988). These stereotypies can be blocked by both typical and atypical antipsychotic drugs, giving additional support to the notion that increased dopaminergic activity is required to produce stereotypical motor behaviour (Tschanz and Rebec, 1988). The different antipsychotics, however, seem to have a variable effect on the different stereotypies. In one study of stereotypies in rats, clozapine selectively blocked oral behaviour, while thioridazine at low doses reduced head bobbing (Tschanz and Rebec, 1988). At high doses, thioridazine also blocked oral movements. Haloperidol abolished all amphetamine-induced stereotypies. Therefore, various neuroleptics seem to have a selective blocking effect on dopamine receptors and the different stereotypies seem to be mediated through unique neurotransmitter receptor systems.

Selective dopamine receptor agonists and antagonists have been used in experimental models to study differential effects of D_1 and D_2 receptors on stereotypical behaviour. SKF 38393, a D_1 agonist, produced no stereotypic behaviour in normal rats, but it did enhance stereotypy induced by apomorphine (mixed D_1 and D_2 agonist) and by PHNO (selected D_2 agonist; Koller and Herbster, 1988). This suggests that the D_2 dopamine receptors mediate stereotypical behaviour, and that activation of the D_1 receptors potentiates these D_2-mediated effects. Additional evidence for the role of D_2 dopamine receptors in the pathogenesis of stereotypies is the observation that upregulation of D_2 receptors (with haloperidol, a selective D_2 antagonist), but not of D_1 receptors (with SCH 23390, a selective D_1 antagonist), enhanced apomorphine-induced stereotypies (Chipkin *et al.*, 1987). While dysfunction in the basal ganglia has been implicated in the pathogenesis of certain stereotypies (Maraganore *et al.*, 1991; Jicha and Salamone, 1991), some studies have also provided evidence for the role of the mesolimbic system, particularly the nucleus accumbens–amygdala neural loop, in the pathogenesis of stereotypical movements (Costall *et al.*, 1977; Hiroi and White, 1989).

Using the technique of *in vivo* microdialysis in freely moving rats, correlation between amphetamine-induced stereotypical behaviour and striatal extracellular release of dopamine was clearly demonstrated (Kuczenski and Segal, 1989). However, this study showed that there was temporal discrepancy between the recorded increase in striatal dopamine and the development of stereotypies. Therefore, some non-dopaminergic neurotransmitters may also play an important role in the pathogenesis of these repetitive movements. Certain aspects of the behavioural response to amphetamine, such as transition from locomotion to focused stereotypy, seemed to correlate better with the relatively brief (20–40 minutes) increase in striatal concentration of serotonin, suggesting that the two neurotransmitters, dopamine and serotonin, exert separate and independent influence on stereotypical behaviour.

Besides the classic neurotransmitters, evidence is accumulating in support of involvement of neuropeptides as modulators of stereotypical behaviour. For example, microinjection of cholecystokinin and neurotensin into the medial nucleus accumbens markedly potentiated apomorphine-induced stereotypy (Blumstein *et al.*, 1987). Since injection of these peptides into the striatum had no effect on the apomorphine-induced stereotypy, these studies provide additional evidence for the involvement of the limbic system in the pathogenesis of this movement disorder.

CLINICAL PHENOMENOLOGY AND AETIOLOGY OF STEREOTYPIES

Stereotypical movements can be classified as either simple (foot tapping, body rocking) or complex (complicated rituals, sitting down and arising from chair). Stereotypies can also be described according to distribution of the predominant site of involvement (orolingual, hand, leg, truncal). The term stereotypy should be used to describe a phenomenological, not an aetiological, category of hyperkinetic movement disorders. However, recognition of stereotypy as a distinct movement disorder can logically lead from a phenomenological to an aetiological diagnosis (Table 25.1).

Table 25.1 Stereotypy

Physiological
Pathological
Mental retardation
Autism (Kanner's infantile autism, Asperger's syndrome)
Rett syndrome
Neuroacanthocytosis
Schizophrenia
Catatonia
Obsessive-compulsive disorder
Tourette's syndrome
Tardive and other dyskinesias
Akathisia
Restless legs syndrome
Epileptic automatism
Psychogenic

Physiological stereotypies

Certain stereotypies, such as tapping of the feet, adduction-abduction and crossing-uncrossing of the legs, may be part of a repertoire of movements seen in otherwise normal individuals. In infants and children there seems to be a progression of normal stereotypies. For example, thumb and hand sucking in infancy is later replaced by body rocking, head rolling and head banging. Head banging, for example, is seen in up to 15% of normal children (Kravitz and Boehm, 1971; Sallustro and Atwell, 1978). Later, some normal children develop bruxism, nail biting and even trichotillomania (hair pulling). *Mannerisms*, which are gestures peculiar or unique to the individual, may at times seem stereotypical. An example of a stereotypical mannerism is the ritualistic movements performed by a baseball pitcher before actually pitching the ball. *Physiological* stereotypies are often more pronounced during periods of anxiety or anticipated stress. However, when stereotypy is accompanied by other behavioural and neurological findings, it usually indicates the presence of a serious underlying neurological and/or psychiatric disorder (Table 25.1).

Mental retardation and autism

Mental retardation and autistic disorders are characteristically associated with stereotypical behaviour. In one study of 102 institutionalized mentally retarded people, mean age 35 (range 21–68) years, 34% exhibited at least one type of stereotypy (rhythmic movement 26%, bizarre posturing 13%, object manipulation 7%, and others; Dura *et al.*, 1987). Although there seems to be an inverse correlation between stereotypies and IQ, stereotypical behaviour may be seen even in the mildly retarded.

Autism is a type of pervasive developmental disorder (PDD) with onset during infancy or childhood, characterized by impairment in reciprocal social and interpersonal interactions, impairment in verbal and non-verbal communication, markedly restricted repertoire of activities and interests, and stereotyped movements (Wing and Attwood, 1987; Allen, 1988; Schreibman, 1988). It has been estimated that over 0.1% of all children are autistic (Sugiyama and Abe, 1989). In children and adults with autism of any cause, stereotypies and other self-stimulatory activities constitute the most recognizable symptoms. Typical stereotypies seen in autistic individuals include facial grimacing, staring at flickering lights, waving objects in front of the eyes, producing repetitive sounds, arm flapping, rhythmic body rocking, repetitive touching, feeling and smelling of objects, jumping, walking on toes, and unusual hand and body postures. The motor manifestations are often associated with insensitivity or excessive sensitivity to sensory stimuli including pain and extremes of temperature, preoccupations with perceptual sensations such as lights or odours, insistence on preservation of sameness, and absence of fear or other emotional reactions. Self-stimulatory and self-injurious behaviours such as self-biting and head banging, are also common. In addition to these and other behavioural and developmental abnormalities, some autistic individuals have isolated areas of remarkable and sometimes spectacular mental skills – the so-called *savant* syndrome (Treffert, 1988; O'Connor and Hermelin, 1989).

There are many causes of autism, including the fragile X syndrome and a variety of eponymically classified types such as Kanner, Heller, Asperger and Rett syndromes (Wing and Attwood, 1987; Burd *et al.*, 1989; Steffenburg *et al.*, 1989; Gillberg, 1989; Percy *et al.*, 1990). Population-based twin studies have suggested that genetic factors are important in many cases of autism and that perinatal stress may play a role in some (Steffenburg *et al.*, 1989). Asperger syndrome is one of the most common forms of autism, found in 1–3/1000 children (Burd *et al.*, 1989; Gillberg, 1989; Steffenburg *et al.*, 1989; Szatmari *et al.*, 1989). Characterized by social isolation in combination with odd and eccentric behaviour, Asperger syndrome shares many features with infantile autism. Several studies have indeed noted an overlap in various clinical and demographic characteristics between Asperger syndrome and infantile autism (Gillberg and Gillberg, 1989; Szatmari *et al.*, 1989). In one study of 23 patients, the Asperger children seemed to have relatively poor motor skills, had a stiff and awkward gait (without arm-swing), and their speech development was delayed, although they acquired better expressive speech as compared with infantile autism. In contrast to infantile autism, Asperger syndrome usually does not become fully manifest until 30–36 months of age, but some may have first symptoms in infancy. A recent study of 7 patients with the combination of Asperger's syndrome and Tourette's syndrome showed MRI evidence of cortical and subcortical abnormalities in 5 of these patients (Berther *et al.*, 1993). Because the Asperger children are generally brighter, it has been suggested that this syndrome merely represents a mild variant of autism.

Dysfunction of the frontal/parietal cortex, neostriatum and thalamus has been demonstrated in autistic patients by cerebral glucose metabolic studies (Horwitz *et al.*, 1988). Imaging studies, including magnetic resonance imaging (MRI), have suggested left frontal and brainstem atrophy in some autistic patients (Hashimoto *et al.*, 1989) but more recent studies have failed to find any characteristic abnormalities on MRI scans of autistic children (Kleiman *et al.*, 1992). Furthermore, decreased neuronal size with immature dendritic pattern in the hippocampus along with cerebellar vermal hypoplasia have been found in brains of patients with idiopathic (infantile) autism (Courchesne *et al.*, 1988). However, the pathogenesis of most autistic disorders is still unknown (Rapin, 1987).

In patients with mental retardation and autism, irrespective of aetiology, stereotypies are often associated with self-injurious behaviour (Robertson, 1992). This is particularly true for patients with body-rocking movements, a stereotypy most often associated with self-hitting (Rojahn, 1986). While head banging and other self-injurious behaviour may occur in normal children (Kravitz and Boehm, 1971; Sallustro and Atwell, 1978), this type of behaviour is usually abnormal and is particularly common in patients who also exhibit stereotypical behaviour (Jankovic, 1988). The observation that self-biting behaviour induced by dopaminergic drugs in 6-hydroxydopamine rats and in monkeys with a unilateral lesion in the ventral medial tegmentum can be blocked by a selective D_1 antagonist SCH 23390 suggests that self-injurious behaviour is mediated primarily by the D_1 receptors (Breese *et al.*, 1984; Goldstein *et al.*, 1985; Schroeder *et al.*, 1991). This is in contrast to stereotypies, which are mediated presumably by the D_2 receptors. Supersensitivity of D_1 receptors, possibly in response to abnormal arborization of dopamine neurons in the striatum, has been postulated as a possible mechanism of self-injurious behaviour in Lesch–Nyhan syndrome (Jankovic, 1988; Jankovic *et al.*, 1988). Self-injurious behaviour also often accompanies stereotypical behaviour in autistic children. Marked improvement in self-injurious behaviour observed in autistic children after administration of the opiate blockers naloxone and naltrexone has been interpreted as evidence for the role of endogenous opiates (e.g. beta-endorphins) in this abnormal behaviour (Sandman, 1988). Additional support for the role of endorphins in self-injurious and stereotypical behaviour is the finding of elevated plasma and cerebrospinal fluid (CSF) levels of beta-endorphins in autistic patients with these behavioural abnormalities (Sandman, 1988).

Rett syndrome

Rett syndrome is an autistic disorder reported only in girls and manifested clinically by stereotypic movements and other movement disorders (Hagberg, 1989; Percy *et al.*, 1988, 1990; Fitzgerald *et al.*, 1990a). In contrast to infantile autism and mental retardation, Rett patients tend to have normal development until 6–18 months of age; this is then followed by gradual regression of both motor and language skills. Usually between the ages of 9 months and 3 years there is a gradual social withdrawal and psychomotor regression with loss of acquired communicative skills. Acquired finger and hand skills are gradually replaced by stereotypical hand movements, including hand clapping, wringing, clenching, washing, patting, and rubbing (Fig. 25.1). Additionally, Rett girls often exhibit body-rocking movements and shifting of weight from one leg to the other. Other motor disturbances include respiratory dysregulation with episodic hyperventilation and breath holding, bruxism, ocular deviations, dystonia, myoclonus, athetosis, tremor, jerky truncal and gait ataxia and

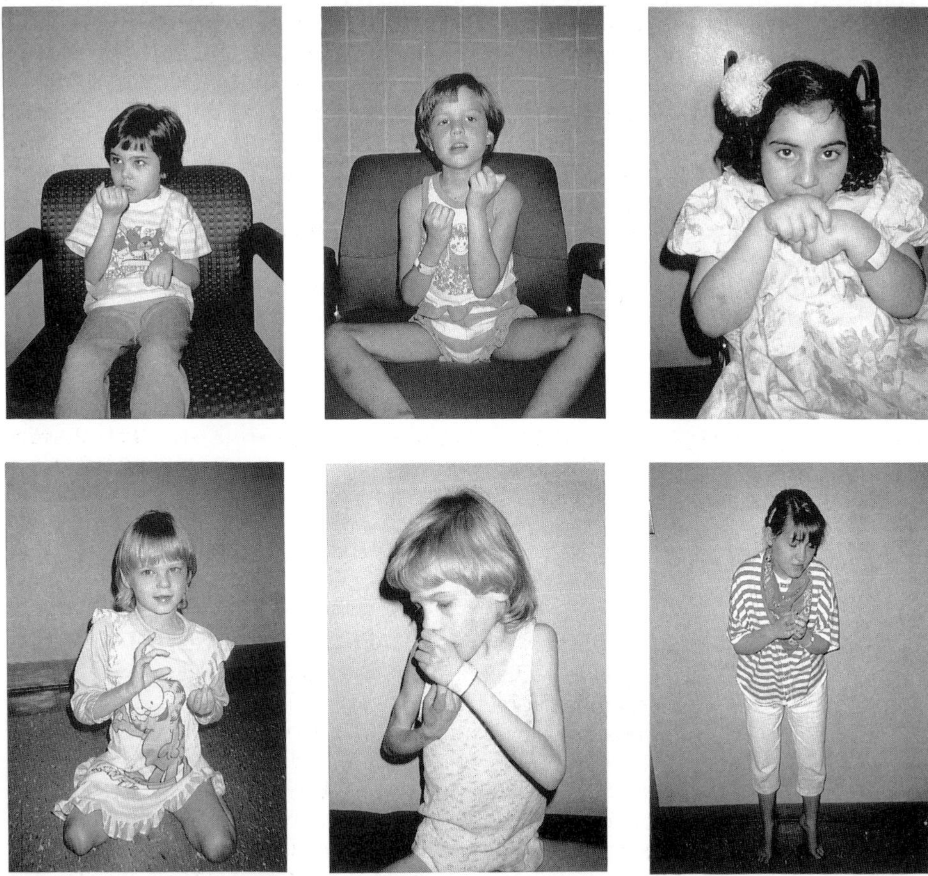

Figure 25.1 A series of Rett girls showing typical hand sterotypies.

parkinsonian findings. In a study of 32 Rett patients, ages 30 months to 28 years, we suggested that the occurrence of the different motor disorders seemed to be age-related (Fitzgerald *et al.*, 1990b). The hyperkinetic disorders were more common in younger girls while bradykinetic disorders seemed more prominent in the older patients.

The pathophysiological basis of the motor disturbances in Rett syndrome has not been elucidated. Magnetic resonance imaging studies have shown generalized brain and bilateral caudate atrophy (Casanova *et al.*, 1991; Reiss *et al.*, 1993). Electroencephalographic recordings show age-related progressive deterioration characterized by slowing, loss of normal sleep characteristics and the appearance of epileptiform activity. In a few postmortem examinations of Rett brains, besides microcephaly, spongy degeneration of cerebral and cerebellar white matter, and deposition of lipofuscin, there was evidence of depigmentation of substantia nigra and locus coeruleus (Hagberg, 1989; Lekman *et al.*, 1989). The monoamine metabolites and biopterin levels were variably and inconsistently decreased in the CSF, while CSF beta-endorphin immunoreactivity was increased (Myer *et al.*, 1988; Perry *et al.*, 1988; Zoghbi *et al.*, 1989). Postmortem biochemical analyses, performed in only a few Rett brains, showed decreased dopamine, noradrenaline, serotonin and choline acetyl transferase activity in most cortical regions, suggesting a defect in the maturation of central monoaminergic and cholinergic systems. However, in one study of 4 brains, the biogenic amines and their metabolites were normal in the striatum and pallidum, but all 3 neurotransmitters and their metabolites, with the exception of the noradrenaline metabolite MHPG (3-methoxy 4-hydroxy phenyl glycol), were markedly reduced in the substantia nigra (Lekman *et al.*, 1989). Various genetic hypotheses, including X-linked dominant mutation or mitochondrial DNA mutation, have been suggested, but further studies are needed before any of these hypotheses can be accepted (Zoghbi, 1988; Eeg-Olofsson *et al.*, 1989).

Neuroacanthocytosis

Progression from a hyperkinetic to a bradykinetic movement disorder, as seen in Rett syndrome, may be also encountered in neuroacanthocytosis, another disorder manifested by stereotypical and self-injurious (e.g. lip and tongue biting) behaviour (Spitz *et al.*, 1985; Jankovic 1988). The onset is usually in the third and fourth decade and the disorder is often inherited in an autosomal recessive pattern. In one report of two brothers with this disorder, the facial and vocal tics, orofacial stereotypies, and lip biting were gradually replaced by evidence of motor neuron disease and parkinsonism (Spitz *et al.*, 1985). Wet blood and Wright-stain fast-dried smear show that at least 15% of red blood cells are in a form of acanthocytes. Other features of neuroacanthocytosis include progressive dementia, chorea, dystonia, ophthalmoparesis, seizures, areflexia, increased cholecystokinin and caudate atrophy on neuroimagining and postmortem examinations. Striatal involvement is also supported by demonstration of marked reduction of glucose metabolism on (^{18}F)-2-fluoro-2-deoxyglucose positron emission tomography scans (Dubinsky *et al.*, 1989). Postmorten biochemical analysis in 2 unrelated patients with this disorder showed marked depletion of dopamine in the striatum, elevation of noradrenaline levels in the putamen and globus pallidus, and marked reduction in levels of substance P in the striatum and substantia nigra (de Yebenes *et al.*, 1988).

Schizophrenia and catatonia

Various stereotypies were described in schizophrenic patients long before neuroleptics were first introduced for the treatment of psychotic disorders. In 1873, Kahlbaum described a motor disorder he termed catatonia in 21 psychotic patients (Kahlbaum, 1873). Half of the patients had facial stereotypies, such as facial grimacing, lip pursing and bruxism, phenomenologically similar to the orofacial tardive dyskinesias. In one study of 100 schizophrenic patients initially evaluated prior to the introduction of neuroleptics in 1954, 77 exhibited some stereotypies (Rogers and Hymas, 1988). These included facial grimacing in 48 patients, inappropriate smiling in 36, and 'facial contortions, habit spasms and manneristic twitching' in 15. The presence of these and other abnormal involuntary movements, the frequent occurrence of 'soft' neurological signs, the response to antidopaminergic drugs, and some subtle anatomical abnormalities (small medial temporal lobes, particularly anterior hippocampi, and enlarged third and lateral ventricles) provide support for the current notion that schizophrenia is a neurological disturbance primarily involving the dopaminergic system (Kovelman and Scheibel, 1986; Carlsson, 1988; Heinrichs and Buchanan, 1988; Roberts, 1990; Suddath *et al.*, 1990).

Although conventionally classified as a subtype of schizophrenia, catatonia is commonly associated with affective disorders and only about 5–10% of catatonics satisfy diagnostic criteria for schizophrenia (Abrams and Taylor, 1976). Thus catatonia should be viewed as a syndrome, caused by a variety of medical, neurological and psychiatric conditions, with abnormal motor behaviour ranging from extreme hyperactivity to akinesia with mutism and stupor (Stoudemire, 1982). Stereotypies, such as shifting position, maintaining unusual postures, tapping or touching objects, repetitively moving mouth and jaw, performing rituals and mannerisms, repeating phrases and sentences (verbigeration) and repeating the examiner's questions (echolalia), are among the most characteristic motor disorders in catatonia. When catatonia is associated with stereotypies, the diagnosis of mania should be considered and a favourable response to treatment should be expected (Abrams *et al.*, 1979).

Obsessive-compulsive disorder

Another psychiatric disorder frequently accompanied by stereotypic movements is the obsessive-compulsive disorder (OCD) (Zohar and Insel, 1987; Rogers and Hymas, 1988). Once considered a rare psychiatric disorder, recent epidemiological studies indicate that the lifetime prevalence of OCD is approximately 2.5% (Karno *et al.*, 1988). Compulsions may be difficult to differentiate from stereotypies. In contrast to stereotypies, compulsions are usually preceded by or associated with feelings of inner tension or anxiety and a need to perform the same act repeatedly in the same manner. Examples of compulsions are ritualistic hand washing, repetitively touching the same place, evening up, arranging, and checking doors, locks and appliances. In one study of 70 child and adolescent patients with OCD, 26% exhibited certain stereotypies such as licking, spitting and other repetitive, patterned and coordinated movements (Rapoport, 1988). Reports of focal striatal lesions giving rise to severe OCD (Croisile *et al.*, 1989; Modell *et al.*, 1989; Weilburg *et al.*, 1989) and the frequent association of OCD with basal ganglia disorders such as Parkinson's disease and Sydenham's chorea (Swedo *et al.*, 1993) provide additional support for the link between abnormal behaviour, such as OCD, and extrapyramidal dysfunction

(Baxter *et al.*, 1987; Croisile *et al.*, 1989; Laplane *et al.*, 1989; Modell *et al.*, 1989; Weilburg *et al.*, 1989; Cummings, 1993).

Tourette's syndrome

Another disorder often associated with OCD and stereotypies is Tourette's syndrome (Jankovic and Rohaidy, 1987). The following criteria are required for its diagnosis:

1. Both multiple motor and one or more vocal/phonic tics must be present at some time during the illness, although not necessarily concurrently.
2. The tics occur many times a day, nearly every day, or intermittently throughout a period of more than 1 year.
3. The anatomical location, number frequency, type, complexity, or severity of tics change over time.
4. Onset before age 21.
5. Involuntary movements and noises cannot be explained by other medical conditions.
6. Motor and/or vocal/phonic tics must be witnessed by a reliable examiner directly at some point during the illness or be recorded by video tape or cinematography (The Tourette Syndrome Study Group, 1993). Motor tics can be subdivided into simple motor tics, which are involuntary, abrupt, sudden, brief and isolated movement, and complex motor tics, which are distinct coordinated, sequential movements. Repetitive complex motor tics, such as repetitive touching, hand gesturing, head shaking, facial grimacing, truncal gyrating and bending movements, may have the characteristics of stereotypies.

In addition to motor and phonic tics, Tourette's syndrome patients exhibit a variety of behavioural disorders including attention deficit disorder with hyperactivity, learning disorders, impulse control problems and OCD (Kurlan, 1989). Because some of the complex motor tics may be repetitive and stereotypic, Tourette's syndrome is occasionally misdiagnosed as autism. Indeed, in one study of 59 patients with infantile autism and other pervasive developmental disorders, 12 patients later developed symptoms consistent with Tourette's syndrome (Burd *et al.*, 1987). That Tourette's syndrome and autism occasionally coexist is now well recognized (Berther *et al.*, 1993). The Tourette's syndrome patients scored significantly higher on measures of IQ and language and seemed to have a better developmental outcome than the other children.

Tardive dyskinesia

Repetitive and patterned movements, phenomenologically identical to stereotypy, are characteristically seen in patients with tardive dyskinesia (Stacy *et al.*, 1993). Because all types of movement disorders, including parkinsonism, chorea, dystonia, tics, myoclonus and stereotypy, can result from the use of dopamine receptor blocking drugs (neuroleptics), the nosology of the movement disorders in tardive dyskinesia is sometimes problematic and controversial (Miller and Jankovic, 1990a). The most typical form of tardive dyskinesia, the orofacial-lingual-masticatory movement, is one of the best examples of a stereotypic movement disorder (Rupniak *et al.*, 1990).

Because of its resemblance to a choreic movement, this and other patterned and repetitive movements typically seen in tardive dyskinesia have been labelled by some as chorea or rhythmic chorea (Fahn, 1989). However, stereotypy, a coordinated, patterned and repetitive movement, differs from chorea, defined as randomly distributed, non-patterned jerks and, therefore, the term stereotypy more accurately describes the hyperkinetic movement disorder typically encountered in tardive dyskinesia. When video tapes of children with stereotypies associated with autism were compared by three experienced raters to neuroleptic-related dyskinesias, no reliable differentiation between the two hyperkinesias could be made (Meiselas *et al.*, 1989). Other stereotypies commonly seen in patients with tardive dyskinesia include body rocking and pelvic-thrusting (copulatory dyskinesia) movements (Kameko *et al.*, 1993).

In an analysis of 125 patients referred to the Baylor College of Medicine Movement Disorders Clinic with a drug-induced movement disorder, 79 (63%) had stereotypical movements, originally classified as chorea (Miller and Jankovic, 1990b). Other hyperkinetic movement disorders included tardive dystonia, seen in 30 (24%), tardive akathisia in 9 (7%), and 2 patients had isolated tardive tremor. Neuroleptic-induced parkinsonism was documented in 38 (30%) patients. The majority (53%) of the patients with tardive stereotypy were in their sixth and seventh decade, while those with parkinsonism were on the average a decade older and those with tardive dystonia tended to be younger. Except for tardive dystonia, women outnumbered men at 4 : 1. Only 44 (43%) of the patients had evidence of psychosis; the others were treated with dopamine receptor blocking drugs for a variety of non-psychotic reasons, including depression (61%), gastrointestinal problems (26%), anxiety (23%) and insomnia (5%). The lower part of the face and trunk were most frequently affected by the drug-induced movement disorders. In another study of 100 patients with tardive dystonia, stereotypy was present in 78; other involuntary movements included dystonia, akathisia, tremor, chorea and myoclonus in descending order (Stacy *et al.*, 1993).

More complex stereotypies, such as hair and face rubbing, picking at clothes, crossing and uncrossing of legs, adduction-abduction and up-and-down pumping of legs, arising and sitting down, marching in place, pacing and shifting weight, often associated with feeling of restlessness, are typically seen in patients with *tardive akathisia* (Burke *et al.*, 1989). In addition to these motor manifestations, many patients with akathisia also exhibit respiratory grunting and moaning, which are believed to represent phonic stereotypies or noises produced by associated respiratory dyskinesia. Tardive akathisia is the most disabling form of tardive dyskinesia (Miller and Jankovic, 1990b).

Akathisia may be caused by neuroleptics, Parkinson's disease or other causes and is sometimes confused with the syndrome of restless legs (Blin *et al.*, 1990; Lang, 1993). Both disorders exhibit stereotypical movements and motor restlessness, but patients with restless legs seem to complain more of paraesthesias, particularly a creeping or crawling sensation in the legs associated with an irresistible urge to keep the limbs in motion. The restless legs syndrome is often worse at night, causing insomnia, and it may be associated with periodic movements of sleep (Walters *et al.*, 1988b). A variety of stereotypies, such as body rocking and marching in place, occur in these patients even while they are awake. While genetic factors play an important pathogenic role in many patients with this syndrome, increased excitability of segmental reflexes and involvement of the dopaminergic striatopallidal system (in parkinsonian patients) have been proposed as possible mechanisms for this movement disorder (Askenasy *et al.*, 1987).

TREATMENT

Treatment of stereotypies is largely determined by its severity, intensity, and by the associated neurological and psychiatric disorders. Some studies of patients with mental retardation or autism suggest that stereotypical behaviour interferes with learning and that a control of this behaviour is essential for any training to be successful (Murphy *et al.*, 1977). However, one study concluded that stereotypy interferes with learning only in people with very profound retardation (Watkins and Konarski, 1987). Besides behavioural interventions, various psychoactive drugs have been used in the treatment of disabling stereotypies (Volkmar and Bregmen, 1988). These include sedative-hypnotics (e.g. diazepam, lorazepam, clonazepam), lithium, baclofen, neuroleptics and opiate antagonists (naloxone and naltrexone). Opioid antagonists may also be useful in patients with self-injurous behaviour (Baumeister *et al.*, 1993). Clonidine, deprenyl and methylphenidate may be useful in the treatment of attention deficit disorder with hyperactivity (Baumeister *et al.*, 1993; Jankovic 1993). However, methodological problems in many of the studies make interpretation of the results difficult. Neuroleptics should be used only as a last resort because of the risk of tardive dyskinesia and akathisia.

In addition to supportive therapy, such as hydration and feeding, treatment of catatonia usually involves the use of sedatives (e.g. barbiturates), tricyclic antidepressants, neuroleptics, lithium and electroconvulsive therapy. Patients with OCD, with or without Tourette's syndrome, often improve with the serotonin uptake inhibitors, including fluoxetine, fluvoxamine and clomipramine (Goodman *et al.*, 1992).

Akathisia associated with parkinsonism may improve with dopaminergic drugs. Beta-blockers, anticholinergics and opioids have also been found effective is some patients with akathisia. In contrast, tardive akathisia is usually resistant to pharmacological therapy. However, in a study of 52 patients with tardive akathisia, reserpine and tetrabenazine produced some improvement in 87% and 58% of patients treated with these drugs, respectively (Burke *et al.*, 1989). Indeed, tetrabenazine is considered to be the most effective agent in the treatment of tardive dyskinesia (Jankovic and Orman, 1988). Regrettably, this drug, which acts through a dual mechanism as a monoamine-depleting and dopamine receptor-blocking agent, is available in the USA only as an investigational agent. Although it has some neuroleptic properties, tetrabenazine has never been demonstrated to cause tardive dyskinesia or dystonia. Reserpine, another monoamine-depleting drug, is less effective than tetrabenazine in the treatment of tardive syndromes. Patients with restless legs syndrome may improve with dopaminergic drugs, opioids (e.g. codeine, propoxyphene, methadone), clonazepam, clonidine, carbamezapine and baclofen (Akpinar, 1987; Brodeur *et al.*, 1988; Sandyk *et al.*, 1987; Walters *et al.*, 1988a).

References

Abrams R and Taylor MA (1976) Catatonia: a prospective clinical study. *Arch Gen Psychiatry*, **33**, 579–81

Abrams R, Taylor MA, and Stolurow KA (1979) Catatonia and mania: patterns of cerebral dysfunction. *Biol Psychiatry*, **14**, 111–17

Akpinar S (1987) Restless legs syndrome treatment with dopaminergic drugs. *Clin Neuropharmacol*, **10**, 69–79

Allen DA (1988) Autistic spectrum disorders: clinical presentation in preschool children. *J Child Neurol*, **3** (suppl), S48–56

Askenasy JJM, Weitzman ED, and Yahr MD (1987) Are periodic movements in sleep a basal ganglia dysfunction? *J Neurol Transm*, **70**, 337–47
Baumeister AA, Todd ME, and Levin JA (1993) Efficacy and specificity of pharmacological therapies for behavioral disorders in persons with mental retardation. *Clin Neuropharmacol*, **16**, 271–94
Baxter LR, Phelps ME, Mazziotta JC, Guze BH, Schwartz JM, and Selin CE (1987) Local cerebral glucose metabolic rates in obsessive-compusive disorder. *Arch Gen Psychiatry*, **44**, 211–18
Berther ML, Bayes A, and Tolosa ES (1993) Magnetic resonance imaging in patients with concurrent Tourette's disorder and Asperger's syndrome. *J Am Acad Child Adolesc Psychiatry*, **32**, 633–9
Blin O, Durup M, Pailhous J, and Serratrice G (1990) Akathisia, mobility and locomotion in healthy volunteers. *Clin Neuropharmacol*, **13**, 426–35
Blumstein LK, Crawley JN, Davis LG, and Baldino F (1987) Neuropeptide modulation of apomorphine-induced stereotyped behavior. *Brain Res*, **404**, 293–300
Breese GR, Baumeister AA, McCown TJ, Emerick SG, Frye GD, and Mueller RA (1984) Neonatal 6-hydroxydopamine: model of susceptibility for self mutilation in the Lesch–Nyhan syndrome. *Pharmacol Biochem Behav*, **21**, 459–61
Brodeur C, Montplaisir J, Godbout R, and Marinier R (1988) Treatment of restless legs syndrome and periodic movements during sleep with L-dopa: a double-blind, controlled study. *Neurology*, **38**, 1845–8
Burd L, Fisher WW, Kerbeshian J, and Arnold ME (1987) Is development of Tourette disorder a marker for improvement in patients with autism and other pervasive developmental disorders? *J Am Acad Child Adol Pyschiatry*, **26**, 162–5
Burd I, Fisher W, and Kerbeshian J (1989) Pervasive disintegrative disorder: are Rett syndrome and Heller dementia infantilis subtypes? *Dev Med Child Neurol*, **31**, 609–16
Burke RE, Kang UJ, Jankovic J, Miller LG, Fahn S *et al.* (1989) Tardive akathisia: an analysis of clinical features and response to open therapeutic trials. *Movement Disorders*, **4**, 157–75
Carlsson A (1988) The current status of the dopamine hypothesis of scizophrenia. *Neuropsychopharmacology*, **1**, 179–86
Casanova MF, Naidu S, Goldberg TE *et al.* (1991) Quantitative magnetic resonance imaging in Rett syndrome. *Clinical and Research Reports*, **3**, 66–72
Chipkin RE, McQuade RD, and Iorio LC (1987) D1 and D2 dopamine binding site up-regulation and apomorphine-induced stereotypy. *Pharmacol Biochem Behav*, **28**, 477–82
Cooper SJ and Dourism DT (eds) (1990) *Neurobiology of stereotyped behaviour*. Oxford, Oxford Science Publications, 1–297
Costall B, Marsden CD, Naylor RJ, and Pycock CJ (1977) Stereotyped behavior patterns and hyperactivity induced by amphetamine and apomorphine after discrete 6-hydroxydopamine lesions of extrapyramidal and mesolimbic nuclei. *Brain Res*, **123**, 89–111
Courchesne E, Yeung-Chourchesne R, Press GA, Hesselink JR, and Jermigan TL (1988) Hypoplasia of cerebellar vermal lobules VI and VII in autism. *N Engl J Med*, **318**, 1349–54
Croisile B, Tourniaire D, Confavreux C, Trillet M, and Aimard G (1989) Bilateral damage to the head of the caudate nuclei. *Ann Neurol*, **25**, 313–14
Cummings JL (1993) Frontal sub-cortical circuits and human behaviour. *Arch Neurol*, **50**, 873–80
Dantzer R (1986) Behavioral, physiological and functional aspects of stereotyped behavior: a review and re-interpretation. *J Animal Sci*, **62**, 1776–86
Day BL, Rothwell JC, Thompson PD, Maertens A, Nakshima K, Shannon K (1989) Delay in the execution of voluntary movement by electrical or magnetic brain stimulation in intact man. *Brain*, **112**, 649–63
de Yebenes JG, Brin MF, Mena MA, de Felipe C, Del Rio RM, Bazan E (1988) Neurochemical findings in neuroacanthocytosis. *Movement Disorders*, **3**, 300–12
Dubinsky RM, Hallett M, Levey R, and Di Chiro G (1979) Regional brain glucose metabolism in neuroacanthocytosis. *Neurology*, **39**, 1253–5
Dura JR, Mullick JA, and Rasnake LK (1987) Prevalance of stereotypy among institutionalized nonambulatory profoundly mentally retarded people. *Am M Ment Defic*, **91**, 548–9
Eeg-Olofsson O, Al-Zuhair AGH, Teebi AS, and Al-Essa MMN (1989) Rett syndrome: genetic clues based on mitochondrial changes in muscle. *AM J Med Genet*, **32**, 142–4
Fahn S (1989) Choreic disorders. *Curr Opin Neurol Neurosurg*, **2**, 319–23
Fahn S and The Tourette Syndrome Study Group (1993) Definitions and classification of tic disorders. *Arch Neurol*, (in press)
Fitzgerald PM, Jankovic J, Glaze DG, Schultz R, and Percy AK (1990a) Extrapyramidal involvement in Rett's syndrome. *Neurology*, **40**, 293–5
Fitzgerald PM, Jankovic J, and Percy AK (1990b) Rett syndrome and associated movement disorders. *Movement Disorders*, **5**, 195–203
Gillberg and Gilberg (1989) Asperger syndrome in 23 Swedish children. *Dev Med Child Neurol*, **31**, 520–31
Goldstein M, Anderson LT, Reuben R, and Dancis (1985) Self-mutilation in Lesch–Nyhan disease is caused by dopaminergic denervation. *Lancet*, **1**, 339–9

Goodman WK, McDougal CJ, and Price LH (1992) Pharmacotherapy of obsessive compulsive disorders. *J Clin Psychiatry*, **53**, (4, suppl) 29–37
Hagberg BA (1989) Rett syndrome: clinical peculiarities, diagnostic approach, and possible cause. *Pediatr Neurol*, **5**, 75–83
Hashimoto T, Tayama M, Mori K, Fujino K, Miyazaki M, Kuroday *et al.* (1989) Magnetic resonance imaging in autism: preliminary report. *Neuropediatrics*, **20**, 142–6
Heinrichs D and Buchanan RW (1988) Significance and meaning of neurologic signs in schizophrenia. *Am J Psychiatry*, **145**, 11–18
Hiroi N and White NM (1989) Conditioned stereotypy: behavioral specification of the UCS and pharmacologic investigation of the neural change. *Pharmacol Biochem Behav*, **32**, 249–58
Horwitz B, Rumsey JM, Grady CL, and Rapoport SI (1988) The cerebral metabolic landscape in autism. Intercorrelations of regional glucose utilization. *Arch Neurol*, **45**, 749–55
Jankovic J (1988) Orofacial and other self-mutilations. In Jankovic J, Tolosa E, eds, *Facial Dyskinesias. Advances in Neurology*, vol 49, New York, Raven Press, 365–81
Jankovic J and Orman J (1988) Tetrabenazine therapy of dystonia, chorea, tics and other dyskinesias. *Neurology*, **38**, 391–4
Jankovic J and Rohaidy H (1987) Motor behavioral and pharmacologic findings in Tourette's syndrome. *Can J Neurol Sci*, **14**, 541–6
Jankovic J, Caskey TC, Stout JT, and Butler I (1988) Lesch–Nyhan syndrome: a study of motor behavior and CSF monoamine turnover. *Ann Neurol*, **23**, 466–9
Jankovic J (1992) Diagnosis and classification of tics and Tourette's syndrome. *Adv Neurol*, **58**, 7–14
Jankovic J (1993) Deprenyl in attention deficit associated with Tourette's syndrome. *Arch Neurol*, **50**, 268–88
Jicha GA and Salamone JD (1991) Vacuous jaw movements and feeding deficits in rats with ventrolateral striatal dopamine depletion: possible relation to parkinsonism symptoms. *J Neurosci*, **11**, 3822–9
Kahlbaum KL (1873) *Catatonia* (Levij Y, Priden T, transl), Baltimore, Johns Hopkins University Press
Kaneko K, Yuasa T, Miyatake T, and Tsuji S (1993) Stereotyped hand clasping: an unusual tardive movement disorder. *Movement Disorders*, **8**, 230–1
Karno M, Golding JM, Sorenson SB, and Burnam A (1988) The epidemiology of obsessive-compulsive disorder in five US communities. *Arch Gen Psychiatry*, **45**, 1094–9
Kleiman MD, Neff S, and Rosman NP (1992) The brain in infantile autism: are posterior fossa structures abnormal? *Neurology*, **42**, 753–60
Koller WC and Biary NM (1989) Volitional control of involuntary movements. *Movement Disorders*, **4**, 153–6
Koller WC and Herbster G (1988) D1 and D2 dopamine receptor mechanisms in dopaminergic behaviors. *Clin Neuropharmacol*, **11**, 221–31
Kovelman JA and Scheibel AB (1986) Biological substrates of schizophrenia. *Acta Neurol Scand*, **73**, 1–32
Kravitz H and Boehm JJ (1971) Rhythmic habit patterns of infancy: their sequence, age of onset, and frequency. *Child Dev*, **42**, 399–413
Kuczenski R and Segal D (1989) Concomitant characterization of behavioral and neurotransmitter response to amphetamine using *in vivo* microdialysis. *J Neurosci*, **9**, 2051–65
Lang AE (1989) Other hyperkinetic and paroxysmal movements. *Curr Opin Neurol Neurosurg*, **2**, 334–42
Lang AE (1993) Akathisia and the restless legs syndrome. In Jankovic J and Tolosa E, eds, Parkinson's disease and movement disorders. Baltimore, Williams and Wilkins, 399–418
Laplane D, Levasseur M, Pillon B, Dubois B, Baulac M, Mazoyer B (1989) Obsessive-compulsive and other behavioral changes with bilateral basal ganglia lesions. A neuropsychological, magnetic resonance imaging and positron tomography study. *Brain*, **112**, 699–726
Lekman A, Witt-Engerstrom I, Gottfries J, Hagberg BA, Percy AK, and Sveerholm L (1989) Rett syndrome: biogenic amines and metabolites in postmorten brain. *Pediatr Neurol*, **5**, 357–62
Maraganore DM, Lees AJ, and Marsden CD (1991) Complex stereotypies after right putaminal infarction: a case report. *Movement Disorders*, **6**, 358–61
Meiselas K, Spencer EK, Oberfield R, Peselow ED, Angrist B, and Campbell M (1989) Differentiation of stereotypies from neuroleptic-related dyskinesias in autistic children. *J Clin Psychopharmacol*, **9**, 207–9
Miller LG and Jankovic J (1990a) Drug-induced dyskinesias. In Appel SH, ed, *Current Neurology*, vol 10, Chicago, Year Book Medical Publishers, 321–55
Miller LG and Jankovic J (1990b) Neurological approach to drug-induced movement disorders: a study of 125 patients. *South Med J*, **83**, 525–35
Modell JG, Mountz JM, Curtis GC, and Greden JF (1989) Neurophysiologic dysfunction in basal ganglia/limbic striatal and thalamocortical circuits as a pathogenetic mechanism of obsessive-compulsive disorder. *J Neuropsychiatry*, **1**, 27–36
Murphy RJ, Nunes DL, and Hutchings-Reprecht M (1977) Reduction of stereotyped behavior in profoundly retarded individuals. *Am J Ment Defic*, **82**, 238–45

Myer EC, Morris DL, Brase DA, and Dewey WL (1988) Hyperendorphonism in Rett syndrome: cause or result? *Ann Neurol*, **24**, 340–1

O'Connor N and Hermelin B (1989) The memory structure of autistic idiot-savant mnemonists. *Br J Psychol*, **80**, 97–111

Papa SM, Artieda J, and Obeso JA (1991) Cortical activity preceding self-initiated and externally triggered voluntary movement. *Movement Disorders*, **6**, 217–24

Percy AK, Zoghbi HY, Lewis KR, and Jankovic J (1988) Rett syndrome: qualitative and quantitative differentiation from autism. *J Child Neurol*, **3** (suppl), S65–7

Percy A, Gillberg C, Hagberg B, and Witt-Engerstrom I (1990) Rett syndrome and the autistic disorders. *Neurol Clin*, **8**, 659–76

Perry TL, Dunn HG, Ho HH, and Crichton JU (1988) Cerebrospinal fluid values for monoamine metabolites, gamma-aminobutyric acid, and other amino compounds in Rett syndrome. *J Pediatr*, **112**, 234–8

Pitman RK (1989) Animal models of compulsive behavior. *Biol Psychiatry*, **26**, 189–98

Rapir I (1987) Searching for the cause of autism: a neurological perspective. In Cohen DJ, Donnelan AM, and Paul R, eds, *Handbook of Autism and Pervasive Developmental Disorders*, New York, NY, John Wiley, 710–17

Rapoport JL (1988) The neurobiology of obsessive-compulsive disorder. *JAMA*, **260**, 2888–90

Reiss AL, Faruque F, Naidu S *et al.* (1993) Neuroanatomy of Rett syndrome: a volumetric imaging study. *Ann Neurol*, **34**, 227–37

Roberts GW (1990) Schizophrenia: the cellular biology of a functional psychosis. *TINS*, **13**, 207–11

Robertson MM (1992) Self injurious behaviour and Tourette's syndrome. *Adv Neurol*, **58**, 105–14

Rogers D and Hymas N (1988) Sporadic facial stereotypies in patients with schizophrenia and compulsive disorders. In Jankovic J and Tolosa E, eds, *Facial Dyskinesias. Advances in Neurology*, vol 49, New York, Raven Press, 383–94

Rojahn J (1986) Self-injurious and stereotypic behavior of noninstitutionalized mentally retarded people: prevalence and classification. *Am J Ment Defic*, **91**, 268–76

Rupinak NMJ, Tye SJ, Steventon MJ, Boyce S, and Iversen SO (1990) Spontaneous orofacial dyskinesia. *Movement Disorders*, **5**, 314–18

Sallustro A and Atwell CW (1978) Body rocking, head banging, and head rolling in normal children. *J Pediatr*, **93**, 704–8

Sandman CA (1988) β-endorphin disregulation in autistic and self-injurious behavior: a neurodevelopmental hypothesis. *Synapse*, **2**, 193–9

Sandyk R, Bamford CR, and Gillman MA (1987) Opiates in the restless legs syndrome. *Int J Neurosci*, **36**, 99–104

Schreibman L (1988) Diagnostic features of autism. *J Child Neurol*, **3** (suppl), S57–64

Schroeder SR, Breese GR, and Mueller RA (1990) Dopaminergic mechanisms in self-injurious behavior. In Routh DK and Wolraich M, eds, *Advances in Developmental and Behavioral Pediatrics*, Greenwich, CT, JAI Press

Silvestri R, De Domenico P, Di Rosa AE, Bramanti P, Serra S, and Di Perri R (1990) The effect of nocturnal physiologic sleep on various movement disorders. *Movement Disorders*, **5**, 8–14

Spitz MC, Jankovic J, and Killian JM (1985) Familial tic disorder, parkinsonism, motor neuron disease, and acanthocytosis: a new syndrome. *Neurology*, **35**, 366–70

Stacy M, Cardoso F, and Jankovic J (1993) Tardive stereotypy and other movement disorders in tardive dyskinesia. *Neurology*, **43**, 937–41

Steffenburg S, Gillberg C, Hellgren I, Andersson I, Gilberg IC, Jakobsson G *et al.* (1989) A twin study of autism in Denmark, Finland, Iceland, Norway and Sweden. *J Child Psychol Psychiatry*, **30**, 405–16

Stoudemire A (1982) The differential diagnosis of catatonic states. *Psychosomatics*, **23**, 245–52

Suddath RL, Christison GE, Torrey EF, Casanova MF, and Weinberger DR (1990) Anatomical abnormalities in the brains of monozygotic twins discordant for schizophrenia. *N Engl J Med*, **322**, 89–94

Sugiyama T and Abe T (1989) The prevalence of autism in Nagoya, Japan: a total population study. *J Autism Dev Dis*, **19**, 87–96

Swedo SE, Rapoport JL, Cheslo WI, Leonard HI, Ayoub EM, Hosier DM *et al.* (1989) High prevalence of obsessive-compulsive symptoms in patients with Sydenham's chorea. *Am J Psychiatry*, **146**, 246–9

Swedo SE, Leonard HL, Schapiro MB *et al* (1993) Sydenham's chorea: physical and psychological symptoms of St Vitus dance. *Pediatrics*, **91**, 706–13

Szatmari P, Bremner R, and Nagy J (1989) Asperger syndrome: a review of clinical features. *Can J Psychiatry*, **34**, 554–60

The Tourette's Syndrome Study Group (1993) Definitions and classification of tic disorders. *Arch Neurol* (in press)

Treffert DA (1988) The idiot savant: a review of the syndrome. *Am J Psychiatry*, **145**, 563–72
Tschanz JT and Rebec GV (1988) Atypical antipsychotic drugs block selective components of amphetamine-induced sterotypy. *Pharmacol Biochem Behav*, **31**, 519–22
Volkmar FR and Bregman JD (1988) Stereotyped and self-injurious behaviors in disorders other than Tourette's syndrome. In Cohen DJ, Bruun RD, Leckman JF, eds, *Tourette's Syndrome and Tic Disorders: Clinical Understanding and Treatment*, New York, NY, John Wiley, 163–76
Walters A, Hening W, Kavey N, Chokroverty S, and Gidro-Frank S (1988a) A double-blind randomized crossover trial of bromocriptine and placebo in restless legs syndrome. *Ann Neurol*, **24**, 455–8
Walters AS, Hening WA, and Chokroverty S (1988b) Frequent occurrence of myoclonus while awake and at rest, body rocking and marching in place in a subpopulation of patients with restless legs syndrome. *Acta Neurol Scand*, **77**, 418–21
Watkins KM and Konarski EA (1987) Effect of mentally retarded persons' level of stereotypy on their learning. *Am J Ment Defic*, **91**, 361–5
Weilburg JB, Mesulam M-M, Weintraub S, Buonano F, Jenke M, Stakes JW (1989) Focal striatal abnormalities in a patient with obsessive-compulsive disorder. *Arch Neurol*, **46**, 233–5
Wing L and Attwood A (1987) Syndromes of autism and atypical development, In Cohen DJ, Donnelan AM, and Paul R, eds, *Handbook of Autism and Pervasive Developmental Disorders*, New York, NY, John Wiley, 3–19
Zoghbi H (1988) Genetic aspects of Rett syndrome. *J Child Neurol*, **3**, 76–8
Zoghbi HY, Milstien S, Butler IJ, Smith EO, Kaufman S, Glaze DG *et al.* (1989) Cerebrospinal fluid biogenic amines and biopterin in Rett's syndrome. *Ann Neurol*, **25**, 56–60
Zohar J and Insel TR (1987) Obsessive-compulsive disorder: psychological approaches to diagnosis, treatment, and pathophysiology. *Biol Psychiatry*, **22**, 667–87

Index